AAOS

First Responder

Your First Response in Emergency Care

1(800)222-1222

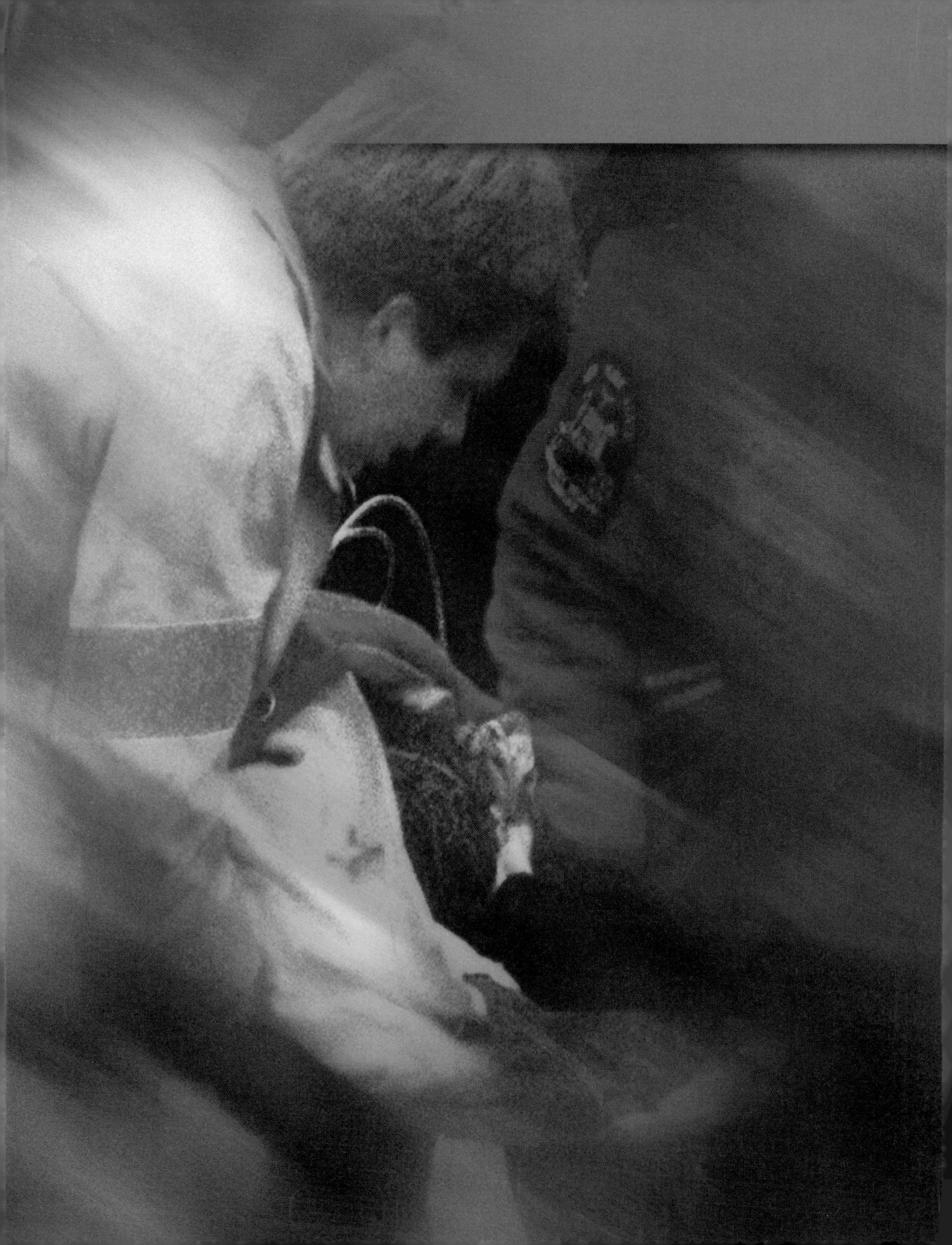

AAOS

First Responder

Your First Response in Emergency Care

Third Edition

David Schottke, RN, NREMT-P, MPH
Washington, D.C.

JONES AND BARTLETT PUBLISHERS
Sudbury, Massachusetts
BOSTON TORONTO LONDON SINGAPORE

Jones and Bartlett Publishers
40 Tall Pine Drive
Sudbury, MA 01776
978-443-5000
www.FirstResponderTraining.com
www.jbpub.com

Jones and Bartlett Publishers Canada
2406 Nikanna Road
Mississauga, ON L5C 2W6
CANADA

Jones and Bartlett Publishers International
Barb House, Barb Mews
London W6 7PA
UK

Production Credits
Chief Executive Officer: Clayton E. Jones
Chief Operating Officer: Donald W. Jones, Jr.
Executive V.P. and Publisher: Tom Manning
V.P., Managing Editor: Judith H. Hauck
V.P., Sales and Marketing: Paul Shepardson
V.P., Production and Design: Anne Spencer
V.P., Manufacturing and Inventory Control: Therese Bräuer
Emergency Care Senior Acquisitions Editor: Tracy Foss
Director of Marketing, EMS and Health Sciences: Kimberly Brophy
Senior Developmental Editor: Dean W. DeChambeau
Emergency Care Associate Editors: Carol Brewer and Jennifer Reed
Senior Production Editor: Linda S. DeBruyn
Director of Media Services: W. Scott Smith
Design and Composition: Studio Montage
Cover Photograph: © Bruce Ayres, Tony Stone Images
Printing and Binding: Courier Company

American Academy of Orthopaedic Surgeons
Vice President, Education Programs: Mark W. Wieting
Director, Department of Publications: Marilyn L. Fox, PhD
Managing Editor: Lynne Roby Shindoll
Senior Editor: Barbara A. Scotese

Library of Congress Cataloging-in-Publication Data

First Responder, Your First Response in Emergency Care. — 3rd ed. / [edited by]
David Schottke
p. cm.
Includes index.
ISBN 0-7637-1471-2 (pbk)
1. Medical emergencies. 2. Emergency medical technicians. 3) First aid in illness and injury. I. Title.
II. Jacobs, Lenworth M. III. American Academy of Orthopaedic Surgeons.
[DNLM: 1 Emergencies—Programmed Instruction. 2. Emergency Medical Technicians. 3. Emergency Treatment—Programmed Instruction. W 18.2 S375f2001]
RC86.7.S35 2001
616.025—21
DNLM/dc21 00-054604
for Library of Congress CIP

Additional credits appear on page 455.

Printed in the United States of America
05 04 10 9 8 7 6 5

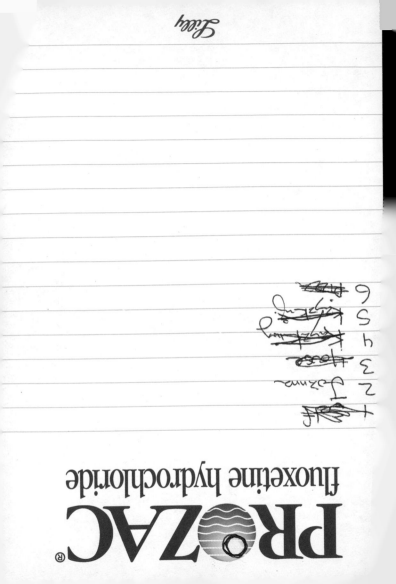

PROZAC®

fluoxetine hydrochloride

Lilly

Brief Contents

First Responder Skill Drills

Contents

Contents

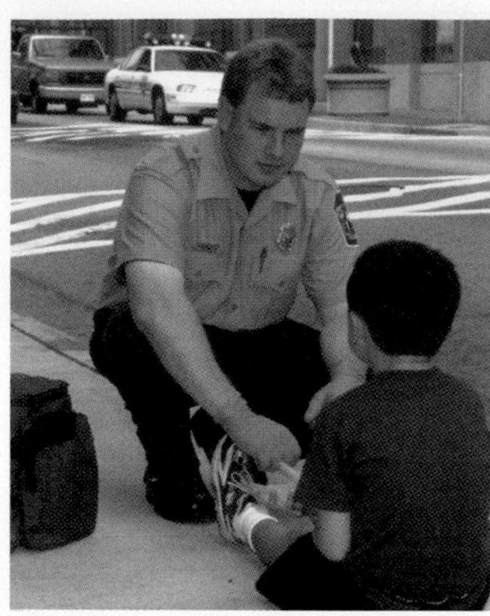

Contents

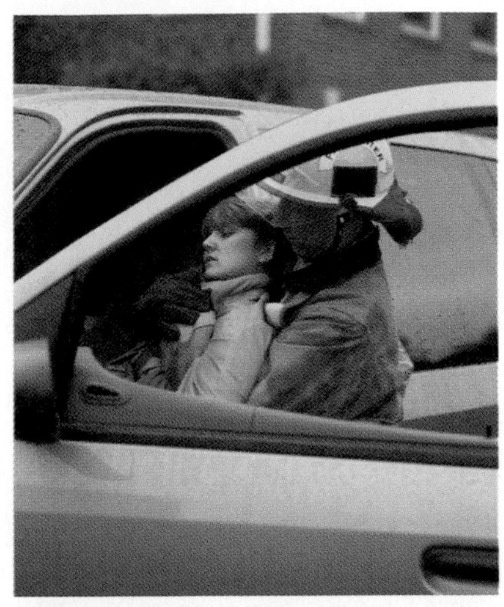

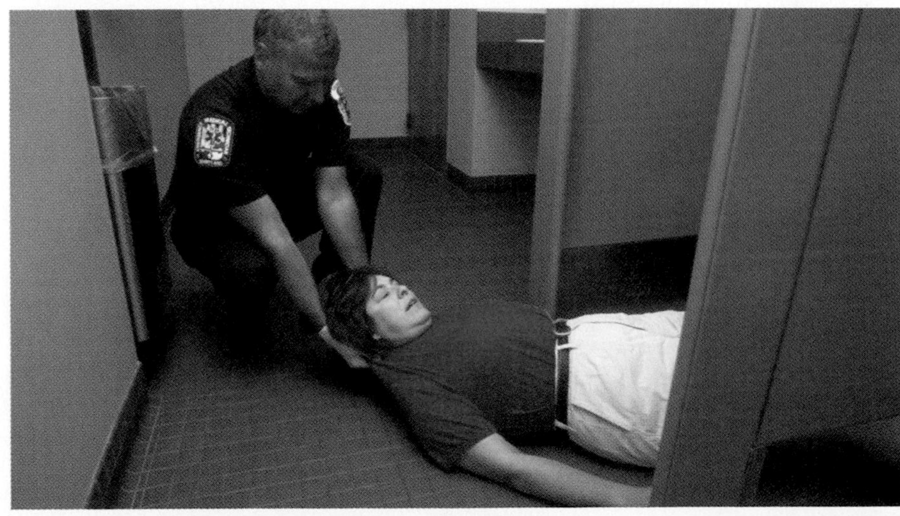

Contents

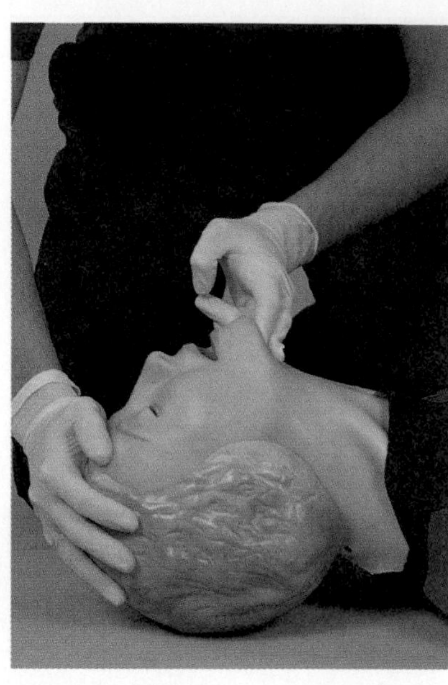

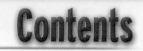

Contents

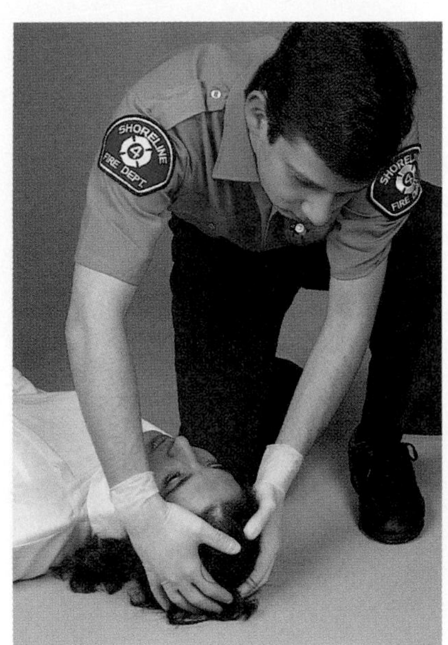

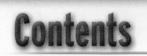

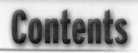

Contents

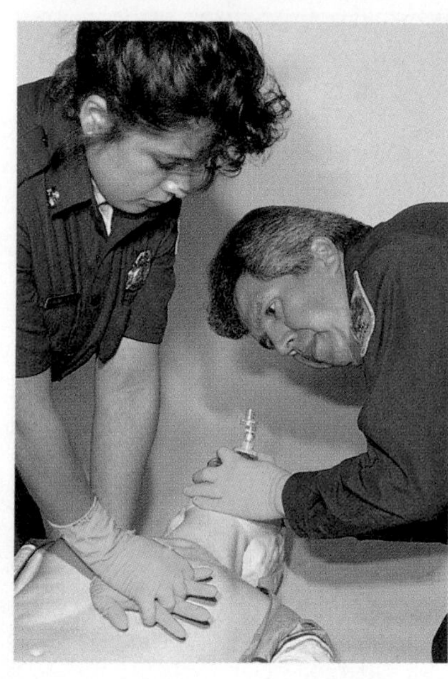

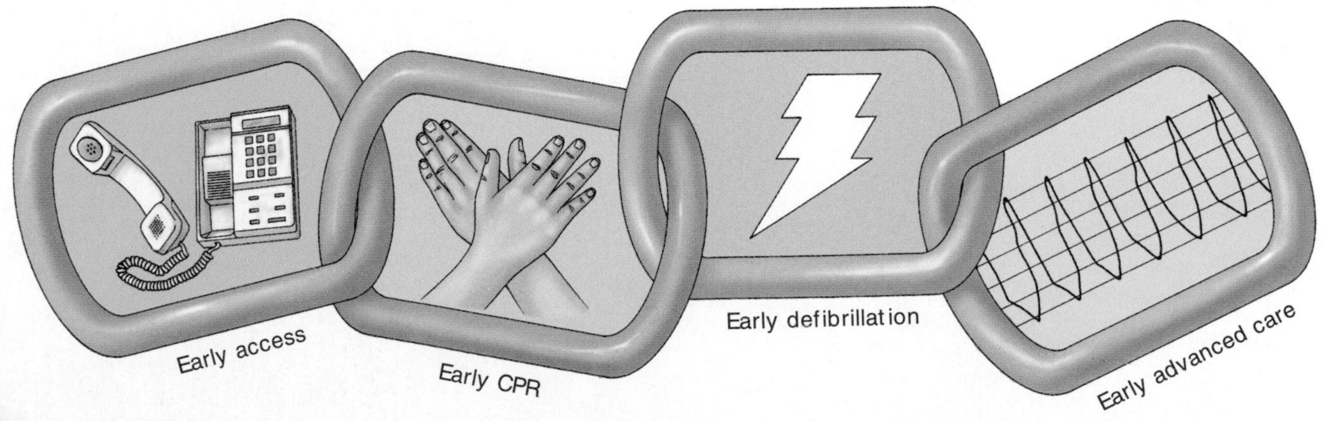

Early access
Early CPR
Early defibrillation
Early advanced care

Contents

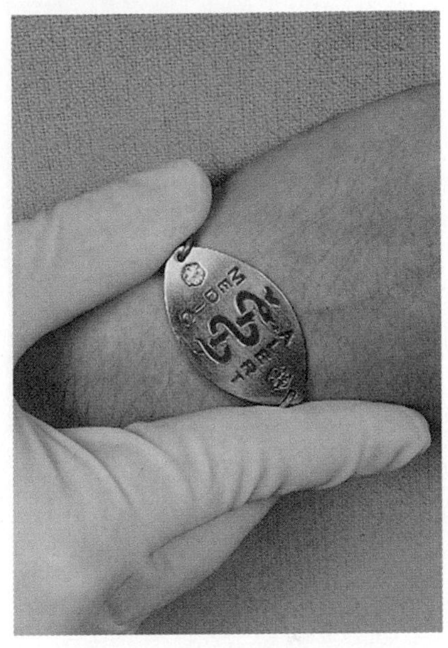

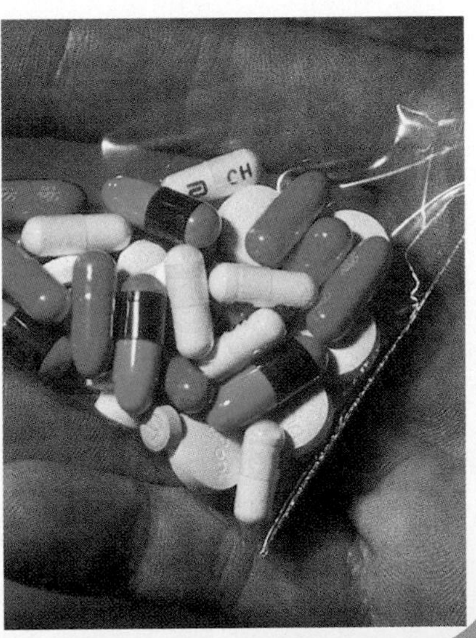

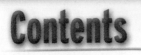

Contents

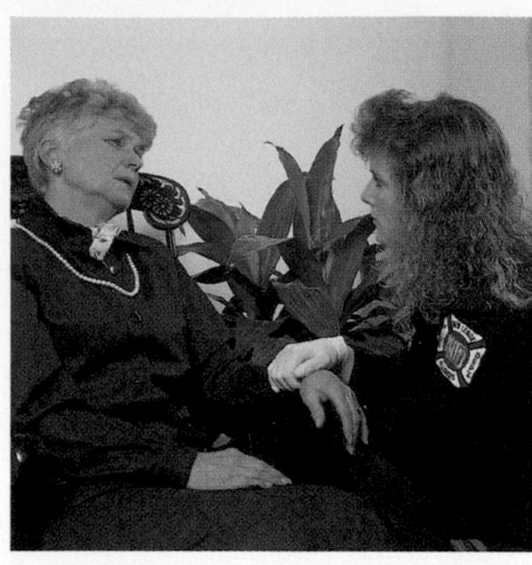

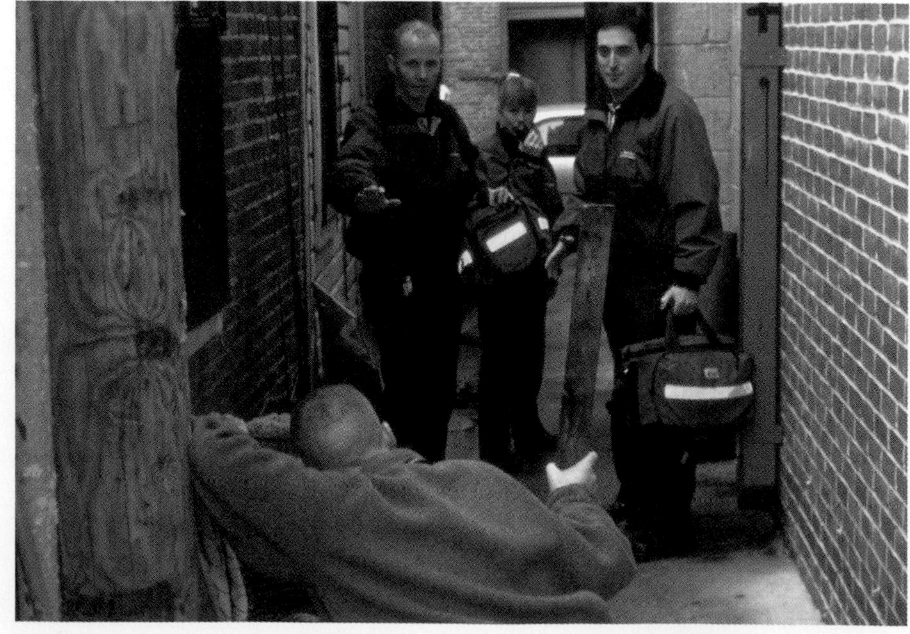

Contents

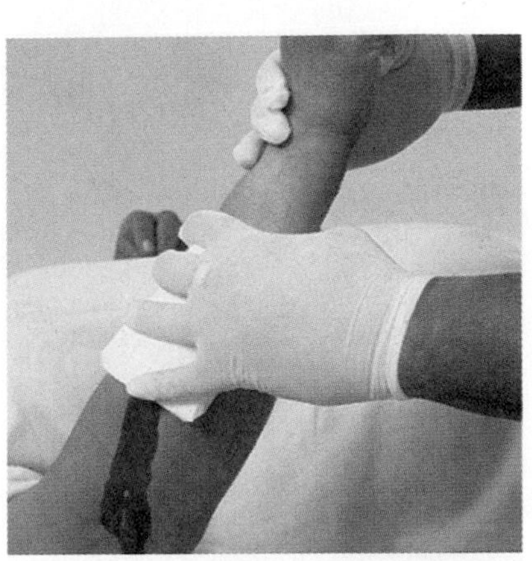

Contents

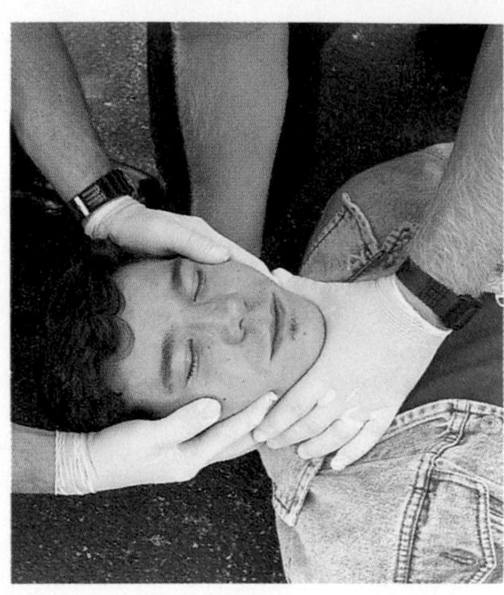

Contents

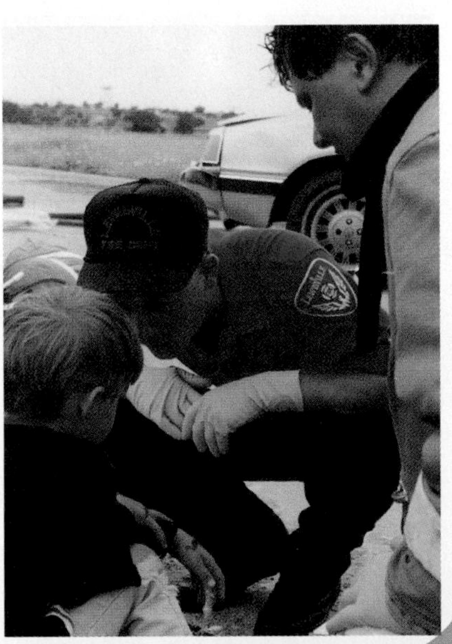

Contents

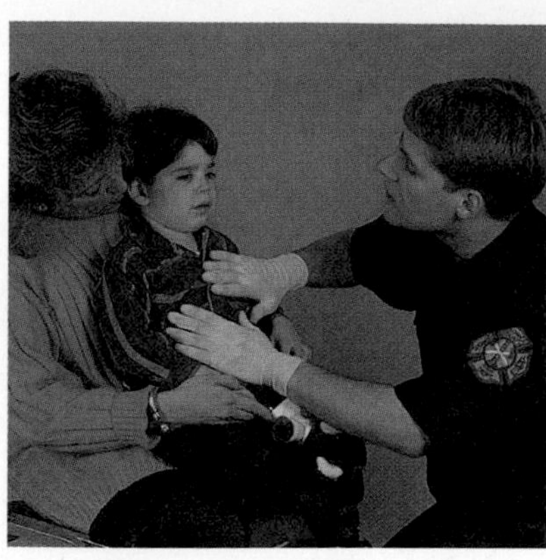

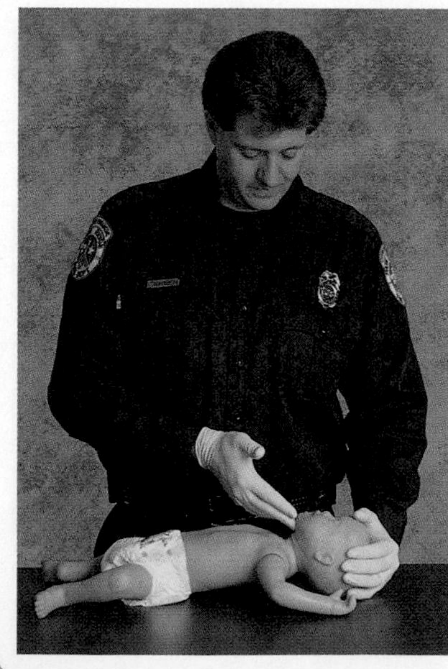

Contents

Contents

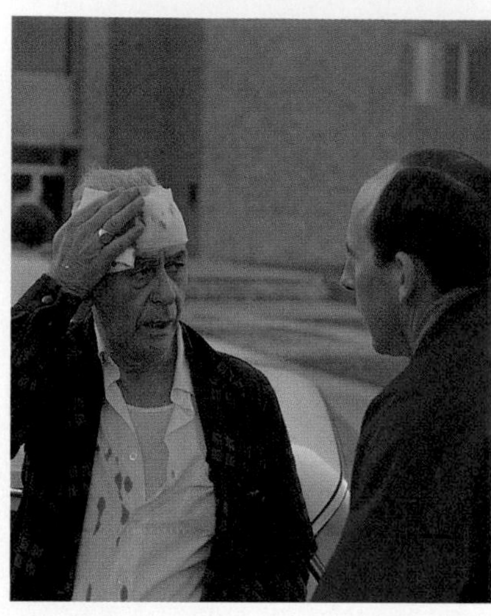

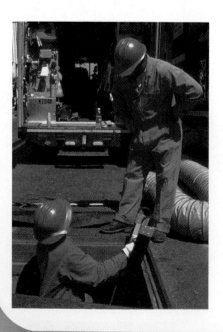

Contents

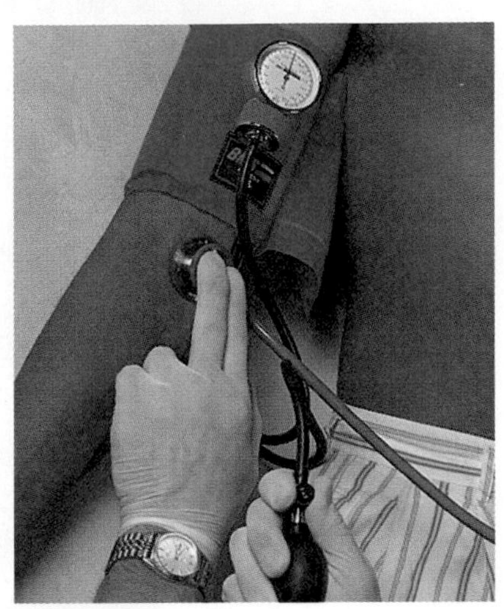

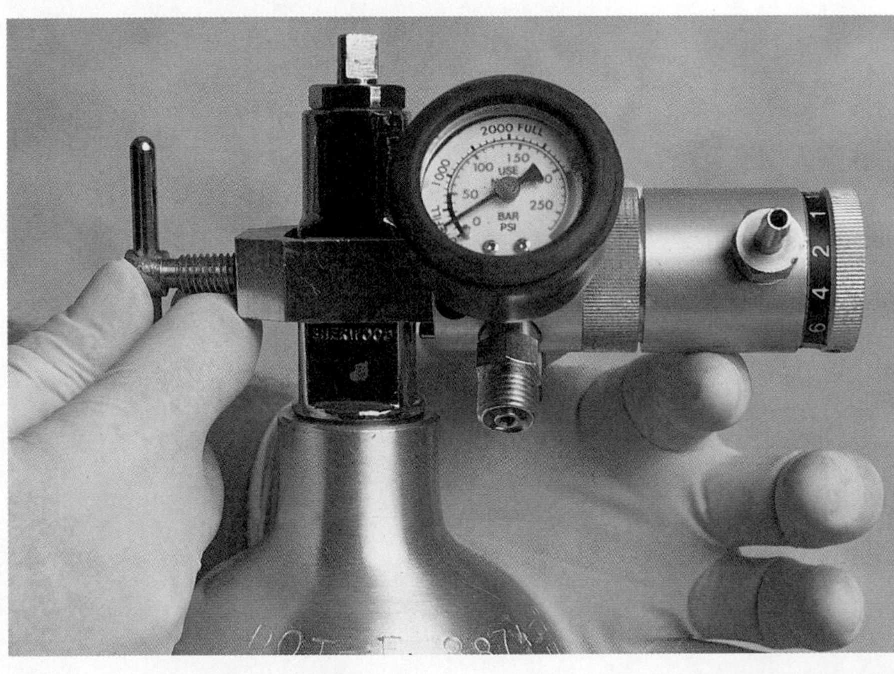

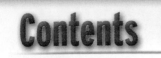

Resource Preview

First Responder

Your First Response in Emergency Care

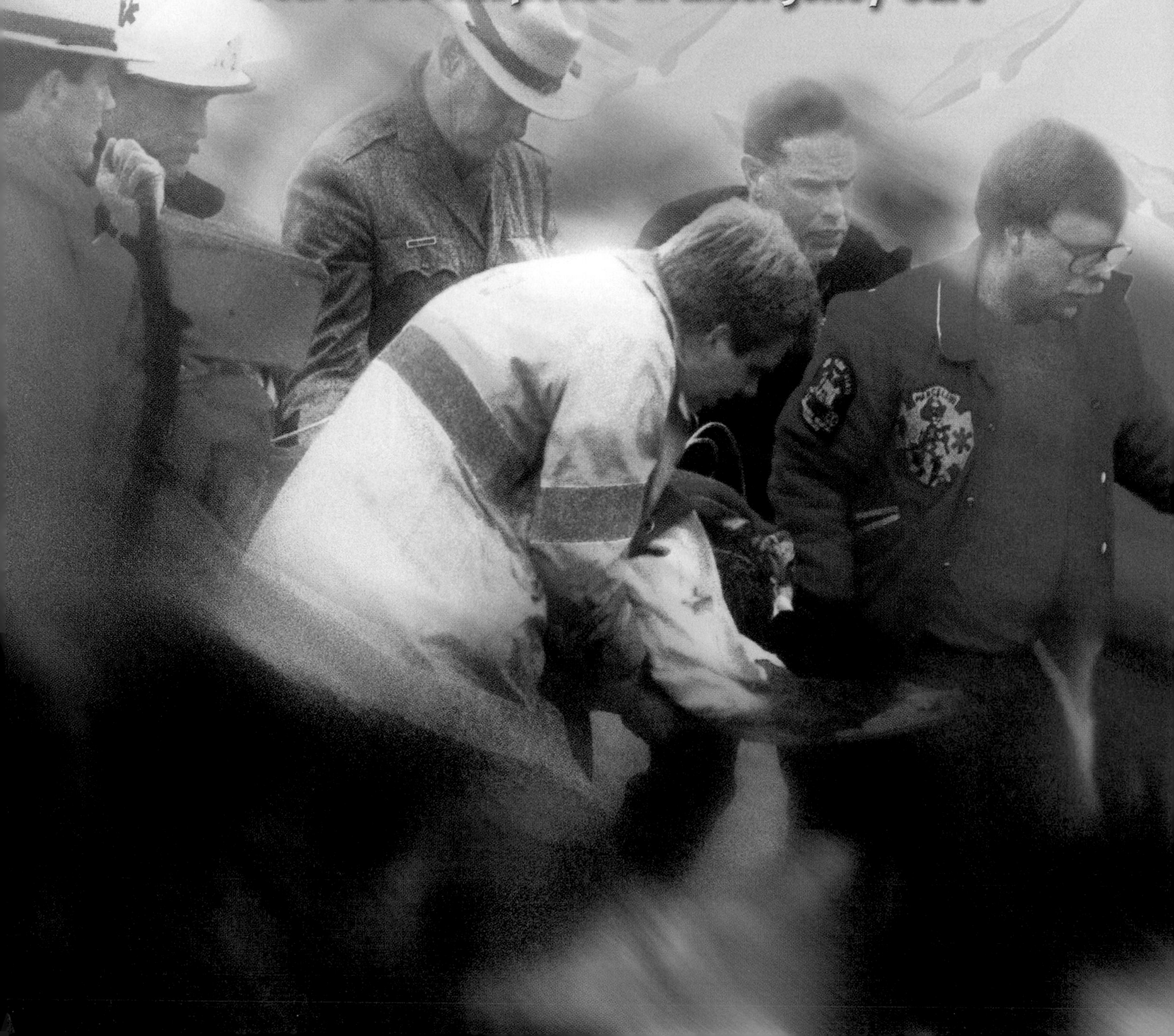

Resource Preview

The third edition of First Responder continues with an assessment-based approach to first responder training and has been revised to reflect the latest Emergency Cardiac Care Guidelines.

First Responder fully integrates the National Standard Curriculum guidelines to provide the knowledge and skills needed to work as a first responder. Additionally, some topics are covered in greater depth and are identified as supplemental material by an FYI icon.

In this era of increased awareness of the incidence and transmission of infectious diseases, first responders need to understand how to protect themselves and their patients from infectious diseases. This text stresses the importance of body substance isolation during the discussion of each type of disease or illness. Practical suggestions for the field are highlighted.

Effective first responders need to understand four basic principles. These are:

1. Know what you should not do.
2. Know how to use your first responder life support kit.
3. Know how to improvise.
4. Know how to assist other emergency medical services providers.

This text has been written with these principles in mind. By continuing to remember the four principles, students will be able to better understand the different roles they will have as first responders.

This new program provides a variety of special technology and features to help students acquire the knowledge and techniques they will need to work as a first responder.

This textbook is the core of the First Responder program with features that will reinforce and expand on the essential information and techniques.

In the beginning of each chapter a ***navigation toolbar*** *will guide you through the technology resources and text features available for that chapter.*

Resource Preview

Knowledge and Attitude Objectives *and* **Skill Objectives** *are drawn from the National Standard Curriculum.*

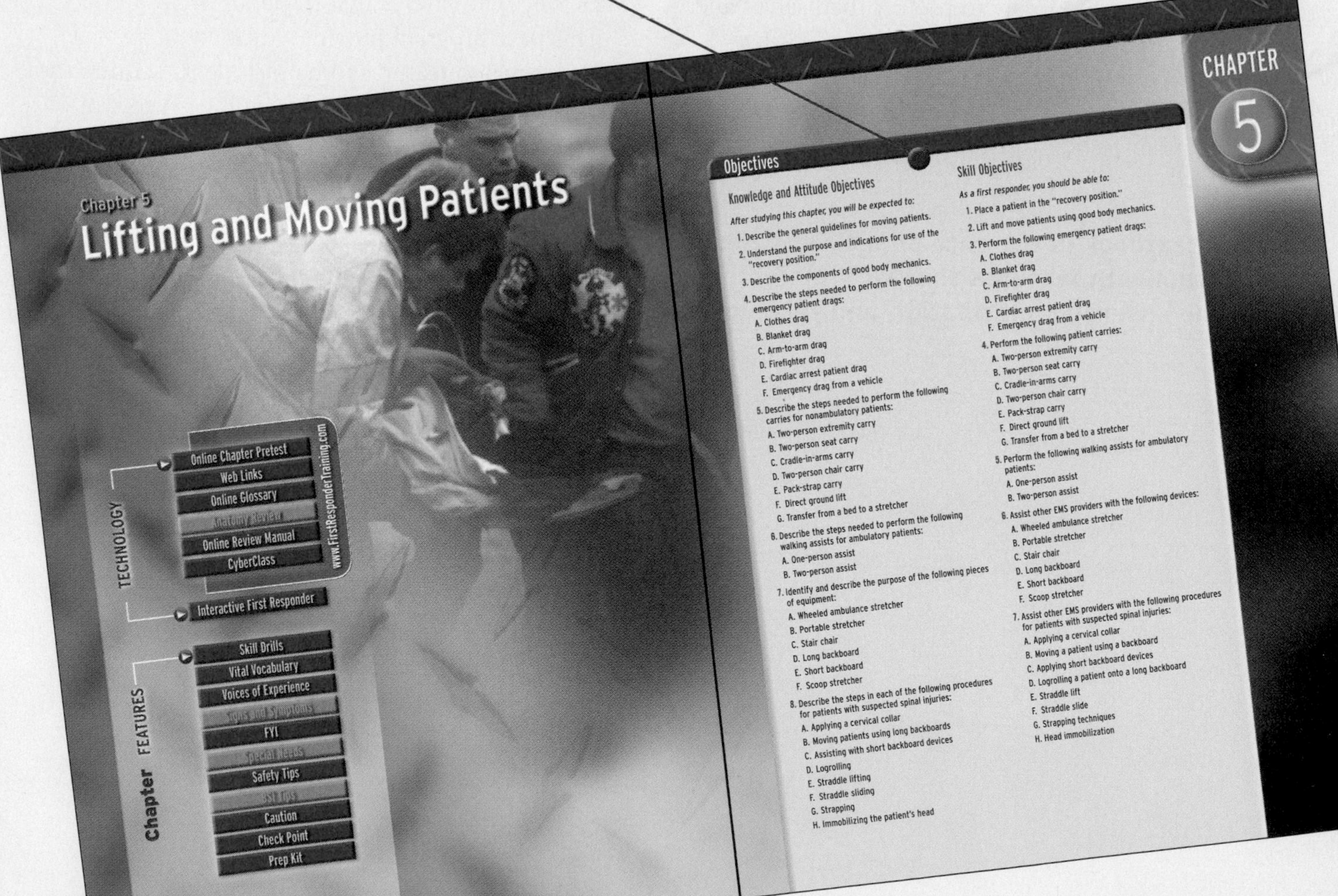

Chapter 5
Lifting and Moving Patients
TECHNOLOGY
Online Chapter Pretest
Web Links
Online Glossary
Online Review Manual
CyberClass
www.FirstResponderTraining.com
Interactive First Responder
Chapter FEATURES
Skill Drills
Vital Vocabulary
Voices of Experience
FYI
Safety Tips
Caution
Check Point
Prep Kit
CHAPTER
5
Objectives
Knowledge and Attitude Objectives
After studying this chapter, you will be expected to:
1. Describe the general guidelines for moving patients.
2. Understand the purpose and indications for use of the "recovery position."
3. Describe the components of good body mechanics.
4. Describe the steps needed to perform the following emergency patient drags:
A. Clothes drag
B. Blanket drag
C. Arm-to-arm drag
D. Firefighter drag
E. Cardiac arrest patient drag
F. Emergency drag from a vehicle
5. Describe the steps needed to perform the following carries for nonambulatory patients:
A. Two-person extremity carry
B. Two-person seat carry
C. Cradle-in-arms carry
D. Two-person chair carry
E. Pack-strap carry
F. Direct ground lift
G. Transfer from a bed to a stretcher
6. Describe the steps needed to perform the following walking assists for ambulatory patients:
A. One-person assist
B. Two-person assist
7. Identify and describe the purpose of the following pieces of equipment:
A. Wheeled ambulance stretcher
B. Portable stretcher
C. Stair chair
D. Long backboard
E. Short backboard
F. Scoop stretcher
8. Describe the steps in each of the following procedures for patients with suspected spinal injuries:
A. Applying a cervical collar
B. Moving patients using long backboards
C. Assisting with short backboard devices
D. Logrolling
E. Straddle lifting
F. Straddle sliding
G. Strapping
H. Immobilizing the patient's head
Skill Objectives
As a first responder, you should be able to:
1. Place a patient in the "recovery position."
2. Lift and move patients using good body mechanics.
3. Perform the following emergency patient drags:
A. Clothes drag
B. Blanket drag
C. Arm-to-arm drag
D. Firefighter drag
E. Cardiac arrest patient drag
F. Emergency drag from a vehicle
4. Perform the following patient carries:
A. Two-person extremity carry
B. Two-person seat carry
C. Cradle-in-arms carry
D. Two-person chair carry
E. Pack-strap carry
F. Direct ground lift
G. Transfer from a bed to a stretcher
5. Perform the following walking assists for ambulatory patients:
A. One-person assist
B. Two-person assist
6. Assist other EMS providers with the following devices:
A. Wheeled ambulance stretcher
B. Portable stretcher
C. Stair chair
D. Long backboard
E. Short backboard
F. Scoop stretcher
7. Assist other EMS providers with the following procedures for patients with suspected spinal injuries:
A. Applying a cervical collar
B. Moving a patient using a backboard
C. Applying short backboard devices
D. Logrolling a patient onto a long backboard
E. Straddle lift
F. Straddle slide
G. Strapping techniques
H. Head immobilization

Resource Preview

Key terms *are defined in the margin at the point at which they are introduced in the text.*

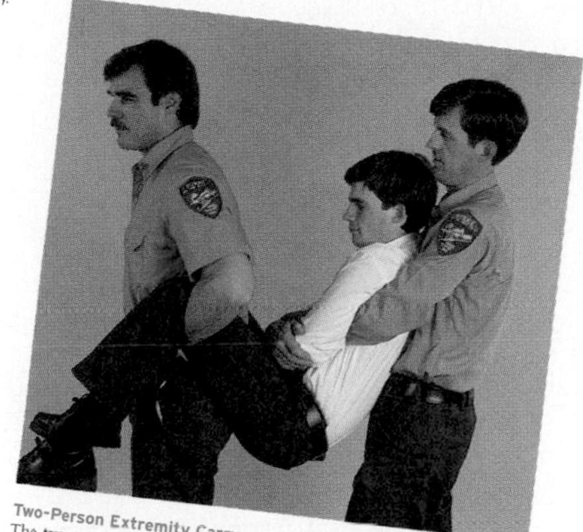

Figure 5.9 Two-person extremity carry.

two-person extremity carry A method of carrying a patient out of tight quarters using two rescuers and no equipment.

extremities The arms and legs.

two-person seat carry A method of carrying a patient in which two rescuers link arms behind the patient's back and under the patient's knees; requires no equipment.

cradle-in-arms carry A one-rescuer patient movement technique used primarily for children. The patient is cradled in the hollow formed by the rescuer's arms and chest.

Two-Person Extremity Carry

The **two-person extremity** carry can be done by two rescuers with no equipment in tight or narrow spaces, such as mobile home corridors, small hallways, and narrow spaces between buildings (**Figure 5.9**). The focus of this carry is on the patient's **extremities**. The rescuers help the patient sit up. Rescuer One kneels behind the patient and reaches under the patient's arms and grasps the patient's wrists. Rescuer Two then backs in between the patient's legs, reaches around, and grasps the patient behind the knees. At a command from Rescuer One, the two rescuers stand up and carry the patient away, walking straight ahead.

Two-Person Seat Carry

FYI

With the **two-person seat carry**, two rescuers use their arms and bodies to form a seat for the patient. The rescuers kneel on opposite sides of the patient near the patient's hips. The rescuers then raise the patient to a sitting position and link arms behind the patient's back. The rescuers then place the other arm under the patient's knees and link with each other. If possible, the patient puts his or her arms around the necks of the rescuers for additional support. Although the two-person seat carry needs two rescuers, it does not require any equipment (**Figure 5.10**).

Cradle-in-Arms Carry

The **cradle-in-arms carry** can be used by one rescuer to carry a child. Kneel beside the patient and place one arm around the child's back and the other arm under the thighs. Lift slightly and roll the child into the hollow formed by your arms and chest. Be sure to use your leg muscles to stand (**Figure 5.11**).

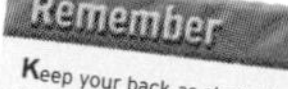

Remember

Keep your back as straight as possible and use the large muscles in your legs to do the lifting!

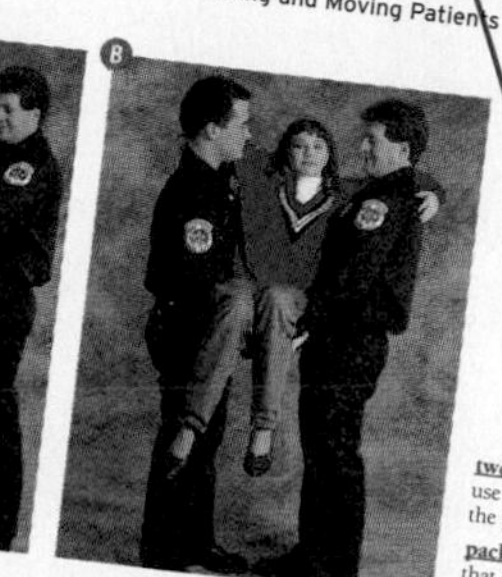

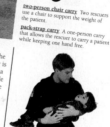

Figure 5.10 Two-person seat carry. **A.** Link arms. **B.** Raise the patient to a sitting position.

two-person chair carry Two rescuers use a chair to support the weight of the patient.

pack-strap carry A one-person carry that allows the rescuer to carry a patient while keeping one hand free.

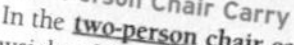

Two-Person Chair Carry

In the **two-person chair carry**, two rescuers use a chair to support the weight of the patient. A folding chair cannot be used. The chair carry is especially useful for taking patients up or down stairways or through a narrow hallway. An additional benefit is that because the patient is able to hold on to the chair (and should be encouraged to do so), he or she feels much more secure than with the two-person seat carry.

Rescuer One stands behind the seated patient, reaches down, and grasps the back of the chair close to the seat. Rescuer Two then tilts the chair slightly backward on its rear legs so that Rescuer Two can back in between the legs of the chair and grasp the tips of the chair's front legs. The patient's legs should be between the legs of the chair. When both rescuers are correctly positioned, Rescuer One gives the command to lift and walk away.

Pack-Strap Carry

The **pack-strap carry** is a one-person carry that allows you to carry a patient while keeping one hand free. Have the patient stand (or have other rescue personnel support the patient) and back into the patient so your shoulders fit into the patient's armpits. Grasp the patient's wrists and cross the arms over your chest (**Figure 5.13**, page 76). Now you can hold both wrists in one hand, and your other hand remains free.

Optimal weight distribution occurs when the patient's armpits are over your shoulders. Squat deeply to avoid potential injury to your back and pull the patient onto your back. Once the patient is positioned correctly, bend forward to lift the patient off the ground, stand up, and walk away.

Direct Ground Lift

The direct ground lift is used to move a patient who is on the ground or the floor to an ambulance cot. It should be used only for those patients who have not suffered a traumatic injury. The direct ground lift requires you to bend over the patient and lift with your back in a bent position. Because the use of the direct ground lift results in poor body mechanics, its use is to be discouraged. Using a long backboard or portable cot is

Figure 5.11 Cradle-in-arms carry.

Note: Because the chair carry may force the patient's head forward, Rescuer One should watch the patient for airway problems.

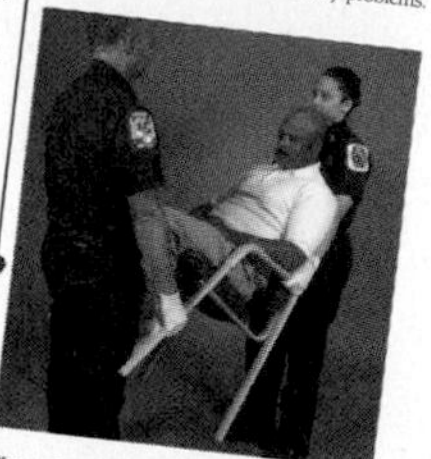

Figure 5.12 Two-person chair carry.

FYI sections *cover additional information for further study. This material goes beyond the scope of the DOT curriculum and may be incorporated at the instructor's discretion.*

Resource Preview

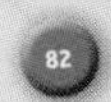

MODULE 1 Preparatory

Voices of Experience

Firefighters Save Patient's Eyesight

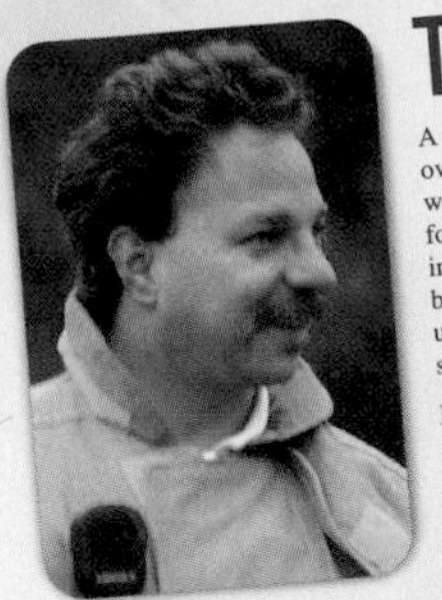

The man inside has a stick in his head!" That's what a bystander told the first arriving units when they reached the scene of a pre-dawn accident on a frigid morning.

A car had crashed through a board fence lined with barbed wire, and overturned in a field. The sole occupant of the car, a 21-year-old male, was conscious but pinned in the automobile. Upon entering the auto, I found the patient with an 18 inch long, 2 inch by 2 inch piece of wood impaled in his right eye socket. In addition, a 1 inch by 4 inch fence board had lacerated his scalp and was, in effect, supporting his head and upper body. The patient's only complaint was that he was cold (the outside temperature was about 15° F).

I assessed the patient while other firefighters began stabilizing the scene. Access to the automobile was made and the auto was stabilized using ropes, shoring, and chocks.

A paramedic firefighter joined me and began ALS care while another firefighter and I worked on stabilizing the patient and the 1 inch by 4 inch board that was supporting him. Other firefighters used b... blankets to "shore up" the p... the board entrapping the pa... removed. Firefighters were... safely remove a rear windo... board out, freeing the vict...

“Upon entering the auto, I found the patient with an 18 inch long, 2 inch by 2 inch piece of wood impaled in his right eye socket.”

As this was going on, we carefully stabilized the impale... Firefighters slid a spine board under the victim as the t... the car lifted him. The patient was loaded into the ALS... was further stabilized and transported to a waiting heli... a trauma center. Evaluation at the trauma center show... injuries, and the patient was taken into surgery. The i... removed, and the wound examined. There was no ... eye socket, and the surgical team was able to replan...

Within a few days, the patient had regained sight i... ophthalmologic surgeon felt a full recovery was lik... ited the rapid and conscientious actions of the fire... patient evaluated, stabilized, extricated, treated, t... gery in less than two hours—with saving the you... ticular importance, he said, was the stabilization... one of the "basics" taught in EMS training. ❖

Gordon M. Sachs, EMT, Deputy Chief Marion County Fir...

In Voices of Experience essays, veteran EMS providers share accounts of memorable incidents and offer advice and encouragement.

MODULE 5 Illness and Injury

This chapter presents the skills you need to recognize and care for patients who are suffering from shock, bleeding, or soft-tissue injuries. Because most soft-tissue injuries result in bleeding, maintaining good body substance isolation (BSI) is important when you are caring for these injuries. The chapter describes four types of wounds: abrasions, lacerations, punctures, and avulsions. Techniques for controlling external bleeding are stressed. It is important that you learn the techniques for dressing and bandaging wounds presented here.

BSI Tip

Most soft-tissue injuries involve some degree of bleeding. Any time you approach a patient with a potential soft-tissue injury, you need to consider your BSI strategy.

Damage to internal soft tissues and organs can cause life-threatening problems. Internal bleeding causes the patient to lose blood in the circulatory system and results in shock. More trauma patients die from shock than any other reason. Your ability to recognize the signs and symptoms of shock and to take simple measures to aid shock patients will give them the best chance for survival. This chapter explains the causes and types of shock using an analogy of a pump, pipes, and fluid. You will learn how a failure of any part of the system can cause shock.

Burns are another type of soft-tissue injury. Burns may be caused by heat, chemicals, or electricity. They may damage any part of the body and are especially harmful if they occur inside the respiratory tract. This chapter examines the extent, depth, and cause of burns. As you study this chapter, keep in mind the importance of maintaining good BSI techniques to prevent the spread of disease-carrying organisms.

Safety Tips

Whatever technique you use for moving patients, keep these rules of good body mechanics in mind:

1. Know your own physical limitations and capabilities. Do not try to lift too heavy a load.
2. Keep yourself balanced when lifting or moving a patient.
3. Maintain a firm footing.
4. Lift and lower the patient by bending your legs, not your back. Keep your back as straight as possible at all times and use your large leg muscles to do the work.
5. Try to keep your arms close to your body for strength and balance.
6. Move the patient as little as possible.

Body Substance Isolation and Soft-Tissue Injuries

The BSI concept assumes that all body fluids are potentially dangerous. Therefore, you must take appropriate measures to prevent contact with the patient's body fluids. When dealing with patients who have soft-tissue injuries, wear gloves to prevent contact with the patient's blood. At times, you may also need to wear a surgical mask and eye protection if there is danger of blood splatter from a massive wound or if the patient is coughing or vomiting bloody material.

Review of the Parts and Function of the Circulatory System

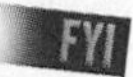

Figure 12.1 presents a schematic illustration of the circulatory system.

The Pump

The heart functions as the human circulatory system's pump. The heart consists of four separate chambers, two on top and two on the bottom.

BSI and Safety Tips are included to reinforce safety concerns for both the responder and the patient.

*Over 30 **Skill Drills** present a step-by-step, visual summary of key skills in a format that enhances student comprehension.*

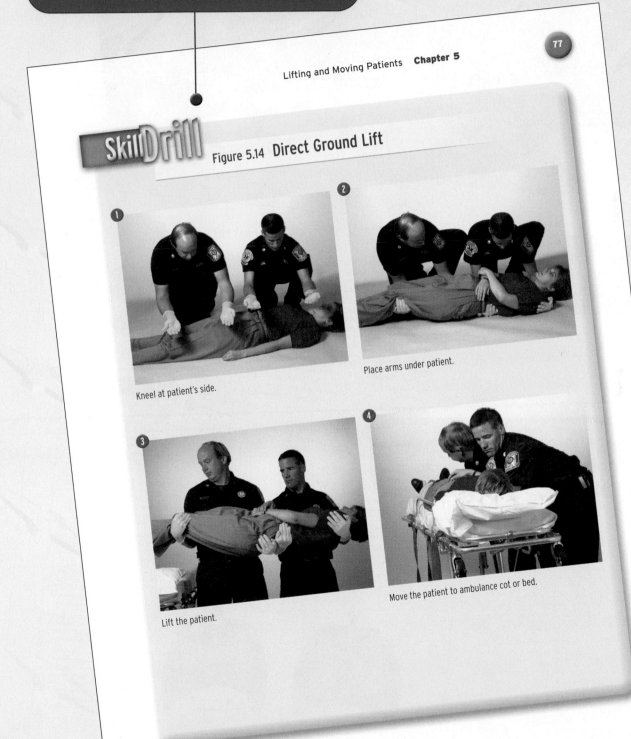

Skill Drill

Figure 5.14 Direct Ground Lift

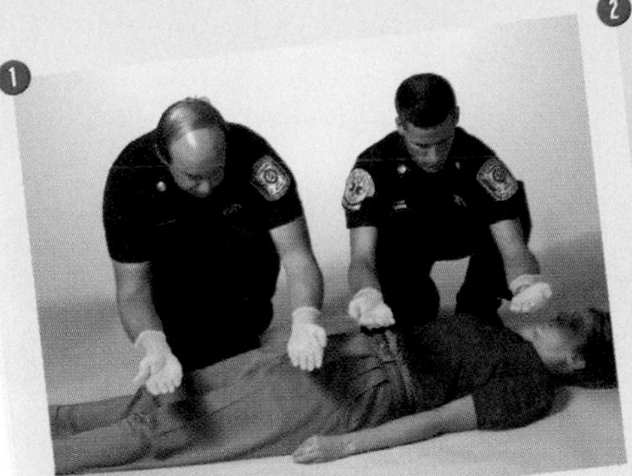

1 Kneel at patient's side.

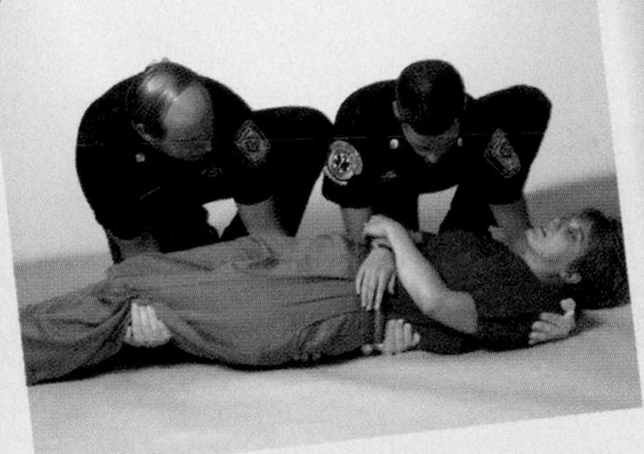

2 Place arms under patient.

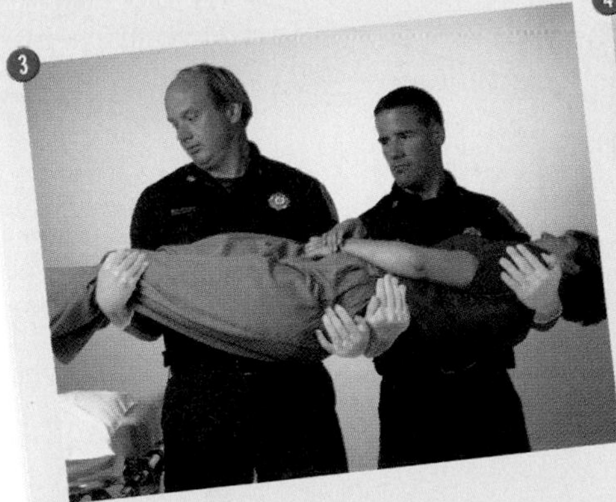

3 Lift the patient.

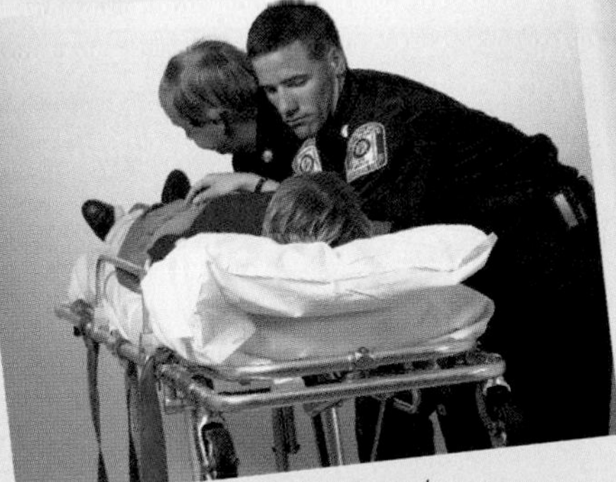

4 Move the patient to ambulance cot or bed.

Resource Preview

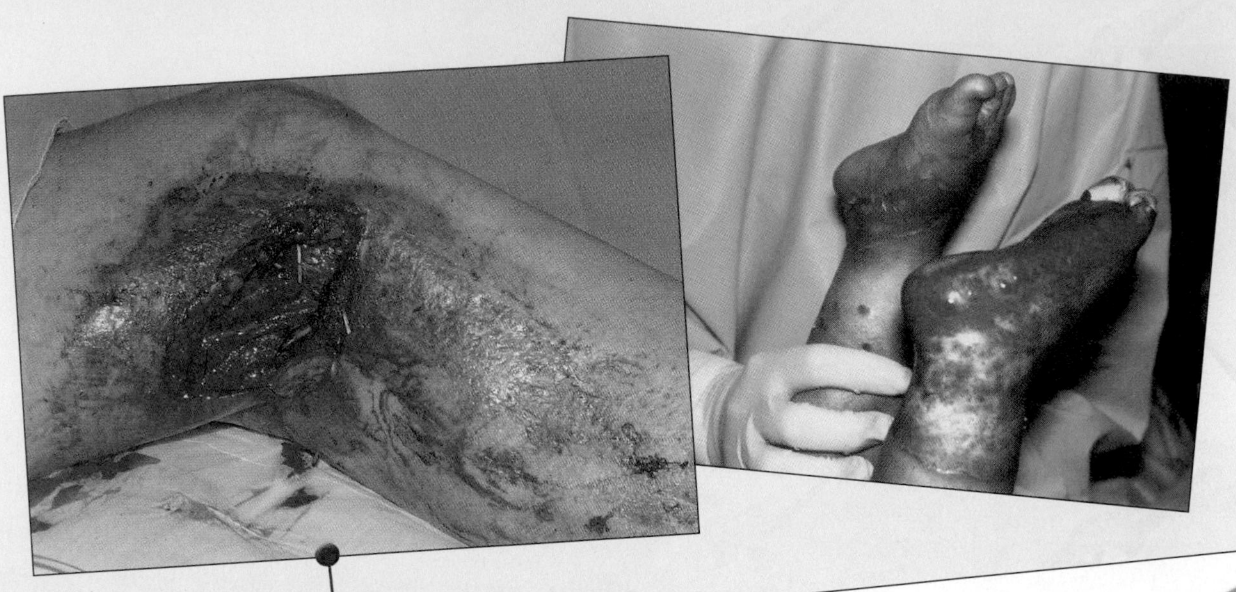

Trauma photos *prepare students to handle an actual real-life emergency.*

pillaries. The actual exchange of gases takes embrane that separates the capillaries of the om the alveoli of the lungs (**Figure 6.4**). The sses from the alveoli into the blood, and the outgoing dioxide passes from the blood into the alveoli.

The lungs consist of soft, spongy tissue with no muscles. Therefore, movement of air into the lungs depends on movement of the rib cage and the diaphragm. As the rib cage expands, air is drawn into the lungs through the trachea. The diaphragm, a muscle that separates the abdominal cavity from the chest, is dome-shaped when it is relaxed. When the diaphragm contracts, it flattens and moves downward. This action increases the size of the chest cavity and draws air into the lungs through the trachea. In normal breathing, the combined actions of the diaphragm and the rib cage automatically produce adequate inhalation and exhalation (**Figure 6.5**).

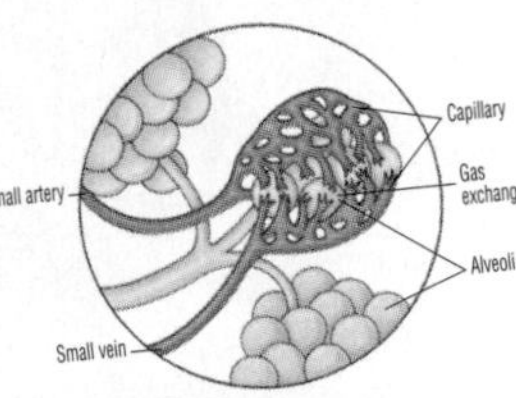

Figure 6.4 The exchange of gases occurs in the alveoli of the lungs.

point

the major structures of the respiratory system?

the function of each structure?

these functions interrelated?

Special Needs *sections highlight specific concerns or procedures for particular groups, such as elderly or pediatric patients.*

Special Needs

INFANTS AND CHILDREN

- The structures of the respiratory systems in children and infants are smaller than they are in adults. Thus the air passages of children and infants may be more easily blocked by secretions or by foreign objects.
- In children and infants, the tongue is proportionally larger than it is in adults. Thus the tongue of these smaller patients is more likely to block their airway than it would in an adult patient.
- Because the trachea of an infant or child is more flexible than that of an adult, it is more likely to become narrowed or blocked than that of an adult.
- The head of a child or an infant is proportionally larger than the head of an adult. You will have to learn slightly different techniques for opening the airway of children.
- Children and infants have smaller lungs than adults. You need to give them smaller breaths when you perform rescue breathing.
- Most children and infants have healthy hearts. When a child or infant suffers cardiac arrest (stoppage of the heart), it is usually because the patient has a blocked airway or has stopped breathing, not because there is a problem with the heart.

"A" Is for Airway

The patient's airway is the pipeline that transports life-giving oxygen from the air to the lungs and transports the waste product, carbon dioxide, from the lungs to the air. In healthy individuals, the airway automatically stays open. An injured or seriously ill person, however, may not be able to protect the airway, and it may become blocked. If a patient cannot protect his or her airway, you, as a first responder, must take certain steps to check the condition of the patient's airway and correct the problem to keep the patient alive.

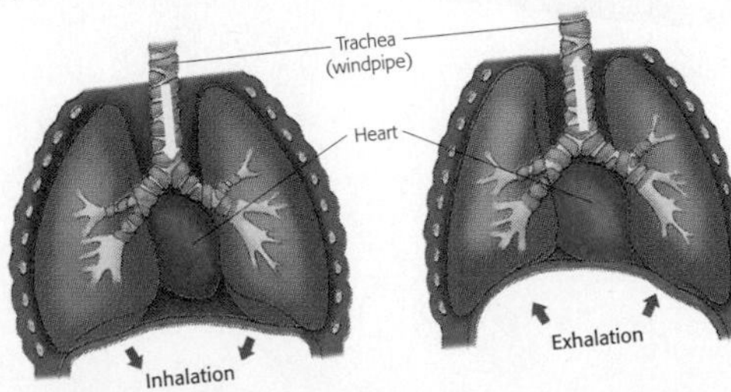

Figure 6.5 Normal mechanical act of breathing.

Resource Preview

16 Prep Kit

Prep Kit, *end of chapter activities, reinforce important concepts and evaluate student mastery of the subject.*

Ready for Review

Ready for Review thoroughly summarizes the chapter.

This chapter covers EMS operations. As a first responder, you need the proper equipment on an emergency call. The chapter covers the five phases of an emergency response and the seven steps of extrication. You should be able to perform the first four steps of extrication and assist other rescuers with steps five through seven. Because you may be the first trained person on the scene of an incident involving hazardous materials, you must be able to identify the potential problem and respond appropriately.

You should also understand the role of a first responder during the first few minutes of a multiple-casualty incident. The START system is a simple triage system that you can use at a multiple-casualty incident. By learning these simple but important skills involving EMS operations, you can become an effective and life-saving member of the EMS system in your community.

Vital Vocabulary

The Vital Vocabulary are the key

casualty sorting—*page 400*
chocking—*page 390*
extrication—*page 385*
fusee—*page 388*

Practice Points

The Practice Points are the key sk
need to know.

1. Performing simple procedures fo to a patient in a wrecked vehicle
2. Using the START system during ple- or mass-casualty incidents.

one-person walking assist A method used if the patient is able to bear his or her own weight.

two-person walking assist Used when a patient cannot bear his or her own weight; two rescuers completely support the patient.

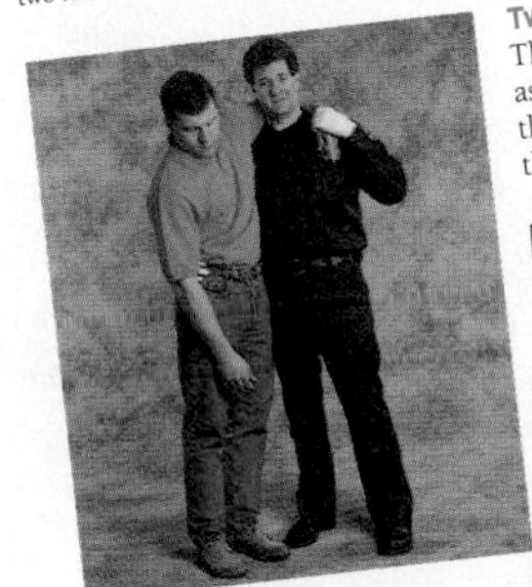

Figure 5.16 One-person walking assist.

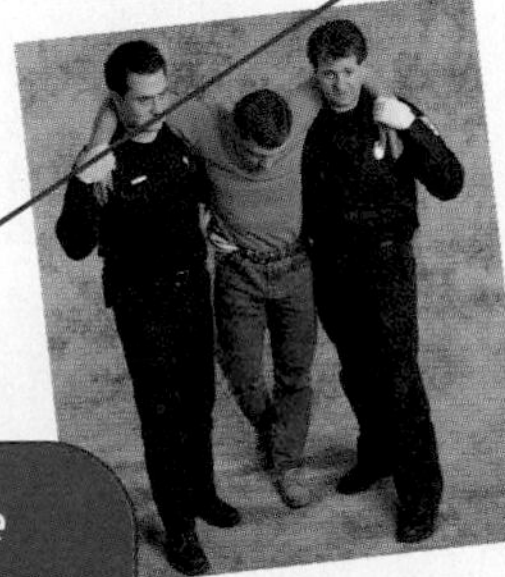

Figure 5.17 Two-person walking assist.

One-Person Walking Assist

The **one-person walking assist** can be used if the patient is able to bear his or her own weight. Help the patient stand. Have the patient place one arm around your neck, and hold the patient's wrist (which should be draped over your shoulder). Put your free arm around the patient's waist and help the patient to walk (**Figure 5.16**).

Two-Person Walking Assist

The **two-person walking assist** is the same as the one-person walking assist, except that two rescuers are needed. This technique is useful if the patient cannot bear weight. The two rescuers completely support the patient (**Figure 5.17**).

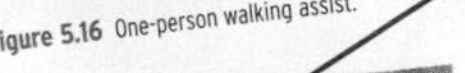

CAUTION

Do not use any of the preceding lifts or carries if you suspect that the patient has a spinal injury, unless, of course, it is necessary to remove the patient from a life-threatening situation.

Check point

- How can you move a patient by yourself if the patient may have suffered a neck injury?
- How can you move a patient by yourself if the patient has not suffered a neck injury?
- When should you remove a patient from a wrecked vehicle if you are by yourself? How would you move this patient?
- Why is it sometimes best to move a patient who has suffered cardiac arrest before you begin CPR?

Check Point *questions, within the chapter, allow students to gauge their own progress.*

Equipment

Most of the lifts and moves described in the previous section are done without any specialized equipment. However, EMS services commonly use various types of patient-moving equipment. To be able to assist other EMS providers, you should be familiar with this equipment.

Wheeled Ambulance Stretchers

Wheeled ambulance stretchers are carried by ambulances and are one of the most commonly used EMS devices (**Figure 5.18**). These stretchers are also called cots. Most of them can be raised or lowered to several different heights. The head end of the cot can be raised to elevate the patient's head. These stretchers have belts to secure the patient. Each type of stretcher has its own set of levers and controls for raising and lowering. If you regularly work with the same EMS unit, it will be helpful to learn how their particular type of stretcher operates.

Online Resources

www.FirstResponderTraining.com

A key component in our program, innovative and interactive activities help students become great First Responders.

Online Pretests *help prepare students for training. Each chapter has an online pretest and provides instant results, feedback on incorrect answers, and page references.*

Online Glossary *expands student's medical vocabulary through an interactive key term review.*

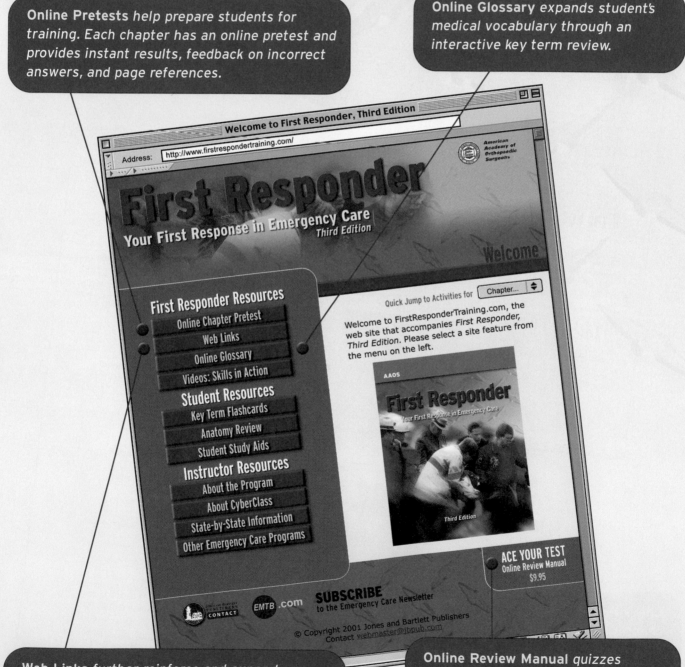

Web Links *further reinforce and expand on topics covered in each chapter. Every link is presented with a description of both the topic and the web site.*

Online Review Manual *quizzes students on chapter material and provides instant feedback.*

www.FirstResponderTraining.com

Online Resources

Ace Your Course! Online Review Manual

The **Online Review Manual** is designed to evaluate mastery of material learned in class and covered in First Responder, Third Edition. Each chapter in the book is supplemented with:

- an exam consisting of multiple-choice questions to test students' knowledge of key concepts and procedures,
- a special grading feature for immediate results and answers to all of the questions,
- a chapter correlation of the question/answer to the Third Edition.

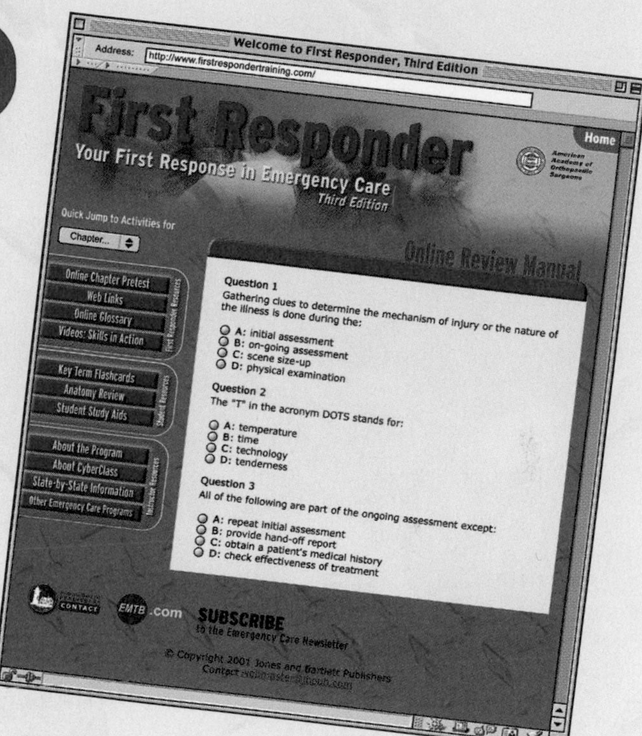

Instructor Resources

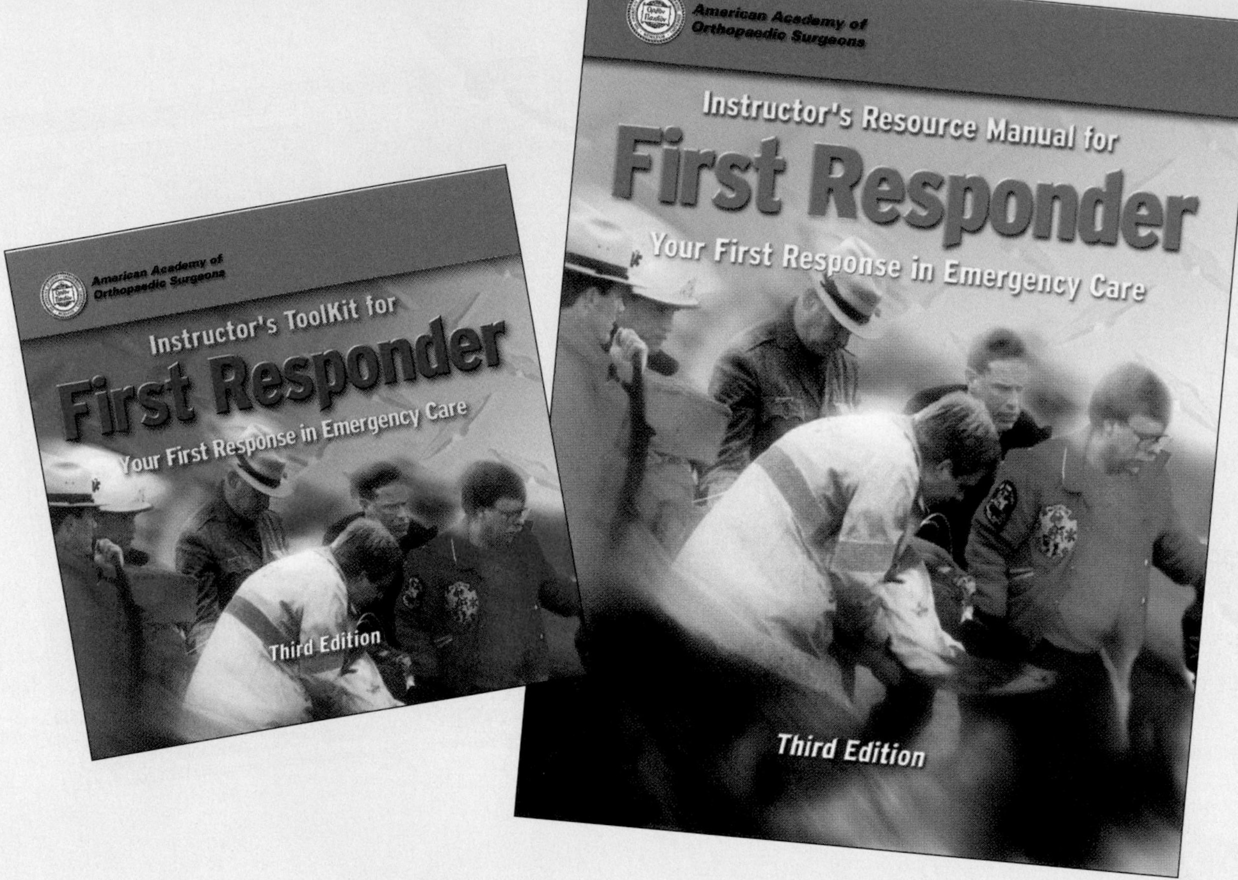

Instructor's ToolKit CD-ROM

We have made it easy for you with fully adaptable:

- *Lecture Outlines*—complete, ready-to-use lesson plans from the Instructor's Resource Manual outlines all of the topics covered in the text.
- *PowerPoint™ Presentations*—provide you with a powerful way to make presentations that are educational and engaging to your students. The slides can be modified and edited to fit your individual presentation.
- *Lecture Success Image Bank*—all images from the book, both photographs and illustrations.
- *Video Clips*—allow you to illustrate the most important skills students need to learn.

ISBN: 0-7637-1759-2

Instructor's Resource Manual

This new manual includes:

- lesson plans
- teaching strategies
- proficiency tests
- supplemental information
- additional scenarios

This manual is designed to be your quick reference guide and helps you to utilize all of the outstanding instructor resources.

ISBN: 0-7637-1755-X

Instructor Resources

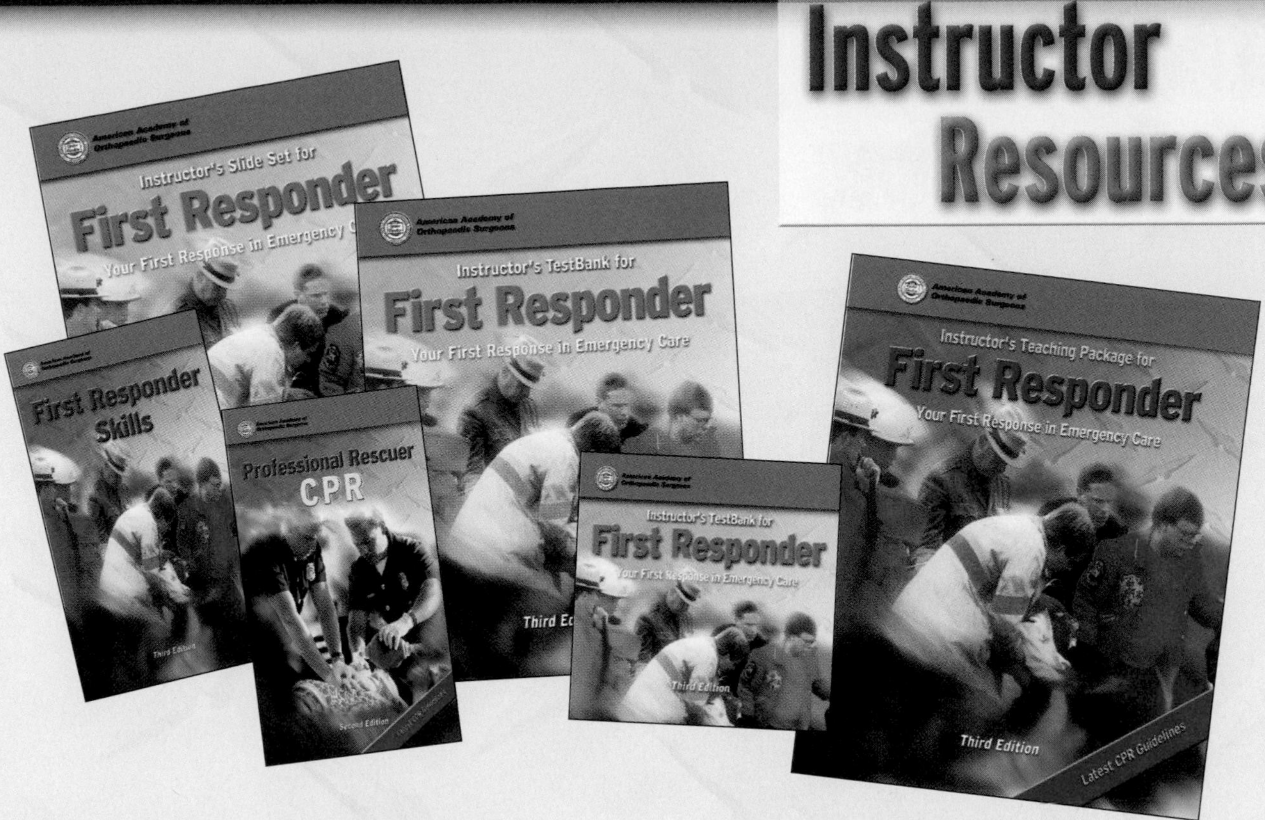

First Responder Skills Video

This new full-feature video, designed in a topical format, corresponds with the material in the text. A combination of dramatic, real-life emergencies with a proven format make this video essential for all courses covering first responder skills.

ISBN: 0-7637-1758-4

Instructor's TestBank

A new 1,000 test question manual corresponds to the chapters in the text and includes scenario-based questions.

ISBN: 0-7637-1752-5

Professional Rescuer CPR Video

This outstanding video applies to all CPR training and follows the latest CPR guidelines.

ISBN: 0-7637-1756-8

Instructor's TestBank on CD-ROM

This computerized test bank allows you to originate tailor-made tests quickly, easily, and error-free by selecting, editing, organizing, and printing a test along with an answer key.

ISBN: 0-7637-1751-7

Instructor's Slide Set

This all-new set of 35mm color slides depicts key first responder topics and actual injuries. The topical slides outline the most important information in the text while the injury slides prepare your students to handle real-life emergencies.

ISBN: 0-7637-1757-6

Teaching Package

In one convenient box, the Teaching Package combines:

- Instructor's Resource Manual
- First Responder Skills Video
- Professional Rescuer CPR Video
- Instructor's Slide Set
- Instructor's TestBank (printed version)

ISBN: 0-7637-1754-1

Please call 1-800-832-0034 for more information.

Student Resources

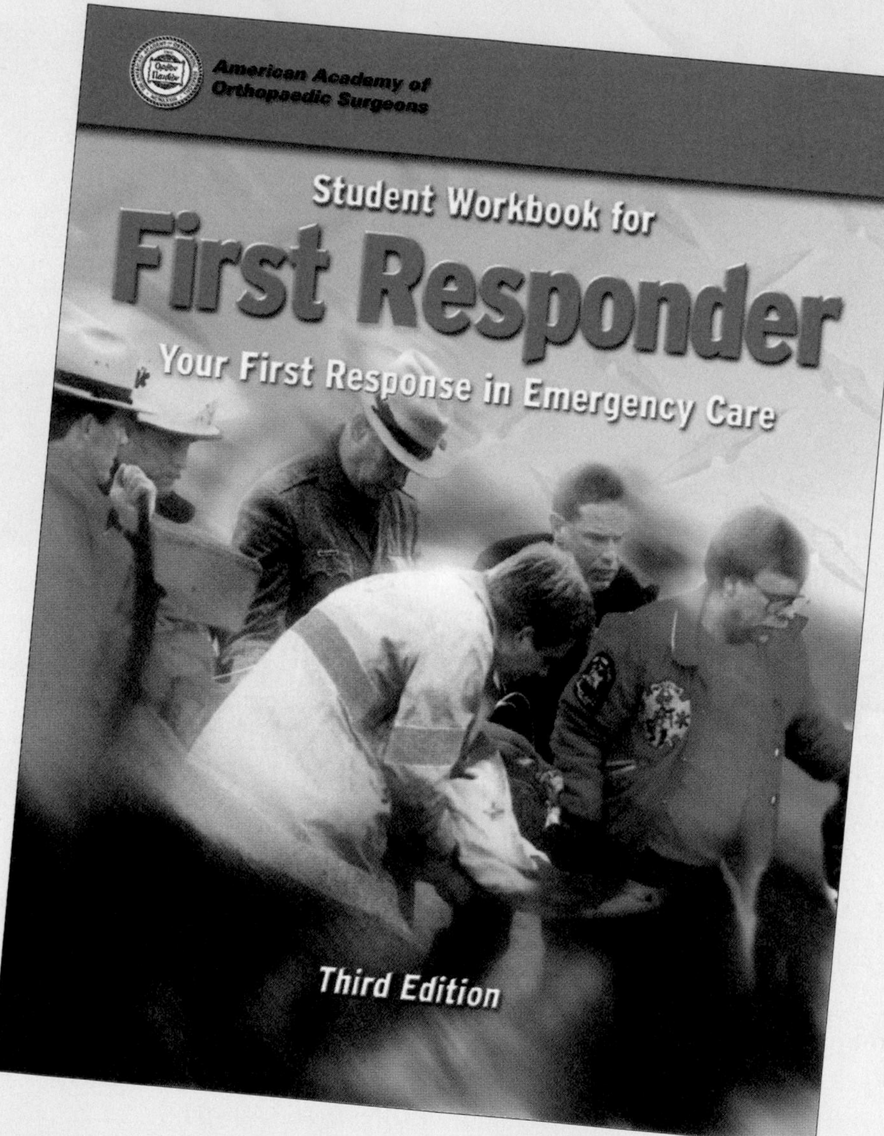

Student Workbook

Designed to encourage critical thinking and aid comprehension of course material, the workbook's organization and content follow the DOT curriculum. A variety of interesting exercises and scenarios reinforce the objectives and concepts found in the text. It will help students achieve a fuller understanding of the role of the first responder in emergency care.

ISBN: 0-7637-1750-9

To The Student

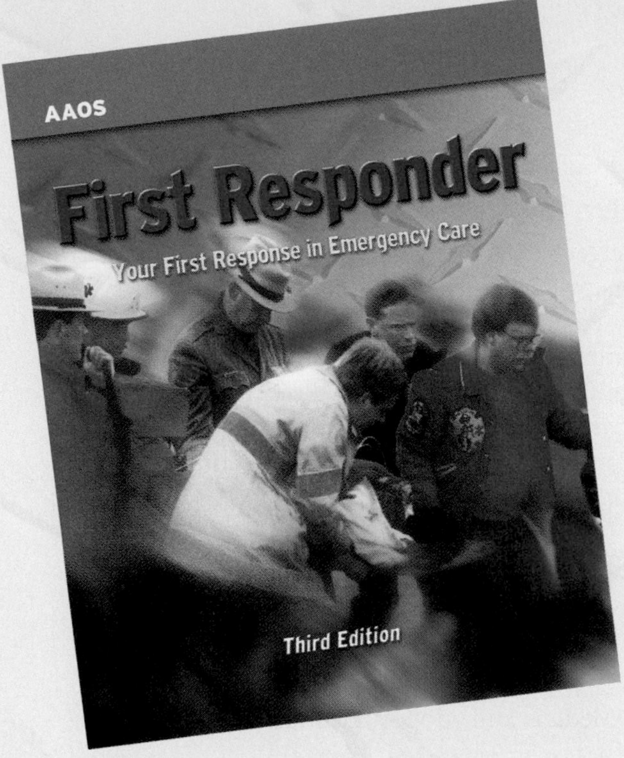

As recently as the mid-1950s there were no commonly used medical techniques that were effective for restarting stopped hearts, and victims often died. Today, simple and advanced techniques can restart a stopped heart. A trained first responder can keep a person alive until advanced techniques can be performed by other medical personnel. Opening a patient's airway, performing rescue breathing, controlling external bleeding, and treating a patient for the signs and symptoms of shock can make a vital difference. Because first responders are often the first medically trained personnel on the scene of an emergency, they supply the first and vital link in a chain of survival. As you study this book, realize that you are about to become a First Responder, an emergency care provider who can make a real difference to patients.

Before studying the knowledge and skills needed to become a medical first responder, it is important to understand more about the following topics:

1. Overview of the First Responder course
2. Criteria for First Responder certification
3. Implications of the Americans with Disabilities Act
4. Ten standard criteria for EMS systems

1. Overview of the First Responder Course

The first responder course presents an exciting opportunity to develop emergency medical skills and knowledge that will enable you to assist people who have sustained an accidental injury or who are suffering from a sudden illness or medical problem. This course follows a national curriculum that was developed by representatives from many federal and state agencies and from professional medical groups. The material you will learn is divided into seven modules, which follow the national standard curriculum. We have added an eighth module, which covers supplemental skills that may be taught to first responders in some communities. The decision about whether to cover this material will be made by course directors. These modules are:

- Module 1 **Preparatory**
- Module 2 **Airway**
- Module 3 **Patient Assessment**
- Module 4 **Circulation**
- Module 5 **Illness and Injury**
- Module 6 **Childbirth and Children**
- Module 7 **EMS Operations**
- Module 8 **Supplemental Skills**

2. Criteria for First Responder Certification

The process of becoming a first responder begins with your thorough study and mastery of the knowledge and skills presented in this book. To practice these skills you must be certified or registered as a first responder in the state where you will be working. Some states require certification or registration through a state agency such as a department of health. Other states may require you to become registered through the National Registry of Emergency Medical Technicians. In either case, you will be required to successfully complete this course and then pass a written and practical test. Your certification or registration is good for a limited period of time. To maintain your certification or recertification, you will be required to complete certain course work to refresh your knowledge and skills and probably take a written and/or practical test. It is important to remember that your ability to function as a first responder depends on maintaining your certification or registration. It is your responsibility to do this even though you may receive help from the agency for which you work.

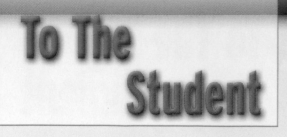

3. Implications of the Americans with Disabilities Act

The Americans with Disabilities Act was passed by Congress in 1990 to protect people with physical or mental disabilities against discrimination. The Act, also known as the ADA, has requirements that affect both you and your patients.

Title I: This section prohibits employment discrimination.

Title II: This section states that no one can be denied access to services provided by local or state governments based on a person's disability. As a public safety employee, you must provide the same level of care for a disabled patient as you provide to a nondisabled patient.

Title III: This section prohibits employers from failing to provide full and equal employment to disabled persons.

Title IV: This section addresses the responsibilities of phone companies to provide special communication features to disabled persons.

Title V: This section explains the implementation of the Americans with Disabilities Act.

As a provider of emergency medical services, it is important that you understand the general purpose of the ADA. Remember, disabled patients are entitled to the same quality care as other patients.

4. Ten Standard Criteria for EMS Systems

Emergency medical services systems can be categorized in many different ways. Different parts of the system may be provided by different agencies in various locations. The National Highway Traffic Safety Administration (NHTSA) of the United States Department of Transportation evaluates EMS systems based on the following ten criteria:

1. Regulation and policy
2. Resource management
3. Human resources and training
4. Transportation equipment and systems
5. Medical and support facilities
6. Communications facilities
7. Public information and education
8. Medical direction
9. Trauma system and development
10. Evaluation

These criteria are used primarily in the administration of an EMS system. There are many ways to categorize an EMS system. A simple model is presented in Chapter 1 and is based on a functional model of an EMS system.

This overview of four topics related to the first responder is designed to familiarize you with some of the background information that will help to make your first responder training more valuable. By giving you some information about the first responder course content, criteria required for certification and recertification, implications of the Americans with Disabilities Act, and ten criteria for evaluating EMS systems, you will have the background to better understand the material presented throughout this book.

Acknowledgments

The American Academy of Orthopaedic Surgeons acknowledges the following individuals for reviewing this text and/or previous editions.

Reviewers

Michael P. Bell
Department of Fire and Rescue Operations
Toledo, OH

Margarita S. Brown
El Paso Community College
El Paso, TX

Steve Brumm
Gulf Coast Community College
Panama City, FL

Raymond W. Burton
Plymouth County Sheriff's Office
Plymouth, MA

Elizabeth Cascio
Fire Department - New York City
Bayside, NY

David C. Cone
Yale University School of Medicine
Newhaven, CT

K. Lee Darnell
North Carolina Office of EMS
Raleigh, NC

Joseph Escobedo
Albuquerque, NM

Judith Guenst
H.K. Carr & Associates
Englishtown, NJ

Paul Guns
Orange County Fire Authority
Orange County, CA

J. Kevin Henson
State of New Mexico
Santa Fe, NM

Victor Robert Hernandez
Sierra College
Rocklin, CA

Wayne Hollis
State of Kansas
Topeka, KS

David M. Magnino
California Highway Patrol
West Sacramento, CA

Gary P. Morris
Phoenix Fire Department
Phoenix, AZ

Robert Pringle
Life Air Rescue
Shreveport, LA

John Reed
Birmingham Regional Emergency Medical Services System
Birmingham, AL

Robb Rehberg
Ramsey, NJ

Gordon M. Sachs
Marion County Fire Rescue
Ocala, FL

David Spiro
St. Mary's Hospital of Brooklyn
Brooklyn, NY

Peggy Stark
Paramedic Instructor
Springfield, NE

Mendee Bayless-Tarrowski
Hennepin County Medical Center - EMS Education
Minneapolis, MN

Alton Thygerson
Brigham Young University
Provo, UT

James Tzitzon
Criminal Justice Training Council
Waltham, MA

Holly Weber
SOLO, Wilderness Emergency Medicine
Conway, NH

Brian Yeaton
SOLO, Wilderness Emergency Medicine
Conway, NH

Aaron W. York
California Highway Patrol
West Sacramento, CA

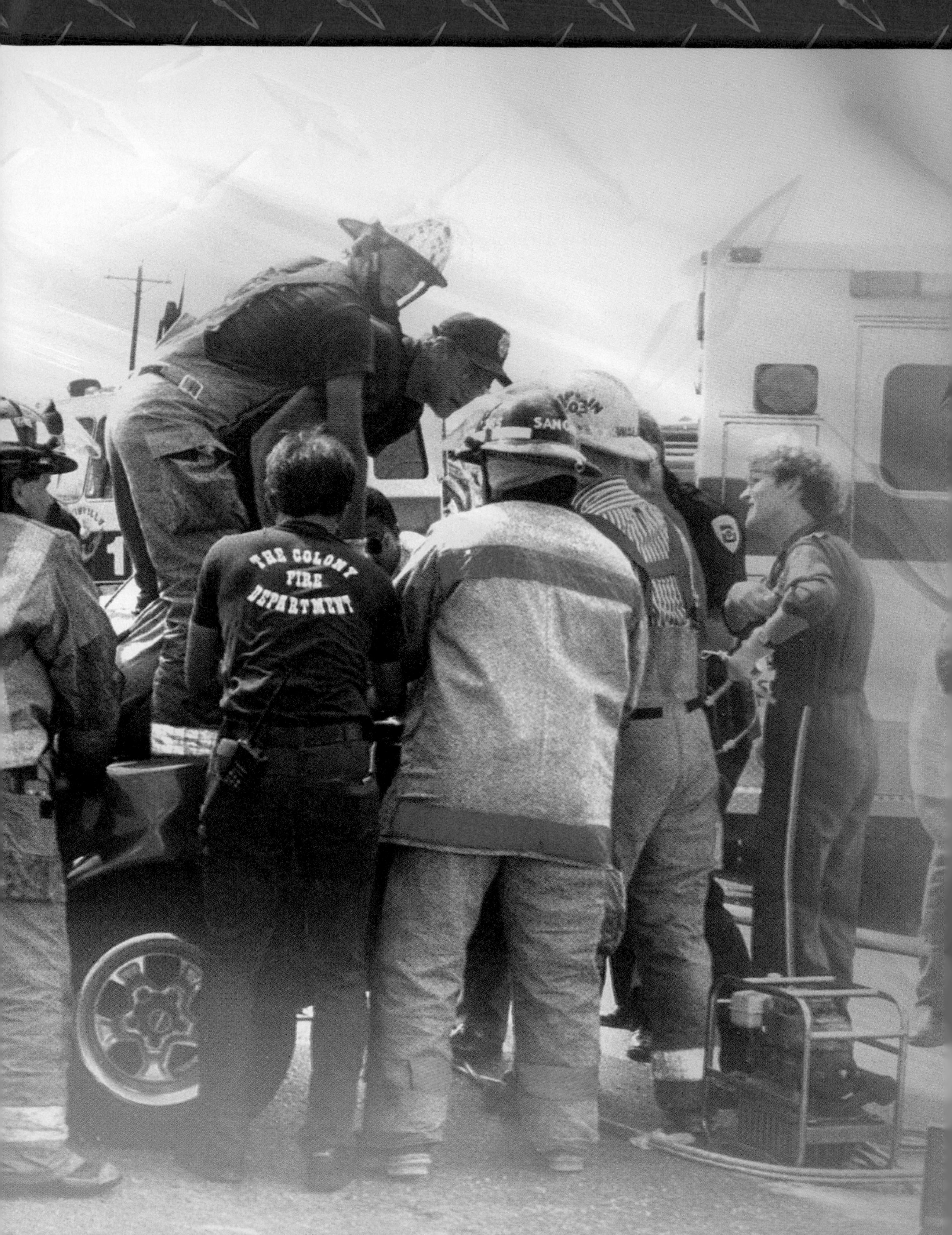
THE COLONY
FIRE
DEPARTMENT

MODULE 1

Preparatory

Module CONTENTS

Chapter 1

Introduction to the EMS System

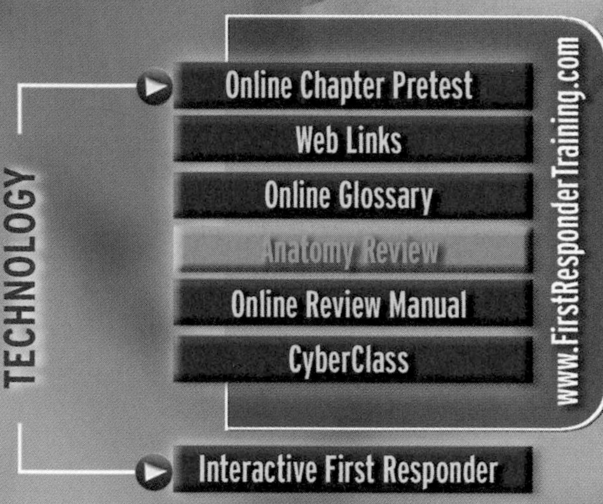

Chapter FEATURES

- Skill Drills
- Vital Vocabulary
- Voices of Experience
- Signs and Symptoms
- FYI
- Special Needs
- Safety Tips
- BSI Tips
- Caution
- Check Point
- Prep Kit

CHAPTER 1

Objectives

Knowledge and Attitude Objectives

After studying this chapter, you will be expected to:

1. Understand and describe the four general goals of your first responder training.
2. Define the components of an emergency medical services (EMS) system.
3. Describe how the seriousness of the patient's condition is used to determine the urgency of transportation to an appropriate medical facility.
4. Define the roles and responsibilities of a first responder.
5. Describe the importance of documentation.
6. Describe the relationship between your attitude and conduct and acceptable patient care.
7. Define medical oversight and discuss the first responder's role in the process.

*The **first responder** is, by definition, the first medically trained person to arrive on the scene. The initial care you give as the first responder is essential because it is available sooner than more advanced emergency medical care and could mean the difference between life and death. Your initial care is usually followed by more sophisticated care given by emergency medical technicians (EMTs), paramedics, nurses, and physicians.*

Did You Know?

In ten minutes, as you read this chapter, two people in the United States will be killed and 350 people will suffer disabling injuries from some type of accident.

First Responder Training

This book has been written for a first responder training course. Although the book alone can teach you some things, it is best to use it as part of an approved first responder course. A first responder course will teach you the basics of good patient care and the skills you will need to deliver appropriate care to the victim of an accident or sudden illness until more highly trained emergency personnel arrive.

The skills and knowledge you will gain from this course provide the foundation for the entire emergency medical services (EMS) system (**Figure 1.1**). Your actions can prevent a minor situation from becoming serious and may even determine whether a patient lives or dies.

In this first responder course, you will learn how to examine patients and how to use basic emergency medical skills. These skills are divided into two main groups: (1) those needed to treat injured **trauma** patients and (2) those needed to care for patients suffering from illness or serious **medical** problems.

You will learn the following skills to stabilize and treat persons who have been injured:

- Controlling airway, breathing, and circulation (Chapters 6 and 8)
- Controlling external bleeding (hemorrhage) (Chapter 12)
- Treating shock (Chapter 12)
- Treating wounds (Chapter 12)
- Splinting injuries to stabilize extremities (Chapter 13)

In addition to these **trauma** skills, you will learn to recognize, stabilize, and provide initial treatment for the following **medical** conditions:

- Heart attacks (Chapter 9)
- Seizures (Chapter 9)
- Problems associated with excessive heat or cold (Chapter 9)
- Alcohol and drug abuse (Chapter 10)
- Poisonings (Chapter 10)
- Bites and stings (Chapter 10)
- Altered mental status (Chapter 11)
- Behavioral or psychological crises (Chapter 11)
- Emergency childbirth (Chapter 14)

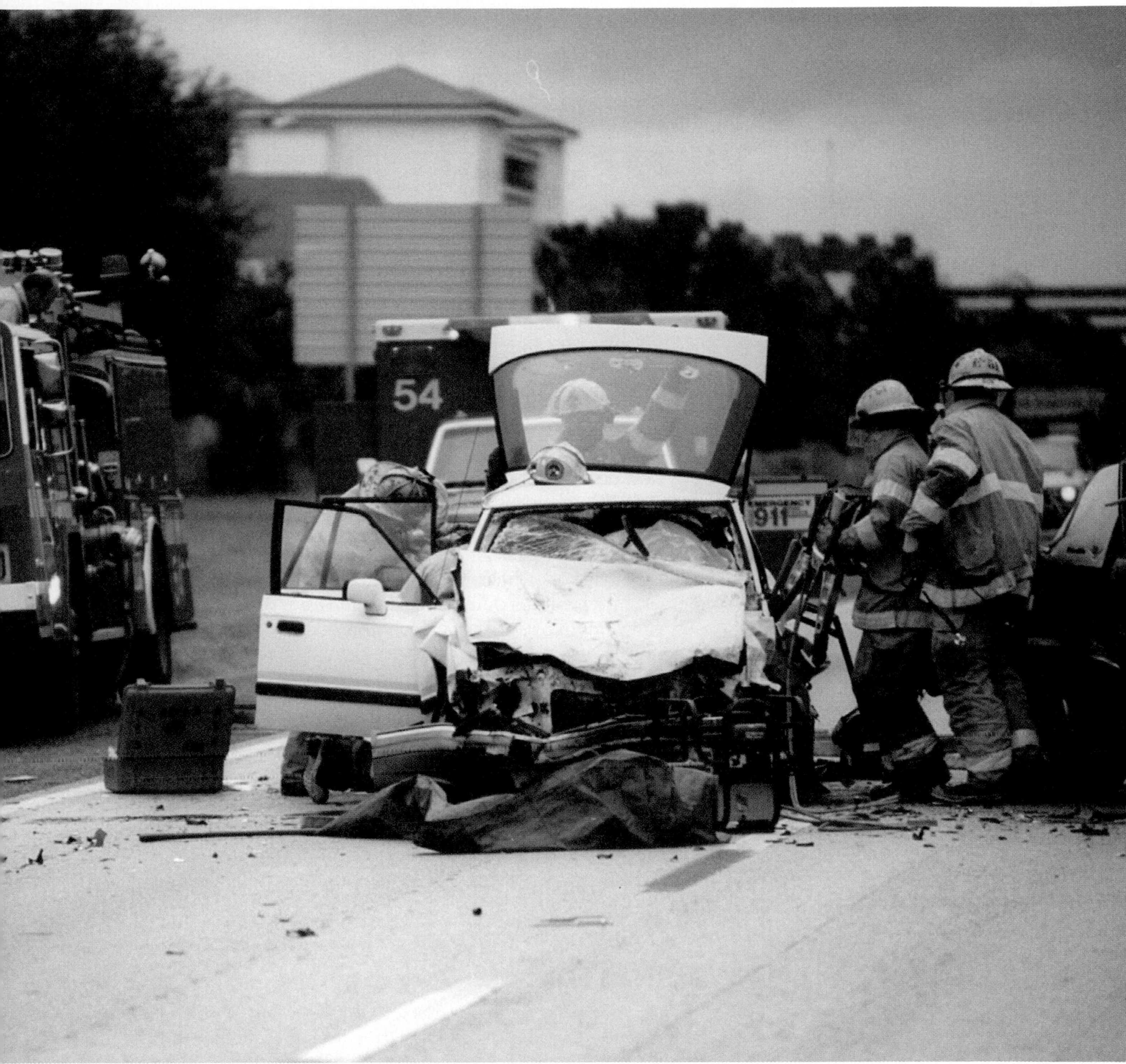

Figure 1.1 A typical emergency scene with injured patients.

Goals of First Responder Training

It is important for you to understand the basic goals of first responder training. This training aims to teach you how to evaluate, stabilize, and treat patients using a minimum of specialized equipment. As a first responder, you will find yourself in situations where little or no emergency medical equipment is readily available, so you must know how to improvise. Finally, first responder training teaches you what you can do to help EMTs and paramedics when they arrive on the scene.

WHAT FIRST RESPONDERS SHOULD KNOW

- *What you should not do*
- *How to use your first responder life support kit*
- *How to improvise*
- *How to assist other EMS providers*

Know What You Should Not Do

The first lesson you must learn as a first responder is what not to do! For example, it may be better for you to leave a patient in the position found rather than attempt to move him or her without the proper equipment or an adequate number of trained personnel.

CAUTION

Above all, do nothing that would further harm the patient!

Know How to Use Your First Responder Life Support Kit

The second goal of first responder training is to teach you to treat patients using limited emergency medical supplies. A first responder life support kit should be small enough to fit in the trunk of an automobile or on almost any police, fire or rescue vehicle. Although the contents of the kit are limited, such supplies are all you need to provide immediate care for most patients you will encounter. The suggested contents of a first responder life support kit are shown in **Figure 1.2** and described in **Table 1.1**.

Know How to Improvise

The third goal of first responder training is to teach you to improvise. As a trained first responder, you will often be in situations with little or no emergency medical equipment. Therefore, it is important that you know how to improvise. Although no course can teach improvisation, this course provides examples that can be applied to real-life situations. You will learn, for example, how to use articles of clothing and handkerchiefs to stop bleeding and how to use wooden boards, magazines, or newspapers to immobilize injured extremities.

Know How to Assist Other EMS Providers

Finally, first responder training teaches you how to assist EMTs and paramedics once they arrive on the scene. Many procedures that EMTs and paramedics use cannot be performed correctly by fewer than three people. Thus you may have to assist with these procedures, and must know what to do.

Additional Skills

First responders operate in a variety of settings. Many problems encountered in urban areas differ sharply from those found in rural settings. In addition, regional variations in climate create conditions that not only affect the situations you encounter but also require you to use different skills and equipment in treating patients.

Certain skills and equipment mentioned in this book are beyond the essential, minimum knowledge level that you need to successfully complete a first responder course. However, these supplemental skills and equipment may be required in your local EMS system. Supplemental skills are identified by the following icon: FYI

Table 1.1

Suggested Contents of a First Responder Life Support Kit

Patient Examination Equipment	1 flashlight
Personal Safety Equipment	5 pairs of gloves 5 face masks
Resuscitation Equipment	1 mouth-to-mask resuscitation device 1 portable hand-powered suction device 1 set oral airways 1 set nasal airways
Bandaging and Dressing Equipment	10 gauze-adhesive strips 1" 10 gauze pads 4" x 4" 5 gauze pads 5" x 9" 2 universal trauma dressings 10" x 30" 1 occlusive dressing for sealing chest wounds 4 conforming gauze rolls 3" x 5 yd 4 rolls 4½" x 5 yd 6 triangular bandages 1 adhesive tape 2" 1 burn sheet
Patient Immobilization Equipment	2 (each) cervical collars: small, medium, large or 2 adjustable cervical collars 3 rigid conforming splints (SAM™ splints) OR 1 set air splints for arm and leg OR 2 (each) cardboard splints 18" and 24"
Extrication Equipment	1 spring-loaded center punch 1 pair heavy leather gloves
Miscellaneous Equipment	2 blankets (disposable) 2 cold packs 1 bandage scissors

Other Equipment:

1 set personal protective clothing (helmet, eye protection, EMS jacket)
1 reflective vest
1 fire extinguisher (5 lb. ABC dry chemical)
1 Emergency Response Guidebook
6 fusees
1 binoculars

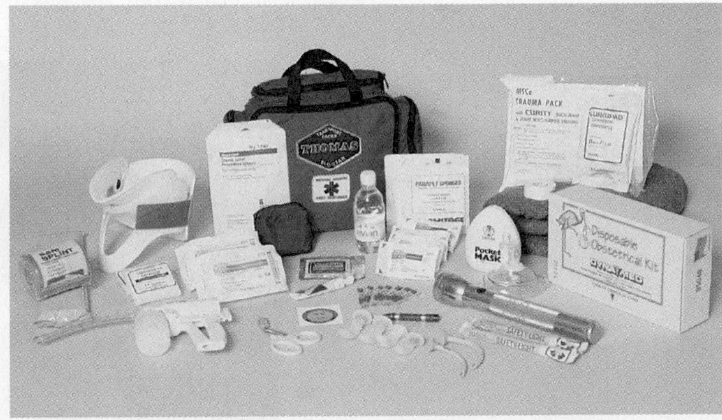

Figure 1.2 Suggested contents of a first responder life support kit.

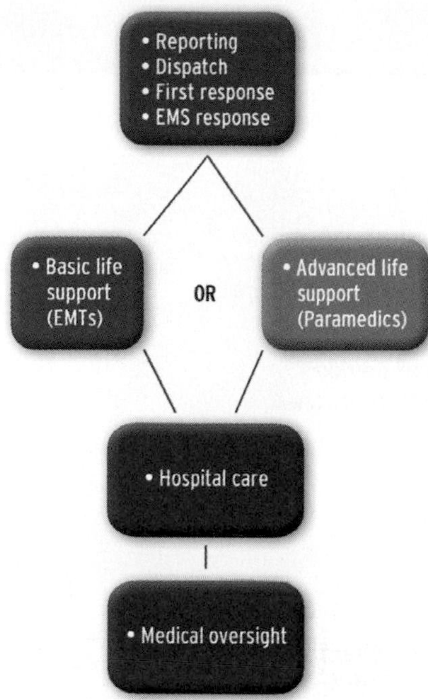

Figure 1.3 The emergency medical services system.

The Emergency Medical Services System

The EMS system was developed because evidence showed that patients who received appropriate emergency medical care before they reached the hospital had a better chance of surviving a major accident or sudden illness than patients who did not receive such care. It is important that you understand the operation and complexity of an EMS system (**Figure 1.3**).

Problems that occur in the "prehospital" phase of the EMS operation often focus on control and coordination of resources and personnel. All agencies and personnel need to share a mutual understanding of their roles for an EMS system to operate smoothly in both "routine" and multiple-casualty situations. This understanding develops through close cooperation, careful planning, and continual effort. You can best understand the EMS system by examining the sequence of events as an injured or ill patient moves through the system.

Reporting

The reporting of the emergency incident activates the EMS system (**Figure 1.4**). An **emergency services dispatch center** usually receives the phone call reporting an incident. The dispatch center may be a fire, police, or EMS agency; a 9-1-1 center; or a seven-digit emergency telephone number used by one or all of the emergency agencies. Enhanced 9-1-1 centers can determine the location of the caller by computer as soon as the telephone in the 9-1-1 center is answered.

emergency services dispatch center A fire, police, or emergency medical services (EMS) agency; a 9-1-1 center; or a seven-digit telephone number used by one or all of the emergency agencies to receive and dispatch requests for emergency care.

Dispatch

Once the emergency services dispatch center is notified of an incident, appropriate equipment and personnel are dispatched to the scene (**Figure 1.5**). How notification occurs (pager, telephone, and so forth) and what agencies, personnel, and equipment are involved in the first response varies by community.

First Response

Because of their location or speed in responding, firefighters (paid or volunteer) or law enforcement personnel are likely to be the first

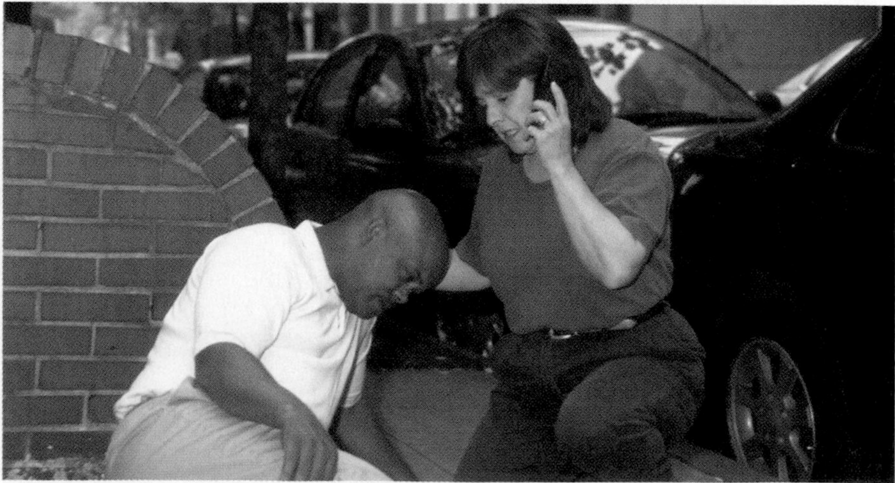

Figure 1.4 Reporting an emergency.

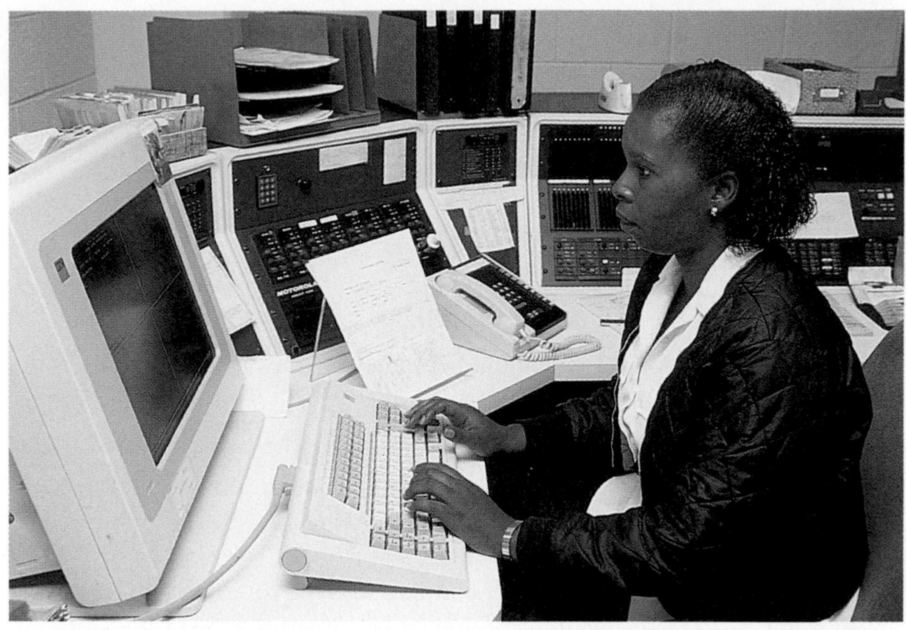

Figure 1.5 A dispatch center receives the call.

responders in most emergencies (**Figure 1.6**). Most communities have many potential first responders, but few EMTs and even fewer paramedics. A community with four or five fire stations may have only two or three ambulances. In some situations, a first responder's actions can mean the difference between life and death. For example, a key survival factor for people in cardiac arrest is the length of time between when the heartbeat stops and when manual cardiopulmonary resuscitation (CPR) starts.

The patient's first and perhaps most crucial contact with the EMS system occurs when the trained first responder arrives. The first responder is a key element in providing emergency care.

EMS Response

The arrival of an emergency medical vehicle (usually an ambulance) (**Figure 1.7**) staffed by **Emergency Medical Technicians-Basic (EMT-Bs)** or paramedics is the patient's second contact with the EMS system. A properly equipped vehicle and the EMTs who staff it make up a **basic life support (BLS)** unit. Each EMT has completed at least 110 hours of training, and many may complete even longer training courses.

EMTs continue the care begun by first responders. EMTs stabilize the patient further and prepare the patient for transport to the emergency

Emergency Medical Technician-Basic (EMT-B) A person who is trained and certified to provide basic life support and certain other noninvasive prehospital medical procedures.

basic life support (BLS) Emergency lifesaving procedures performed without advanced emergency procedures to stabilize patients who have experienced sudden illness or injury.

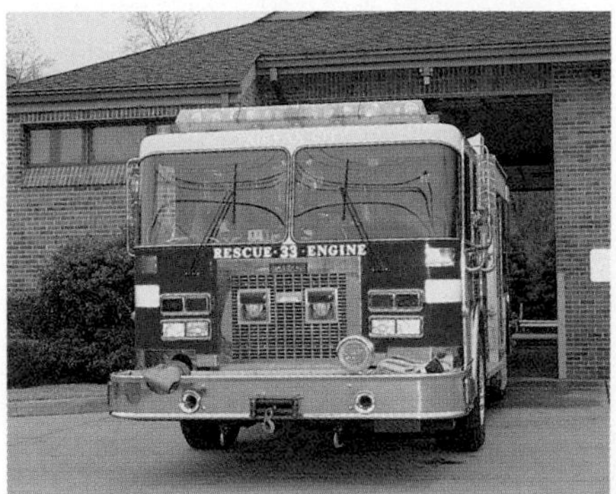

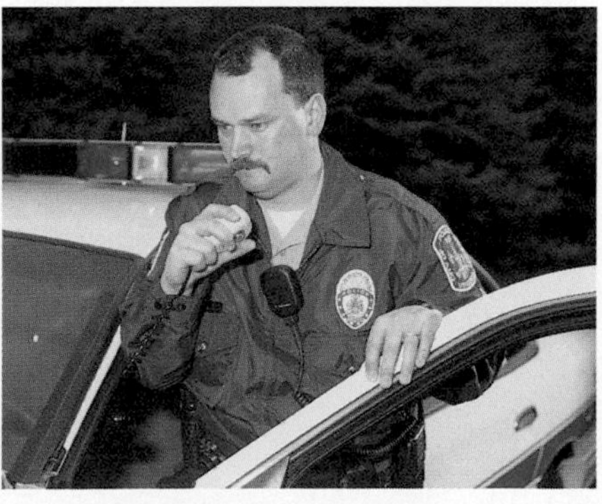

Figure 1.6 Firefighters and law enforcement personnel are first responders in many emergencies.

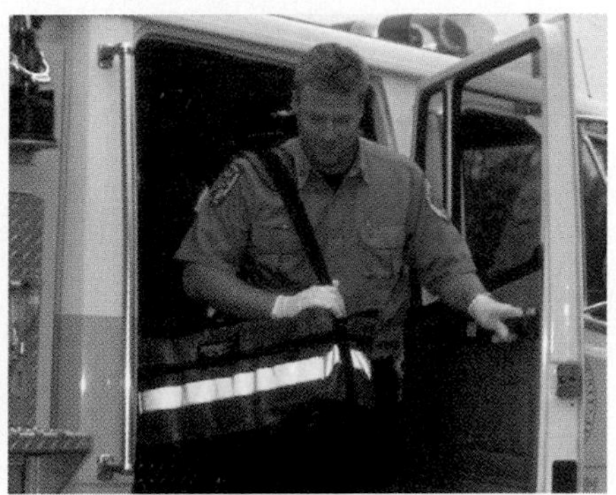

Figure 1.7 EMS responds.

Voices of Experience

A Normal Response to Stress

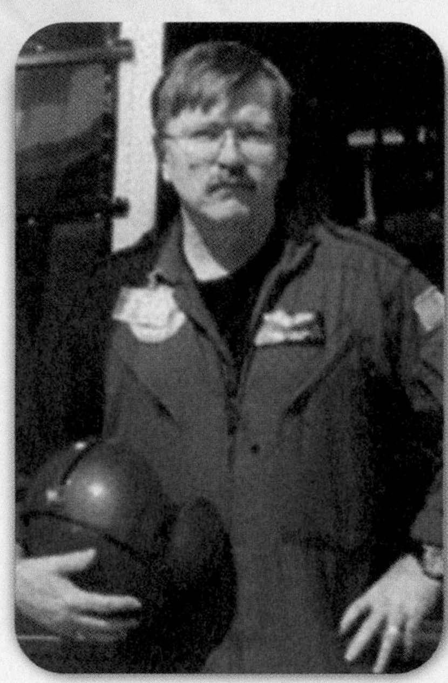

A normal response to a patient death is self-questioning such as, "What could I have done differently?", "What did I do wrong?", and "What will my partner think of me?" These are thoughts that all emergency personnel have at one time or another. It is normal to experience these thoughts.

It is also normal to suddenly find yourself in over your head on a bad call. This is especially likely to occur when something about the call strikes a personal note. For example, the abused child looks like your son, the woman reminds you of a girl you knew, the motorcyclist reminds you of an old boyfriend, or something else about the scene clicks. When this happens, the wall of professional distancing you have worked so hard to build crumbles in a split second, preventing you from being able to think straight. In such a situation, you cannot remember what to do, and may not want to be there at all. This kind of experience is called critical incident stress. Sooner or later, it happens to each and every one of us. The good news is that it is a normal response to an abnormal situation. It does not mean you are weak, crazy, or not cut out for the job. It means that you are human. Always make your best effort to save lives, but also remember and accept that you can only do your best, regardless of the outcome. ❖

"Sooner or later, critical incident stress happens to each and every one of us. The good news is that it is a normal response to an abnormal situation."

Michael Cox, EMT-P, RN, MA, CEN, NCC, CCRN
Florida Flight 1
Florida Hospital Medical Center
Orlando, Florida

department of the hospital. Well-trained emergency personnel who can carefully move the patient and provide proper treatment increase the chance that the patient will arrive at the emergency department in the best possible condition.

In addition to BLS services provided by EMTs, patients may receive **advanced life support (ALS)** services from paramedics. **Paramedics** have more than the BLS skills and knowledge of EMTs. They have received additional training so they can administer intravenous (IV) fluids and certain medications, and monitor and treat heart conditions with medications and **defibrillation**. Defibrillation is the administration of an electric shock to the heart of a patient who is suffering from a highly irregular heartbeat. This may also be done by specialty trained EMT-B and First Responders. Paramedics are also trained to place special airway tubes (endotracheal tubes) to keep the patient's airway open.

Emergency Medical Technicians-Intermediate (EMT-Is) are able to perform limited ALS skills. They may work alone or they may work with a paramedic on an ALS unit.

Each level of skill builds upon the one that precedes it: the paramedic's skills originate from those of the EMT-B, and the techniques used by the EMT-B depend on those of the first responder. All skill levels are based on what you will learn in the first responder course: airway maintenance, control of bleeding, and prevention, recognition, and treatment of shock.

The EMS system involves more than emergency medical care. For example, law enforcement personnel are often a crucial part of the system because they may provide protection and control at the scene of an incident. Fire units provide fire protection, specialized rescue, and patient extrication.

advanced life support (ALS) The use of specialized equipment such as cardiac monitors, defibrillators, intravenous fluids, drug infusion, and endotracheal intubation to stabilize patients who have experienced sudden illness or injury.

paramedic An emergency medical technician who has completed an extensive course of 800 or more hours and who can perform advanced life support skills.

defibrillation Delivery of an electric current through a person's chest wall and heart for the purpose of ending lethal heart rhythms such as ventricular fibrillation.

Hospital Care

The patient's third contact with the EMS system occurs in the hospital, primarily in the emergency department. After being treated at the scene, the patient is transported to an appropriate hospital, where definitive treatment can be given (**Figure 1.8**).

It may be necessary for the patient to be transported to the closest appropriate medical facility first, for stabilization, and then to a hospital that provides specialized treatment. Special facilities include burn centers, pediatric centers, poison control centers, perinatal centers, and trauma centers. You must learn and follow your local patient transportation protocols.

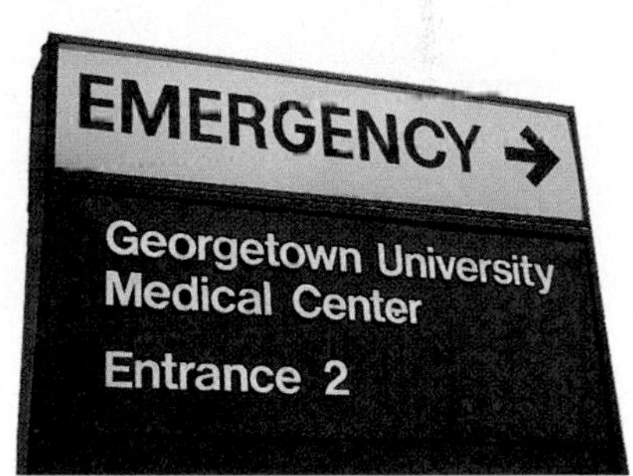

Figure 1.8 Hospital emergency care.

Ten Standard Components of an EMS System

Emergency medical services systems can be categorized in many different ways. Depending on location, the same part of the system may be provided by different agencies. The National Highway Traffic

Checkpoint

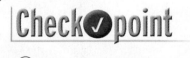

- ○ Why is it important to understand the sequence of events in the emergency medical services system?

Safety Administration (NHTSA) of the United States Department of Transportation evaluates EMS systems based on the following ten criteria, which are used primarily in the administration of an EMS system.

1. Regulation and policy
2. Resource management
3. Human resources and training
4. Transportation equipment and system
5. Medical and support facilities
6. Communications system
7. Public information and education
8. Medical direction
9. Trauma system and development
10. Evaluation

FYI

A Word about Transportation

As a first responder, your primary goal is to provide immediate care for a sick or injured patient. As more highly trained emergency medical service personnel (EMTs or paramedics) arrive on the scene, you will assist them in treating and preparing the patient for transportation. Although other EMS personnel usually provide patient transportation, it is important that you understand when a patient must be transported quickly to a hospital or other medical facility (**Figure 1.9**).

This book uses three terms to describe proper patient transportation:

- Ⓣ *Transport* Transportation to an appropriate medical facility. This phrase means that a patient's condition requires care by medical professionals, but speed in getting the patient to a medical facility is not the most important factor. For example, this might describe the transportation needed by a patient who has sustained an isolated injury to an extremity but whose condition is otherwise stable.

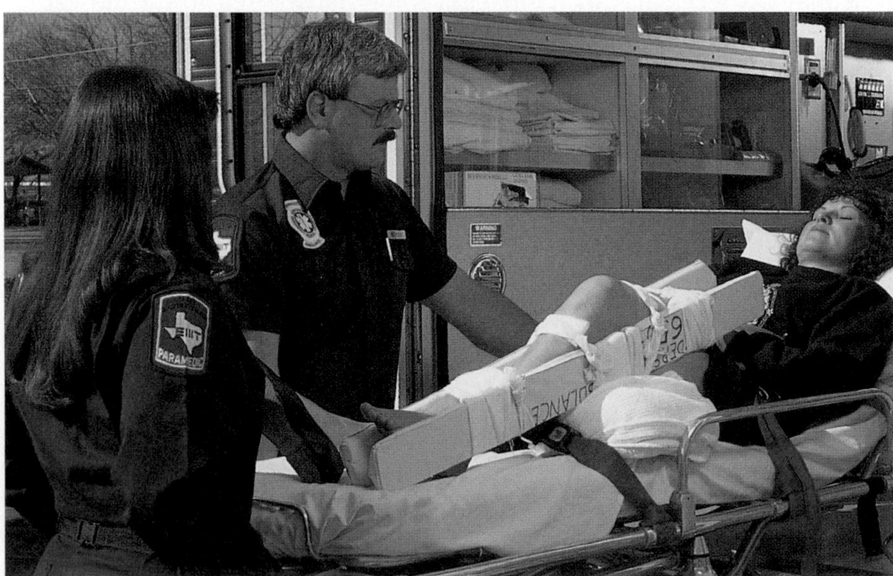

Figure 1.9 Ambulance transport to a hospital or medical facility.

- Ⓣ ***Prompt Transport*** Prompt transportation to an appropriate medical facility. This phrase is used when a patient's condition is serious enough that the patient needs to be taken to an appropriate medical facility in a fairly short period of time. If the patient is not transported fairly quickly, the condition may get worse and the patient may die.
- Ⓣ ***Rapid Transport*** Rapid transportation to an appropriate medical facility. This phrase is used for the few cases when EMS personnel are unable to give the patient adequate lifesaving care in the field. This patient may die unless he or she is transported immediately to an appropriate medical facility. This phrase is rarely used in this book.

Each of these three phrases refers to transportation to an **appropriate medical facility**. An appropriate medical facility may be a hospital, trauma center, or medical clinic. It is essential that you be familiar with the services provided by the medical facilities in your community. EMS personnel must work closely with their medical director to establish transportation protocols that ensure that patients are transported to the closest medical facility capable of providing adequate care.

appropriate medical facility A hospital with adequate medical resources to provide continuing care to sick or injured patients who are transported after field treatment by first responders.

To provide the best possible care for the patient, all members of the EMS team must remember that they are key components in the total system. Smooth operation of the team ensures the best care for the patient.

Roles and Responsibilities of the First Responder

As a first responder, you have several roles and responsibilities.

Depending on the emergency situation, you may need to:

- Respond promptly to the scene of an accident or sudden illness.
- Protect yourself.
- Protect the incident scene and patients from further harm.
- Summon appropriate assistance (EMTs, fire department, rescue squad).
- Gain access to the patient.
- Perform patient assessment.
- Administer emergency medical care and reassurance.
- Move patients only when necessary.
- Seek and then direct help from bystanders, if necessary.
- Control activities of bystanders.
- Assist EMTs and paramedics, as necessary.
- Document your care.
- Keep your knowledge and skills up to date.

Concern for the patient is primary; you should perform all activities with the patient's well-being in mind.

Prompt response to the scene is essential if you are to provide quality care to the patient. It is important that you know your response area well so you can quickly determine the most efficient route to the emergency scene.

When you reach the emergency scene, park your vehicle so that it does not create an additional hazard. The emergency scene should be protected with the least possible disruption of traffic. Do not block the roadway unnecessarily. As first responder, you should assess the scene to determine whether any hazards are present, such as downed electrical wires, gasoline spills, or unstable vehicles. This assessment is necessary to ensure that patients suffer no further injuries and that rescuers, other EMS personnel, and bystanders are not hurt.

If the equipment and personnel already dispatched to the scene cannot cope with the incident, you must immediately summon additional help. It may take some time for additional equipment and personnel to reach the scene, especially in rural areas or communities with systems staffed by volunteers.

Once you have taken the preceding steps, you must gain access to the patient. This may be as simple as opening the door to a car or house, or as difficult as squeezing through the back window of a wrecked automobile.

Next, examine the patient to determine the extent of the injury or illness. This initial assessment of a patient is called the patient assessment sequence. Once the patient assessment is completed, you must stabilize the patient's condition to prevent it from getting worse. The techniques you use to do this are limited by your training and the equipment available. Correctly applying these techniques can have a positive effect on the patient's condition.

When EMTs or paramedics arrive to assist, it is important to tell them what you have discovered about the patient's condition and what you have done so far to stabilize or treat it. Your next task is to assist the EMTs or paramedics.

In some communities or situations, you may be asked to accompany the patient in the ambulance. If CPR is being performed, you may need to assist or relieve the EMT or paramedic, especially if the hospital is far from the scene. In some EMS systems, you may be asked to drive the ambulance to the hospital so EMS personnel with more advanced training can devote all their efforts to patient care.

The Importance of Documentation

Once your role in treating the patient is finished, it is important that you record your observations about the scene, the patient's condition, and the treatment you provided. Documentation should be clear, concise, accurate, and according to the accepted policies of your organization. This documentation is important because you will not be able to remember the treatment you give to all patients. It also serves as a legal record of your treatment and may be required in the event of a lawsuit. Documentation also provides a basis to evaluate the quality of care given.

Documentation should include:

- Condition of the patient when found.
- The patient's description of the injury or illness.
- The initial and later vital signs.
- The treatment you gave the patient.
- The agency and personnel who took over treatment of the patient.
- Any other helpful facts.

Attitude and Conduct

As a first responder, you will be judged by your attitude and conduct, as well as by the medical care you administer. It is important to understand that professional behavior has a positive impact on your patients.

Because you will often be the first medically trained person to arrive on the scene of an emergency, it is important for you to act in a calm and caring way. You will gain the confidence of both patient and bystanders more easily by using a courteous and caring tone of voice. Show an interest in your patient. Avoid embarrassing your patient and help protect his or her privacy. Talk with your patient and tell him or her what you are doing.

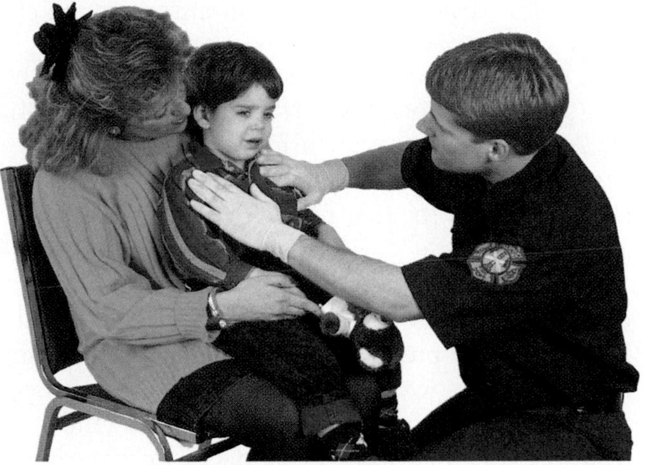

Figure 1.10 A professional attitude and neat appearance provide reassurance to the patient.

Remember that medical information about a patient is confidential and do not discuss it with your family or friends. This information should be shared only with other medical personnel who are involved in the care of that particular patient.

Your appearance should be neat and professional at all times. You should be well groomed and clean. A uniform helps identify you as a first responder. If you are a volunteer who responds from home, always identify yourself as a first responder. Your professional attitude and neat appearance help provide much needed reassurance to the patient (**Figure 1.10**).

Medical Oversight

The overall leader of the medical care team is the physician. To ensure that the patient receives appropriate medical treatment, it is important that first responders receive direction from a physician. Each first responder agency should have a physician who directs training courses, helps set medical policies, and assures quality management of the EMS system. This type of medical direction is known as indirect, or off-line, medical control.

A second type of medical control is known as direct, or on-line, medical control. On-line medical control is provided by a physician who is in contact with prehospital EMS providers, usually paramedics or EMTs, by two-way radio or wireless telephone (**Figure 1.11**). In cases where large numbers of people are injured, physicians may respond to the scene of the incident to provide on-scene medical control.

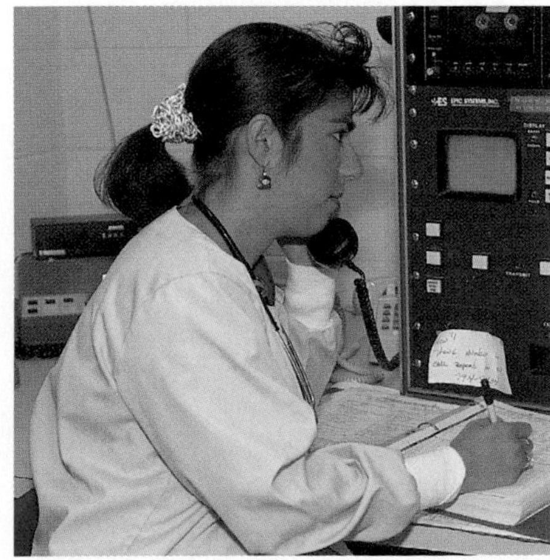

Figure 1.11 A physician providing on-scene medical control.

1

Prep Kit

Ready for Review

Ready for Review thoroughly summarizes the chapter.

This chapter provides an introduction to the first responder course and an overview of the operation of an EMS system, the legal principles guiding prehospital emergency care, and the role of the first responder in prehospital emergency care.

The introduction to first responder training outlines the types of skills you will learn as a first responder and presents four goals of first responder training: know what not to do, know how to use your first responder life support kit, know how to improvise, and know how to assist other EMS providers. First responders should understand their roles in the EMS system. The typical sequence of events of the EMS system are reporting, dispatch, first response, EMS response, hospital care, and medical oversight. Although most first responders do not provide patient transportation, a brief section on patient transportation covers the information you need to determine how rapidly a patient needs to be transported to the hospital. The chapter also presents the roles and responsibilities of the first responder, and stresses the importance of documentation and appropriate attitudes and conduct. After you have mastered this introductory material, you are ready to proceed to Chapter 2.

Vital Vocabulary

The Vital Vocabulary are the key terms for this chapter.

advanced life support (ALS)—*page 11*
appropriate medical facility—*page 13*
basic life support (BLS)—*page 9*
defibrillation—*page 11*
Emergency Medical Technician-Basic (EMT-B)—*page 9*
emergency services dispatch center—*page 8*
paramedic—*page 11*

Ready to Respond

Ready to Respond presents a fictitious scenario to help you review what you learned in this chapter.

As a first responder, you are dispatched for a reported automobile collision. You have just completed your first responder course.

1. Most calls for emergency medical care are made using?

A. Citizen band radios

B. Telephones

C. Emergency alarm boxes

D. Other means

2. When an emergency medical call is received in your community, how does the dispatcher notify you?

____

____

____

3. All but which one of the following agencies might regularly be dispatched when a motor vehicle collision is reported?

A. First responder

B. Law enforcement personnel

C. Utility company

D. Specialized rescue units

4. In your community, which level of emergency medical personnel would be dispatched for a motor vehicle collision?

A. First responder

B. Emergency Medical Technician-Basic (EMT-B)

C. EMT-Intermediate

D. Paramedic

Chapter 2

The Well-Being of the First Responder

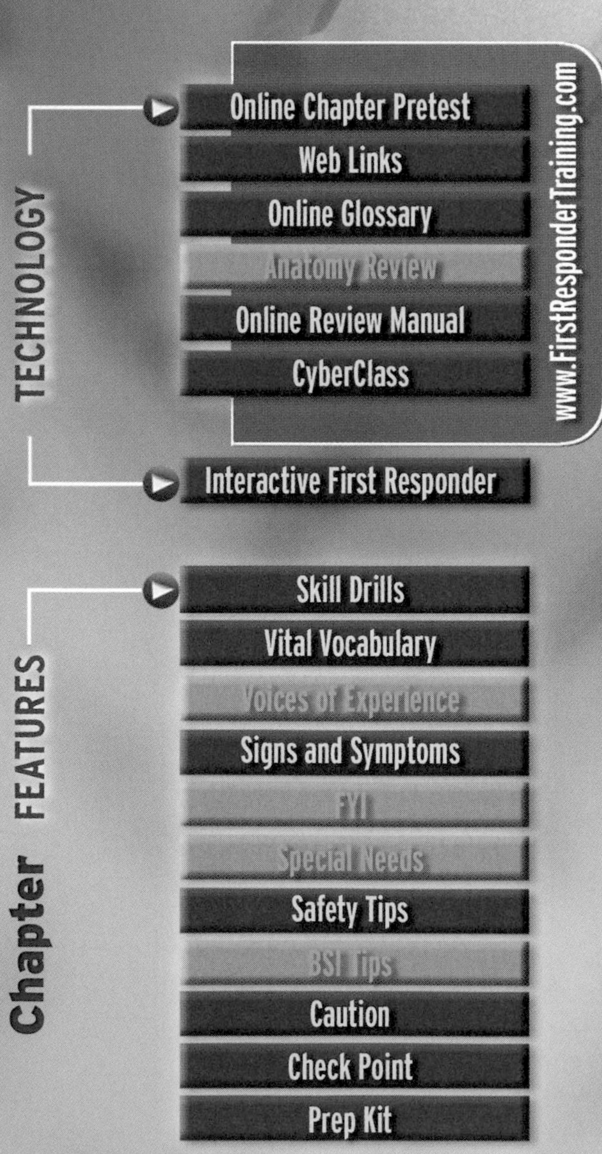

CHAPTER 2

Objectives

Knowledge and Attitude Objectives

After studying this chapter, you will be expected to:

1. Define the emotional aspects of emergency care encountered by patients, patients' families, and first responders.
2. Define the five stages in the normal reaction to death and dying.
3. Explain at least six signs and symptoms of stress.
4. Explain the type of actions a first responder can take to reduce or alleviate stress.
5. Describe the following three phases in critical incident stress reduction:
   a. Pre-incident stress education
   b. On-scene peer support
   c. Critical incident stress debriefing (CISD)
6. Discuss the importance of body substance isolation.
7. Describe the universal precautions for preventing infectious diseases from bloodborne and air-borne pathogens.
8. Describe three phases of scene safety.
9. Describe ten types of hazards to look for when assessing the scene for unsafe conditions.
10. Describe the safety equipment that first responders should have available for their protection.

Skill Objectives

As a first responder, you should be able to:

1. Put on and remove medical gloves safely.
2. Assess the scene of a real or simulated rescue event for safety hazards.
3. Properly use the safety equipment needed for first responders.

This chapter is designed to help you understand the factors that may affect your physical or emotional well-being as a first responder. You, your patients, and their families will all experience stress, so this chapter addresses methods for preventing and reducing stress. It also discusses hazards you may encounter from infectious diseases and presents methods you must follow to reduce your risk of infection. Finally, this chapter covers scene safety and how to prevent injury to yourself and further injury to your patients.

Emotional Aspects of Emergency Medical Care

Providing emergency medical care as a first responder is a stress-producing experience. You will feel the stress, as well as your patients, their families and friends, and bystanders. Because stress cannot be completely eliminated, you must learn how to avoid unnecessary stress and how to prevent your stress level from getting too high. Some of the same stress-reduction techniques that you will learn can also be used by your patients and their families and friends.

Though all emergency medical calls produce a certain level of stress, some types of calls are more stressful than others. Your past experiences may make it difficult for you to deal with certain types of calls. For example, if a patient with severe injuries reminds you of a close family member, you may have difficulty treating the patient without experiencing a high level of stress. This is especially true if an emergency call involves a very young patient or a very old patient (**Figure 2.1**). Calls involving death, violence, mass casualties or pediatric patients are also likely to produce high levels of stress.

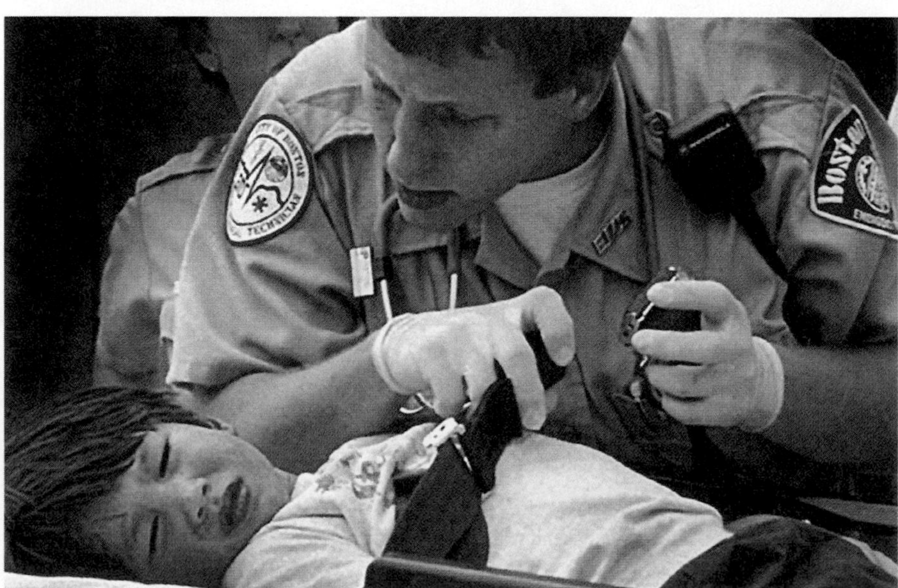

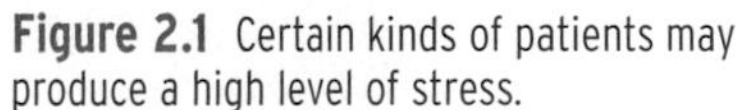

Figure 2.1 Certain kinds of patients may produce a high level of stress.

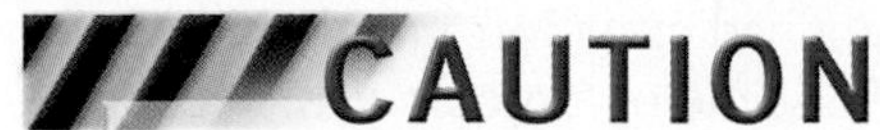

Do not underestimate the effect that stress can have on you. A firefighter, EMS provider, or law enforcement official in a busy department can see much more suffering in a year than many people will see in their entire lifetimes.

Because you work in a stressful environment, you must make a conscious effort to prevent and reduce unnecessary stress. You can do this in several different ways: learn to recognize the signs and symptoms of stress, adjust your lifestyle to include stress-reducing activities, and learn what services and resources are available to help you.

Normal Reactions to Stress

You need to understand how stress can affect you and the people for whom you provide emergency medical services. Because death/dying is one of the most intense types of stress that people experience, the grief reaction to death and dying provides a basis for looking at stress. Everyone who is involved with a death or with a dying patient—the patient, the family, and the caregivers—goes through this grief process, even though each is involved with the patient in different ways.

One well-recognized model for people's reaction to death and dying defines five stages: denial, anger, bargaining, depression, and acceptance. But not all people move through the grief process in exactly the same way and at the same pace. When you first encounter someone, he or she may be experiencing any stage of grief.

1. *Denial ("Not me!").* The first stage in the grief process is **denial**. A person experiencing denial cannot believe what is happening. This stage may serve as a protection for the person experiencing the situation, and it may also serve as a protection for you as the caregiver. Realize that this reaction is normal.
2. *Anger ("Why me?").* The second stage of the grief process is **anger**. Understanding that anger is a normal reaction to stress can also help you deal with anger that is directed toward you by a patient or by a patient's family. Do not get defensive because this anger is a result of the situation, and not a result of anything you do. This realization can enable you to tolerate the situation without letting the patient's anger distract you from performing your duties as an emergency medical provider.

   As you go through this phase of the process, you may direct your anger at the patient, the patient's family, your co-workers, or your own family. Anger is a normal reaction to unpleasant events. Sometimes it helps to talk out your anger with co-workers, family, members, or a counselor. By talking through your anger, you avoid keeping it bottled up inside where it can cause unhealthy physical symptoms or emotional reactions. Directing the energy from your

denial The first stage of a grief reaction, when the person suffering grief rejects the grief-causing event.

anger The second stage of the grief reaction, when the person suffering grief becomes upset at the grief-causing event or other situation.

bargaining The third stage of the grief reaction, when the person experiencing grief barters to change the grief-causing event.

depression The fourth stage of the grief reaction, when the person expresses despair—an absence of cheerfulness and hope—as a result of the grief-causing event.

acceptance The fifth stage of the grief process, when the person experiencing grief recognizes the finality of the grief-causing event.

anger in positive ways to alleviate a bad situation may help you move forward. For example, at the scene of a motor vehicle crash, you may be angry that a child has been injured. Focusing your energy on providing the best medical care for the injured child may help you work through your feelings.

3. ***Bargaining ("Okay, but . . .").*** The third stage of the grief process is **bargaining**. Bargaining is the act of trying to make a deal to postpone death and dying. If you encounter a patient who is in this stage, try to respond with a truthful and helpful comment such as, "We are doing everything we can and the paramedics will be here in 5 to 7 minutes." Remember that bargaining is a normal part of the grief process.
4. ***Depression.*** The fourth stage of the grief process is **depression**. Depression is often characterized by sadness or despair. A person who is unusually silent, or who seems to retreat into his or her own world may have reached this stage. This may also be the point a person begins to accept the situation. It is not surprising that patients and their families get depressed about a situation that involves death and dying. Nor is it surprising that you as a rescuer also get depressed. American society tends to consider death a failure of medical care rather than a natural event that will happen to everyone. A certain amount of depression is a natural reaction to a major threat or loss. The depression can be mild or severe; it can be of short duration or long lasting. If depression continues, it is important to contact qualified professionals who can help you.
5. ***Acceptance.*** The final stage of the grief process is **acceptance**. Acceptance does not mean that you are satisfied with the situation. It means that you understand that death and dying cannot be changed. It may require a lot of time to work through the grief process and arrive at this stage. As an emergency medical provider, you may see acceptance in family members who have had time to realize that their loved one's illness is a terminal event and that the patient is not going to recover. But not all people who experience grief are able to work through it and accept the loss.

By understanding these five stages, you can better understand the grief reaction experienced by patients, their families, and their friends. You can also better understand your reaction to stressful situations. Some helpful techniques for dealing with patients in stressful situations are presented in Chapter 11. These techniques will help you to develop more comfort and skill when dealing with stressful situations.

Stress Management

Stress management has three components: recognizing stress, preventing stress, and reducing stress.

Recognizing Stress

An important step in managing stress in yourself and others is the ability to recognize its signs and symptoms. Then you can take steps to prevent or reduce stress.

Signs & Symptoms

STRESS

The following warning signs should help you recognize stress in co-workers or friends or in yourself:

- Irritability (often directed at co-workers, family, and friends)
- Inability to concentrate
- Change in normal disposition
- Difficulty in sleeping or nightmares (may be hard to recognize because many emergency care workers work a pattern of rotating hours that makes normal sleep patterns hard to maintain)
- Anxiety
- Indecisiveness
- Guilt
- Loss of appetite
- Loss of interest in sexual relations
- Loss of interest in work
- Isolation

Knowing these signs of stress should help you recognize it in co-workers, friends, or yourself.

Preventing Stress

Three simple-to-remember techniques that can prevent stress are: eat, drink, and be merry (in a healthy, stress-reducing manner).

1. ***Eat.*** A healthy well-balanced diet helps prevent and reduce stress. A healthy daily diet should include 6 to 11 servings of bread, cereal, rice, and pasta; 3 to 5 servings of vegetables; 2 to 4 servings of fruits; 2 to 4 servings of milk, yogurt, and cheese; 2 to 3 servings of meat, poultry, fish, and eggs; and a limited amount of fats, oils, and sweets. This healthy diet is illustrated by the Food Guide Pyramid (**Figure 2.2**). Many people need to cut down on the amount of fat and sweets in their diet. Eating large quantities of sweets puts your energy level on a roller coaster. Your blood sugar quickly rises, but in a couple of hours, the blood sugar drops and you crave more sweets. It is much better to eat an adequate amount of breads, cereals, rice, and pasta. These provide energy over a longer period of time and help to reduce the highs and lows brought onby excess sugars.

   EMS providers often find it hard to maintain regular meal schedules. By planning your food intake and having healthy food available, you can improve your eating habits. Healthy eating not only helps to cut down on your stress level, it also helps reduce your risk of heart and blood vessel diseases, which are the most common causes of death in public safety workers. Keeping your weight at recommended levels helps your body deal better with stress.

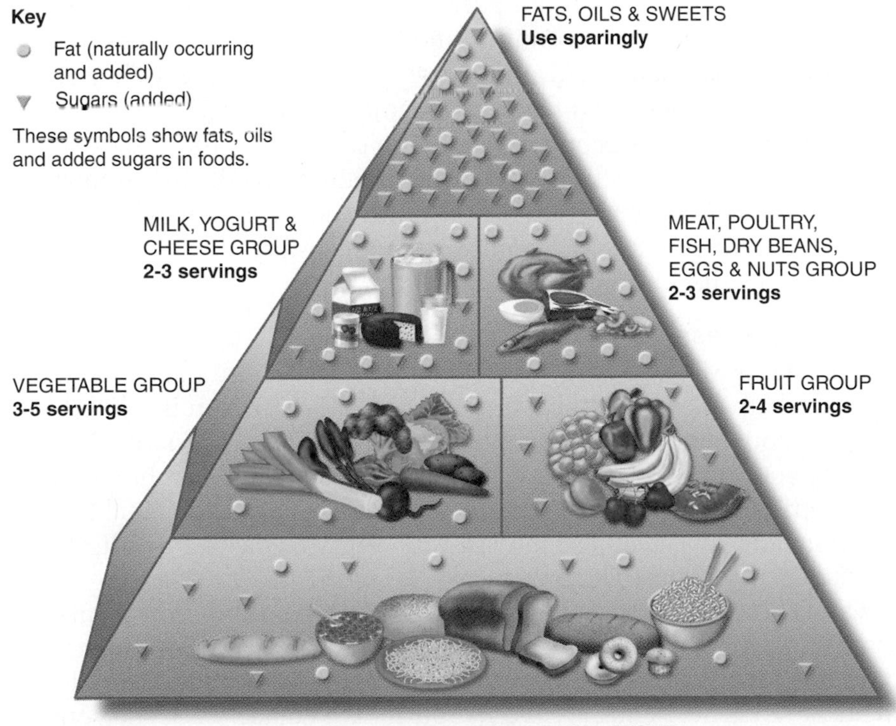

Figure 2.2 A healthy diet is illustrated by the USDA food guide pyramid.

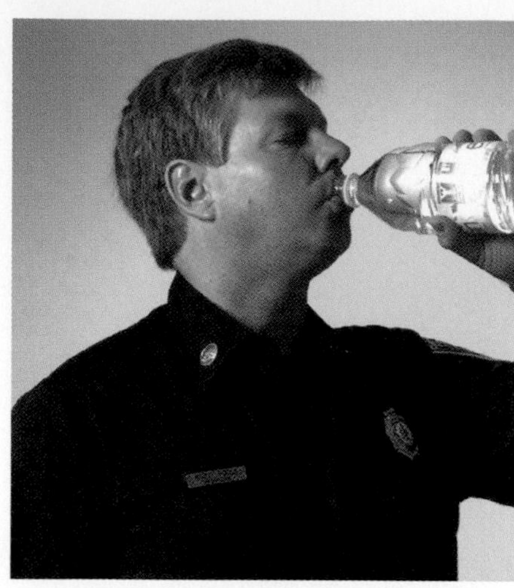

Figure 2.3 Drinking adequate quantities of water and juice is important.

2. ***Drink.*** Active EMS providers need to drink adequate amounts of fluids every day (**Figure 2.3**). Dehydration is a special risk for law enforcement officers, firefighters, and EMS providers who wear hot bunker gear or ballistic vests. The average adult loses about eight glasses of water a day through sweat, exhaling, and elimination. Water in adequate quantities is essential for maintaining proper body processes. Natural fruit juices are another good source of fluids.

   Avoid consuming excessive amounts of caffeine and alcohol. Caffeine is a drug that causes adrenaline to be released in your body; adrenaline raises your blood pressure and increases your stress level. By limiting your intake of caffeine-containing beverages such as coffee and cola drinks, you can reduce your tendency toward stress. Caffeine and alcohol also cause dehydration. Drinking alcoholic beverages is to be discouraged. Though alcoholic drinks seem to relax you, they cause depression and reduce your ability to deal with stress.

3. ***Be merry.*** A happy person is not suffering from elevated stress. It is important to balance your lifestyle. Assess both your work environment and your home environment. At work, address problems promptly before they produce major stress. Try to schedule your work to allow adequate off-duty time for sleep and personal activities. If you are working in a volunteer agency, avoid having everyone on call all the time.

Try to create a stress-reducing environment away from work. Spend time with your friends and family. In your recreational activities, include friends who are not co-workers. Develop hobbies or activities that are not related to your job. Exercise regularly. Exercise is a great stress reliever. Swimming, running, and bicycling are three types of excellent aerobic exercise. Avoid the use of tobacco products; they are stress producers, not stress relievers . Meditation or religious activities reduce stress for some people. People who can balance the pressures of work with relaxing activities at home usually enjoy life much more than people who can never leave the stories and stress of work behind. If you are feeling stress away from your job, consider seeking assistance from a mental health care professional.

Note: Because public safety services must be provided 24 hours a day, many law enforcement, fire, EMS, and security personnel work rotating shifts. Firefighters may work 24-hour shifts with a variety of days off. Law enforcement personnel may be required to alternate between day and night shifts. These work schedules disrupt normal sleep patterns. In addition, many people in public safety work overtime shifts or a second job. This combination of factors means that many public safety providers don't get an adequate amount of sleep.

Scientific studies have documented that most people need about eight hours of uninterrupted sleep per night. If you are not meeting this need, your mental and physical health may suffer and you will be less able to deal with stress. It is important to establish adequate sleep as a priority in your life.

Reducing Stress

If pressures at work or home cause continual stress, you may benefit from the help of a mental health professional. This person is trained to listen nonjudgmentally and to help you resolve the issues that are causing your stress. Mental health professionals include psychologists, psychiatrists, social workers, and specially trained clergy. A mental health professional may be connected with your department. Your medical insurance may cover this type of care.

Critical Incident Stress Management is a comprehensive program that is available through many public safety departments. It consists of pre-incident stress education, on-scene peer support, and critical incident stress debriefings (CISDs). You should contact CISD personnel whenever you are exhibiting signs or symptoms of stress.

1. **Pre-incident stress education** provides information about the stresses that you will encounter and the reactions you may experience. It helps emergency responders understand the normal stress responses to the abnormal emergency situations they encounter.
2. **On-scene peer support** and disaster support services provide aid for you on the scene of especially stressful incidents such as major disasters or and situations that involve the death of a co-worker or a child.
3. **Critical incident stress debriefings (CISDs)** are used to alleviate the stress reactions caused by high-stress emergency situations. Debriefings are meetings between emergency responders and specially trained leaders. The purpose of a debriefing is to allow an open discussion of feelings, fears, and reactions to the high-stress situation.

   A debriefing is not an investigation or an interrogation. Debriefings are usually held within 24 to 72 hours after a major incident. The CISD leaders offer suggestions and information on overcoming stress (**Figure 2.4**).

Find out if your department has a critical incident stress debriefing program. Contact this team if you are involved in a high stress incident such as a call that involves a very young or a very old patient, a mass casualty incident, or a situation that involves unusual violence. If you think you might be experiencing signs or symptoms of stress from such an incident, contact your supervisor or a stress counselor. More information about critical incident stress debriefing is available in Chapter 11.

pre-incident stress education Training about stress and stress reactions conducted for public safety providers before they are exposed to stressful situations.

on-scene peer support Stress counselors at the scene of stressful incidents to deal with stress reduction.

critical incident stress debriefing (CISD) A system of psychological support designed to reduce stress on emergency personnel after a major stress-producing incident.

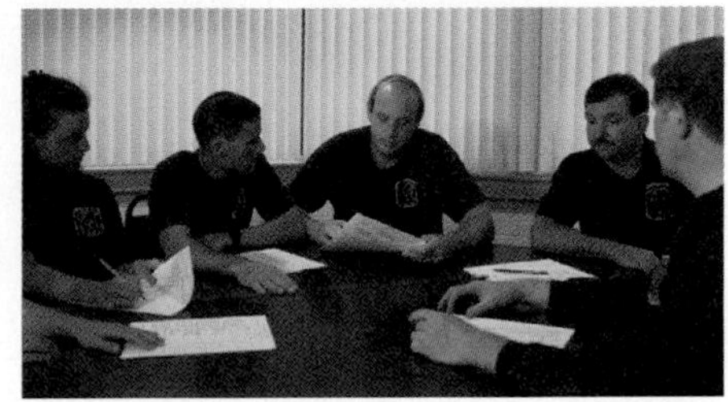

Figure 2.4 Critical incident stress debriefings (CISD) are important to relieve stress.

Checkpoint

- ○ List six signs and symptoms of stress.
- ○ Are you experiencing any of these signs or symptoms of stress?
- ○ What actions or changes in your lifestyle might help you reduce stress?
- ○ What calls have you or your department experienced recently that might have caused critical incident stress?
- ○ How do you access the CISD system in your department?

Scene Safety

Infectious Diseases and Body Substance Isolation (BSI)

In recent years, the acquired immunodeficiency syndrome (AIDS) epidemic and the growing concern about tuberculosis and hepatitis have increased awareness of infectious diseases. Some understanding of the most common infectious diseases is important so you can protect yourself from unnecessary exposure to these diseases and so you do not become unduly alarmed about them.

Federal regulations require all health care workers, including first responders, to assume that all patients in all settings are potentially infected with human immunodeficiency virus (HIV), the virus that can lead to AIDS; hepatitis B virus (HBV); or other bloodborne **pathogens**. These regulations require that all health care workers use protective equipment to prevent possible exposure to blood and certain bodily fluids of patients. This concept is known as **body substance isolation (BSI)**.

pathogens Microorganisms that are capable of causing disease.

body substance isolation (BSI) An infection control concept that treats all bodily fluids as potentially infectious.

HIV is transmitted by direct contact with infected blood, semen, or vaginal secretions. There is no scientific documentation that the virus is transmitted by contact with sweat, saliva, tears, sputum, urine, feces, vomitus, or nasal secretions, unless these fluids contain visible signs of blood.

Hepatitis B is also spread by direct contact with infected blood. First responders should follow the universal precautions described in the next section to reduce their chance of contracting hepatitis B. Check with your medical director about receiving injections of hepatitis vaccine to protect you against this infection. This vaccine should be made available to you at no cost.

Tuberculosis is also becoming a common problem, and the presence of drug-resistant strains makes this disease very dangerous to first responders. Tuberculosis is spread through the air whenever an infected person coughs or sneezes. Wear a face mask or a high-efficiency particulate air (HEPA) respirator (**Figure 2.5**) and put an oxygen mask on the patient to minimize your exposure. If no oxygen mask is available, place a face mask on the patient. First responders should have a skin test for tuberculosis every year.

Universal Precautions

You will not always be able to tell whether a patient's bodily fluids contain blood. Therefore, the Centers for Disease Control and Prevention (CDC) recommend that all health care workers use universal precautions, based on the assumption that all patients are potential carriers of bloodborne pathogens.

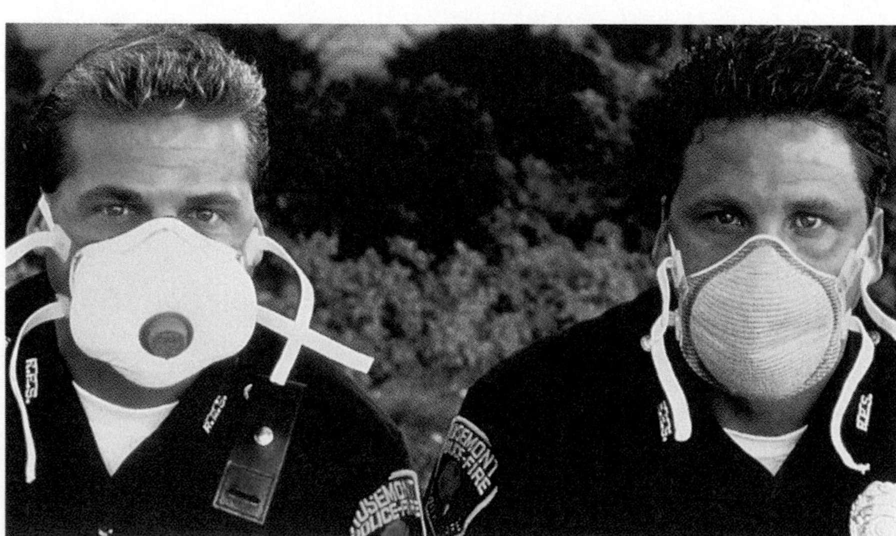

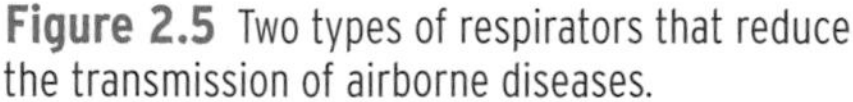

Figure 2.5 Two types of respirators that reduce the transmission of airborne diseases.

The CDC recommends that all health care workers use the following **universal precautions**:

1. Always wear gloves when handling patients, and change gloves after contact with each patient (**Figure 2.6**, page 28). Wash your hands immediately after removing gloves. (Note that leather gloves are not considered safe—leather is porous and traps fluids.)
2. Always wear protective eye wear or a face shield when you anticipate that blood or other bodily fluids may splatter. Wear a gown or apron if you anticipate splashes of blood or other bodily fluids such as those that occur with childbirth and major trauma.
3. Wash your hands and other skin surfaces immediately and thoroughly if they become contaminated with blood and other bodily fluids (**Figure 2.7**, page 29). Change contaminated clothes and wash exposed skin thoroughly.
4. Do not recap, cut, or bend used needles. Place them directly in a puncture-resistant container designed for "sharps."
5. Even though saliva has not been proven to transmit HIV, you should use a face shield, pocket mask, or other airway adjunct if the patient needs resuscitation.

universal precautions Procedures for infection control that treat blood and certain bodily fluids as capable of transmitting bloodborne diseases.

Federal agencies such as the Occupational Safety and Health Administration (OSHA) and state agencies such as state public health departments have regulations about body substance isolation. Because these regulations are constantly changing, it is important for your department to keep up to date on these regulations.

Immunizations

Certain immunizations are recommended for emergency medical care providers. These include tetanus prophylaxis and hepatitis B vaccine. Tuberculin testing is also recommended. Your medical director can determine what immunizations and tests are needed for members of your department.

Responding to the Scene

Scene safety is a most important consideration to you as a first responder. Safety considerations need to include your own safety and the safety of all the other people present at the scene of an emergency. An injured or killed first responder cannot help those in need, and becomes someone who needs help, increasing the difficulty of a rescue. Close attention to factors involving safety can prevent unnecessary illness, injuries, and death.

Dispatch

Safety begins when you are dispatched to an emergency. Use your dispatch information to anticipate what hazards may be present and to determine how to approach the scene of the emergency.

Safety Tips

Simple, portable safety equipment can help prevent injuries and illnesses.

- **Medical gloves, masks, and eye protection** prevent the spread of infectious diseases.
- **Brightly colored clothing or vests** make you more visible to traffic in the daytime; reflective striping or vests make you more visible in the dark.
- **Heavy gloves** can help prevent cuts at a motor vehicle accident scene.
- **A hard hat or helmet** is needed when you are at an industrial or motor vehicle accident scene.

Some situations require additional safety equipment. Do not hesitate to call for additional equipment as needed.

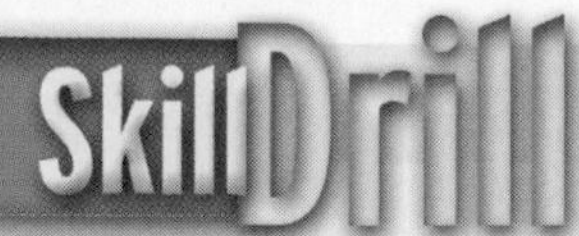

Figure 2.6 Proper Removal of Medical Gloves

Proper removal of gloves is important to minimize the spread of pathogens.

1

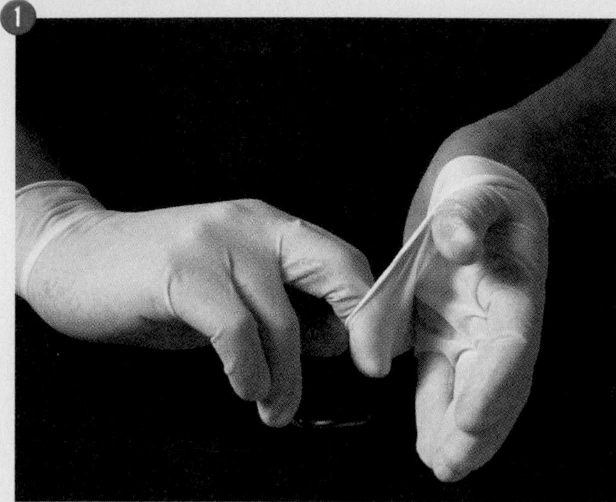

Insert a finger inside the glove.

2

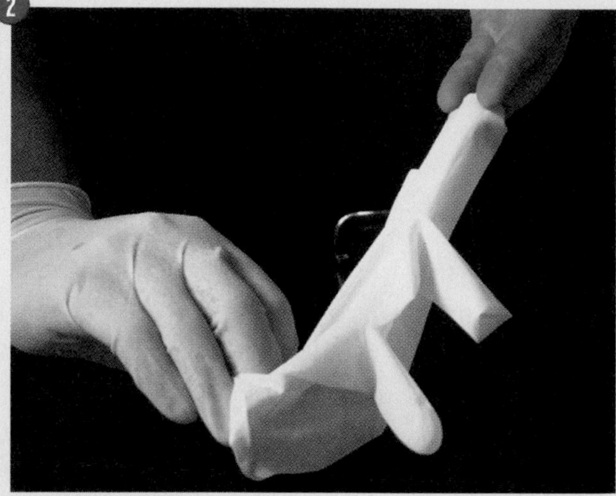

Pull off the first glove inside out.

3

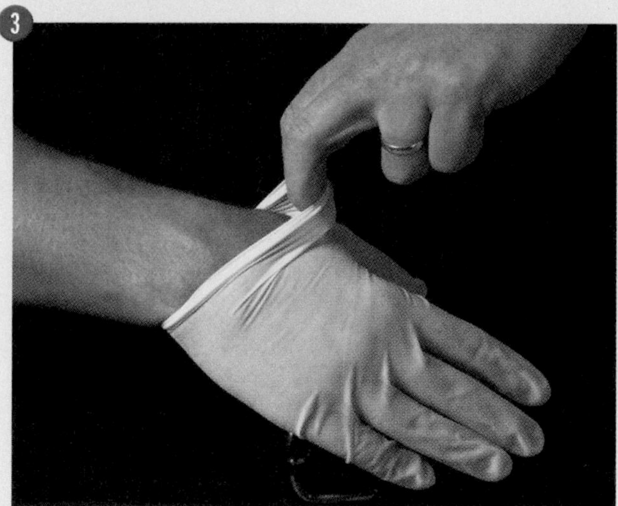

Avoid touching the outside of the glove.

4

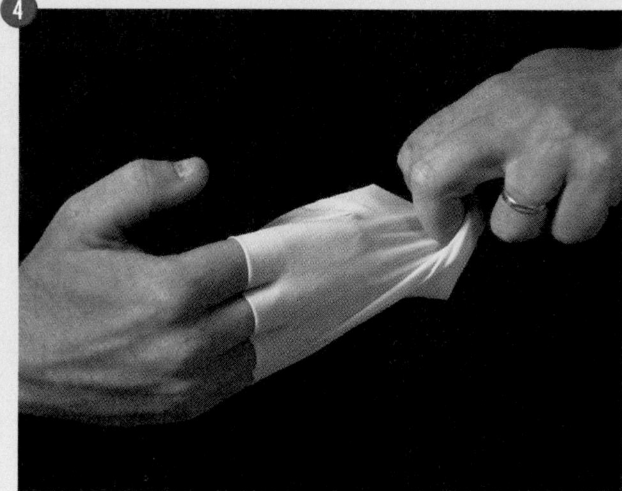

Pull off the second glove inside out.

Remember

If you are injured or killed, you lose your ability to help those in need.

Response

Vehicle accidents are a major cause of death and disability of both law enforcement officials and firefighters. As you respond to the scene of an emergency, remember the safety information that you have been taught in your driving courses. Fasten your safety belt, plan the best route, and drive quickly but safely to the scene.

Parking Your Vehicle

When you arrive at the emergency scene, park your vehicle so that it protects the area from traffic hazards. Check to be sure that the emergency warning lights are operating correctly. Be careful when getting out of your vehicle, especially if you must step into a traffic area. Brightly colored uniforms or vests enhance your visibility in the daytime; reflective material on your uniform or on a safety vest helps make you more visible in the dark (**Figure 2.8**). If your vehicle is not needed to protect the incident scene, park it out of the way of traffic. Leave room for other arriving vehicles such as ambulances to be positioned near the patient. Above all else, make sure that you have protected the emergency scene from further accidents.

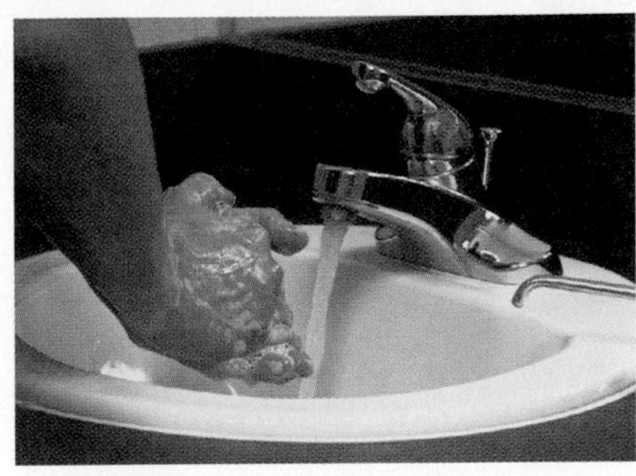

Figure 2.7 Wash your hands thoroughly if you are contaminated with blood or other bodily fluids.

Assessing the Scene

As you approach the emergency scene, scan the area carefully to determine what hazards are present. Consider the following hazards based on the type of emergency; address them in whatever order is most appropriate. For example, you should assess the scene of a motor vehicle accident for downed electrical wires before you check for broken glass.

Traffic

Is traffic a problem? Sometimes (for example, on a busy highway) your first action should be to control the flow of traffic so that additional accidents do not make the situation any worse. If you need more help to handle traffic, call for assistance before you get out of your vehicle.

Crime or Violence

If your dispatch information leads you to believe that the incident involves violence or a crime, approach carefully. If you are trained in law enforcement procedures, follow your local protocols. If you are not a law enforcement official, proceed very carefully. If you have any doubts about the safety of the scene, it is better to wait at a safe distance and request help from law enforcement officials. If the scene involves a crime, remember to take a mental picture of the scene and avoid disturbing anything at the scene unless it is absolutely necessary to move objects to provide patient care.

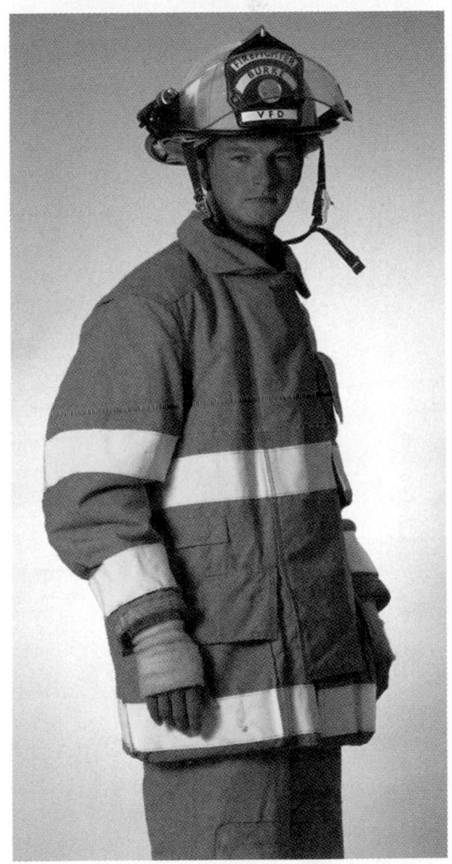

Figure 2.8 Reflective clothing helps to make you more visible.

Crowds

Crowds come in all sizes and have different personalities. Friendly neighborhood crowds may interfere very little with your duties. Unfriendly crowds may require a police presence before you are able to treat the patient. Assess the feeling of the crowd before you get in a position from which there is no exit. Request help from law enforcement officials before the crowd is out of control. Safety considerations may require you to wait for the arrival of police before you approach the patient.

Electrical Hazards

Electrical hazards can be present at many different types of emergency scenes. Patients located inside buildings may be in contact with a wide variety of electrical hazards, ranging from a faulty extension cord in a house to a high voltage feeder line in an industrial setting. Patients located outside may be in contact with high voltage electrical power lines that have fallen because of a motor vehicle accident or a storm.

Did You Know?

In a recent year, 97 police cars, 20 fire trucks, and 28 ambulances were involved in fatal traffic accidents in the United States. In the same year, 32,398 emergency vehicles were involved in nonfatal accidents.

You must assess the emergency scene for any indications of electrical problems. Inside a building, look for cords, electrical wires, or electrical appliances near or in contact with the patient; outside, look for damaged electrical poles and downed electrical wires. Do not approach an emergency scene if there are indications of electrical problems. Keep all other people away from the source of the hazard, too. Because electricity is invisible, make sure that the electrical current has been turned off by a qualified person before you get close to the source of the current.

Fire

Fire is a hazard that can result in injury or death to you and to the patient. If there appears to be a fire, call at once for fire department assistance. If you are a trained firefighter, follow rescue and fire-fighting procedures for your department. If you are not a trained firefighter, do not exceed the limits of your training. Entering a burning building without proper turnout gear and self-contained breathing apparatus is an unwise course of action. Any attempt to rescue someone from a burning building is a high risk undertaking. Vehicles that have been involved in accidents also may present a fire hazard from fuel or other spilled fluids. Keep all ignition sources such as cigarettes and road flares away. Carefully assess the fire hazard before you determine your course of action.

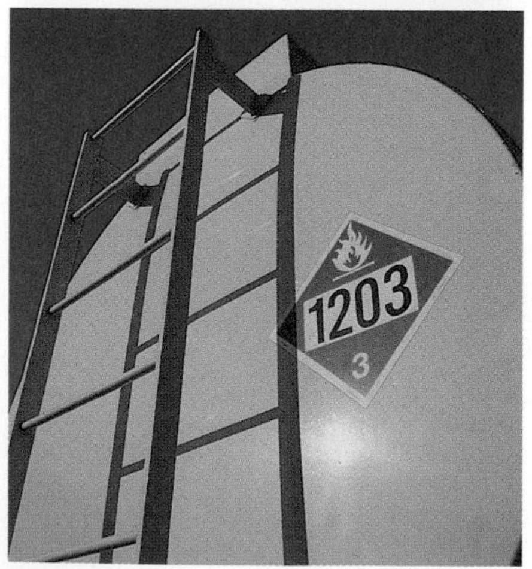

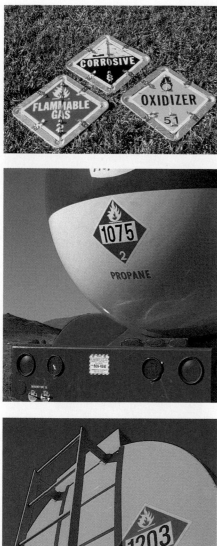

Figure 2.9 Hazardous materials placards.

Hazardous Materials

Hazardous materials (sometimes referred to as "haz mats") may be found almost anywhere. Some transportation accidents involve hazardous materials. They may also be found in homes, businesses, and industries. Federal regulations require vehicles that are transporting hazardous materials to be marked with specific placards (**Figure 2.9**). If you believe that an accident may involve hazardous materials, stop at some distance from the accident and determine if the vehicle is marked with a placard. A pair of binoculars in the life support kit is helpful for this. The placard indicates the class of material that is being carried. You should carry an emergency response guide book to assist you in determining the hazard involved. The presence of odors or fumes may be the first indication of hazardous materials located in buildings. If you believe that a hazardous material is present, call for assistance from the agency that handles hazardous materials in your community. Remain far enough away from a suspected haz-mat incident that you do not become an additional casualty. (See Chapter 16 for more information on handling hazardous materials incidents.)

Unstable Objects

Unstable objects may include vehicles, trees, poles, buildings, cliffs, and piles of materials. After an accident, a motor vehicle may be located in an unstable position. You may need to stabilize the vehicle before you can begin patient extrication. Do not attempt to enter or get under an unstable vehicle. Motor vehicle accidents may result in other unstable objects, including trees or poles that were hit in the accident. Fires and explosions can result in unstable buildings. Assess a building for stability before attempting to enter it. If you are in doubt about the safety of the building, call for trained personnel rather than attempt to enter an unsafe building alone.

Sharp Objects

Sharp objects are frequently present at an emergency scene. These range from broken glass at the scene of a motor vehicle crash to hypodermic needles in the pocket of a drug addict. Being aware of sharp objects can reduce the chance of injury to yourself and to your patients. Vinyl or latex medical gloves can help prevent the spread of disease from blood contamination, but they provide no protection against sharp objects. When glass or other sharp objects are present, you should wear heavy leather or fire-fighting gloves over your gloves to prevent injuries.

Animals

Animals, whether they are pets, farm stock, or wild, are present in a wide variety of indoor and outdoor settings. Pets can become very upset in the confusion of a medical emergency. If you need to enter a house to take care of a patient, be sure excited pets have been secured in a part of the house away from the patient. People travel with their pets, so pets can be part of the scene of a motor vehicle crash. Guide dogs may be possessive of their owners. Farm animals can be a safety hazard, too. Be careful when entering a field that may contain livestock. Animals may present other hazards such as bites or stings. Careful assessment of the incident scene can prevent unnecessary injuries.

Environmental Conditions

Weather is one part of life that cannot be changed or controlled. Therefore, you should consider the effect it will have on rescue operations. Dress appropriately for the expected weather. Keep patients dry and at a comfortable temperature. Be prepared for temperature extremes. Avoid getting too hot or too cold. Be prepared for precipitation. Be alert to possible damage from high winds. Darkness makes it hard for you to see all the hazards that may be present. Use any emergency lighting that is present. A flashlight is a valuable tool to have in many rescue situations.

Special Rescue Situations

Special safety considerations are required in situations involving water rescue, ice rescue, confined space or below grade rescue, terrorism, and mass casualty incidents. These situations are covered in Chapters 16 and 18. Do not enter an emergency situation that is unsafe unless you have the proper training and equipment.

Airborne and Bloodborne Pathogens

Because airborne and bloodborne pathogens cannot be seen directly, you should always remember the universal precautions described earlier and apply them as appropriate.

2 Prep Kit

Ready for Review

Ready for Review thoroughly summarizes the chapter.

This chapter covers the topics needed to help you understand the role stress plays in the lives of emergency care providers and patients who have suffered a sudden illness or accident. Stress is a normal part of our lives. The five stages of the grief process that occur as a result of the grief of death or dying are: denial, anger, bargaining, depression, and acceptance. Patients and rescuers move through these stages at different rates. Stress management consists of recognizing, preventing, and reducing critical incident stress.

Scene safety is an important part of your job. You should understand how airborne and bloodborne infectious diseases are spread and how body substance isolation prevents their spread. As you arrive on the scene of an accident or illness, you must assess the scene for a wide variety of hazards, including traffic, crime, crowds, unstable objects, sharp objects, electrical problems, fire, hazardous materials, animals, environmental conditions, special rescue situations, and infectious disease exposure. You should understand the safety equipment that is needed for first responder rescue situations.

Vital Vocabulary

The Vital Vocabulary are the key terms for this chapter.

acceptance—*page 22*
anger—*page 21*
bargaining—*page 22*
body substance isolation (BSI)—*page 26*
critical incident stress debriefing (CISD)—*page 25*
denial—*page 21*
depression—*page 22*
on-scene peer support—*page 25*
pathogens—*page 26*
pre-incident stress education—*page 25*
universal precautions—*page 27*

Practice Points

The Practice Points are the key skills you need to know.

1. Putting on and removing medical gloves.

2. Assessing the scene of a real or simulated rescue scene for safety hazards.

3. Using the safety equipment needed for first responders' safety.

Skill Drills

The Skill Drills provide a visual summary of some of the more complex skills from the skills objectives.

2.6 Proper Removal of Medical Gloves—*page 28*

Ready to Respond

Ready to Respond presents a fictitious scenario to help you review what you learned in this chapter.

You and your partner have just returned from a call involving a motor vehicle collision. A two-year-old child was seriously injured and a 67-year-old man was killed.

1. Your partner seems to be angry. Is this
   A. A normal part of the grief process
   B. An unusual response to this type of call

2. What other signs might help you recognize that your partner is suffering from stress?
   1. Anxiety
   2 Change in normal disposition
   3. Overly quick decision-making
   4. Loss of interest in work
      A. 1,2,3
      B. 2,3,4
      C. 1,2,4
      D. 1,3,4

3. Which of the following should be avoided to prevent unnecessary stress?
   A. Fruits and vegetables
   B. Coffee and cola drinks
   C. Fats and oils
   D. Pasta and cereals

The following questions are not related to the scenario above.

4. Hepatitis B:
   A. Is a disease that is easily treated
   B. Cannot be prevented
   C. Is spread by direct contact
   D. Poses no risk to the first responder

5. Critical incident stress debriefings are usually held
   A. During an incident
   B. 10 to 20 days after an incident
   C. 1 to 3 days after an incident

6. Electricity should be treated as a hazard
   A. Only if it is sparking
   B. Only if a wire is in contact with an auto
   C. Until the electrical company has turned it off
   D. Except when the switch is off

Chapter 3

Legal and Ethical Issues

TECHNOLOGY

- Online Chapter Pretest
- Web Links
- Online Glossary
- Anatomy Review
- Online Review Manual
- CyberClass

www.FirstResponderTraining.com

- Interactive First Responder

Chapter FEATURES

- Skill Drills
- Vital Vocabulary
- Voices of Experience
- Signs and Symptoms
- FYI
- Special Needs
- Safety Tips
- BSI Tips
- Caution
- Check Point
- Prep Kit

CHAPTER 3

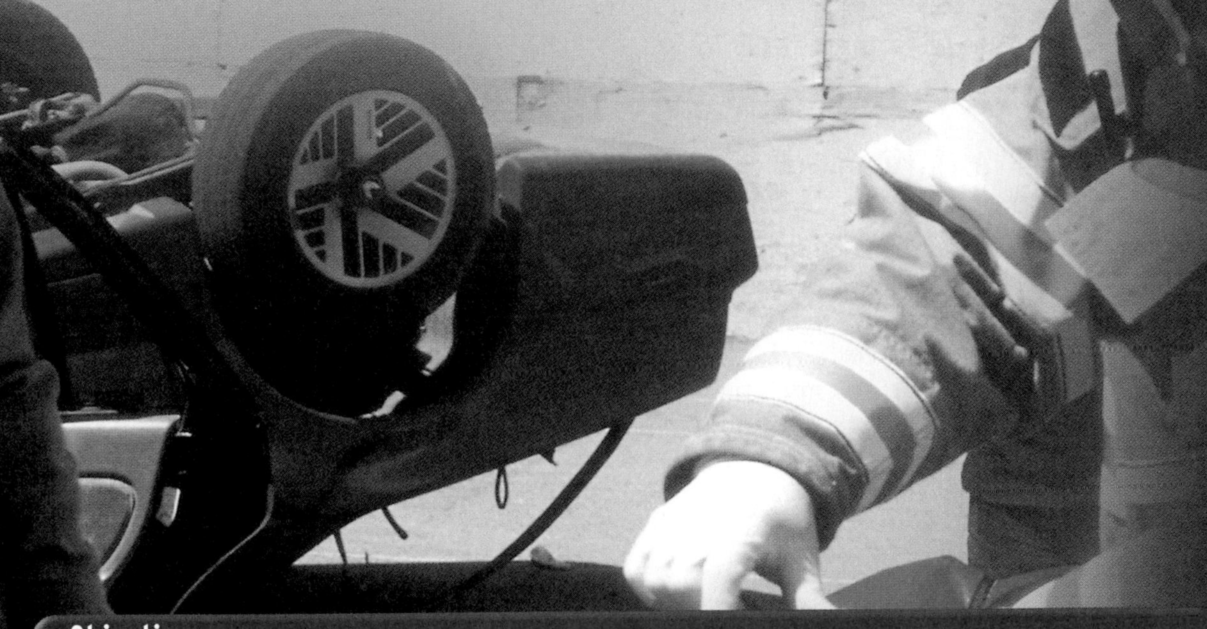

Objectives

Knowledge and Attitude Objectives

After studying this chapter, you will be expected to:

1. Define "duty to act" as it relates to a first responder.
2. Describe the standard of care and the scope of care for a first responder.
3. Describe and compare the following types of consent:
   a. Expressed consent
   b. Implied consent
   c. Consent for minors
   d. Consent of mentally ill patients
   e. Refusal of care
4. Explain the purpose of living wills and advance directives.
5. Describe the importance of the following legal concepts:
   a. Abandonment
   b. Death on the scene
   c. Negligence
   d. Confidentiality
6. Explain the purpose of Good Samaritan laws.
7. Describe the federal, state, and local regulations that apply to first responders.
8. Describe reportable events in your local area.
9. Describe the steps to be taken at a crime scene.
10. Explain the reasons for documentation.

First responders need to know some basic legal principles that govern the way they provide care to patients. Knowing these principles can help you provide the best care for patients and prevent situations that could result in legal difficulties for you, your agency, or your department. Because some laws differ from one location to another, you will need to learn the specific laws of your state and your local jurisdiction.

Duty to Act

duty to act A first responder's legal responsibility to respond promptly to an emergency scene and provide medical care (within the limits of training and available equipment).

standard of care The manner in which an individual must act or behave when giving care.

The first legal principle to consider is the **duty to act**. A citizen arriving on the scene of an automobile accident is not required by law to stop and give emergency care to victims. However, if you are employed by an agency that has designated you as a first responder and you are dispatched to the scene of an accident or illness, you do have a duty to act. You must proceed promptly to the scene and render emergency medical care within the limits of your training and available equipment (**Figure 3.1**). Any failure to respond or render necessary emergency medical care leaves both you and your agency vulnerable to legal action.

Standard of Care

What level of care are you expected to give to a patient? As a first responder, you obviously cannot provide the same level of care as a physician, but you are responsible for providing the level of care that a person with similar training would provide under similar circumstances. As a trained first responder, you are expected to use your knowledge and skills to the best of your ability under the circumstances.

The circumstances under which you must provide care may affect the **standard of care**. For example, if you are called out on a cold, dark, rainy night, you may not be able to perform as well as when you are

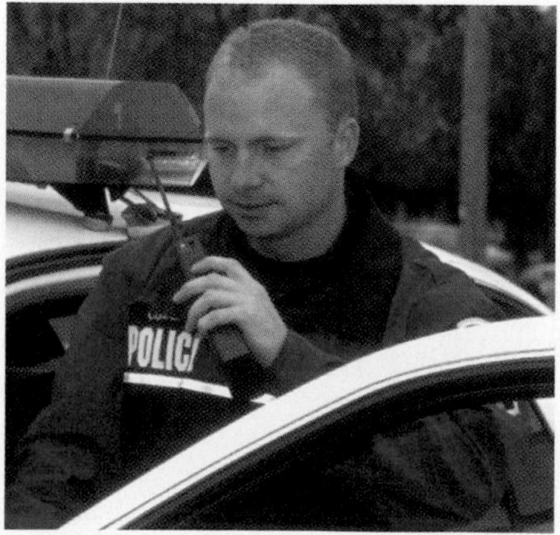

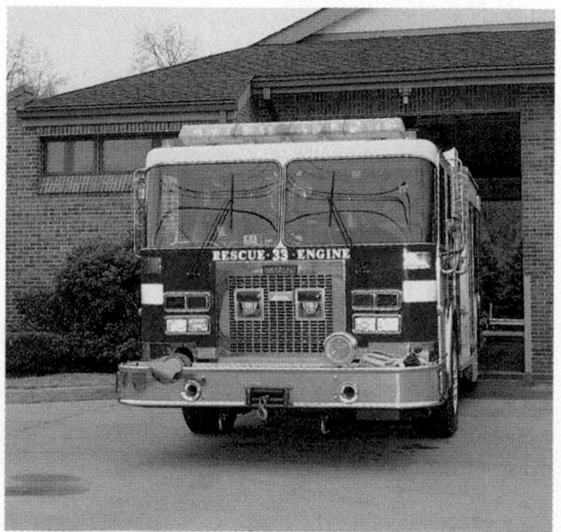

Figure 3.1 First responders being dispatched to an emergency scene.

working in a well-lighted room. To comply with the standard of care, you must meet two criteria. You must treat the patient to the best of your ability and you must provide care that a reasonable, prudent person with similar training would provide under similar circumstances. It is important to know exactly what the local standards of care are and what statutes pertain to your community.

Scope of Care

The scope of care you give as a first responder is defined on several levels. The National Curriculum for First Responders, developed by the United States Department of Transportation, specifies the skills taught in this course and the way those skills should be performed. States also have scope of care laws that may modify parts of the specifications in the National Curriculum. The medical director for your department may use medical protocols or standing orders to specify your scope of care. In some cases, on-line medical direction is provided by two-way radio or wireless telephone.

Ethical Responsibilities and Competence

Your community and your department have entrusted you, as a first responder, with certain ethical responsibilities. You have a responsibility to conform to accepted professional standards of conduct. These include staying up to date on the first responder skills and knowledge needed to provide good patient care. You are also responsible for reviewing your performance and assessing the techniques you use. You should evaluate your response times and try to follow up patient care outcomes with your medical director or hospital personnel. Always look for ways to improve your performance. Continuing education classes and refresher courses are designed to keep you up to date; make the most of them. Participate in quality improvement activities within your department.

Ethical behavior requires honesty. Your reports should accurately reflect the conditions found. Give complete and correct reports to other EMS providers. If you make a mistake, document it. Never change a report except to correct an error. Remember that the actions you take in the first few minutes of an emergency may make the difference between life or death for a patient. Your competence and your ethical behavior are valuable to you and to the patient.

Consent for Treatment

Consent simply means approval or permission. Legally, however, there are several types of consent. In **expressed consent**, the patient actually lets you know—verbally or nonverbally—that he or she is willing to accept the treatment you provide. Expressed consent is based on the assumption that the patient has the right to determine what will be done to his or her body. The patient must be of legal age and able

expressed consent Consent actually given by a person authorizing the first responder to provide care or transportation.

to make a rational decision. As you approach a patient, be sure the patient understands who you are, tell them what you are going to do and be sure they agree to treatment. For example, if you say, "You have a cut on your arm. I need to bandage it to stop the bleeding," and the response is "OK," the patient has given you expressed consent. Expressed consent is sometimes called actual consent or informed consent.

implied consent Consent to receive emergency care that is assumed because the individual is unconscious, underage, or so badly injured or ill that he or she cannot respond.

Any patient who does not specifically refuse emergency care can be treated under the principle of **implied consent**. The principle of implied consent is best understood in the situation of an unconscious patient. Because this patient is unable to communicate, the principles of law assume consent for treatment. Therefore, a first responder should never hesitate to treat an unconscious patient.

Consent for Minors

A minor is a person who has not yet reached the legal age designated by a particular state. Under the law, minors (who may be as old as 18) are not considered capable of speaking for themselves. In most cases, emergency treatment of a minor by a physician must wait until a parent or legal guardian consents to the treatment. If a minor requires emergency medical care in the field (out of the hospital) and the permission of a parent or legal guardian cannot be quickly obtained, do not hesitate to give appropriate emergency medical care. Emergency medical treatment for a minor should never be delayed or withheld just to obtain permission from a parent or legal guardian (**Figure 3.2**). Let hospital officials determine what treatment can be postponed until permission is obtained. Remember that good prehospital patient care is your first responsibility. By following the course of action that is best for the patient, you will stand on firm legal ground.

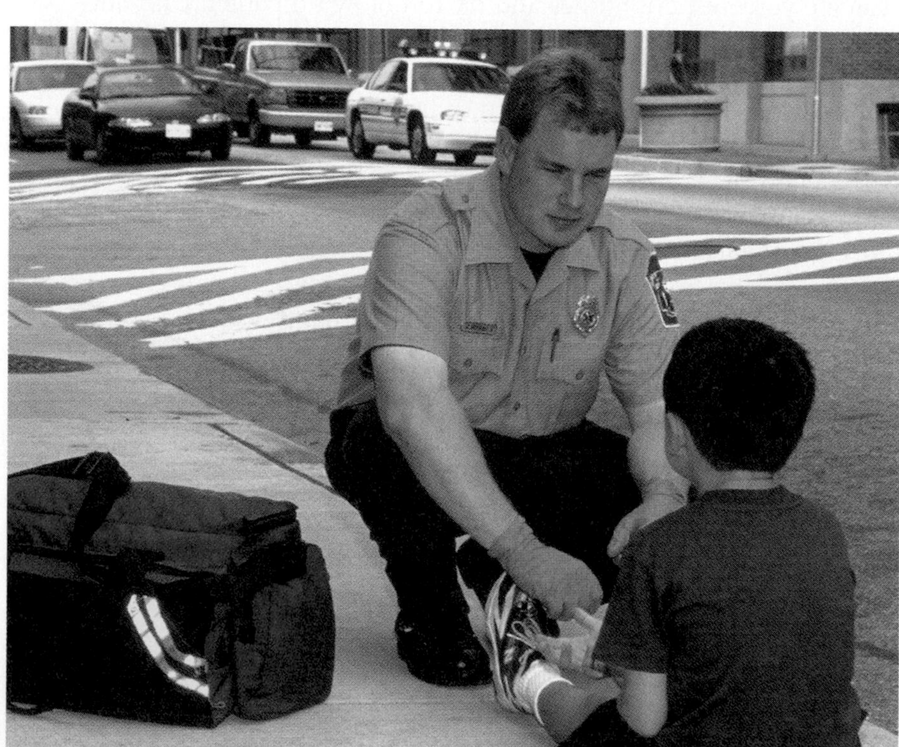

Figure 3.2 Do not withhold treatment from a patient who is a minor.

Consent of Mentally Ill

A rational adult may legally refuse to be treated. The legal issues are more complicated if the patient who refuses to be treated appears to be out of touch with reality and is a danger to self or others. The difficult part, even for highly trained medical personnel, is determining whether such a patient is rational. Generally, if the person appears to be a threat to self or to others, arrangements need to be made to place this person under medical care. The legal means by which these arrangements are made vary from state to state. You and other members of the EMS system should know your state's legal mechanism for handling patients who refuse to be treated and who do not appear to be making rational and reasonable decisions. Do not hesitate to involve law enforcement agencies, because this process may require the issuance of a warrant or an order of protective custody.

Patient Refusal of Care

Remember that any person who is mentally "in control," or **competent**, has a legal right to refuse treatment from emergency medical personnel at any time. You can continue to talk with a person who refuses treatment and try to help him or her understand the consequences of this action. Sometimes another EMS provider or a law enforcement officer may have more success in convincing a patient that he or she needs to receive treatment.

competent Able to make rational decisions about personal well-being.

living wills Legal documents with specific instructions that the patient does not want to be resuscitated or kept alive by mechanical support systems.

Checkpoint

What are the differences between the following types of consent:

- Expressed consent
- Implied consent
- Consent for minors
- Consent of mentally ill patients
- Lack of consent or refusal of care

Living Wills

A **living will** is a written document drawn up by a patient, a physician, and a lawyer. Similar documents are also called advance directives, advance directives to physicians, durable power of attorney for health care, or do not attempt resuscitation (DNR) orders. Living wills are often written when a patient has a terminal condition. For example, a terminally ill patient may request that no CPR be performed. If you are not able determine if a living will or advance directive is legally valid, you should begin appropriate medical care and leave the questions about living wills and advance directives to physicians. Some states have systems, such as bracelets, to identify patients with advance directives. You should know your local policies and protocols.

Legal Concepts

Abandonment

abandonment Failure of the first responder to continue emergency medical treatment until relieved by someone with the same or higher level of training.

Abandonment occurs when a trained person begins emergency care and then leaves the patient before another trained person arrives to take over. Once you have started treatment, you must continue that treatment until a person who has the same or at least as much training arrives on the scene and takes over. Never leave a patient without care after you begin treatment.

The most common abandonment scenario occurs when an EMS provider responds to a call, examines the patient, assesses the patient's condition, fails to transport the patient to a hospital, and finds out later that the patient died. Treatment began, but the patient was abandoned.

FOUR LEGAL CONCEPTS YOU SHOULD UNDERSTAND

- *Abandonment*
- *Persons dead at the scene*
- *Negligence*
- *Confidentiality*

Persons Dead at the Scene

If there is any indication that a person is alive when you arrive on the scene, you should begin providing necessary care. Persons who are obviously dead should be handled according to the laws of your state and the protocols of your service. Generally, you cannot assume a person is dead unless one or more of the following conditions exist:

1. ***Decapitation.*** Decapitation means that the head is separated from the body. When this occurs, there is obviously no chance of saving the patient.

2. ***Rigor mortis.*** Rigor mortis is the temporary stiffening of muscles that occurs several hours after death. The presence of this stiffening indicates that the patient is dead and cannot be resuscitated.

3. ***Tissue decomposition.*** Body tissue begin to decompose and flesh begins to decay only after a person has been dead for more than a day.

4. ***Dependent lividity.*** Dependent lividity is the red or purple color that occurs on the parts of the patient's body that are closest to the ground. It is caused by blood seeping into the tissues on the dependent, or lower, part of the person's body. Dependent lividity occurs after a person has been dead for several hours.

If any of these signs is present, you can usually consider the patient to be dead. It is important that you know the protocol your department uses in dealing with patients who are dead on the scene (**Figure 3.3**). Chapter 8 covers these criteria as they relate to starting CPR.

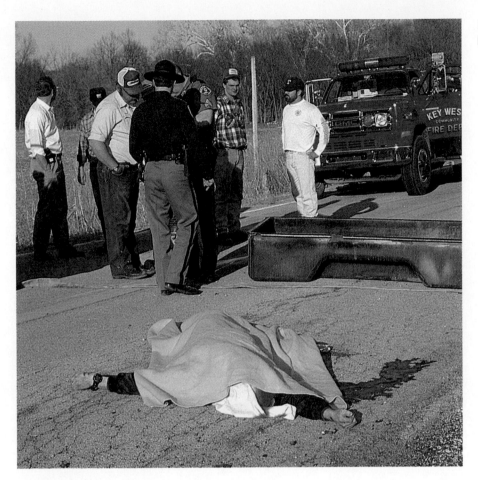

Figure 3.3 Learn the protocol for dealing with patients who are obviously dead at the scene.

Negligence

Negligence occurs when a patient suffers further injury or harm because the care that was administered did not meet the standards expected from a person with similar training in a similar situation.

negligence Deviation from the accepted standard of care resulting in further injury to the patient.

> For negligence to occur, four conditions must be present:
> 1. Duty to act
> 2. Breech of duty
> 3. Resulting injuries
> 4. Proximate cause

As a first responder who has been called to a scene to provide patient care, you have a duty to help the patient. If you fail to provide care according to the level of your training, this could constitute a breech of duty. For negligence to be proved, the patient must sustain injuries as a result of your improper care. Injuries related to your negligent actions or failure to act properly constitute proximate cause. Examples of negligence include reckless or careless performance or care that does not meet the accepted standard for a first responder.

Confidentiality

Most patient information is confidential. Confidential information includes patient circumstances, patient history, assessment findings, and patient care given. This information should be shared only with other medical or law enforcement personnel who are involved in the patient's care. You must not discuss this privileged information with your family or friends.

Some information about a patient's care may be classified as public information. Public information includes the type of incident and the patient's name. You should learn what patient information is considered public information in your state. Public information can be released to the news media through your department's approved process.

Good Samaritan Laws

Good Samaritan laws Laws that encourage individuals to voluntarily help an injured or suddenly ill person by minimizing the liability for any errors or omissions in rendering good faith emergency care.

Good Samaritan laws were passed in an effort to reduce the liability of persons who stop at accidents or emergency situations to give emergency medical care. These laws vary considerably from state to state, and they may or may not apply to first responders in your state. Recently, legal experts have noted that Good Samaritan laws may no longer be needed because they provide little or no legal protection for a rescuer or EMS provider.

Any properly trained first responder who practices the skills and procedures learned in a first responder course should not be overly concerned about lack of protection under Good Samaritan statutes.

Regulations

As a first responder, you are subject to a variety of federal, state, local, and agency regulations. You should become familiar with these regulations so you can follow them. The most important regulations govern your ability to work as a first responder. You may have to become registered or certified as a first responder through a state agency or you may have to register through the National Registry of Emergency Medical Technicians. It is your responsibility to keep any required certifications or registrations up to date.

Reportable Events

State and federal agencies have requirements for reporting certain events, including crimes and infectious diseases. Reportable crimes include knife wounds, gunshot wounds, auto accidents, suspected child abuse, domestic violence, elder abuse, and rape. You must learn which crimes are reportable in your area. You also need to know your agency's procedures on reporting these crimes.

Certain infectious diseases are also reportable. It is important that you learn how this process is handled in your agency and what you are required to do.

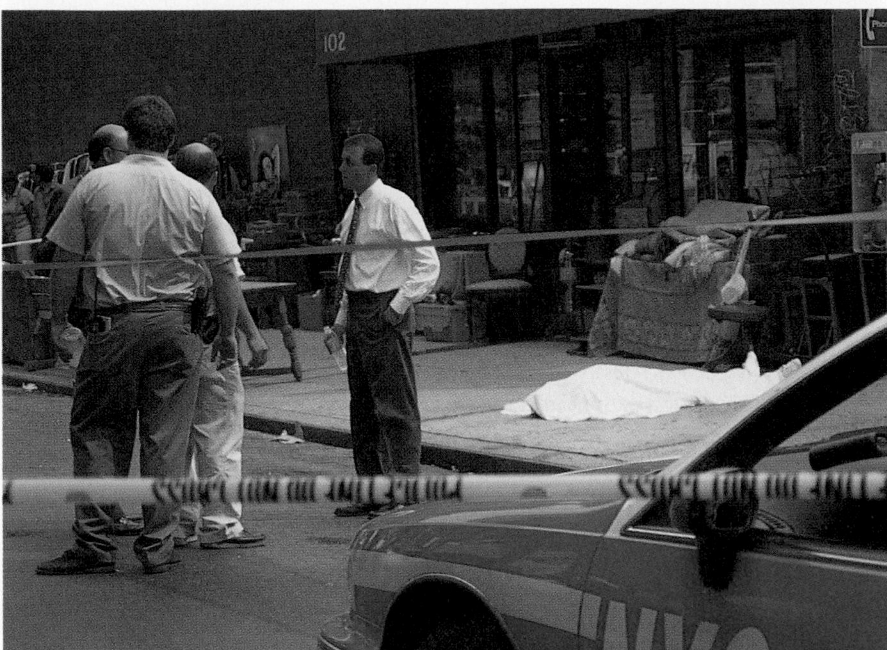

Figure 3.4 Crime scene operations require you to change the scene as little as possible

Crime Scene Operations

Many emergency medical situations are also crime scenes. As a first responder, you should keep the following considerations in mind:

1. Protect yourself. Be sure the scene is safe before you try to enter.
2. If you determine that a crime scene is unsafe, wait until law enforcement personnel signal that the scene is safe for entry.
3. Your first priority is patient care. Nothing except your personal safety should interfere with that effort.
4. Move the patient only if necessary, such as for rapid transport to the hospital, for administration of CPR, or for treatment of severe shock. If you must move the patient, take a mental "snapshot" of the scene.
5. Touch only what you need to touch to gain access to the patient.
6. Preserve the crime scene for further investigation. Do not move furniture unless it interferes with your ability to provide care. If you must move anything out of the way, move it no further than necessary to provide care (**Figure 3.4**).
7. Be careful where you put your equipment. You could alter or destroy evidence if you put your equipment on top of it.
8. Keep nonessential personnel such as curious neighbors away from the scene.
9. After you have attended to a patient at a crime scene, write a short report about the incident and make a sketch of the scene that shows how and where you found the patient. This may be useful if you are required to recall the incident two or three years later.

Voices of Experience

Rescuers Provide Crucial Evidence

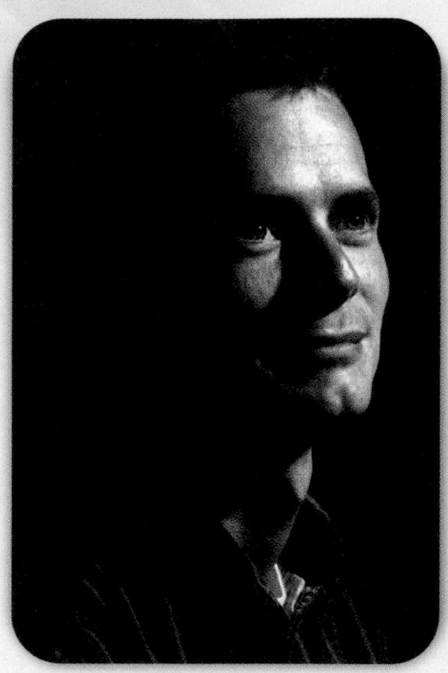

On May 2, 1997, shortly after 1700 hours, our rural volunteer agency was dispatched for a patient in cardiac arrest. The dispatch information confirmed a 4-year-old child in cardiac arrest and the nature of the illness or injury was unknown. Since it was a pediatric cardiac arrest with an unknown origin, the responding unit requested that police be dispatched.

We arrived on the scene prior to police arrival to find a 4-year-old in cardiac arrest. CPR was in progress by a neighbor trained in CPR. Initial assessment confirmed that the patient was unconscious, apneic (not breathing), and pulseless. The mother stated that she felt the child had choked on something, since the child had vomited.The child had been like this for about 15 minutes according to bystanders. This timeframe seemed to correspond with our agency dispatch/response time. However, we noticed several things on further assessment. The child's face had multiple bruising. Her scalp had puncture wounds. There were linear scars on her extremities. Her legs had puncture wounds. The overall skin condition revealed cyanosis to the face, mottling to the back, and a cold temperature. When asked about the bruising, the mother reported that the child had been falling a lot and had fallen from the bed. With these signs and symptoms, we suspected that this was not the truth. Such factors as the severe trauma, mottling, and cold skin indicated that death had occurred earlier than 15 minutes ago. In addition, the mother's unusual calmness, her ever-changing description of injury pattern, and a mechanism that did not match the extensive injuries put red flags up for the suspicion of abuse.

“Our assessments and observations played an important role in the prosecution of those charged with the criminal death of this child.”

As an experienced provider, many key factors were important in this call. Our assessments and observations played an important role in the prosecution of those charged with the criminal death of this child. By observing the scene and the actions of bystanders while providing care to the patient, we were able to provide valuable information that assisted in the conviction.

Some questions that were important in this case during the criminal investigations included: “What was the mother's demeanor/ reaction during resuscitation attempts of the child?” “What did you see at the scene when you arrived?” (remember the unit was there prior to the police), “Was the stepfather present?” “Do you know who the mother was talking to on the phone?” “Who else was present at the scene?” and, “What did you do for the child?”

If you are the first responder, it is important that you protect crime scenes as much as possible. Altering a crime scene can hamper criminal investigations. If you must alter a crime scene for patient care, please note the scene prior to your changes, and include this information in your documentation. In addition to your role as a caregiver, you are a patient advocate. It is important for the responder to remember that suspected child abuse is also a reporting requirement in most states. ❖

Paul Arthur Phillips, RN, BSN, NREMT-P
Captain
Dante Rescue Squad
Dante, Virgina
Flight Nurse/Paramedic
Med Flight II
Abingdon, Virginia

Documentation

After you have finished treating the patient, record your observations about the scene, the patient's condition, and the treatment you provided. Documentation should be done according to the policies of your organization. These policies should follow appropriate local and state laws. Your documentation is important because it is the initial account describing the patient's condition and the care administered. You will not be able to remember the treatment you provide to each patient without documentation. It also serves as a legal record of your treatment and will be required in the event of a lawsuit. Documentation also provides a basis for evaluating the quality of care provided.

Documentation should be clear, concise, accurate, and readable.

Documentation should include the following information:

1. The condition of the patient when found.
2. The patient's description of the injury or illness.
3. The patient's initial and repeat vital signs.
4. The treatment you gave the patient.
5. The agency and personnel who took over treatment of the patient.
6. Any other helpful facts.
7. Any reportable conditions present.
8. Any infectious disease exposure.
9. Anything unusual regarding the case.

3

Prep Kit

Ready for Review

Ready for Review thoroughly summarizes the chapter.

This chapter introduces the legal principles you need to know as a first responder. As a first responder, you have a duty to act when you are dispatched on a medical call as a part of your official duties. You are held to a certain standard of care, which is related to your level of training, and you are expected to perform to the level a similarly trained person would perform under similar circumstances.

You should understand the differences between expressed consent, implied consent, consent for minors, consent of mentally ill persons, and the right to refuse care. Living wills and advance directives give a patient the right to have care withheld. Because first responders cannot determine the validity of these documents, it is best to begin treatment for these patients. This chapter also covers the concepts of abandonment, negligence, and confidentiality, as well as the purpose of Good Samaritan laws, even though they are not needed for first responders.

You must understand the importance of federal and state regulations that govern your performance as a first responder. You must also understand your department's operational regulations. Certain events that deal with contagious diseases or with illegal acts must be reported to the proper authorities. You should know how to deal with these reportable events. Crime scene operations are a complex environment. Following proper procedures assures that the patient receives good medical care and that the crime scene is not compromised for the law enforcement investigation.

Your job is not complete until the paperwork is done. It is important that first responders document their findings and treatment. This provides good patient care and adequate legal documentation.

By understanding and following these legal concepts, you will build the foundation for the skills you need to be a good first responder.

Vital Vocabulary

The Vital Vocabulary are the key terms for this chapter.

abandonment—*page 40*
competent—*page 39*
duty to act—*page 36*
expressed consent—*page 37*
Good Samaritan laws—*page 42*
implied consent—*page 38*
living wills—*page 39*
negligence—*page 41*
standard of care—*page 36*

Ready to Respond

Ready to Respond presents a fictitious scenario to help you review what you learned in this chapter.

You are dispatched to a public school to care for a sick fifth-grade student. When you arrive, you are met by a teacher who says that the child suddenly developed severe pain in her abdomen. The student is lying on a cot in a room near the principal's office. The teacher tells you the school nurse is at another school today.

1. You have a duty to act because

A. The child is under 18 years of age

B. The teacher called you to the school

C. Your agency has been designated as first responders

D. You have been trained as first responder

2. The standard of care you are expected to give is

1. The same a reasonable person with similar training would do under the same circumstances
2. To the best of your ability
3. The same as any other first responder
4. Better than the care the teacher could give

A. 1 and 2

B. 1 and 3

C. 2 and 4

D. 3 and 4

3. The type of consent you would expect from this patient is

A. Expressed consent

B. Implied consent

C. Consent for minors

D. None of the above

4. If you and the teacher are not able to reach the student's parents or guardian, you should

A. Wait until you get their permission

B. Ask to see a school permission form

C. Treat the patient and let the hospital handle the permission

D. Ask the teacher what to do

5. If you left the student because you got a more important call, you might be found guilty of

A. Negligence

B. Lack of confidentiality

C. Failing to act

D. Abandonment

Chapter 4

The Human Body: Anatomy and Function of Body Systems

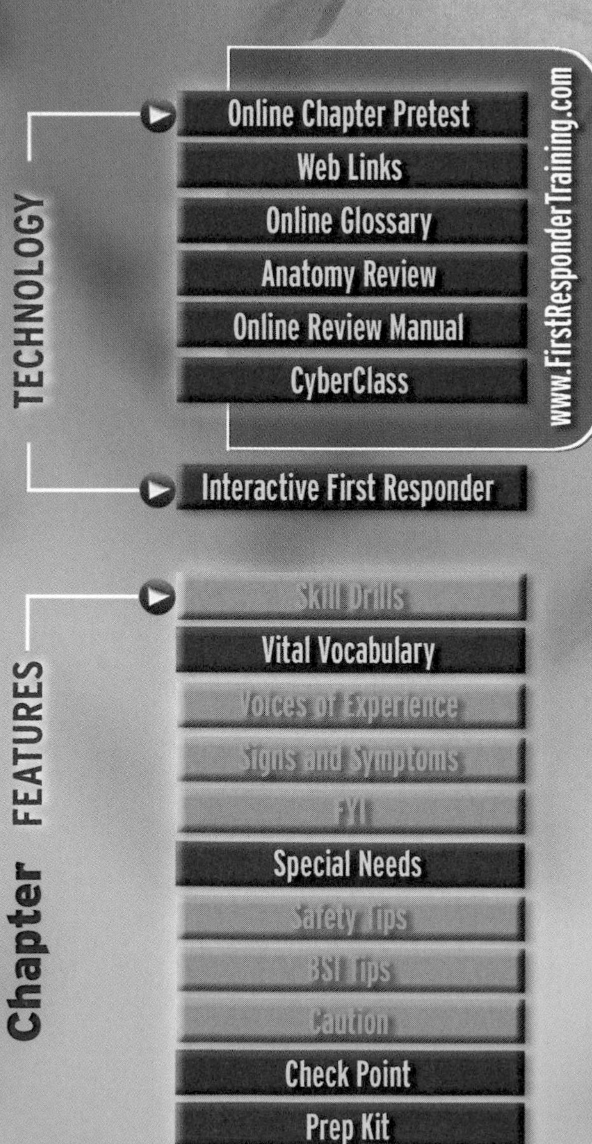

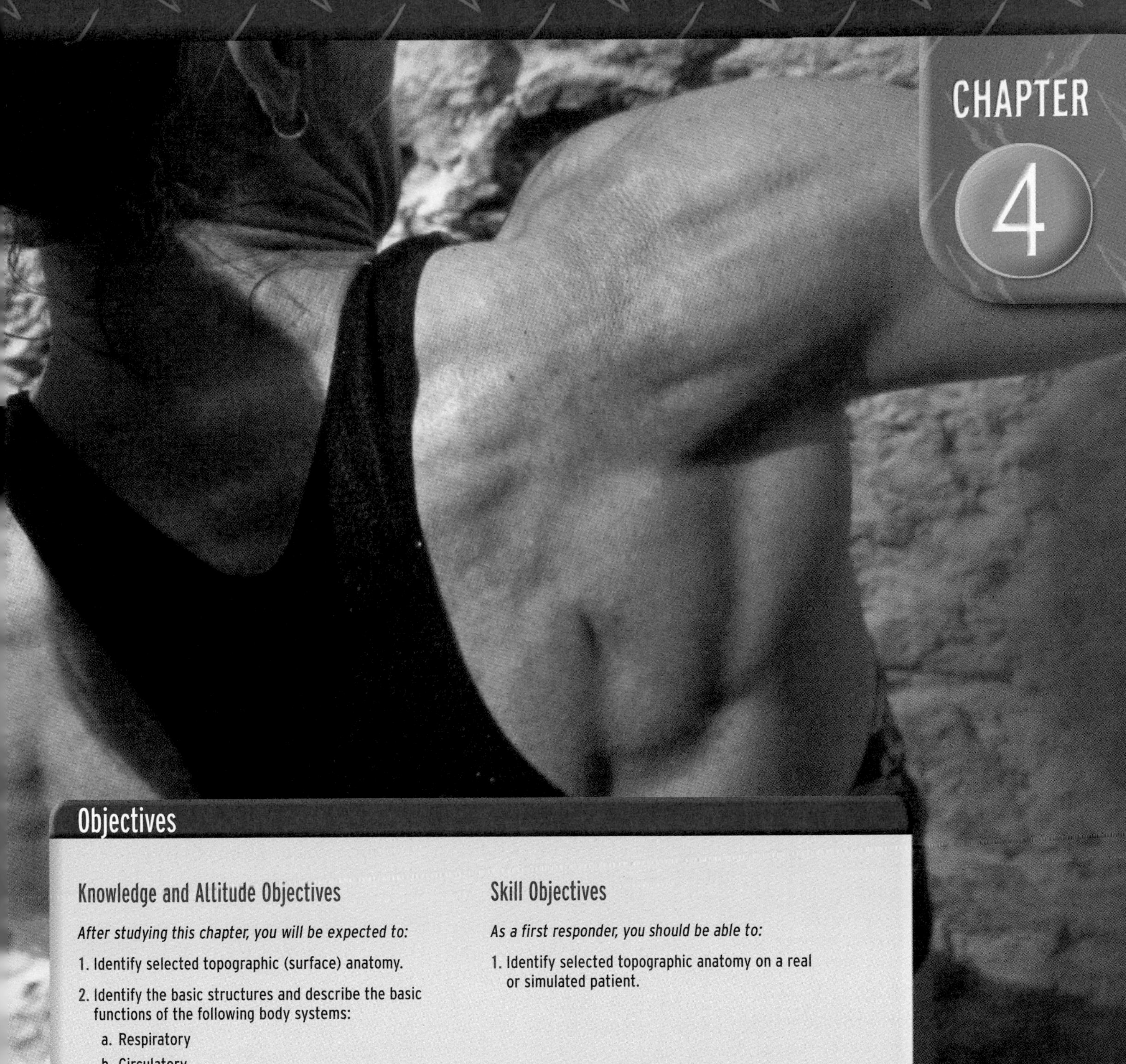

Objectives

Knowledge and Attitude Objectives

After studying this chapter, you will be expected to:

1. Identify selected topographic (surface) anatomy.
2. Identify the basic structures and describe the basic functions of the following body systems:
   a. Respiratory
   b. Circulatory
   c. Skeletal
   d. Muscular
   e. Nervous
   f. Digestive
   g. Genitourinary
   h. Skin

Skill Objectives

As a first responder, you should be able to:

1. Identify selected topographic anatomy on a real or simulated patient.

To be an effective first responder, you must understand the basic structure and functions of the human body. This knowledge will help you understand the problem the patient is experiencing, perform an adequate patient examination, communicate your findings to the other members of the emergency medical team, and provide appropriate emergency treatment for the patient's condition. This chapter describes human anatomy and the relationships among eight body systems

Topographic Anatomy

The anatomic terms in this section are used to describe the location of injury or pain. Knowing the basic anatomic terms for human body parts is important because all members of the emergency medical team must be able to speak the same language when treating a patient. However, if you cannot remember the proper anatomic term for a certain body location, you can use lay terms.

Visualize a person standing and facing you, with arms at the sides and thumbs pointing outward (palms toward you). This is the standard anatomic position; you should keep it in mind when describing a location on the body. **Figure 4.1** identifies **topographic anatomy**.

The first terms that should be clarified are left and right. These terms always refer to the patient's left and right. **Anterior** and **posterior** simply mean front (anterior) and back (posterior). The **midline** refers to an imaginary vertical line drawn from head to toe that separates the body into a left half and a right half.

Two other useful terms are medial and lateral. **Medial** means closer to the midline of the body; lateral means away from the midline. In this context, the eyes are lateral to the nose.

The term **proximal** means close, and **distal** means distant. On the body, proximal means close to the point where an arm or leg is attached. Distal means distant from the point of attachment. For example, if the thigh bone (femur) is broken, the break can be either proximal (the end closer to the hip) or distal (the end farther away from the hip).

The term **superior** means closer to the head, and **inferior** means closer to the feet. For example, the hips are inferior to the chest, and the chest is superior to the hip.

topographic anatomy The superficial landmarks on the body that serve as location guides to the structures that lie beneath them.

anterior The front surface of the body.

posterior The back surface of the body.

midline An imaginary vertical line drawn from the midforehead through the nose and the navel to the floor.

medial Toward the midline of the body.

lateral Away from the midline of the body.

proximal Describing structures that are closer to the trunk.

distal Describing structures that are nearer to the free end of an extremity; any location that is farther from the midline than the point of reference named.

superior Toward the head; lying higher in the body.

inferior That portion of the body or body part that lies nearer the feet than the head.

Body Systems

Body systems work together to perform common functions. By studying these body systems, you will have a better background for understanding illnesses and injuries.

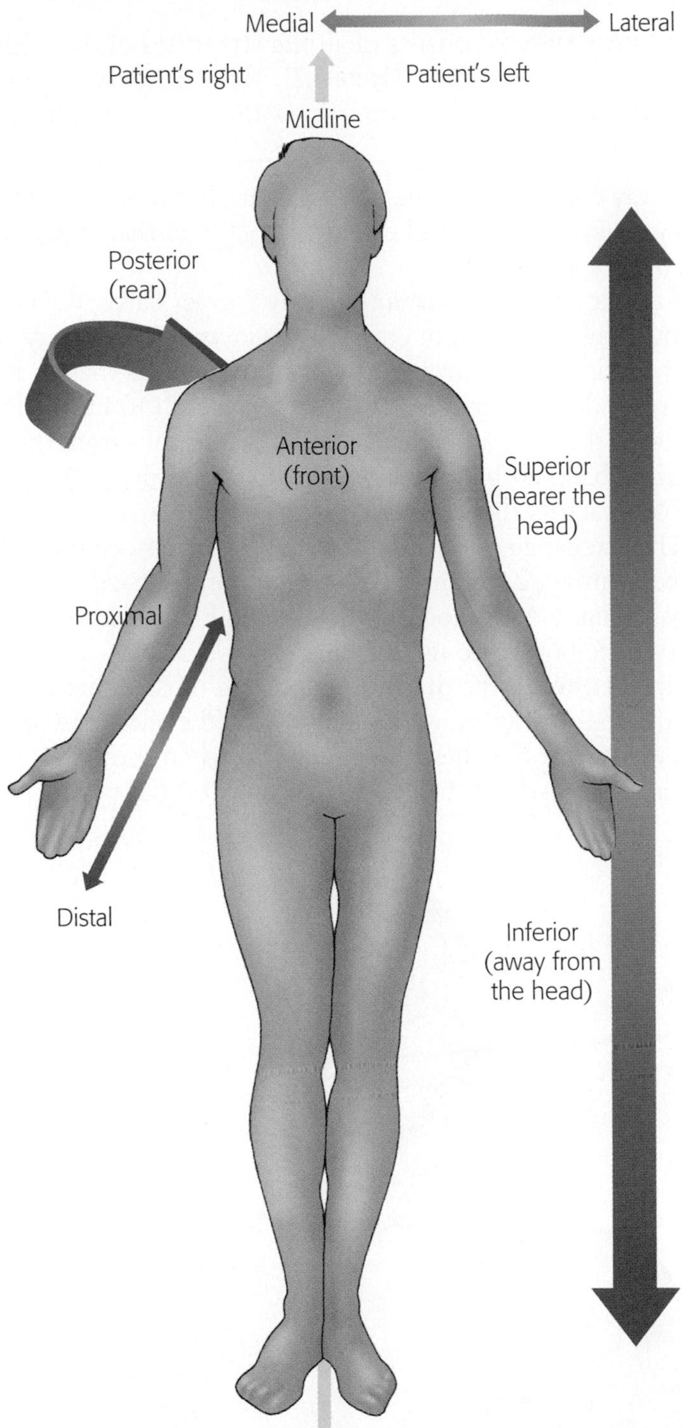

Figure 4.1 Topographic anatomy terms for describing a location on the body.

The Respiratory System

Because airway maintenance is one of the most important skills you will learn as a first responder, the **respiratory system** is the first of the body systems we will study.

respiratory system All body structures that contribute to normal breathing.

The respiratory system consists of all the structures of the body that contribute to normal breathing (**Figure 4.2**). The respiratory system brings oxygen into the body and removes the waste gas, carbon dioxide.

larynx A structure composed of cartilage in the neck that guards the entrance to the windpipe and functions as the organ of voice. Also called the voice box.

epiglottis The valve located at the upper end of the voice box that prevents food from entering the larynx.

carbon dioxide (CO_2) The gas formed in respiration and exhaled in breathing.

diaphragm A muscular dome that separates the chest from the abdominal cavity. Contraction of the diaphragm and the chest wall muscles brings air into the lungs; relaxation expels air from the lungs.

The airway consists of the nose (nasopharynx), mouth (oropharynx), throat, **larynx** (voice box), trachea (windpipe), and the passages within the lungs (**Figure 4.3**).

At the upper end of the larynx is a tiny flapper valve, the **epiglottis**. The epiglottis keeps food from entering the larynx. The airway within the lungs branch into narrower and narrower passages that end in tiny air sacs surrounded by tiny blood vessels. Oxygen (O_2) in inhaled air passes through the thin walls that separate the air sacs from the blood vessels and is absorbed by the blood. **Carbon dioxide (CO_2)** passes from the blood across the same thin walls into the air sacs and is exhaled. This exchange of carbon dioxide for oxygen occurs 12 to 16 times per minute, 24 hours a day, without any conscious effort on your part (**Figure 4.4**). Blood transports the inhaled oxygen to all parts of the body through the circulatory system.

Air is inhaled when the **diaphragm**, a large muscle that forms the bottom of the chest cavity, moves downward and the chest muscles contract to expand the size of the chest. Air is exhaled when these muscles relax, thus decreasing the size of the chest (**Figure 4.5** on page 54).

Special Needs

CHILDREN

Infants and children have somewhat different respiratory systems than adults:

- A child's airway is smaller and more flexible. When you perform rescue breathing on a child, you do not need to apply as much force as for an adult.
- Because of its smaller size, a child's airway is more easily blocked by a foreign object.
- Very young infants can breathe only through their noses. Therefore, if an infant's nose becomes blocked, the infant will show signs of respiratory distress.

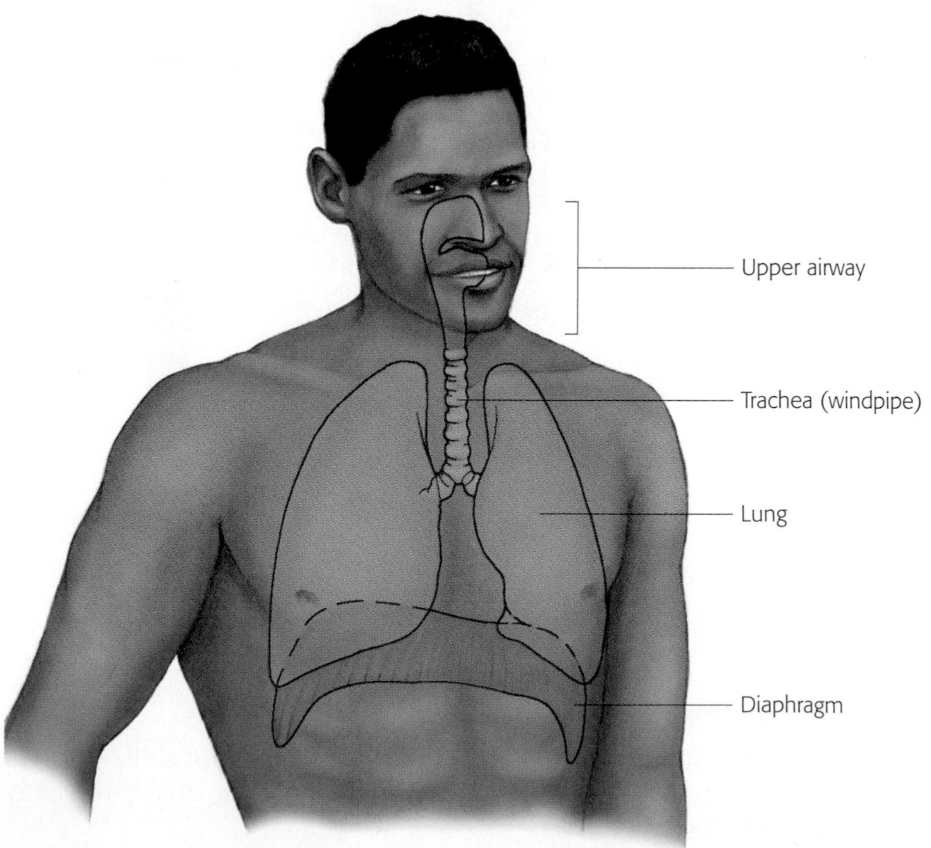

Figure 4.2 The respiratory system.

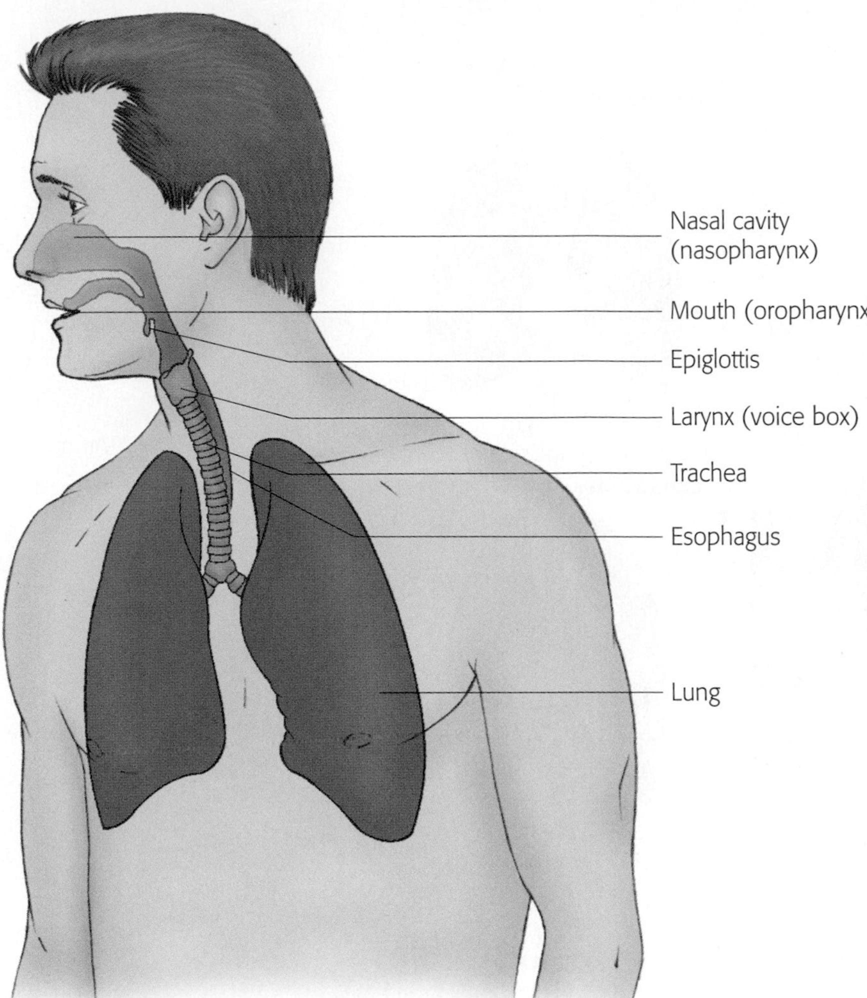

Figure 4.3 The airway consists of these structures.

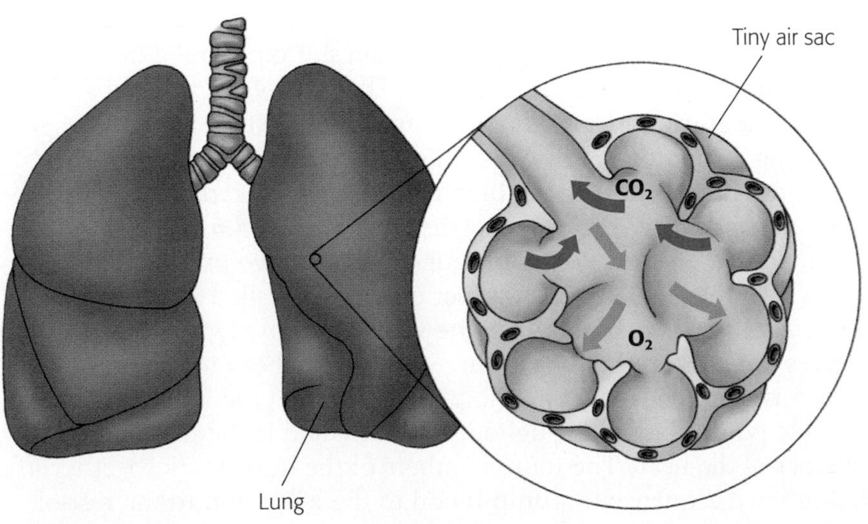

Figure 4.4 The exchange of carbon dioxide (CO_2) and oxygen (O_2) in the lungs.

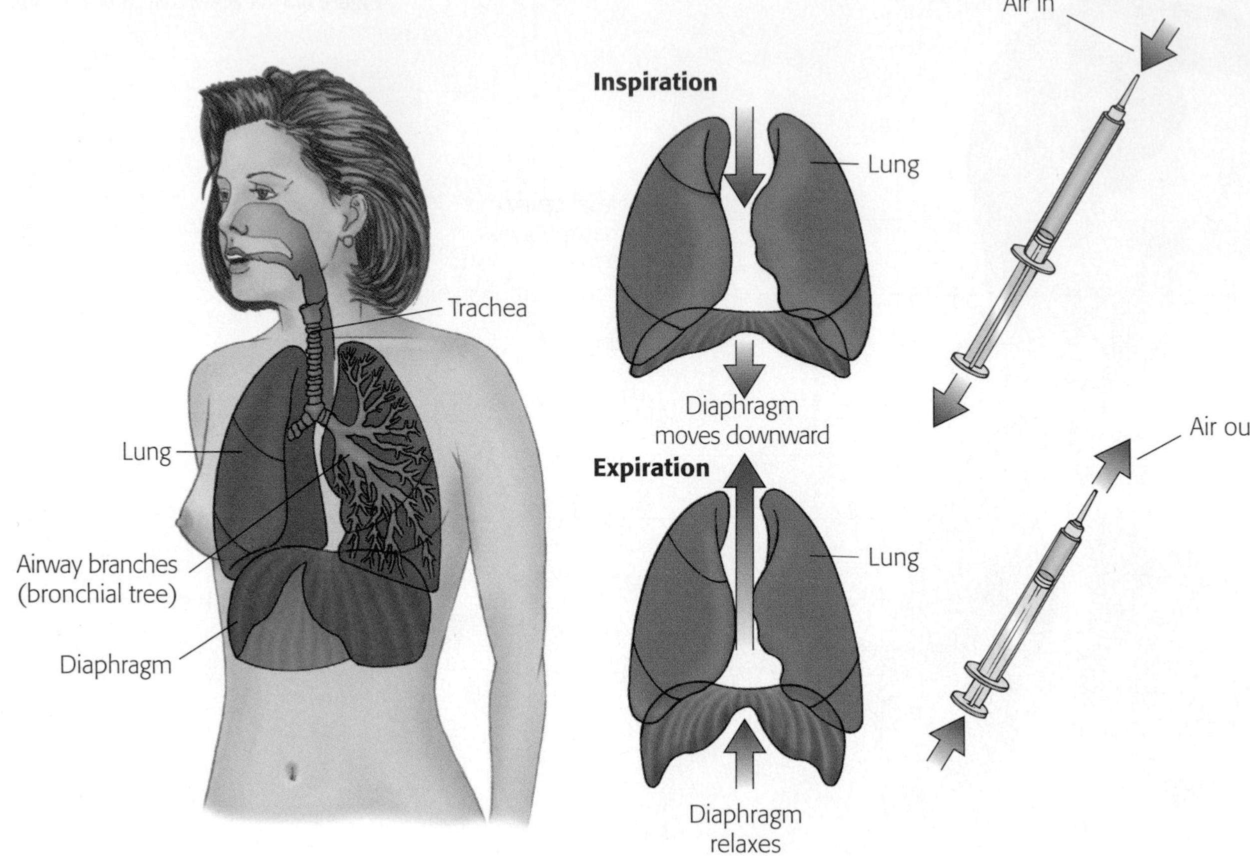

Figure 4.5 Mechanism of breathing.

The Circulatory System

circulatory system The heart and blood vessels, which together are responsible for the continuous flow of blood throughout the body.

The **circulatory system** is responsible for pumping blood through the body. The circulatory system can be compared to a city water system with a central pumping station (the heart), a network of pipes (the blood vessels) that reaches into all parts of the system (the body), and fluid (blood).

After blood picks up oxygen in the lungs, it goes to the heart, which pumps it to the rest of the body. The cells of the body absorb oxygen and nutrients from the blood and release waste products (including carbon dioxide), which the blood carries back to the lungs and kidneys. In the lungs, the blood exchanges the carbon dioxide for more oxygen and the cycle begins again (**Figure 4.6**).

The human heart consists of four chambers, two on the right side and two on the left side. Each upper chamber is called an atrium. The right atrium receives blood from the veins of the body; the left atrium receives blood from the lungs. The bottom chambers are the right and left ventricles. The right ventricle pumps blood to the lungs; the left ventricle pumps blood throughout the body, and is the most muscular chamber of the heart The four chambers of the heart work together in a well-ordered sequence to pump blood to the lungs and to the rest of the body (**Figure 4.7**).

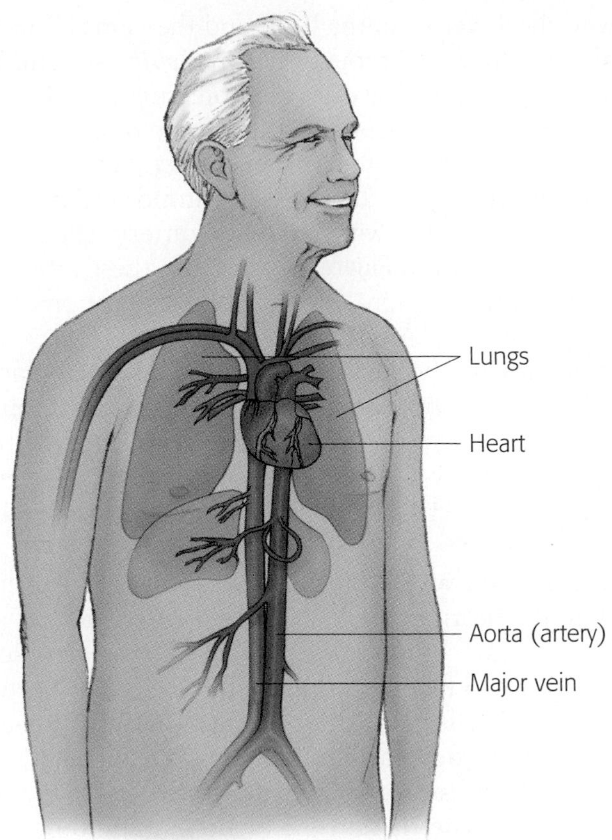

Figure 4.6 The circulatory system.

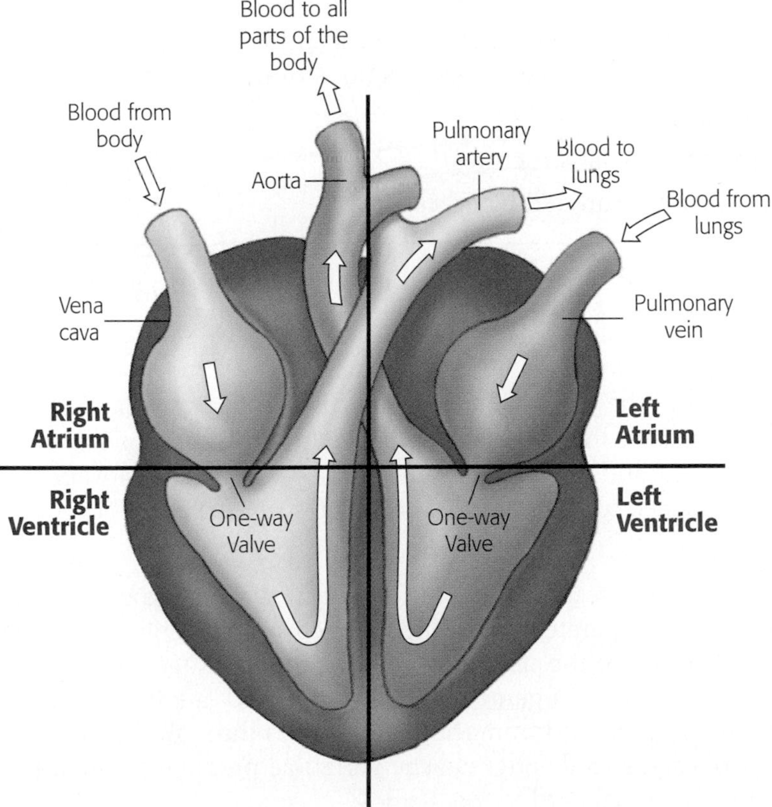

Figure 4.7 Schematic representation of the functions of the four chambers of the heart.

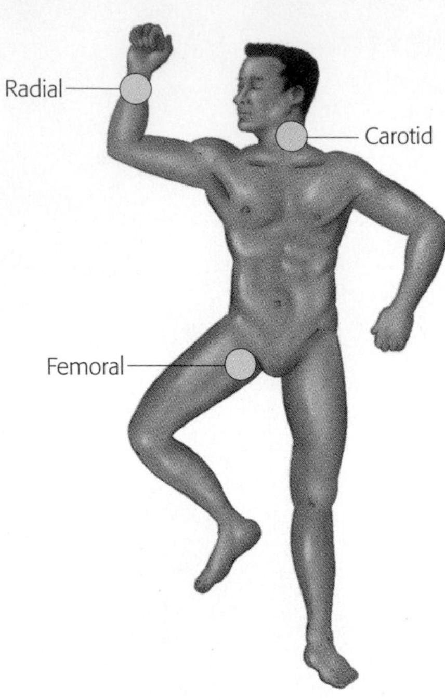

Figure 4.8 The location of the carotid, radial, and femoral pulses.

One-way check valves in the heart and the veins allow the blood to flow in only one direction through the circulatory system. The arteries carry blood away from the heart at high pressure and therefore have thick walls. The arteries closest to the heart are quite large (about 1 inch in diameter) but become smaller farther away from the heart.

Three major arteries are the neck (or carotid) artery, the groin (or femoral) artery, and the wrist (or radial) artery. The locations of these arteries are shown in **Figure 4.8**. Because these arteries lie between a bony structure and the skin, they are used as locations to measure the patient's **pulse**.

The capillaries are the smallest pipes in the system. Some capillaries are so small that only one blood cell at a time can go through them. At the capillary level, oxygen and nutrients pass from the blood cells into the cells of body tissues, and carbon dioxide and other waste products pass from the tissue cells to the blood cells, which then return to the lungs.

Veins are the thin-walled pipes of the circulatory system that carry blood back to the heart.

Blood has several components: **plasma** (a clear, straw-colored fluid), red blood cells, white blood cells, and **platelets**. Blood gets its red color from the red blood cells, which carry oxygen from the lungs to the body and bring carbon dioxide back to the lungs. The white blood cells are called "infection fighters" because they devour bacteria and other disease-causing organisms. Platelets start the blood-clotting process.

pulse The wave of pressure that is created by the heart as it contracts and forces blood out of the heart and into the major arteries.

plasma The fluid part of the blood that carries blood cells, transports nutrients, and removes cellular waste materials.

platelets Microscopic disk-shaped elements in the blood that are essential to the process of blood clot formation; the mechanism that stops bleeding.

skull The bones of the head, collectively; serves as the protective structure for the brain.

vertebrae The 33 bones of the spinal column: 7 cervical, 12 thoracic, 5 lumbar, 5 sacral, and 4 coccygeal vertebrae.

tendons Tough, rope-like cords of fibrous tissue that attach muscles to bones.

ligaments Fibrous bands that connect bones to bones and support and strengthen joints.

The Skeletal System

The skeletal system consists of bones and is the supporting framework for the body. The three functions of the skeletal system are:

- To support the body
- To protect vital structures
- To manufacture red blood cells

The skeletal system is divided into seven areas beginning with the head (**Figure 4.9**).

The Skull

The bones of the head include the **skull** and the lower jawbone. The skull consists of many bones fused together to form a hollow sphere that contains and protects the brain. The jawbone is a movable bone that is attached to the skull and completes the structure of the head.

The Spine

The spine is the second area of the skeletal system and consists of a series of 33 separate bones called **vertebrae**. The spinal vertebrae are stacked up on top of each other and are held together by muscles, **tendons**, disks, and **ligaments**. The spinal cord, a group of nerves that carry messages to and from the brain, passes through the hole in the center of each spinal vertebra. The vertebrae provide excellent protection for the spinal cord.

In addition to protecting the spinal cord, the spine is the primary support structure for the entire body.

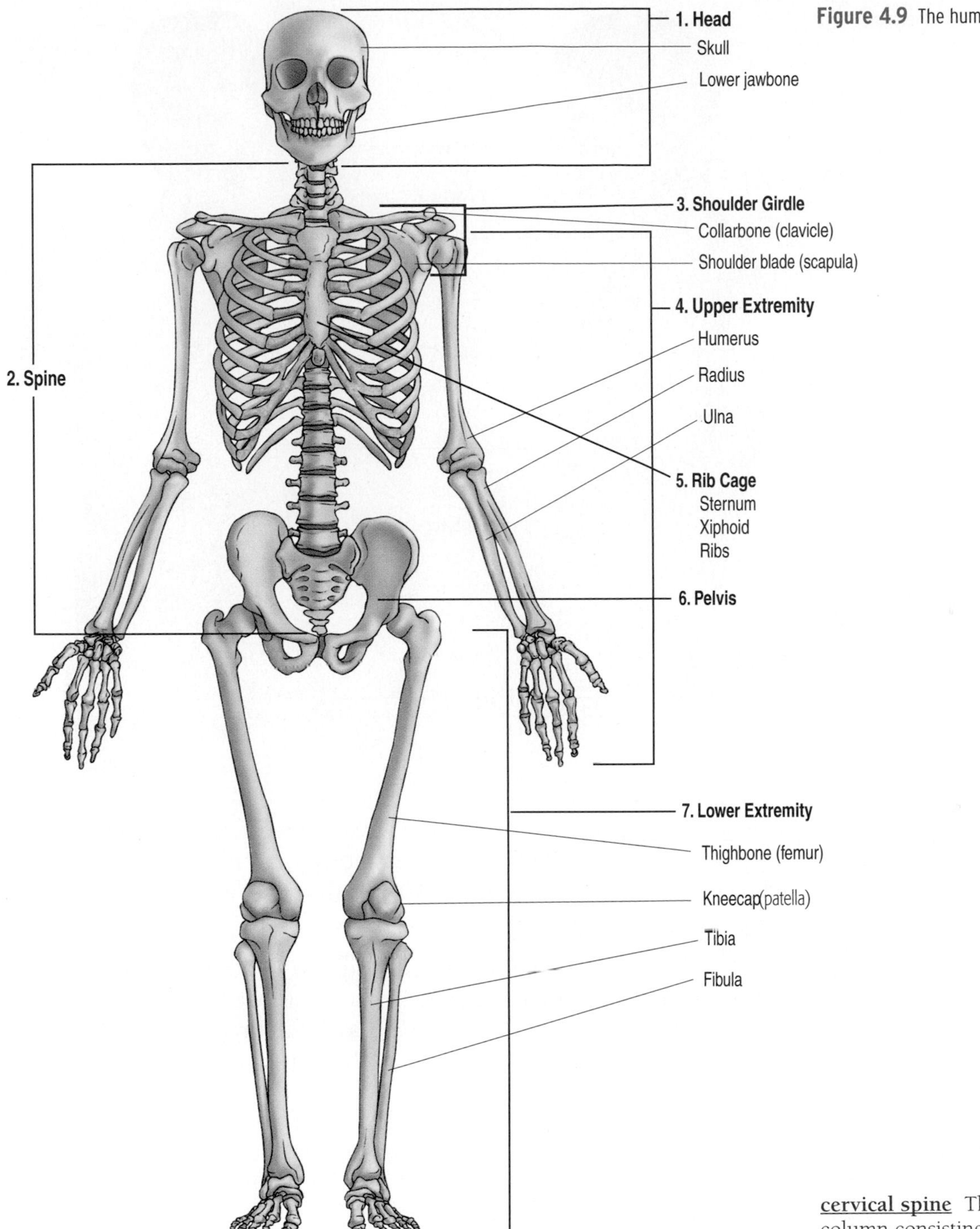

Figure 4.9 The human skeleton.

The spine has five sections (**Figure 4.10**, page 58):

- Cervical spine (neck)
- Thoracic spine (upper back)
- Lumbar spine (lower back)
- Sacrum (base of spine)
- Coccyx (tailbone)

cervical spine That portion of the spinal column consisting of the 7 vertebrae located in the neck.

thoracic spine The 12 vertebrae that attach to the 12 ribs; the upper part of the back.

lumbar spine The lower part of the back formed by the lowest 5 nonfused vertebrae.

sacrum One of 3 bones (sacrum and 2 pelvic bones) that make up the pelvic ring; forms the base of the spine.

coccyx The tailbone; the small bone below the sacrum formed by the final 4 vertebrae.

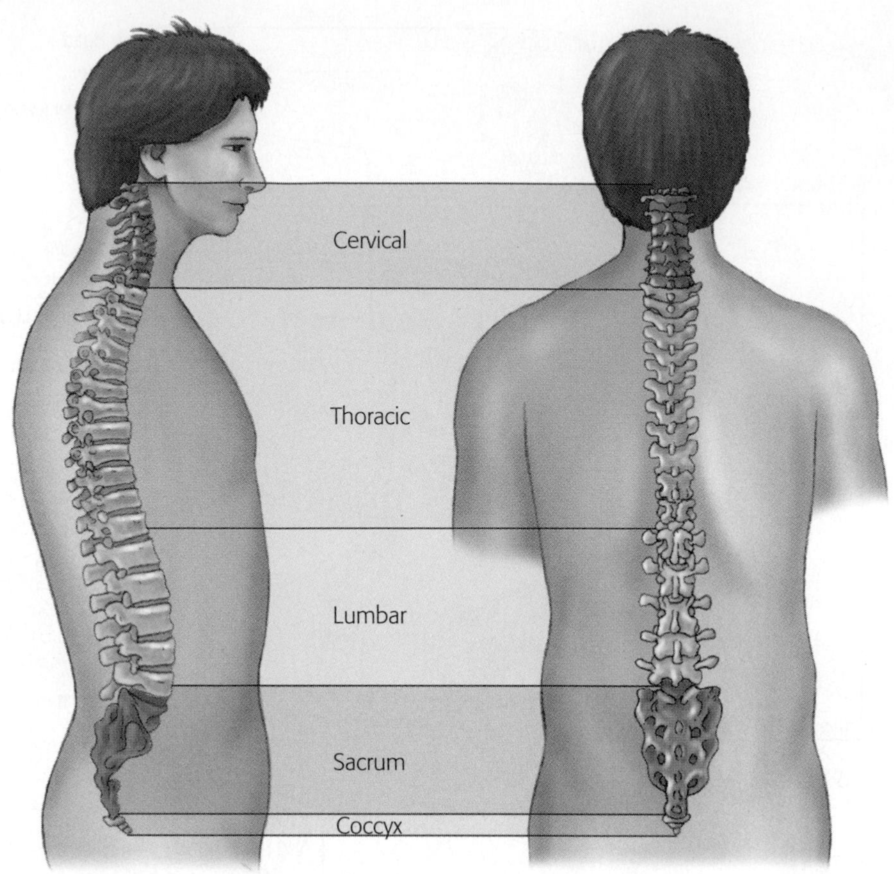

Figure 4.10 The five sections of the spine.

shoulder girdle The proximal portion of the upper extremity; made up of the clavicle, the scapula, and the humerus.

ulna The bone on the little-finger side of the forearm.

radius The bone on the thumb side of the forearm.

ribs The paired arches of bone, 12 on either side, that extend from the thoracic vertebrae toward the anterior midline of the trunk.

sternum The breastbone.

cartilage A tough, elastic form of connective tissue that covers the ends of most bones to form joints. Also found in some specific areas such as the nose and ear.

floating ribs The eleventh and twelfth ribs, which do not connect to the sternum.

xiphoid process The flexible cartilage at the lower tip of the sternum; a key landmark in the administration of CPR and the Heimlich maneuver.

The Shoulder Girdles

The **shoulder girdles** form the third area of the skeletal system. Each shoulder girdle supports an arm and consists of the collarbone (clavicle), the shoulder blade (scapula), and the upper arm bone (humerus).

The Upper Extremity

The fourth major area of the skeletal system is the upper extremity, which consists of three major bones. The arm has one bone (the humerus), and the forearm has two bones (the **ulna** and the **radius**). The radius is located on the thumb side or lateral of the arm, and the ulna is located on the little-finger or medial side.

The wrist and hand are considered part of the upper extremity and consist of several bones, whose names you do not need to learn. You can consider these bones as one unit for the purposes of emergency treatment.

The Rib Cage

The fifth area of the skeletal system is the rib cage (chest). The twelve sets of **ribs** protect the heart, lungs, liver, and spleen. All of the ribs attach to the spine (**Figure 4.11**). The upper five sets of ribs connect directly to the **sternum** (breastbone). The ends of the sixth through tenth rib sets are connected to each other and to the sternum by a bridge of **cartilage**. The eleventh and twelfth rib sets are attached to the spine but not attached to the sternum in any way and are called **floating ribs**.

The sternum is located in the front of the chest. The pointed structure at the bottom of the sternum is called the **xiphoid process**.

The Pelvis

The sixth area of the skeletal system is the **pelvis**. The pelvis serves as the link between the body and the lower extremities. In addition, the pelvis protects the reproductive organs and the other organs located in the lower abdominal cavity.

pelvis The closed bony ring, consisting of the sacrum and the pelvic bones, that connects the trunk to the lower extremities.

You can see that a protective bony structure encases each of the essential organs of the body:

- The skull protects the brain
- The vertebrae protect the spinal cord
- The ribs protect the heart and lungs
- The pelvic bones protect the lower abdominal and reproductive organs

The Lower Extremities

The lower extremities form the seventh area of the skeletal system. Each lower extremity consists of the thigh and the leg. The thighbone (femur) is the longest and strongest bone in the entire body. The leg has two bones, the tibia and fibula. The kneecap (patella) is a small, relatively flat bone that protects the front of the knee joint. Like the wrist and hand, the ankle and foot contain a large number of smaller bones that you can consider as one unit.

Note: The xiphoid process is an important location to remember because it is used to determine proper hand placement during cardiopulmonary resuscitation

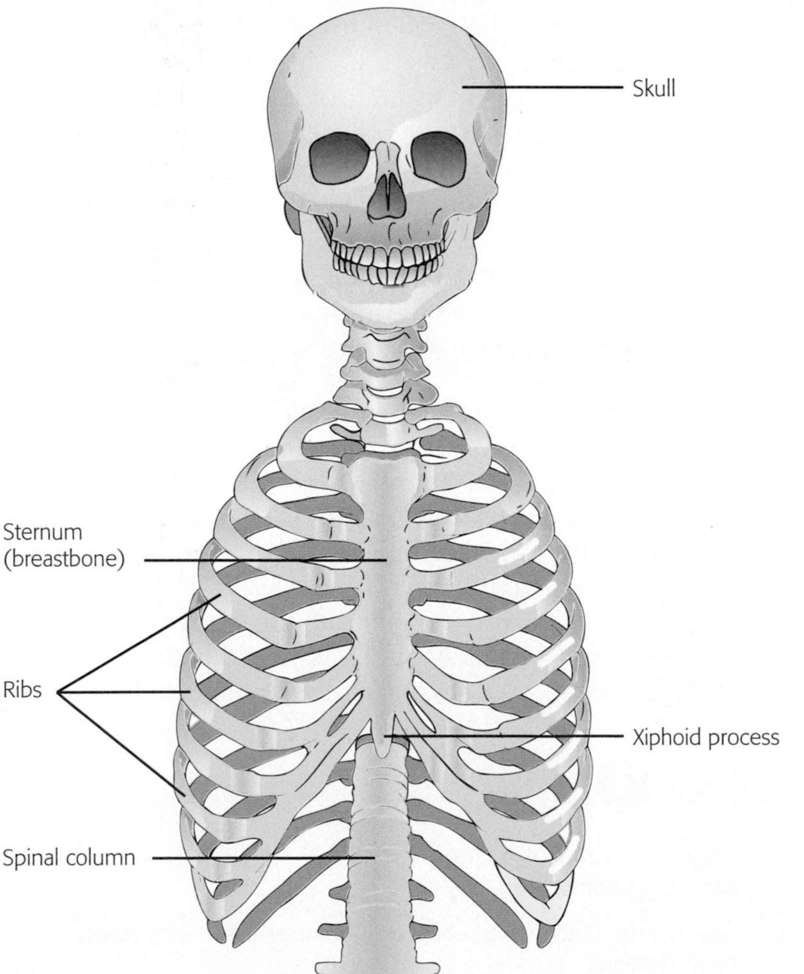

Figure 4.11 The rib cage.

The Muscular System

Your body contains three different types of muscles: skeletal, smooth, and cardiac.

Skeletal muscles provide both support and movement. They are attached to bones by tendons. These muscles cause movement by alternately contracting (shortening) and relaxing (lengthening). To move bones, skeletal muscles are usually paired in opposition: as one member of the pair contracts, the other relaxes. This mechanical opposition enables you to open and close your hand, turn your head, and bend and straighten your elbow. For example, when the biceps relaxes, an opposing muscle on the back of the arm contracts, straightening the elbow. Because skeletal muscles can be contracted or relaxed whenever you want, they are also called voluntary muscles.

Smooth muscles carry out many of the automatic functions of the body, such as propelling food through the digestive system. You have no control over smooth muscles, so they are also called involuntary muscles.

Cardiac muscle is found only in the heart. Cardiac muscle is adapted to its special function of working all the time. It has a rich blood supply and can live only a few minutes without an adequate supply of oxygen.

Sometimes the skeletal and muscular systems are considered together. In this case, the two systems are referred to as the musculoskeletal system.

The Nervous System

nervous system The brain, spinal cord, and nerves.

nerves Fiber tracts or pathways that carry messages from the spinal cord and brain to all body parts and back; sensory, motor, or a combination of both.

The **nervous system** governs the body's functioning. The nervous system consists of the brain, the spinal cord, and the individual **nerves** that extend throughout the body (**Figure 4.12**).

The brain is the body's "central computer" and controls the functions of thinking, voluntary actions (things you do consciously), and involuntary (automatic) functions such as breathing, heartbeat, and digestion.

The spinal cord is like the "trunk line" for a complex network of nerves that make up a two-way communication system between the brain and the rest of the body. Nerves branch out from the spinal cord to every part of the body (like telephone lines, internet connections, and television cables going into houses and individual rooms). Some nerves send signals to the brain about what is happening to the body, for example, whether it is feeling heat, cold, pain, or pleasure. Other nerves carry signals to muscles that cause the body to move in response to the sensory signals it has received. Without the nervous system, you would not have such sensations, nor would you be able to control the movement of your muscles.

Checkpoint

- What are the functions of the respiratory, skeletal, muscular, and nervous systems?
- How are the functions of each system interrelated with other body systems?

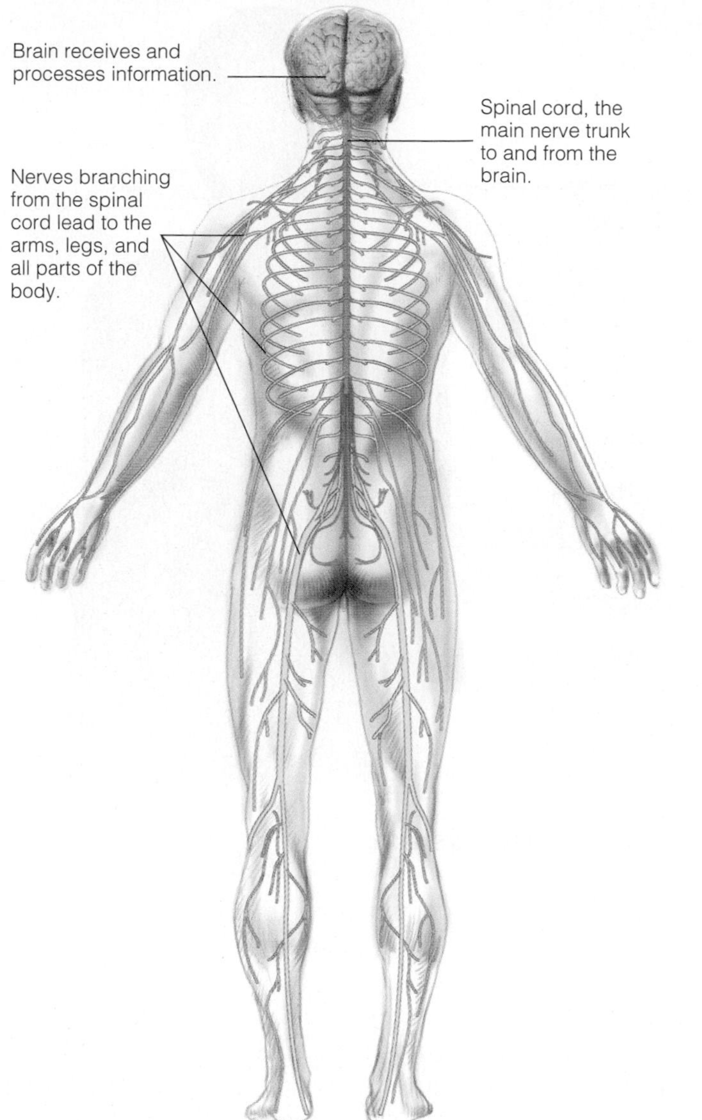
Brain receives and processes information.
Spinal cord, the main nerve trunk to and from the brain.
Nerves branching from the spinal cord lead to the arms, legs, and all parts of the body.

Figure 4.12 The nervous system.

The Digestive System

The **digestive system** breaks down food into a form that can be carried by the circulatory system to the cells of the body. Food that is not used is eliminated as solid waste from the body.

The major organs of the digestive system are located in the abdomen. The digestive tract is about 35 feet long. It begins at the mouth and continues through the throat, esophagus (food tube), stomach, small intestine, large intestine, rectum, and anus. Besides the digestive tract, the digestive system also includes the liver, gallbladder, and pancreas (**Figure 4.13**, page 62).

The liver performs several digestive functions, including the production of bile. Bile is stored in the gallbladder and released into the small intestine to help digest fats.

The pancreas also has several digestive functions. Probably its best known function is the production of **insulin**. Insulin is released directly into the bloodstream and aids in the body's use of sugar. Disruption of insulin production causes diabetes.

digestive system The gastrointestinal tract (stomach and intestines), mouth, salivary glands, pharynx, esophagus, liver, gallbladder, pancreas, rectum, and anus, which together are responsible for the absorption of food and the elimination of solid waste from the body.

insulin A hormone produced by the pancreas that enables sugar in the blood to be used by the cells of the body; insulin is used in the treatment and control of diabetes mellitus.

Figure 4.13 The digestive system.

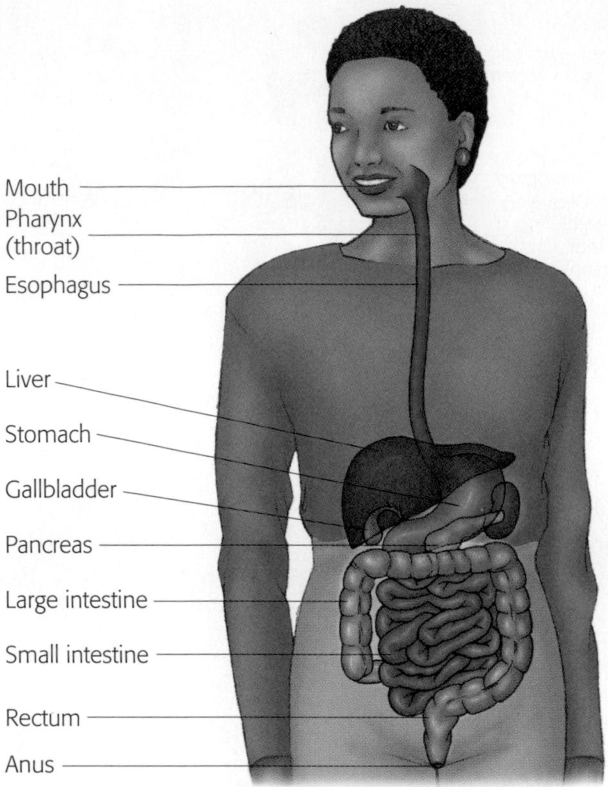

The Genitourinary System

genitourinary system The organs of reproduction, together with the organs involved in the production and excretion of urine.

The **genitourinary system** is responsible for the body's reproductive functions and for the removal of waste products from the bloodstream.

The major organs of male reproduction are the testes, which produce sperm, and the penis, which delivers sperm to fertilize the female egg. The major female reproductive organs are the ovaries, which produce eggs, and the uterus, which holds the fertilized egg as it develops during pregnancy. The ovaries and the uterus are connected by the fallopian tubes. The external opening of the female reproductive system is called the birth canal (vagina).

The removal of waste products by the genitourinary system begins in the kidneys, which filter the blood to form urine. The urine flows down from the kidneys through tubes (ureters) into the bladder. The bladder collects and stores the urine before it passes out of the body through the urethra.

Skin

Skin covers all parts of our body, and has three major functions:

- Protecting against harmful substances
- Regulating temperature
- Receiving information from the outside environment.

Figure 4.14 identifies the layers of the skin.

Skin protects our body from the environment. Because skin provides an intact layer of cells that serves as a barrier to most foreign substances, it prevents harmful materials from getting into the body. The skin is an effective barrier to bacteria and viruses as long as it is not damaged.

Skin regulates the internal temperature of the body. If the body gets too hot, the small blood vessels close to the skin open up (dilate) and bring more body heat to the surface of the skin, where the heat can be transferred to the air. Another source of cooling occurs as the sweat released by the skin evaporates. If the body becomes cold, the blood vessels near the skin surface constrict, transferring more body heat to the inside or core part of the body.

Skin receives information from the environment. Your skin can perceive touch, pressure, and pain. It can sense degrees of heat or cold. These perceptions are picked up by special sensors in the skin and transmitted through the nerves and the spinal cord to the brain. The brain serves as the computer to interpret these sensations.

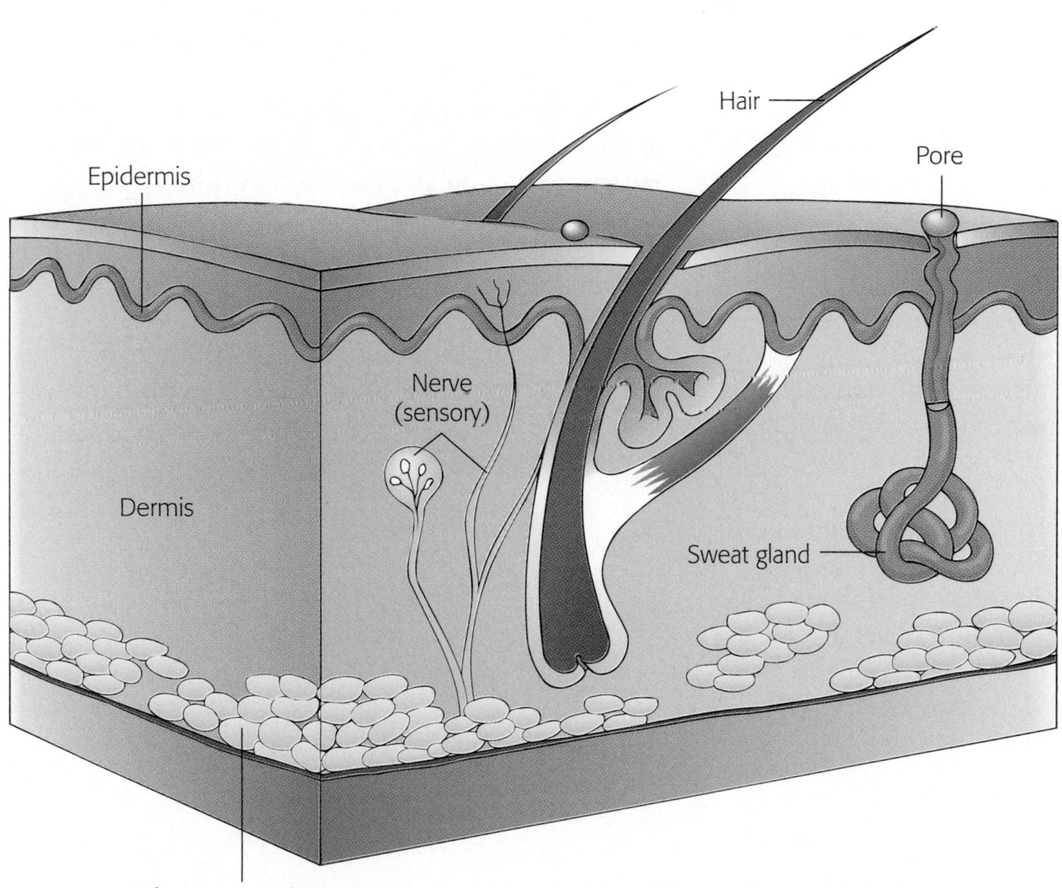

Figure 4.14 The skin.

4

Prep Kit

Ready for Review

Ready for Review thoroughly summarizes the chapter.

This chapter covers human anatomy and the function of body systems. To understand the location of specific signs or symptoms, it is necessary to examine topographic anatomy.

The chapter presents a brief explanation of body systems. The respiratory system consists of the lungs and the airway. This system functions to take in air through the airway and transport it to the lungs. In the lungs, red blood cells absorb the oxygen and release carbon dioxide so it can be expelled from the body.

The circulatory system consists of the heart (the pump), the blood vessels (the pipes), and blood (the fluid). Its role is to transport oxygenated blood to all parts of the body and to remove waste products, including carbon dioxide.

The skeletal system consists of the bones of your body. These bones function to provide support, to protect vital structures, and to manufacture red blood cells.

The muscular system consists of three kinds of muscles: voluntary (skeletal) muscles, smooth (involuntary) muscles, and cardiac (heart) muscles. Muscles provide both support and movement. The skeletal system works with the muscular system to provide motion. Sometimes these two systems together are called the musculoskeletal system.

The nervous system consists of the brain, the spinal cord, and individual nerves. The brain serves as the central computer and the nerves transmit messages between the brain and the body.

The digestive system consists of the mouth, esophagus, stomach, intestines, liver, gallbladder, and pancreas. It breaks down usable food and eliminates solid waste.

The genitourinary system consists of the organs of reproduction together with the organs involved in the production and excretion of urine.

The skin covers all parts of the body. It protects the body from the environment, regulates the internal temperature of the body, and transmits sensations from the skin to the nervous system.

A basic understanding of the body systems provides you with the background you need to treat the illnesses and injuries you will encounter as a first responder.

Vital Vocabulary

The Vital Vocabulary are the key terms for this chapter.

anterior—*page 50*
carbon dioxide (CO_2)—*page 52*
cartilage—*page 58*
cervical spine—*page 57*
circulatory system—*page 54*
coccyx—*page 57*
diaphragm—*page 52*
digestive system—*page 61*
distal—*page 50*
epiglottis—*page 52*
floating ribs—*page 58*
genitourinary system—*page 62*
inferior—*page 50*
insulin—*page 61*
larynx—*page 52*
lateral—*page 50*
ligaments—*page 56*
lumbar spine—*page 57*
medial—*page 50*
midline—*page 50*
nerves—*page 60*
nervous system—*page 60*
pelvis—*page 59*
plasma—*page 56*
platelets—*page 56*
posterior—*page 50*
proximal—*page 50*
pulse—*page 56*
radius—*page 58*
respiratory system—*page 51*
ribs—*page 58*
sacrum—*page 57*
shoulder girdle—*page 58*
skull—*page 56*
sternum—*page 58*
superior—*page 50*
tendons—*page 56*
thoracic spine—*page 57*
topographic anatomy–*page 50*
ulna—*page 58*
vertebrae—*page 56*
xiphoid process—*page 58*

Practice Points

The Practice Points are the key skills you need to know.

1. Identify the location of the major body components, systems, and organs, using a diagram, chart, or patient.

Ready to Respond

Ready to Respond presents a fictitious scenario to help you review what you learned in this chapter.

You are dispatched to a residence for a reported gunshot wound. The scene has been secured by the police officers. As you examine the 31-year-old male patient, you find a small gunshot wound close to the patient's navel. There is a larger wound on the patient's back.

1. Which body systems could be damaged by this injury?
   A. Respiratory system
   B. Digestive system
   C. Skeletal system
   D. Circulatory system

2. What structures of the respiratory system might be damaged?

3. What structures of the circulatory system might be damaged?

4. Which part of the circulatory system has the highest pressure and would probably cause the most bleeding?
   A. Vein
   B. Artery
   C. Capillary

5. Which regions of the skeletal system might be damaged by this type of gunshot wound?
   A. Shoulder girdles
   B. Rib cage
   C. Spine
   D. Upper extremity

Chapter 5

Lifting and Moving Patients

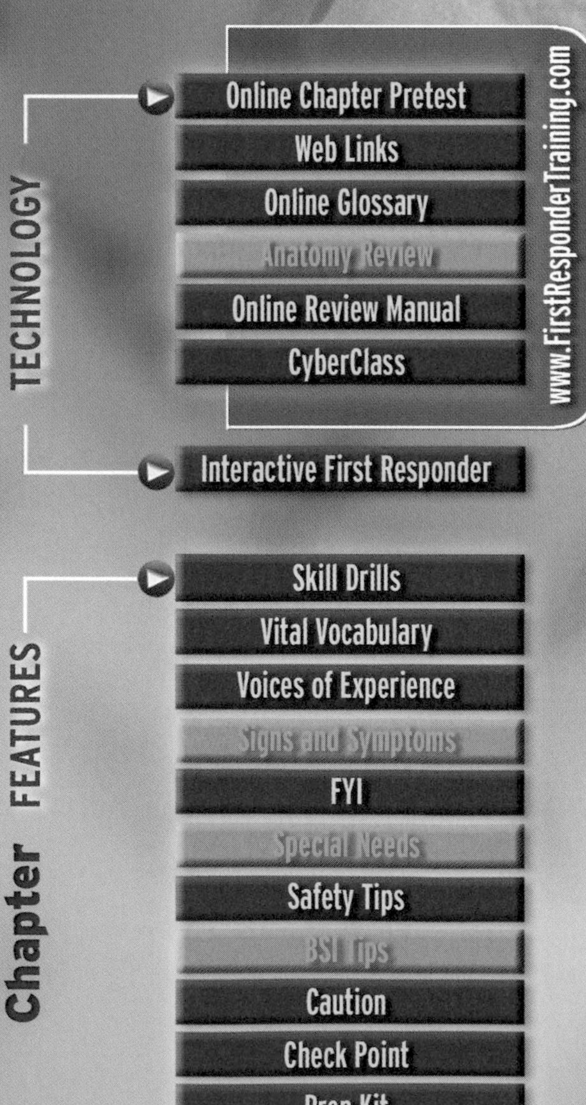

CHAPTER 5

Objectives

Knowledge and Attitude Objectives

After studying this chapter, you will be expected to:

1. Describe the general guidelines for moving patients.
2. Understand the purpose and indications for use of the "recovery position."
3. Describe the components of good body mechanics.
4. Describe the steps needed to perform the following emergency patient drags:
   A. Clothes drag
   B. Blanket drag
   C. Arm-to-arm drag
   D. Firefighter drag
   E. Cardiac arrest patient drag
   F. Emergency drag from a vehicle
5. Describe the steps needed to perform the following carries for nonambulatory patients:
   A. Two-person extremity carry
   B. Two-person seat carry
   C. Cradle-in-arms carry
   D. Two-person chair carry
   E. Pack-strap carry
   F. Direct ground lift
   G. Transfer from a bed to a stretcher
6. Describe the steps needed to perform the following walking assists for ambulatory patients:
   A. One-person assist
   B. Two-person assist
7. Identify and describe the purpose of the following pieces of equipment:
   A. Wheeled ambulance stretcher
   B. Portable stretcher
   C. Stair chair
   D. Long backboard
   E. Short backboard
   F. Scoop stretcher
8. Describe the steps in each of the following procedures for patients with suspected spinal injuries:
   A. Applying a cervical collar
   B. Moving patients using long backboards
   C. Assisting with short backboard devices
   D. Logrolling
   E. Straddle lifting
   F. Straddle sliding
   G. Strapping
   H. Immobilizing the patient's head

Skill Objectives

As a first responder, you should be able to:

1. Place a patient in the "recovery position."
2. Lift and move patients using good body mechanics.
3. Perform the following emergency patient drags:
   A. Clothes drag
   B. Blanket drag
   C. Arm-to-arm drag
   D. Firefighter drag
   E. Cardiac arrest patient drag
   F. Emergency drag from a vehicle
4. Perform the following patient carries:
   A. Two-person extremity carry
   B. Two-person seat carry
   C. Cradle-in-arms carry
   D. Two-person chair carry
   E. Pack-strap carry
   F. Direct ground lift
   G. Transfer from a bed to a stretcher
5. Perform the following walking assists for ambulatory patients:
   A. One-person assist
   B. Two-person assist
6. Assist other EMS providers with the following devices:
   A. Wheeled ambulance stretcher
   B. Portable stretcher
   C. Stair chair
   D. Long backboard
   E. Short backboard
   F. Scoop stretcher
7. Assist other EMS providers with the following procedures for patients with suspected spinal injuries:
   A. Applying a cervical collar
   B. Moving a patient using a backboard
   C. Applying short backboard devices
   D. Logrolling a patient onto a long backboard
   E. Straddle lift
   F. Straddle slide
   G. Strapping techniques
   H. Head immobilization

As a first responder, you must analyze a situation, quickly evaluate a patient's condition (under stressful circumstances and often by yourself) and carry out effective, lifesaving emergency medical procedures. These procedures sometimes include lifting, moving, or positioning patients as well as assisting other EMS providers in moving patients and preparing them for transport.

AUTHOR'S NOTE:

Some instructors may prefer to cover the material in this chapter after presenting the skills in Module 5.

Usually you will not have to move patients. In most situations, you can treat the patient in the position found and later assist other EMS personnel in moving the patient. In some cases, however, the patient's survival may depend on your knowledge of emergency movement techniques. You may have to move patients for their own protection (for example, to remove a patient from a burning building), or you may have to move patients before you can provide needed emergency care (for example, to administer CPR to a cardiac arrest patient found in a bathroom).

General Principles

Every time you move a patient, keep the following general guidelines in mind:

1. Do no further harm to the patient.
2. Move the patient only when necessary.
3. Move the patient as little as possible.
4. Move the patient's body as a unit.
5. Use proper lifting and moving technques to assure your own safety.
6. Have one rescuer give commands when moving a patient (usually the rescuer at the patient's head)

You should also consider the following recommendations:

- Delay moving the patient, if possible, until additional EMS personnel arrive.
- Treat the patient before moving him or her unless the patient is in an unsafe environment.
- Try not to step over the patient (your shoes may drop sand, dirt, or mud onto the patient).
- Explain to the patient what you are going to do and how. If the patient's condition permits, he or she may be able to assist you.
- Move the patient as few times as possible.

Unless you must move patients for treatment or protection, leave them in the position you found them. There is usually no reason to hurry the

Safety Tips

Whatever technique you use for moving patients, keep these rules of good body mechanics in mind:

1. Know your own physical limitations and capabilities. Do not try to lift too heavy a load.
2. Keep yourself balanced when lifting or moving a patient.
3. Maintain a firm footing.
4. Lift and lower the patient by bending your legs, not your back. Keep your back as straight as possible at all times and use your large leg muscles to do the work.
5. Try to keep your arms close to your body for strength and balance.
6. Move the patient as little as possible.

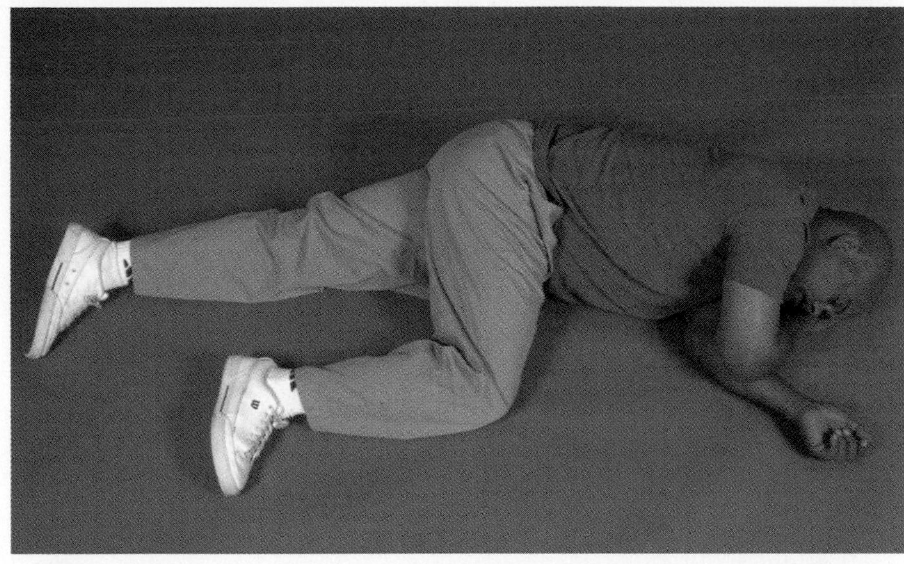

Figure 5.1 A patient in the recovery position.

moving process. If you suspect the patient has suffered from trauma to the head or spine, keep the patient's head and spine immobilized so he or she does not move.

Recovery Position

Unconscious patients who have not suffered trauma should be placed in a sidelying or **recovery position** to help keep the airway open. This position is shown in **Figure 5.1**.

recovery position A sidelying position that helps an unconscious patient maintain an open airway.

Body Mechanics

Your top priority as a first responder is to ensure your own safety. Improperly lifting or moving a patient can result in injury to you or to the patient. By exercising good body mechanics, you reduce the possibility of injuring yourself (**Figure 5.2**). Good body mechanics means using the strength in the the large muscles in your legs to lift patients instead of your back muscles. This prevents strains and injuries to weaker muscles, especially in your back. Get as close to the patient as possible so that your back is in a straight and upright position, and keep your back straight as you lift. Do not lift when your back is bent over a patient. Lift without twisting your body. Keep your feet in a secure position and be sure you have a firm footing before you start to lift or move a patient.

To lift safely, you must keep certain guidelines in mind. Before attempting to move a patient, assess the weight of the patient. Know your physical limitations and do not attempt to lift or move a patient who is too heavy for you to handle safely. Call for additional personnel if needed for your safety and the safety of the patient. Because you will sometimes need to assist other EMS providers, you should practice with them so that lifts are handled in a coordinated and helpful manner. As you are lifting, make sure you communicate with the other members

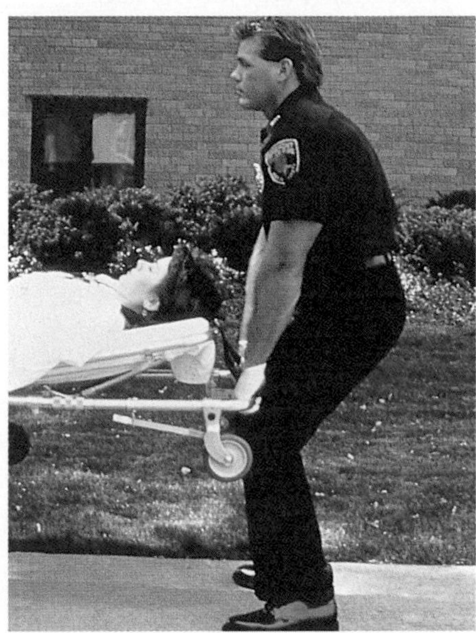

Figure 5.2 A first responder demonstrates good body mechanics while lifting a patient. His back is straight and he is lifting using his leg muscles

of the lifting team. Failure to give clear commands or failure to lift at the same time can result in serious injuries to rescuers and patients. Practice makes perfect! Practice lifts and moves until they become smooth for you and for the patient.

Emergency Movement of Patients

When is emergency movement of a patient necessary?

Move a patient immediately in the following situations:

- Danger of fire, explosion, or structural collapse exists.
- Hazardous materials are present.
- The accident scene cannot be protected.
- It is otherwise impossible to gain access to other patients who need lifesaving care.
- The patient has suffered cardiac arrest and must be moved so that you can begin CPR.

clothes drag An emergency patient move used to remove a patient from a hazardous environment. Performed by grasping the patient's clothes and moving the patient head first from the unsafe area.

FIVE TYPES OF EMERGENCY PATIENT DRAGS:

1. *Clothes drag*
2. *Blanket drag*
3. *Arm-to-arm drag*
4. *Firefighter drag*
5. *Emergency drag from a vehicle*

Emergency Drags

If the patient is on the floor or ground during an emergency situation, you may have to drag the person away from the scene instead of trying to lift and carry. Make every effort to pull the patient in the direction of the long axis of the body in order to provide as much spinal protection for the patient as possible.

Clothes Drag

The **clothes drag** is the simplest way to move the patient in an emergency (**Figure 5.3**). If the patient is too heavy for you to lift and carry, grasp the clothes just behind the collar, rest the patient's head on your arm for protection, and drag the patient out of danger.

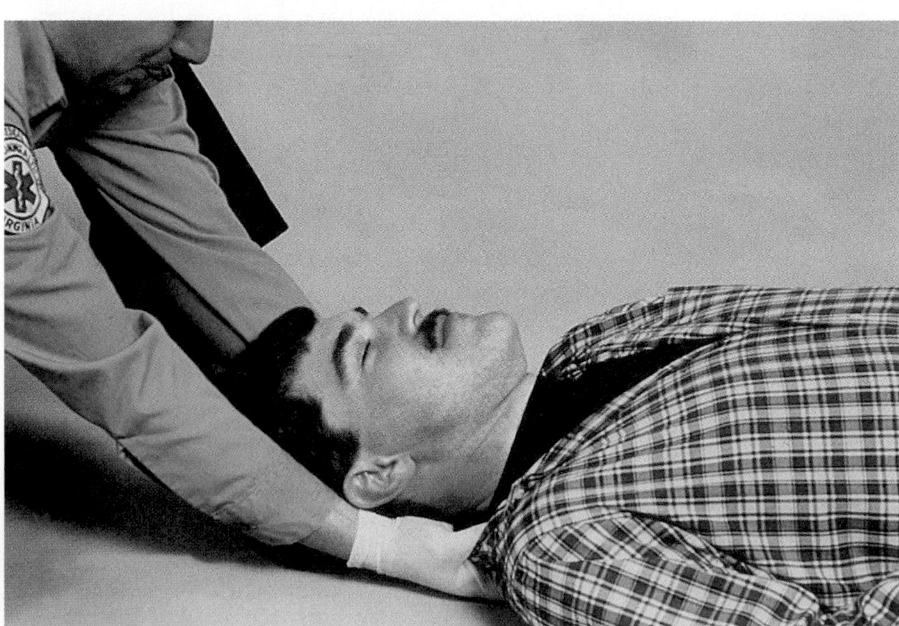

Figure 5.3 Emergency clothes drag.

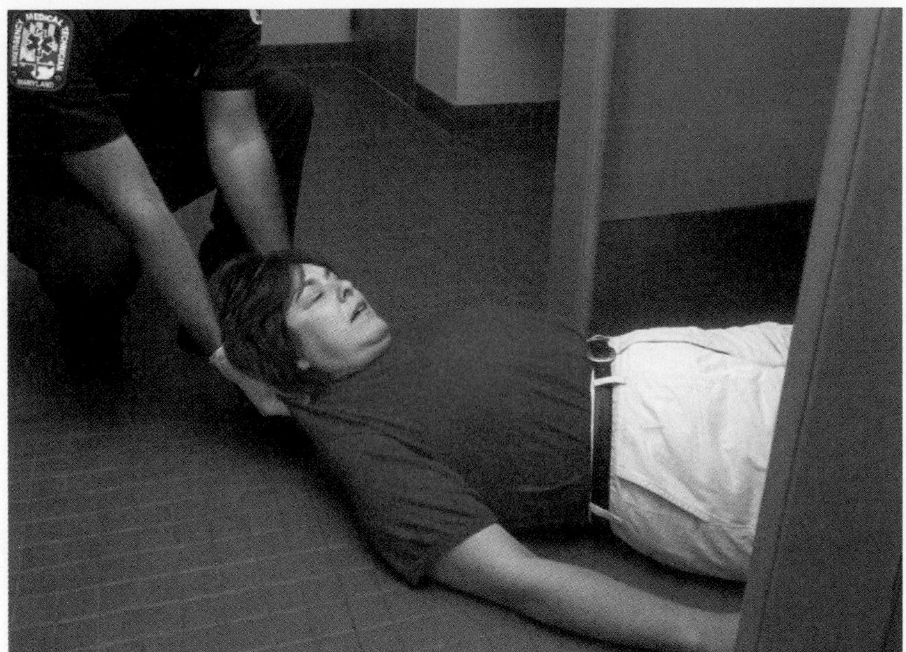

Figure 5.4 Remove the patient from a tight space to administer CPR.

FYI

Cardiac Patients and the Clothes Drag. In most situations, you can easily determine whether emergency movement is necessary. Cases of cardiac arrest are the exception. Cardiac arrest patients are often found in a bathroom or small bedroom. You will have to judge whether basic life support (BLS) or advanced life support (ALS) can be adequately provided in that space. If the room is not large enough, you should move the patient as soon as you have determined that he or she has suffered cardiac arrest.

Drag the cardiac arrest patient from the tight space to a larger room (such as a living or dining room) that has space for two people to perform CPR and ALS procedures (**Figure 5.4**). Quickly move furniture out of the way so you have room to work. You'll be able to deliver BLS and ALS with increased efficiency, more than making up for the time it took to move the patient. Take time to provide adequate room before you begin CPR!

Blanket Drag

If the patient is not dressed or is dressed in clothing that could tear easily during the clothes drag (for example, a nightgown), move the patient by using a large sheet, blanket, or rug. Place the blanket, rug, sheet, or similar item on the floor and roll the patient onto it. Pull the patient to safety by dragging the sheet or blanket. The **blanket drag** can be used to move a patient who weighs more than you do (**Figure 5.5**, page 72).

blanket drag An emergency patient move technique in which a rescuer encloses a patient in a blanket and drags the patient to safety.

Arm-to-Arm Drag

If the patient is on the floor, you can place your hands under the patient's armpits from the back of the patient and grasp the patient's forearms. The **arm-to-arm drag** allows you to move the patient by carrying the weight of the upper part of the patient's body as the lower trunk and legs drag on the floor (**Figure 5.6**, page 72). This drag can be used to move a heavy patient with some protection for the patient's head and neck.

arm-to-arm drag An emergency patient move that consists of the rescuer grasping the patient's arms from behind; used to remove a patient from a hazardous place.

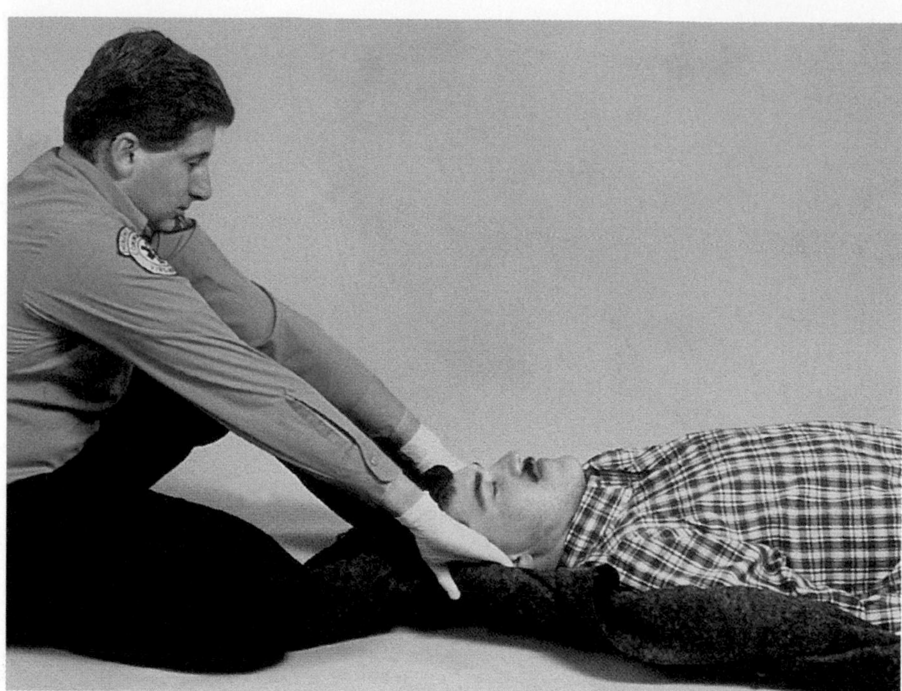

Figure 5.5 Blanket drag.

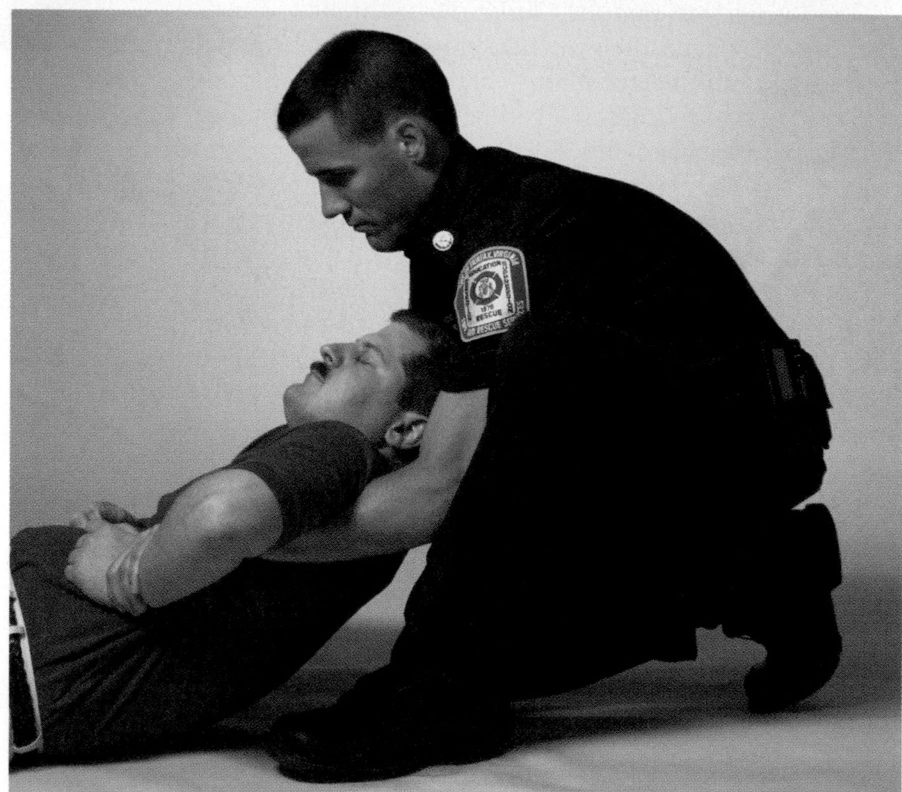

Figure 5.6 Arm-to-arm drag.

firefighter drag A method of moving a patient without lifting or carrying him or her; used when the patient is heavier than the rescuer.

Firefighter Drag

FYI

The **firefighter drag** enables you to move a patient who is heavier than you are because you do not have to lift or carry the patient. Tie the patient's wrists together with anything that is handy: a cravat (a folded triangular bandage), gauze, belt, or necktie, being careful not to impair circulation. Then get down on your hands and

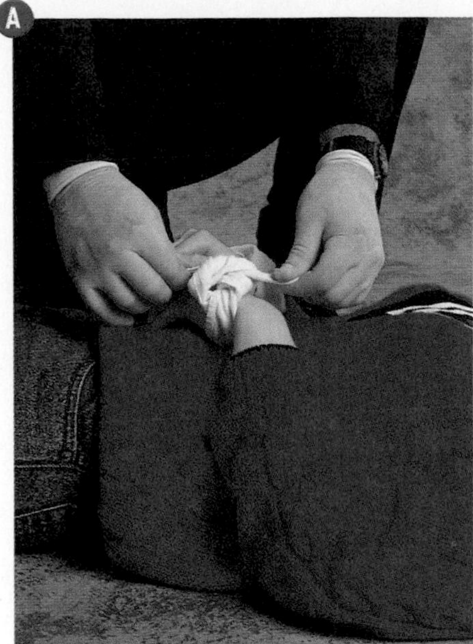

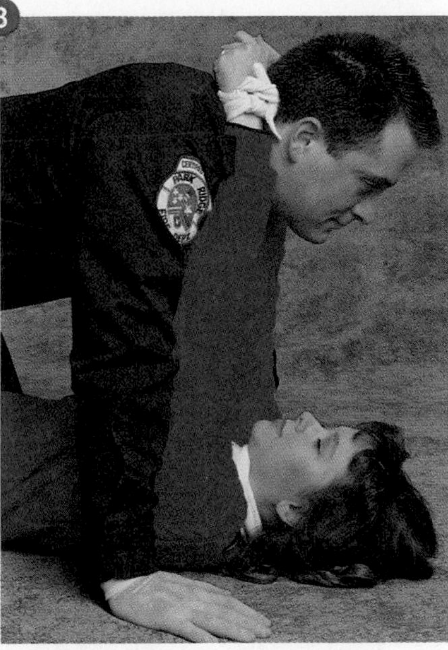

Figure 5.7 Firefighter drag. **A.** Tie the patient's wrists together. **B.** Drag the patient across the floor by crawling on your hands and knees.

knees and straddle the patient. Pass the patient's tied hands around your neck, straighten your arms, and drag the patient across the floor by crawling on your hands and knees (**Figure 5.7**).

Emergency Drag from a Vehicle

One Rescuer Sometimes you have to use emergency movement techniques to remove a patient from a wrecked vehicle (for example, when the vehicle is on fire or the patient needs CPR). All the basic movement principles apply, but the techniques need to be slightly modified because the patient is not lying down.

Grasp the patient under the arms and cradle the patient's head between your arms (**Figure 5.8**). Pull the patient down into a horizontal position as you ease him or her from the vehicle. Although there is no effective way to remove a patient from a vehicle by yourself without causing some movement, it is important to prevent excess movement of the patient's neck.

Two or More Rescuers If you must immediately remove a patient from a vehicle and two or more rescuers are present, have one rescuer support the patient's head and neck, while the second rescuer moves the patient by lifting under the arms. The patient can then be removed in line with the long axis of the body, with the head and neck stabilized in a neutral position. If time permits and if you have one available, use a long backboard for patient removal. Procedures for using a long backboard are covered later in this chapter.

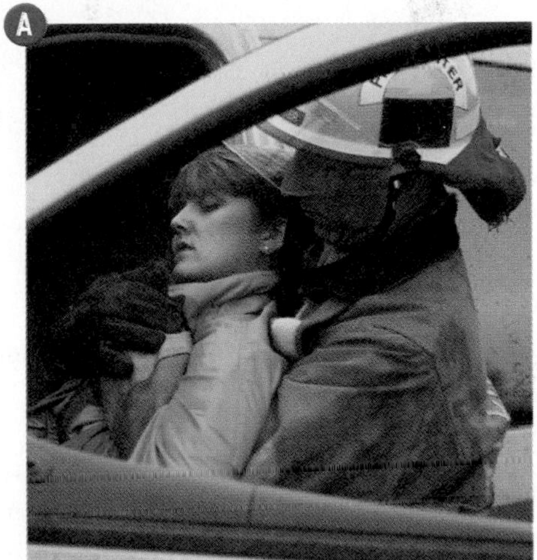

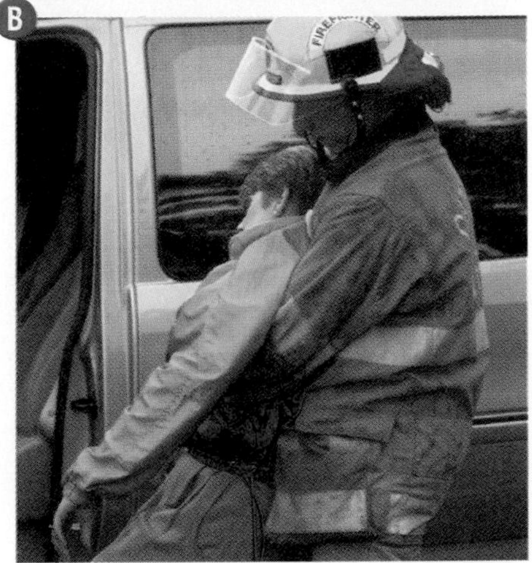

Figure 5.8 Emergency removal from a vehicle. **A.** Grasp the patient under the arms. **B.** Pull the patient down into a horizontal position.

Carries for Nonambulatory Patients

Many patients are not able or should not be allowed to move without your assistance. Patients who are unable to move because of injury or illness must be carried to safety. This section describes several useful carrying techniques for nonambulatory patients. Whatever technique you use, remember to follow the rules of good body mechanics.

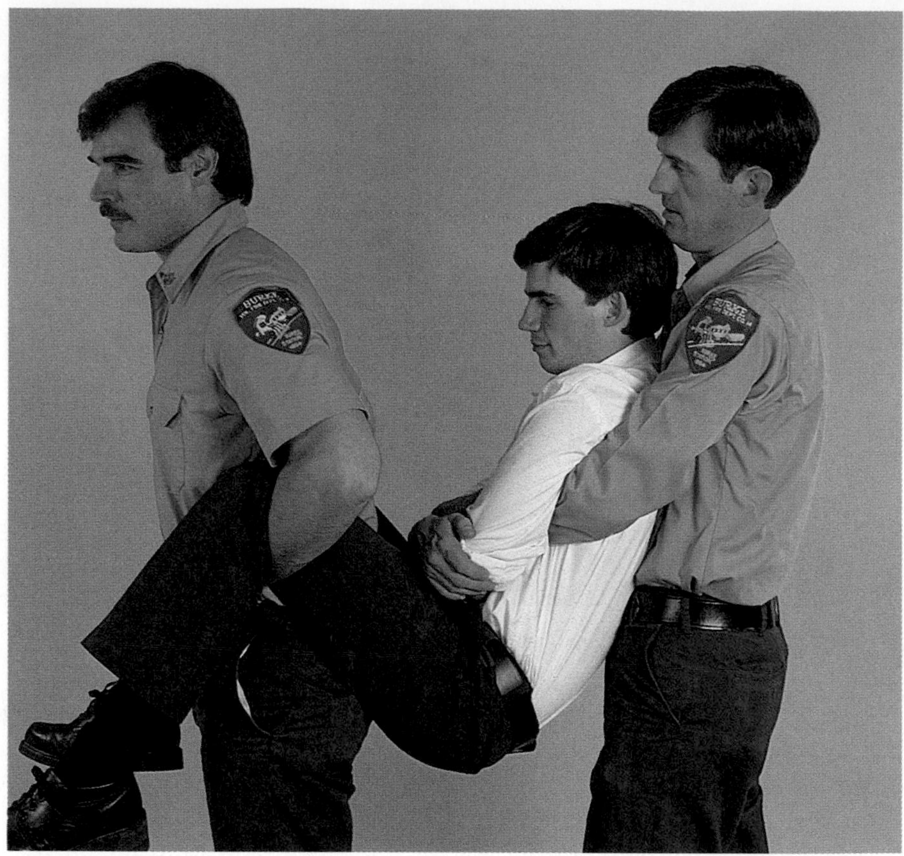

Figure 5.9 Two-person extremity carry.

two-person extremity carry A method of carrying a patient out of tight quarters using two rescuers and no equipment.

extremities The arms and legs.

two-person seat carry A method of carrying a patient in which two rescuers link arms behind the patient's back and under the patient's knees; requires no equipment.

cradle-in-arms carry A one-rescuer patient movement technique used primarily for children. The patient is cradled in the hollow formed by the rescuer's arms and chest.

Two-Person Extremity Carry

The **two-person extremity** carry can be done by two rescuers with no equipment in tight or narrow spaces, such as mobile home corridors, small hallways, and narrow spaces between buildings (**Figure 5.9**). The focus of this carry is on the patient's **extremities**. The rescuers help the patient sit up. Rescuer One kneels behind the patient and reaches under the patient's arms and grasps the patient's wrists. Rescuer Two then backs in between the patient's legs, reaches around, and grasps the patient behind the knees. At a command from Rescuer One, the two rescuers stand up and carry the patient away, walking straight ahead.

Two-Person Seat Carry

FYI

With the **two-person seat carry**, two rescuers use their arms and bodies to form a seat for the patient. The rescuers kneel on opposite sides of the patient near the patient's hips. The rescuers then raise the patient to a sitting position and link arms behind the patient's back. The rescuers then place the other arm under the patient's knees and link with each other. If possible, the patient puts his or her arms around the necks of the rescuers for additional support. Although the two-person seat carry needs two rescuers, it does not require any equipment (**Figure 5.10**).

Cradle-in-Arms Carry

The **cradle-in-arms carry** can be used by one rescuer to carry a child. Kneel beside the patient and place one arm around the child's back and the other arm under the thighs. Lift slightly and roll the child into the hollow formed by your arms and chest. Be sure to use your leg muscles to stand (**Figure 5.11**).

Remember

Keep your back as straight as possible and use the large muscles in your legs to do the lifting!

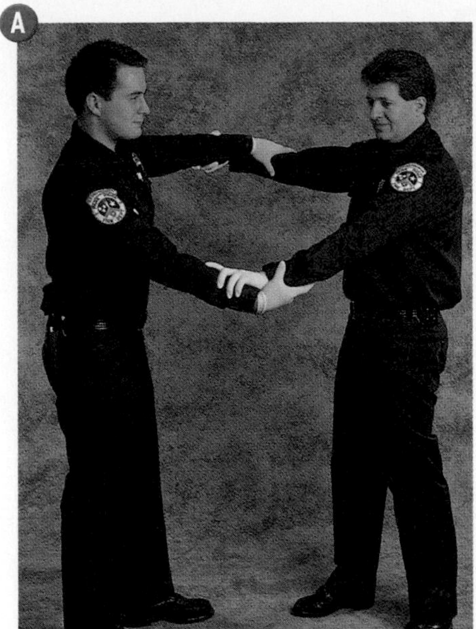

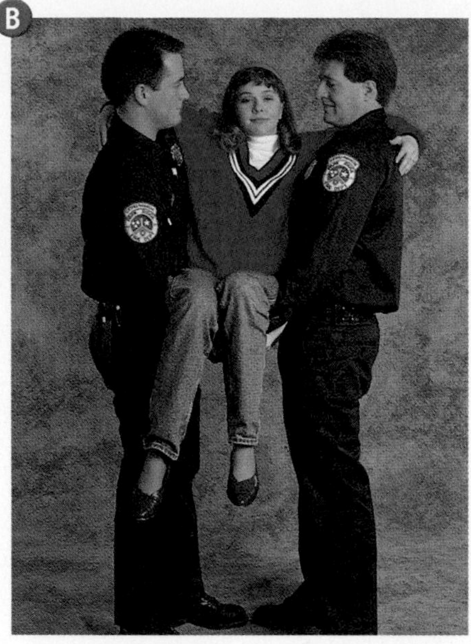

Figure 5.10 Two-person seat carry. **A.** Link arms. **B.** Raise the patient to a sitting position.

two-person chair carry Two rescuers use a chair to support the weight of the patient.

pack-strap carry A one-person carry that allows the rescuer to carry a patient while keeping one hand free.

Two-Person Chair Carry

In the **two-person chair carry**, two rescuers use a chair to support the weight of the patient. A folding chair cannot be used. The chair carry is especially useful for taking patients up or down stairways or through a narrow hallway. An additional benefit is that because the patient is able to hold on to the chair (and should be encouraged to do so), he or she feels much more secure than with the two-person seat carry.

Rescuer One stands behind the seated patient, reaches down, and grasps the back of the chair close to the seat, as shown in **Figure 5.12**. Rescuer One then tilts the chair slightly backward on its rear legs so that Rescuer Two can back in between the legs of the chair and grasp the tips of the chair's front legs. The patient's legs should be between the legs of the chair. When both rescuers are correctly positioned, Rescuer One gives the command to lift and walk away.

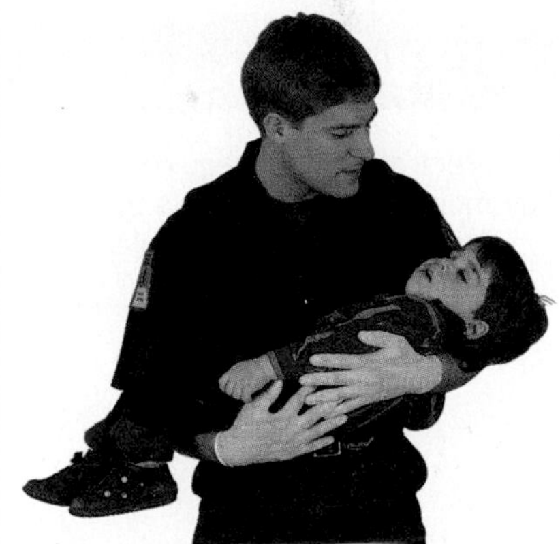

Figure 5.11 Cradle-in-arms carry.

Note: Because the chair carry may force the patient's head forward, Rescuer One should watch the patient for airway problems.

Pack-Strap Carry

The **pack-strap carry** is a one-person carry that allows you to carry a patient while keeping one hand free. Have the patient stand (or have other rescue personnel support the patient) and back into the patient so your shoulders fit into the patient's armpits. Grasp the patient's wrists and cross the arms over your chest (**Figure 5.13**, page 76). Now you can hold both wrists in one hand, and your other hand remains free.

Optimal weight distribution occurs when the patient's armpits are over your shoulders. Squat deeply to avoid potential injury to your back and pull the patient onto your back. Once the patient is positioned correctly, bend forward to lift the patient off the ground, stand up, and walk away.

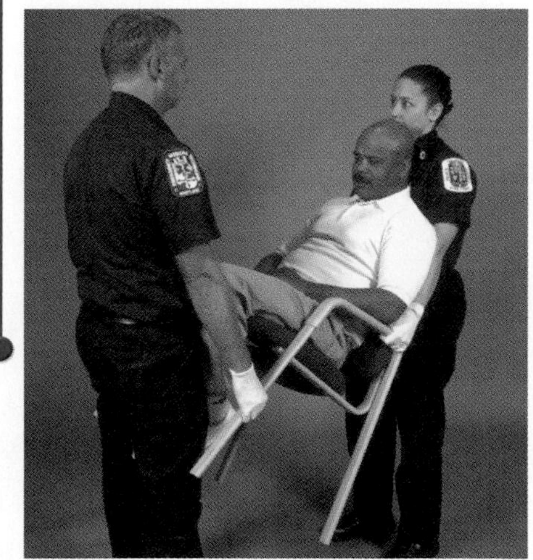

Figure 5.12 Two-person chair carry.

Direct Ground Lift

The direct ground lift is used to move a patient who is on the ground or the floor to an ambulance cot. It should be used only for those patients who have not suffered a traumatic injury. The direct ground lift requires you to bend over the patient and lift with your back in a bent position. Because the use of the direct ground lift results in poor body mechanics, its use is to be discouraged. Using a long backboard or portable cot is

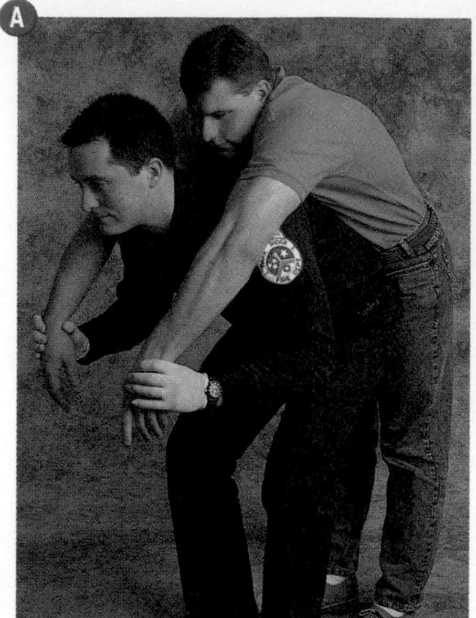

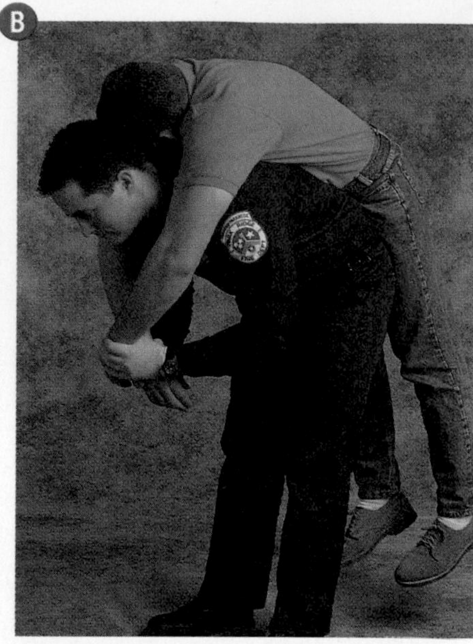

Figure 5.13 Pack-strap carry. **A.** Grasp the patient's wrists. **B.** Cross the patient's arms over your chest.

Safety Tips

The direct ground lift requires poor body mechanics so its use is to be discouraged whenever possible.

much better for your back and may be more comfortable for the patient. The steps for performing the direct ground lift (**Figure 5.14**) are as follows:

1. Assess the patient. Do not use this lift if there is any chance of head, spine, or leg injuries.
2. Rescuer One kneels at the patient's chest on the right or left side.
3. Rescuer Two kneels at the patient's hips on the same side as Rescuer One.
4. Place the patient's arms on the chest.
5. Rescuer One places one arm under the patient's neck and shoulder to cradle the patient's head and then places the other arm under the patient's lower back.
6. Rescuer Two places one arm under the patient's knees and the other arm above the buttocks.
7. Rescuer One gives the command: "Ready? Roll!" and both rescuers roll their forearms up so that the patient is as close to them as possible.
8. Rescuer One gives the command: "Ready? Lift!" and both rescuers lift the patient to their knees and roll the patient as close to their bodies as possible.
9. Rescuer One gives the command: "Ready? Stand!" and both rescuers stand and move the patient to the ambulance cot or bed.
10. To lower the patient to the cot or bed, the rescuers reverse the steps listed above.

CAUTION

The direct ground lift should never be considered for any patient who may have suffered any injury to the head, spine, or legs.

Skill Drill

Figure 5.14 Direct Ground Lift

1
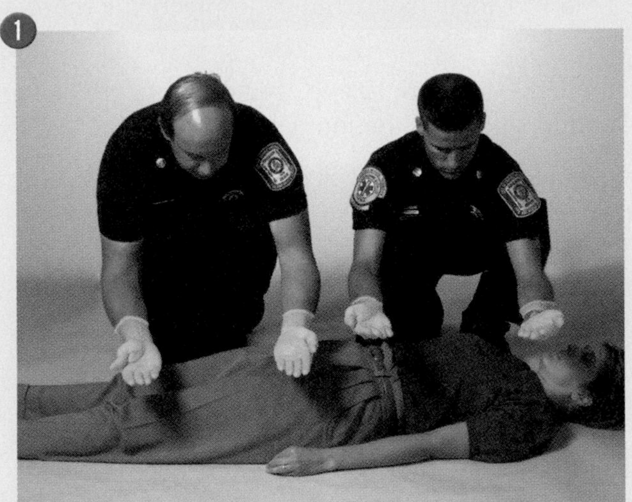
Kneel at patient's side.

2
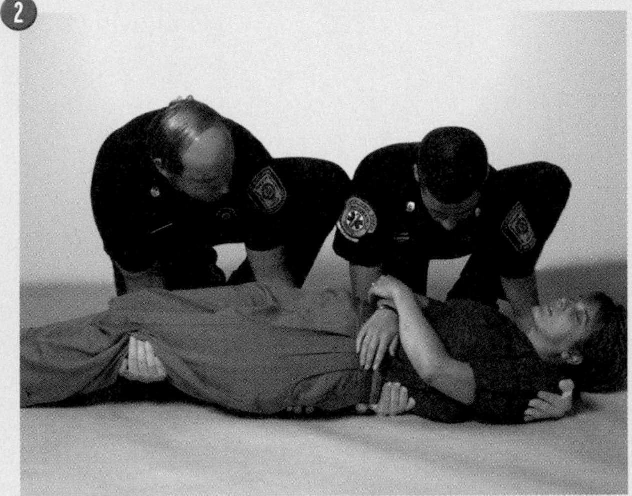
Place arms under patient.

3
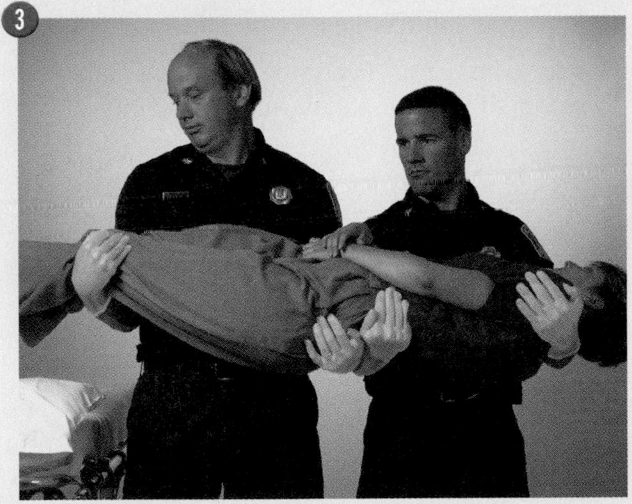
Lift the patient.

4
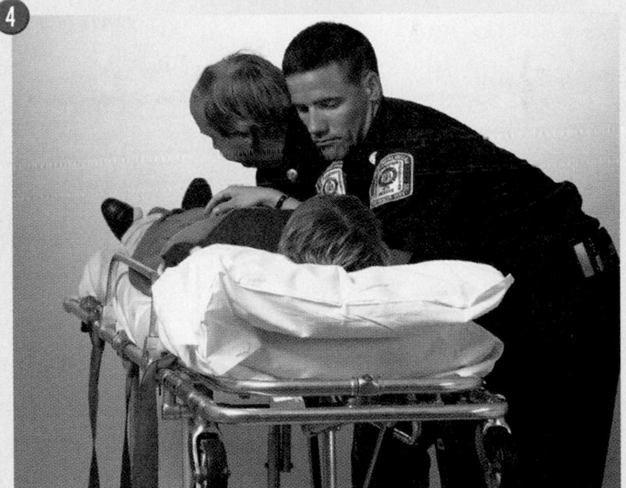
Move the patient to ambulance cot or bed.

Transferring a Patient from Bed to Stretcher

Many times patients who are ill will be found in their beds. If the EMS personnel need to transport these patients to the hospital, they may request your assistance with a patient transfer from the bed to the ambulance cot (**Figure 5.15**).

You can assist the EMS providers by learning and practicing the following steps:

1. Position the ambulance cot at right angles to the patient's bed with the head end of the cot at the foot end of the bed.
2. Prepare the cot by unfastening the belt buckles and folding back the sheets.
3. Rescuer One assumes a position beside the patient's chest and head.
4. Rescuer Two stands next to Rescuer One, beside the patient's hips.
5. Rescuer One slides one arm under the patient's neck, cupping the patient's shoulder, and slides the other arm under the patient's back.
6. Rescuer Two slides one hand under the patient's hip and lifts slightly, then places the second arm underneath the patient's calves.
7. Both rescuers slide the patient to the edge of the bed.
8. Rescuer One gives the command: "Ready? Roll!" and both rescuers contract their forearms to roll the patient toward them.
9. Rescuer One gives the command: "Ready? Lift!" and both rescuers lift the patient.
10. The rescuers turn and rotate so that the patient is positioned properly above the ambulance cot.
11. Rescuer One gives the command: "Ready? Lower!" and both rescuers lower the patient to the ambulance cot.

An alternate method for moving a patient is to loosen the bottom sheet of the patient's bed, place the ambulance cot parallel to the bed, and reach across the cot to pull the sheet and the patient onto the cot. This method must be used with caution because it requires the rescuers to reach across the cot to get to the patient. This results in poor body mechanics and therefore is to be discouraged.

Walking Assists for Ambulatory Patients

Frequently many patients simply need assistance to walk to safety. Either one or two rescuers can do this. Choose a technique after you have assessed the patient's condition and the incident scene. The technique you might use to help a patient to a chair is probably not appropriate to help a patient up a highway embankment.

Skill Drill

Figure 5.15 Transferring a Patient from a Bed to a Stretcher

1

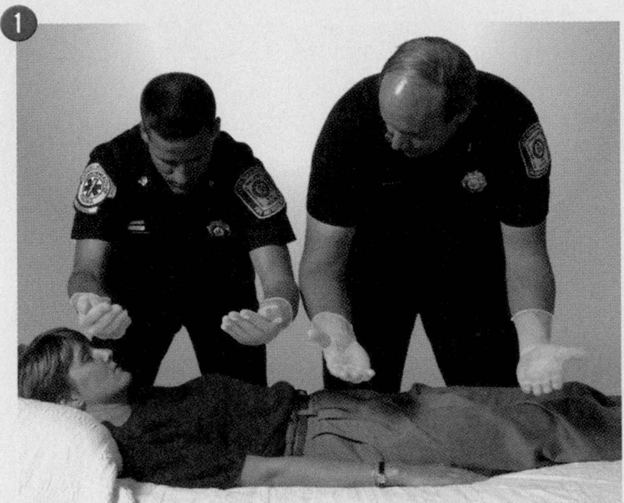

Place your hands under the patient.

2

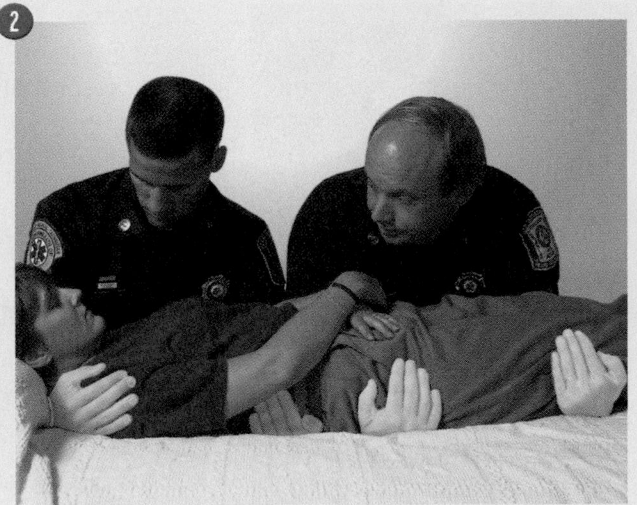

Slide the patient to the edge of the bed.

3

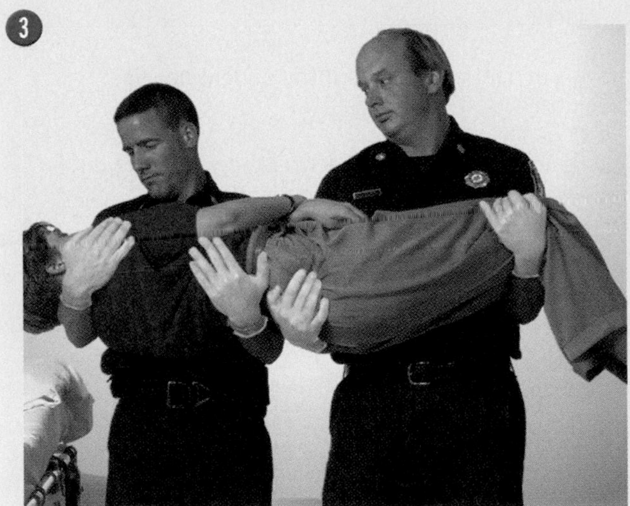

Roll and lift the patient and rotate to the cot.

4

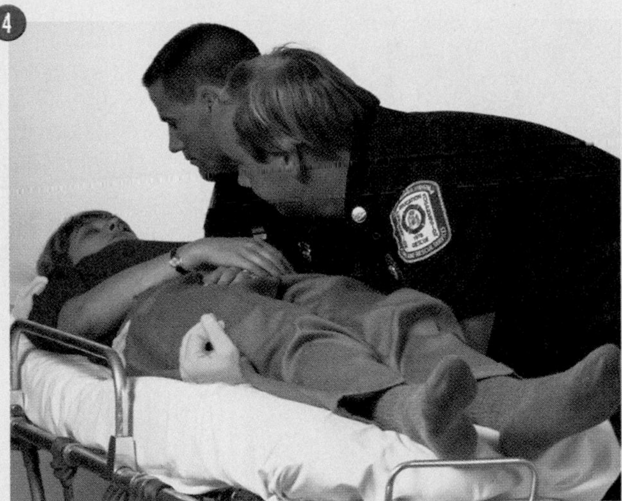

Place the patient on the stretcher.

one-person walking assist A method used if the patient is able to bear his or her own weight.

two-person walking assist Used when a patient cannot bear his or her own weight; two rescuers completely support the patient.

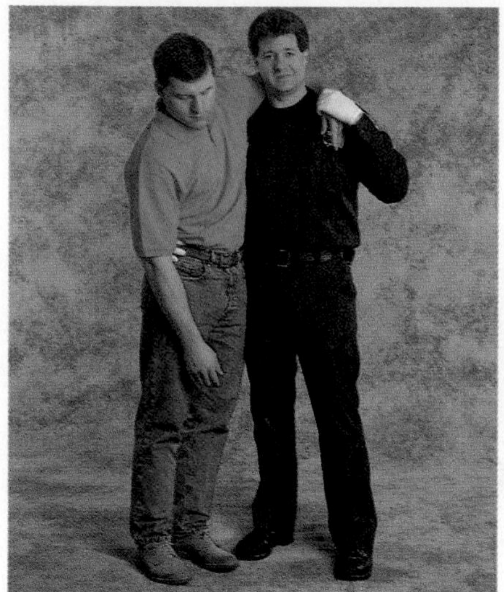

Figure 5.16 One-person walking assist.

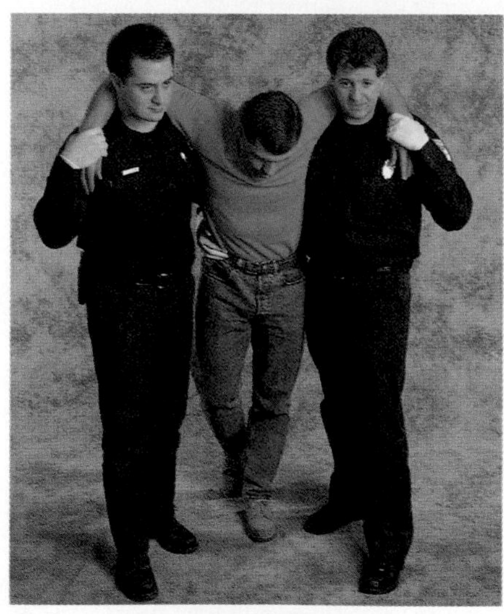

Figure 5.17 Two-person walking assist.

One-Person Walking Assist

The **one-person walking assist** can be used if the patient is able to bear his or her own weight. Help the patient stand. Have the patient place one arm around your neck, and hold the patient's wrist (which should be draped over your shoulder). Put your free arm around the patient's waist and help the patient to walk (**Figure 5.16**).

Two-Person Walking Assist

The **two-person walking assist** is the same as the one-person walking assist, except that two rescuers are needed. This technique is useful if the patient cannot bear weight. The two rescuers completely support the patient (**Figure 5.17**).

CAUTION

Do not use any of the preceding lifts or carries if you suspect that the patient has a spinal injury, unless, of course, it is necessary to remove the patient from a life-threatening situation.

Checkpoint

- How can you move a patient by yourself if the patient may have suffered a neck injury?
- How can you move a patient by yourself if the patient has not suffered a neck injury?
- When should you remove a patient from a wrecked vehicle if you are by yourself? How would you move this patient?
- Why is it sometimes best to move a patient who has suffered cardiac arrest before you begin CPR?

Equipment

Most of the lifts and moves described in the previous section are done without any specialized equipment. However, EMS services commonly use various types of patient-moving equipment. To be able to assist other EMS providers, you should be familiar with this equipment.

Wheeled Ambulance Stretchers

Wheeled ambulance stretchers are carried by ambulances and are one of the most commonly used EMS devices (**Figure 5.18**). These stretchers are also called cots. Most of them can be raised or lowered to several different heights. The head end of the cot can be raised to elevate the patient's head. These stretchers have belts to secure the patient. Each type of stretcher has its own set of levers and controls for raising and lowering. If you regularly work with the same EMS unit, it will be helpful to learn how their particular type of stretcher operates.

Stretchers can be rolled or they can be carried by two or four people. If the surface is smooth, a wheeled stretcher can be rolled with one person guiding the head end and one person pulling the foot end. If the loaded stretcher must be carried, it is best to use four people, one person at each corner. This gives stability and requires less strength than carrying with fewer people. If the stretcher must be carried through a narrow area, only two people will be able to carry it. The two rescuers should face each other from opposite ends of the stretcher. Carrying with two people requires that each be stronger, and it is harder to balance the stretcher than when carrying with four people.

You may also be asked to assist with loading a patient into the ambulance. You need to learn the method of loading ambulance stretchers that your EMS provider uses and practice this procedure with the EMS provider unit. It is important to lift as a team in a uniform way, or else you can injure yourself or the other rescuers.

PATIENT-MOVING EQUIPMENT

- *Wheeled Ambulance Stretcher*
- *Portable Stretcher*
- *Stair Chair*
- *Long Backboard*
- *Short Backboard*
- *Scoop Stretcher*

Portable Stretchers

Portable stretchers are used when the wheeled cot cannot be moved into a small space. They are smaller and lighter to carry than wheeled stretchers. Portable cots can be carried in the same ways that a wheeled cot is carried. An example of one type of portable stretcher is shown in **Figure 5.19**.

portable stretcher A lightweight non-wheeled device for transporting a patient. Used in small spaces where the wheeled ambulance stretcher cannot be used.

stair chair A small portable device used for transporting patients in a sitting position.

Stair Chair

Stair chairs are portable moving devices used to carry patients in a sitting position. They are good for patients who are short of breath or who are more comfortable in a sitting position. They are small, light and easy to carry in narrow spaces. The stair chair is not intended for use with patients who have suffered any type of trauma. When carrying a stair chair, the rescuers must face each other and lift on a set command. If you are going to be assisting your local EMS provider with this device, you should learn how to unfold it and how to assist with carrying it. One type of stair chair is shown in **Figure 5.20**.

Backboards

Long Backboards

Long backboards are used for moving patients who have suffered trauma, especially if they may have

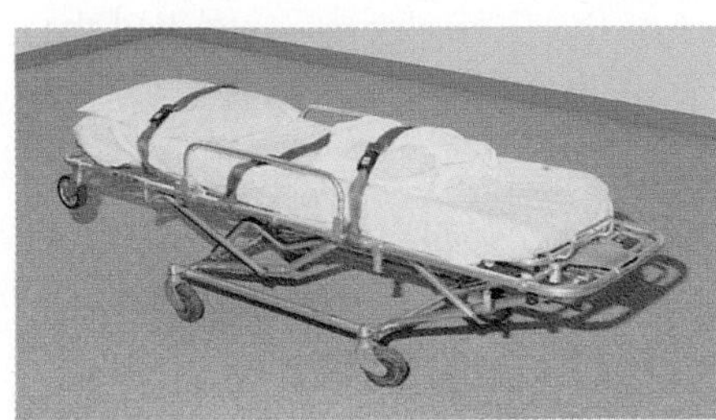

Figure 5.18 A wheeled ambulance stretcher.

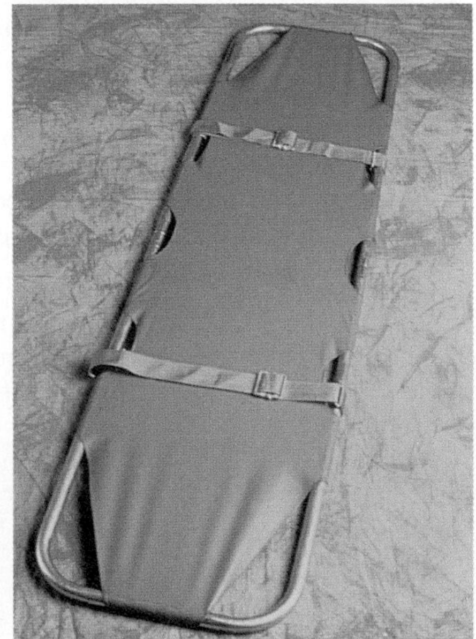

Figure 5.19 A portable stretcher.

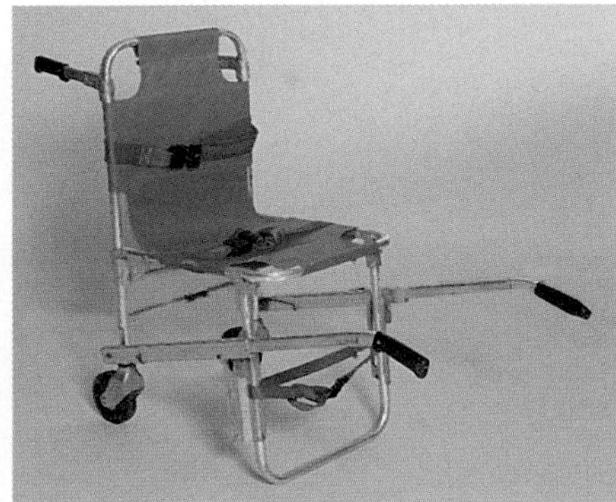

Figure 5.20 A stair chair.

Voices of Experience

Firefighters Save Patient's Eyesight

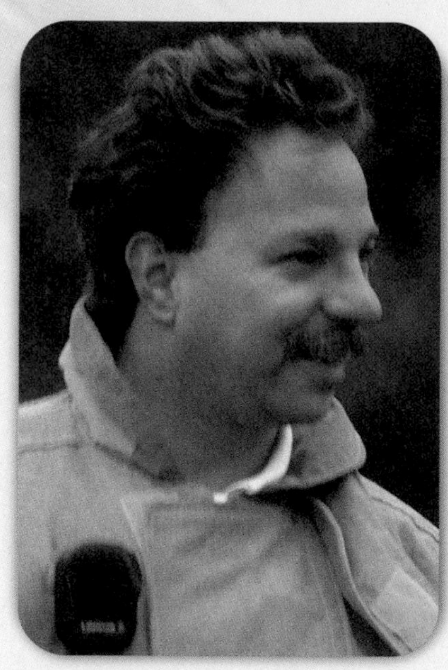

The man inside has a stick in his head!" That's what a bystander told the first arriving units when they reached the scene of a pre-dawn accident on a frigid morning.

A car had crashed through a board fence lined with barbed wire, and overturned in a field. The sole occupant of the car, a 21-year-old male, was conscious but pinned in the automobile. Upon entering the auto, I found the patient with an 18-inch long, 2-inch by 2-inch piece of wood impaled in his right eye socket. In addition, a 1-inch by 4-inch fence board had lacerated his scalp and was, in effect, supporting his head and upper body. The patient's only complaint was that he was cold (the outside temperature was about 15° F).

I assessed the patient while other firefighters began stabilizing the scene. Access to the automobile was made and the auto was stabilized using ropes, shoring, and chocks.

A paramedic firefighter joined me and began ALS care while another firefighter and I worked on stabilizing the patient and the 1-inch by 4-inch board that was supporting him. Other firefighters used helmets and blankets to "shore up" the patient so that the board entrapping the patient could be removed. Firefighters were finally able to safely remove a rear window and slide the board out, freeing the victim.

" Upon entering the auto, I found the patient with an 18-inch long, 2-inch by 2-inch piece of wood impaled in his right eye socket. "

As this was going on, we carefully stabilized the impaled wood. Firefighters slid a spine board under the victim as the three of us inside the car lifted him. The patient was loaded into the ALS ambulance. He was further stabilized and transported to a waiting helicopter for airlift to a trauma center. Evaluation at the trauma center showed no other injuries, and the patient was taken into surgery. The impaled board was removed, and the wound examined. There was no damage beyond the eye socket, and the surgical team was able to replant the eye.

Within a few days, the patient had regained sight in his right eye. The ophthalmologic surgeon felt a full recovery was likely. The surgeon credited the rapid and conscientious actions of the firefighters—who had the patient evaluated, stabilized, extricated, treated, transported, and into surgery in less than two hours—with saving the young man's sight. Of particular importance, he said, was the stabilization of the impaled object: one of the "basics" taught in EMS training. ❖

Gordon M. Sachs, EMT
Deputy Chief
Marion County Fire Department
Ocalo, Florida

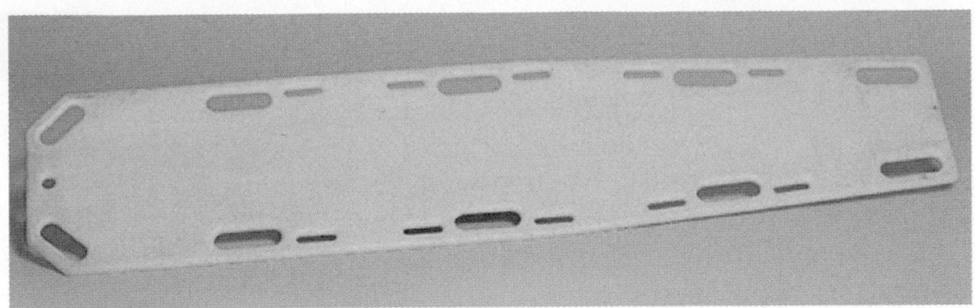

Figure 5.21 A long backboard.

suffered neck or back injuries. They are also useful for lifting and moving patients who are in small places or who need to be moved off the ground or floor. Long backboards are often used because they make lifting a patient much easier for the rescuers. Long backboards are made of varnished plywood or various types of plastic. Patients placed on long backboards must be secured with straps; if the patient has suffered back or neck injuries, the head should be immobilized. Procedures for assisting EMS providers with these devices are covered later in this chapter. One type of long backboard is pictured in **Figure 5.21**.

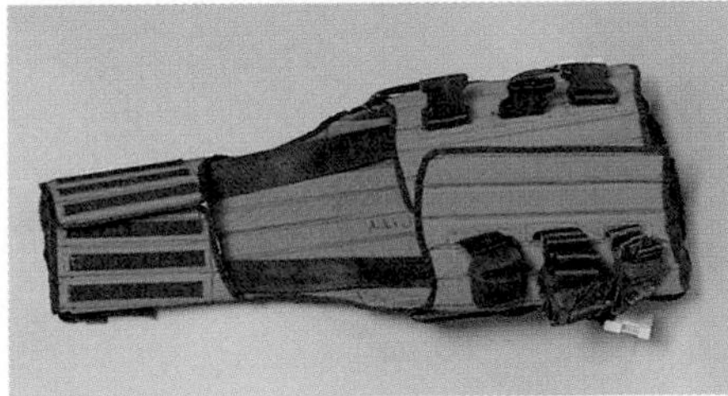

Figure 5.22 A short backboard device.

Short Backboard Devices

Short backboard devices are used to immobilize the head and spine of a patients found in a sitting posistion who may have suffered possible head or spine injuries. Short backboard devices are made of wood or plastic. Some of these devices are in the form of a vest-like garment that wraps around the patient. Procedures to help you assist other EMS providers in applying these devices are covered later in this chapter. A short backboard device is pictured in **Figure 5.22**.

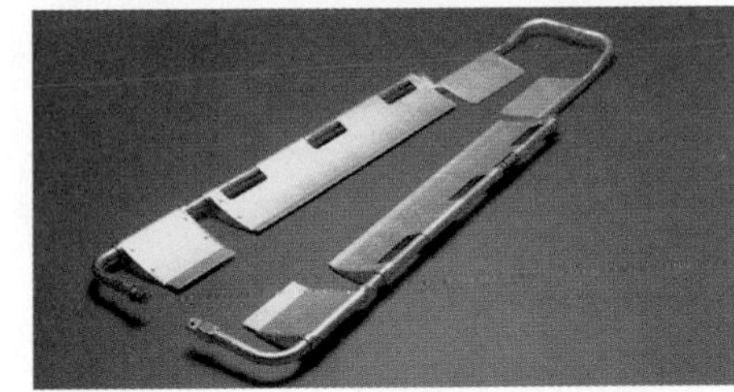

Figure 5.23 A scoop stretcher.

Scoop Stretchers

Scoop stretchers or orthopaedic stretchers are rigid devices that separate into a right half and a left half. These devices are applied by placing one half on each side of the patient and then attaching the two halves together. These devices are helpful in moving patients out of small spaces. They should not be used if the patient has suffered head or spine injuries. You should practice using these devices if you will be assisting your local EMS provider with them. One type of scoop stretcher is shown in **Figure 5.23**.

scoop stretcher A firm patient-carrying device that can be split into halves and applied to the patient from both sides.

Treatment of Patients with Suspected Head or Spine Injury

Any time a patient has suffered a traumatic injury, you should suspect injury to the head, neck, or spine. Improper treatment can lead to permanent damage or paralysis. The patient's head should be kept in a neutral position and immobilized. It is also important that you be able to assist other EMS personnel in caring for patients who may have suffered head or spine injuries. The following sections show you how to immobilize a patient's head and neck, and how to assist other EMS providers in placing a patient on a backboard. More information on spinal cord injuries is presented in Chapter 13.

Applying a Cervical Collar

FYI

cervical collar A neck brace that partially stabilizes the neck following injury.

Cervical collars are used to prevent excess movement of the head and neck (**Figure 5.24**). These collars do not prevent head and neck movement; rather they minimize the movement. When cervical collars are used, it is still necessary to immobilize the head and neck with your hands, a blanket roll, or foam blocks.

Soft cervical collars do not provide sufficient support for trauma patients. Many different types of rigid cervical collars for trauma patients are available. **Figure 5.25** shows how one common style of rigid cervical collar is applied. A cervical collar should be applied before the patient is placed on a backboard.

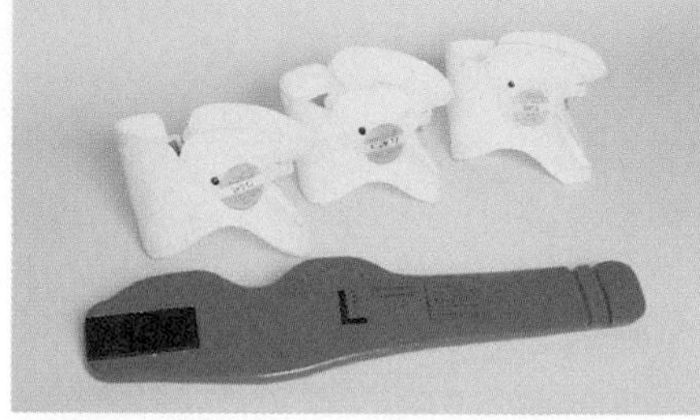

Figure 5.24 Types of cervical collars.

Movement of Patients Using Backboards

Placing a patient on a backboard is not your primary responsibility, but you may be required to assist other EMS personnel. Therefore, you must be familiar with the proper handling of patients who must be moved on backboards. Any patient who has suffered spinal trauma in an auto accident or fall and any victim of gunshot wounds to the trunk should be transported on a backboard. Although the specific technique used depends on the circumstances, the general principles described in the remainder of this chapter are relevant in nearly all cases.

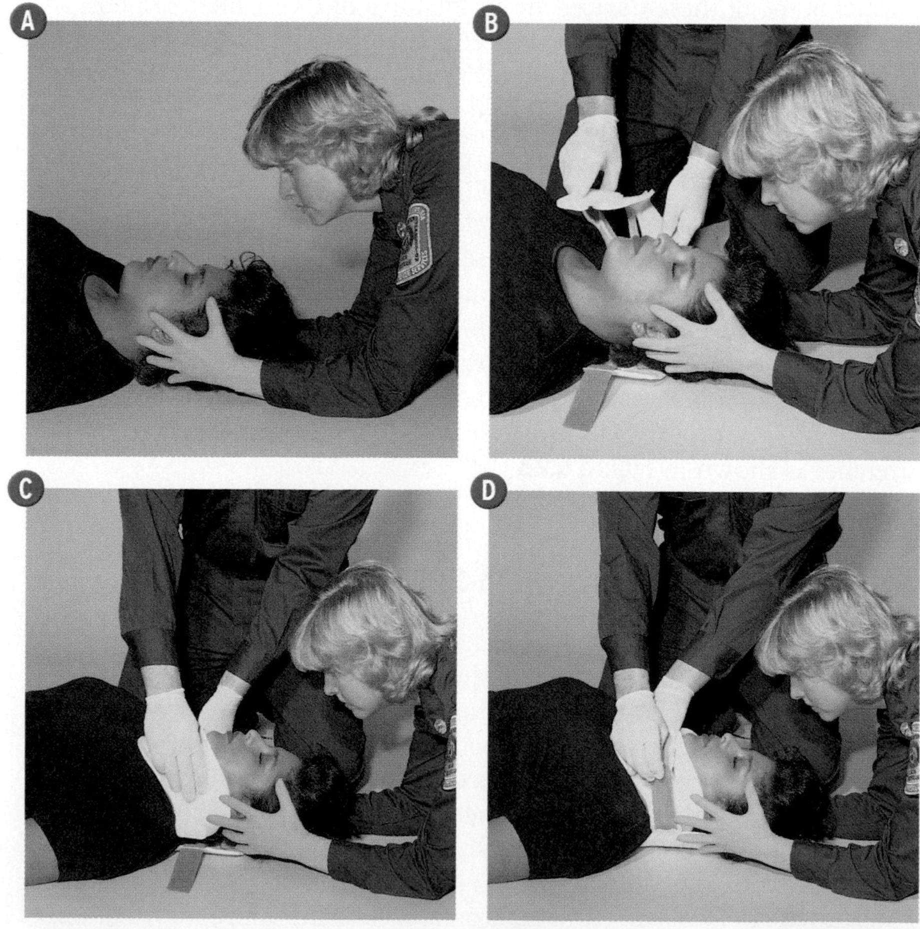

Figure 5.25 Applying a cervical collar. **A.** Stabilize head and neck. **B.** Insert back part of collar. **C.** Apply front part of collar. **D.** Secure collar together.

The following principles of patient movement are especially important if you suspect spinal injury:

1. Move the patient as a unit.
2. Transport the patient face up (supine), the only position that gives adequate spinal stabilization. However, because patients secured to backboards often vomit, be prepared to turn the patient and backboard quickly as a unit to permit the vomitus to drain from the patient's mouth.
3. Keep the patient's head and neck in the neutral position.
4. Be sure that all rescuers understand what is to be done before attempting any movement.
5. Be sure that one rescuer is responsible for giving commands.

Assisting with Short Backboard Devices

Short backboard devices are used to immobilize patients found in a sitting position who have suffered trauma to the head, neck, or spine. Short backboard devices allow rescuers to immobilize the patient before moving. After the short backboard device is applied, the patient is carefully placed on a long backboard. As a first responder, you will not be applying a short backboard device by yourself. However, you may need to assist with the application of this device. **Figure 5.26** illustrates how one common short backboard device is applied.

Figure 5.26 Applying a short backboard device. **A.** Stabilize the head. **B.** Apply a cervical collar. **C.** Insert the device head first. **D.** Apply the middle strap. **E.** Apply the other straps. **F.** Place wings around head. **G.** Secure the head strap.

A
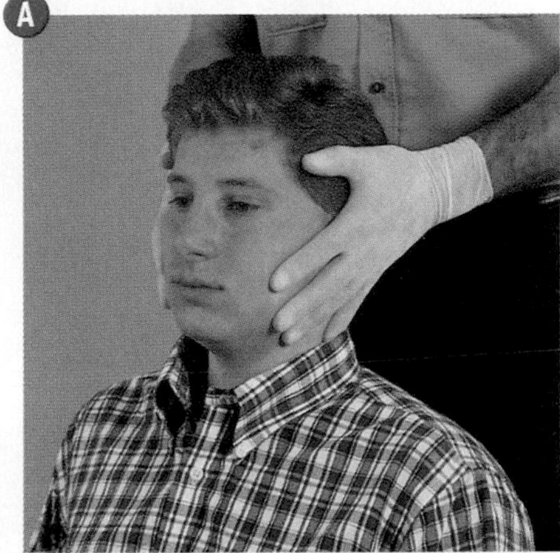

B
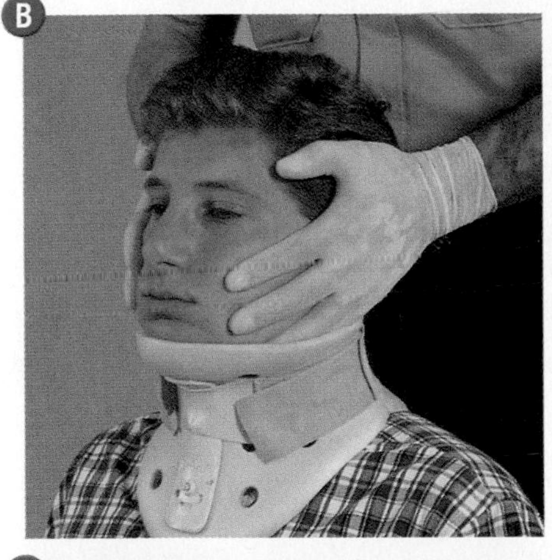

C
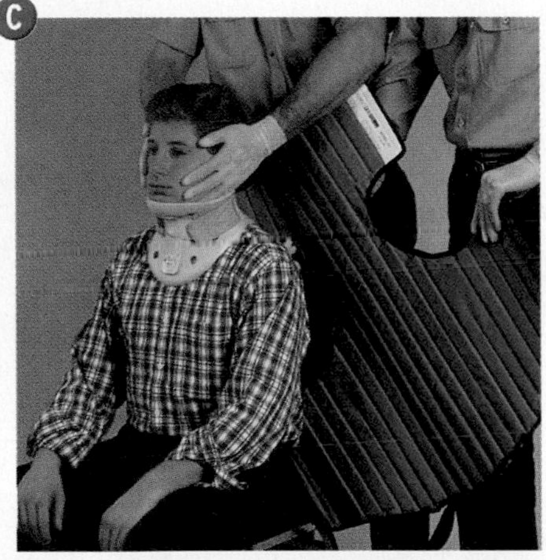

D
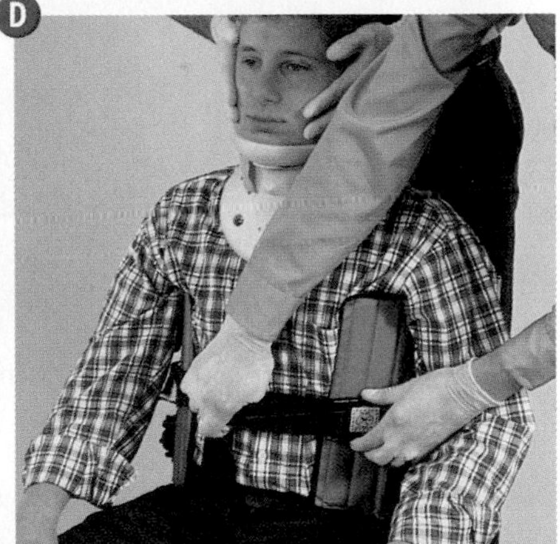

E
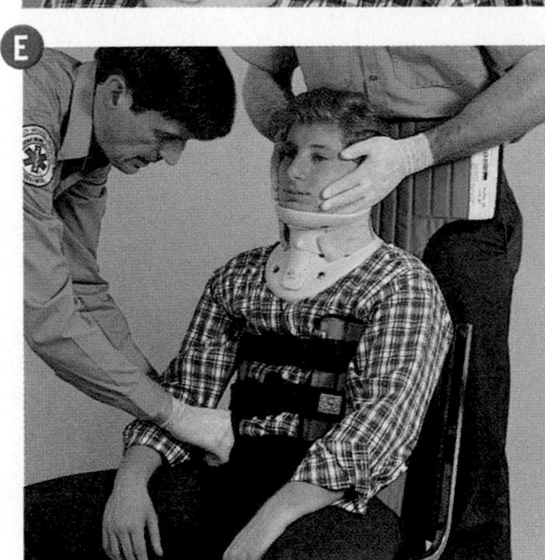

F
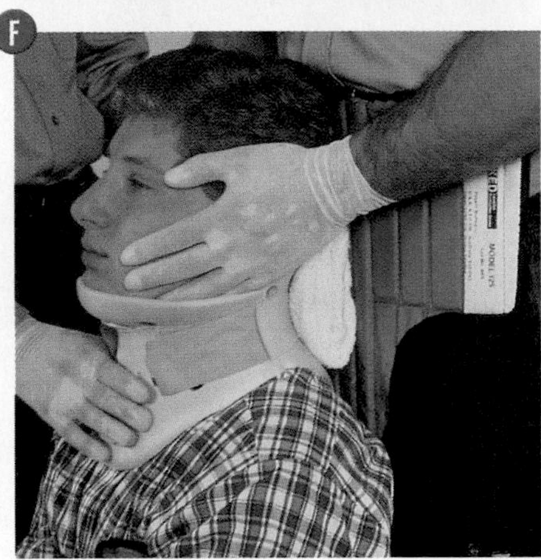

G
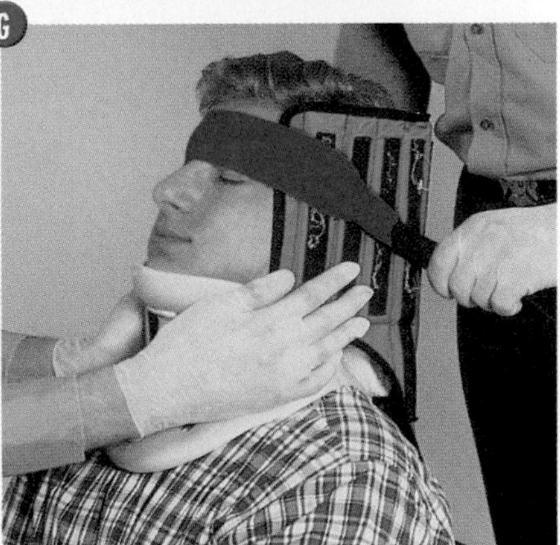

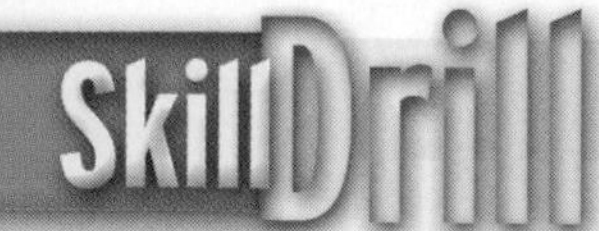

Figure 5.27 Five-person Logroll

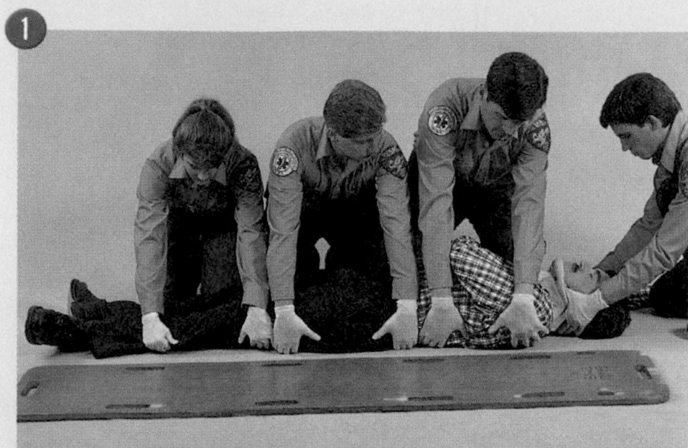

1 In position to roll the patient.

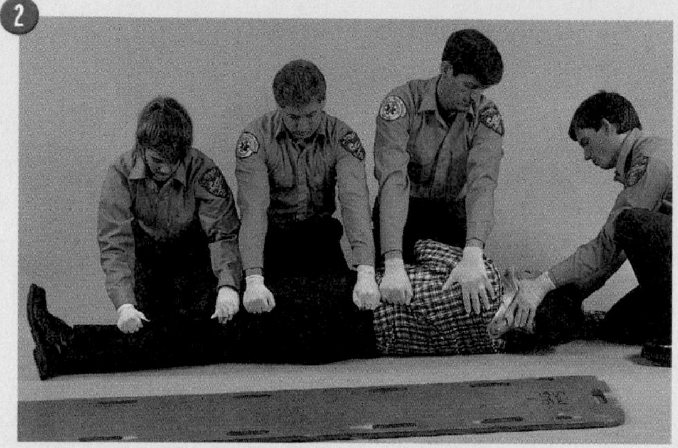

2 Roll the patient onto side.

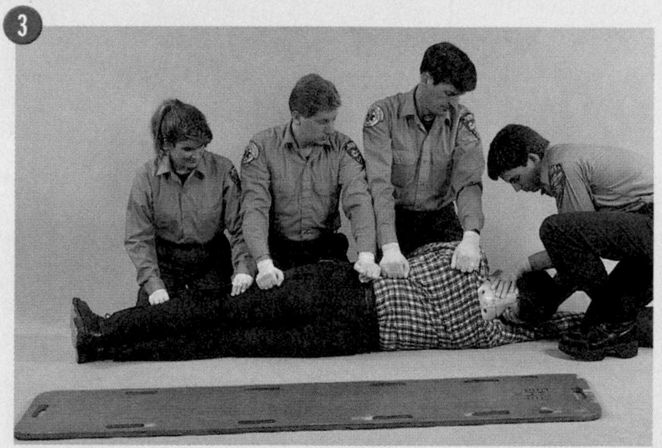

3 The fifth person (not shown) slides the backboard toward the patient.

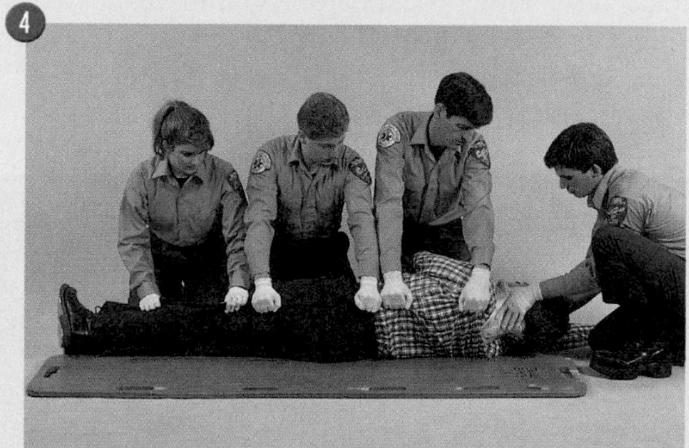

4 Roll patient onto backboard.

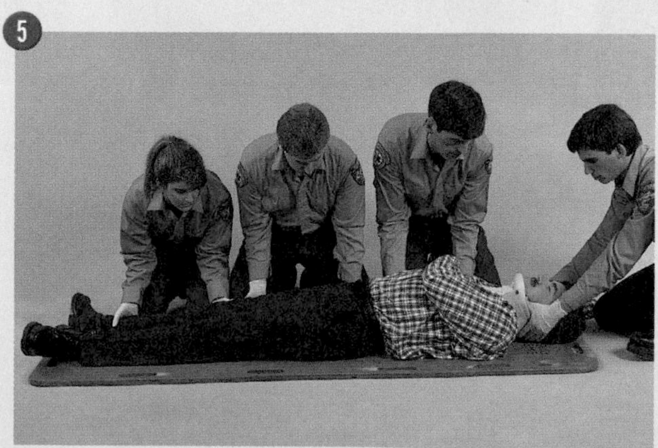

5 Center patient on backboard. Secure patient before moving.

Logrolling

Logrolling is the primary technique used to move a patient onto a long backboard. It is usually easy to accomplish, but it requires a team of five rescuers for safety and effectiveness—four to move the patient and one (not shown here) to maneuver the backboard. Logrolling is the movement technique of choice in all cases of suspected spinal injury. Because the logrolling maneuver requires sufficient space for five rescuers, it is not always possible to perform it correctly. That is why the principles of movement rather than specific rules are stressed here. The five-person logroll is shown in **Figure 5.27**.

In any patient movement technique, and especially if spinal injury is suspected, everyone must understand who is directing the maneuver. The rescuer holding the patient's head (Rescuer One) should always give the commands so that all rescuers can better coordinate their actions. The specific wording of the command is not important, as long as every team member understands what the command is. Each member of the team must understand his or her specific position and function.

All patient movement commands have two parts, a question and the order for movement. Rescuer One says, "The command will be 'Ready? Roll!'" When everyone is ready to roll the patient, Rescuer One says, "Ready? (short pause, to allow for response from the team) Roll!"

In any logrolling technique, you must move the patient as a unit. Keep the patient's head in a neutral position at all times. Do not allow the head to rotate, move backward (extend), or move forward (flex). Sometimes this is simply stated as, "Keep the nose in line with the belly button at all times."

logrolling A technique used to move a patient onto a long backboard.

straddle lift A method used to place a patient on a backboard if there is not enough space to perform a logroll.

Straddle Lift

The **straddle lift** can be used to place a patient on a backboard if you do not have enough space to perform a logroll. Modified versions of the straddle lift are commonly used to remove patients from automobiles. Like logrolling, the straddle lift requires five rescuers: one at the head and neck, one to straddle the shoulders and chest, one to straddle the hips and thighs, one to straddle the legs, and one to insert the backboard under the patient after the other four have lifted the patient ½ inch to 1 inch off the ground (**Figure 5.28**).

The hardest part of the straddle lift technique is coordinating the lifting so that the patient is raised just enough to slide the backboard under the patient. Because such team coordination can be difficult, it is important to practice frequently.

Note: Lift the patient just enough to slide in the backboard.

A
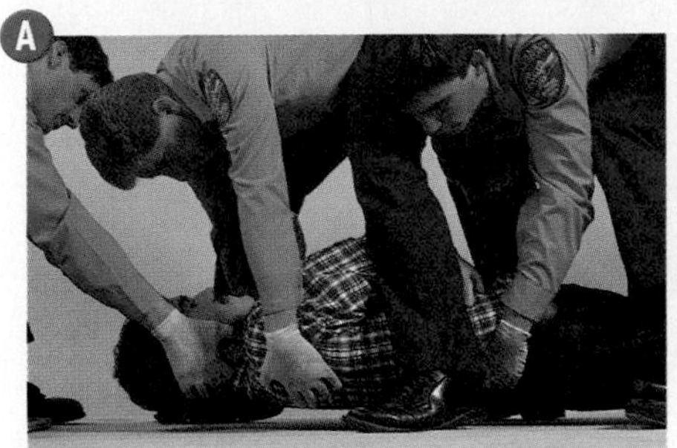

B
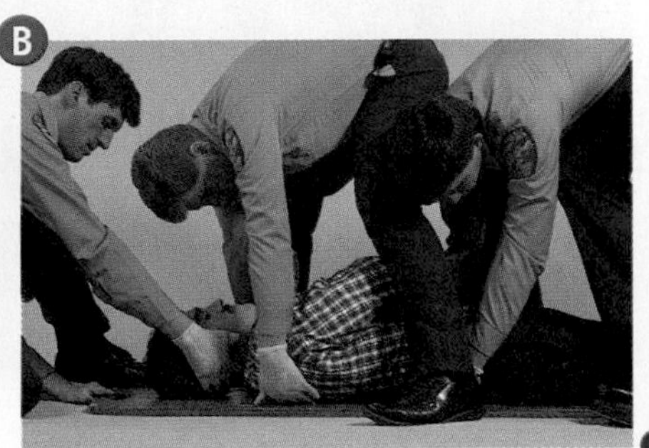

Figure 5.28 Straddle lift. **A.** Lift patient as a unit. **B.** Slide backboard under patient.

Straddle Slide

straddle slide A method of placing a patient on a long backboard by straddling both the board and patient and sliding the patient onto the board.

In the **straddle slide**, a modification of the straddle lift technique, the patient, rather than the backboard, is moved (**Figure 5.29**). The rescuers' positions are the same as for the straddle lift. Each rescuer should have a firm grip on the patient (or the patient's clothing). Lift the patient as a unit just enough to be able to slide (break the resistance with the ground) him or her forward onto the waiting backboard. Slide the patient forward about 10 inches each time. Distances greater than 10 inches to 12 inches cause team coordination problems.

Do not lift the patient off the ground. Rather, slide the patient along the ground and onto the backboard. Each rescuer should lean forward slightly and use a swinging motion to bring the patient onto the board. Rescuer One (who is at the patient's head) faces the other rescuers and moves backward during each movement. Rescuer One must not allow the patient's head to be driven into his or her knees!

Safety Tips

Make the up-and-forward movement in a single, smooth action. Lifting the patient up and then forward can strain your muscles.

A

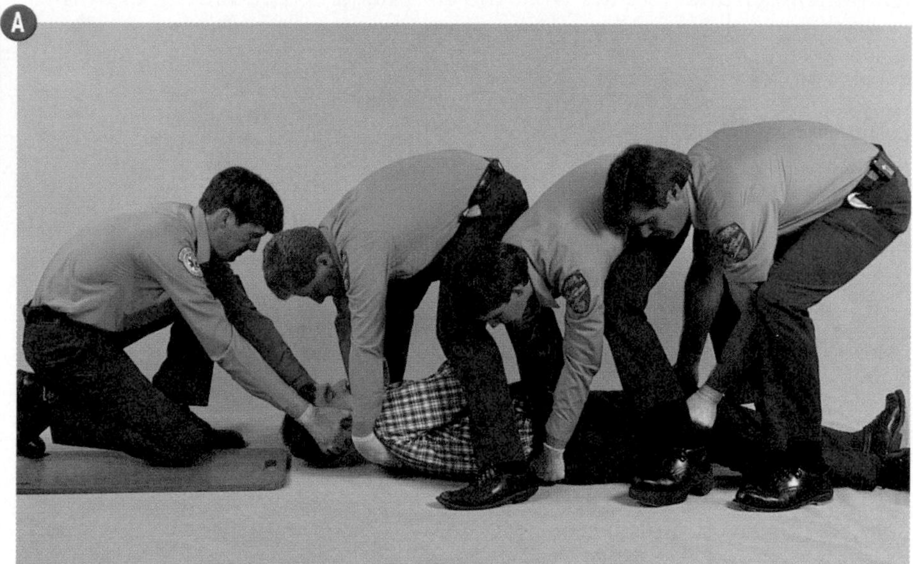

B

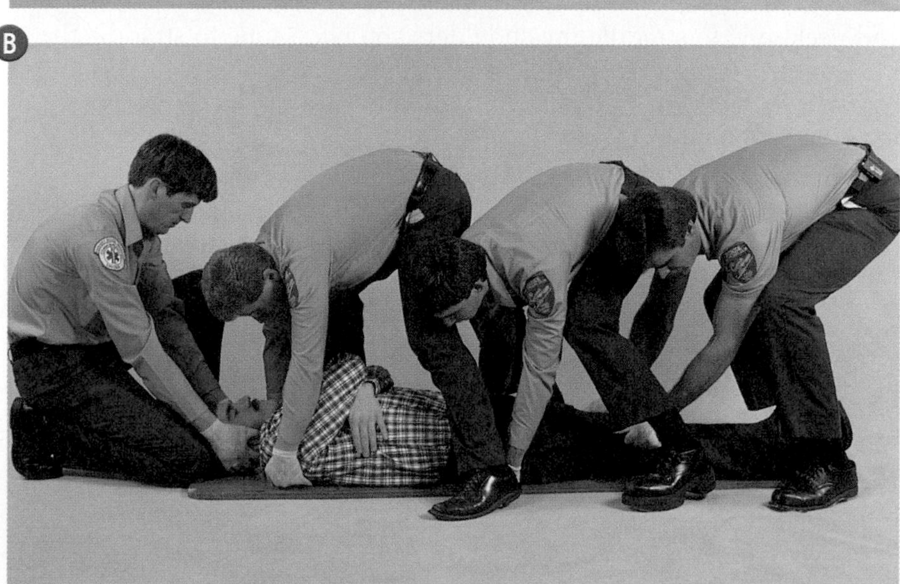

Figure 5.29 Straddle slide. **A.** Slide the patient about 10 inches at a time onto the backboard. **B.** Center the patient on the backboard.

Straps and Strapping Techniques

Every patient who is on a backboard should be strapped down to avoid sliding or slipping off the backboard. There are many ways to strap a patient to a backboard. The method described here is simple to learn and effective in securing the patient.

Around-the-board strapping works best and is easiest to understand and apply. The straps should be long enough to go around the entire board and a large patient. Straps 6 feet to 9 feet long with seat belt–type buckles work well (**Figure 5.30**). Do not loop the straps through the handholes on the sides of the backboard but pass them around both the backboard and the patient. Use three straps, placed around the upper arm area, the wrist and hip area, and just above the knees. This placement affords maximum stabilization of the heaviest parts of the patient's body. When immobilizing a patient to a backboard, secure the straps around the wrist and hip area and the knees before securing the head to the backboard. This reduces the chance of head movement. Strap placement is shown in **Figure 5.31**. Since there are many different types of straps and strapping techniques, learn the method used by your EMS system.

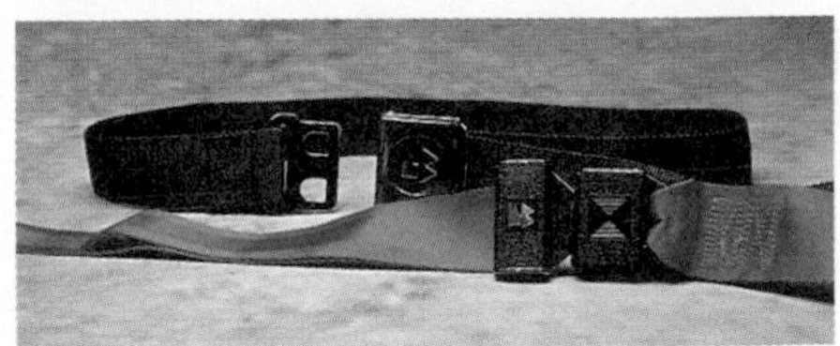

Figure 5.30 Seat-belt-type straps.

Head Immobilization

Once a patient has been secure to the backboard, the head and neck must be immobilized using commercially prepared devices (such as foam blocks) or improvised devices (such as a blanket roll). The use of a blanket roll is explained here because it works well and because a blanket is almost always available. The blanket roll should be assembled ahead of time. Fold and roll the blanket (with towels as bulk filler) as shown in **Figure 5.32**, page 90, since there are many different types of straps and strapping techniques, learn the method used by your EMS system.

To place the blanket roll under a patient's head, one rescuer should unroll it enough to fit around the head as another rescuer maintains head stabilization. The of the rescuer holding the patient's head (Rescuer One) carefully slides his or her hands out from between the blanket, and stabilization is maintained by the blanket roll (**Figure 5.33**, page 91). Head stabilization must be maintained throughout the entire procedure (first by manually stabilizing the patient's head, then by using the blanket roll).

The blanket roll must be fitted securely against the patient's shoulders in order to widen the base of support for the patient's head. Secure the blanket roll to the head with two cravats tied around the blanket roll, one over the patient's forehead and the other under the chin. Use two more cravats in the same positions to bind the head and the blanket roll to the backboard. The patient's head and neck are now adequately stabilized against the backboard. This head immobilization technique, coupled with proper placement of straps around the backboard, adequately immobilizes the spine of an injured patient and packages the patient for movement as a unit.

Foam blocks are quick to apply and provide good stabilization of the patient's head and neck. The use of one type of foam blocks is shown in **Figure 5.34**, page 92.

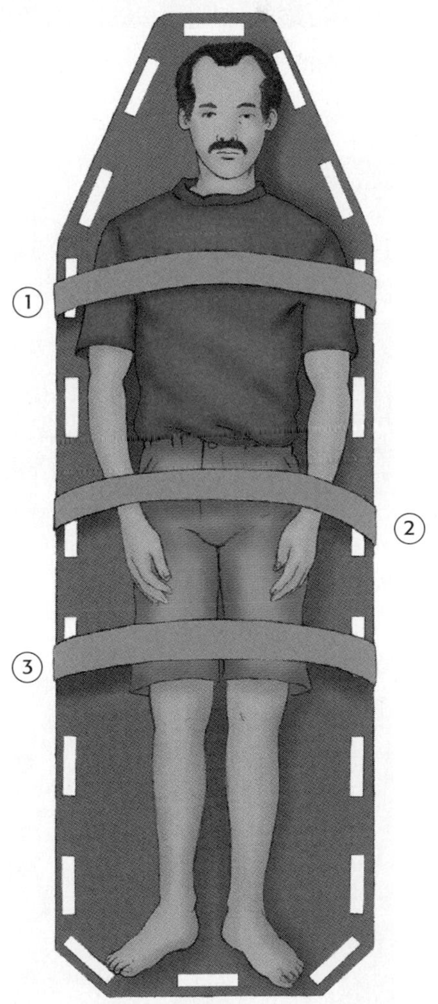

Figure 5.31 Strap placement for effective immobilization on a backboard. **1.** Upper arms. **2.** Wrists and hips. **3.** Above the knees.

Skill Drill

Figure 5.32 Preparing a Blanket Roll

1

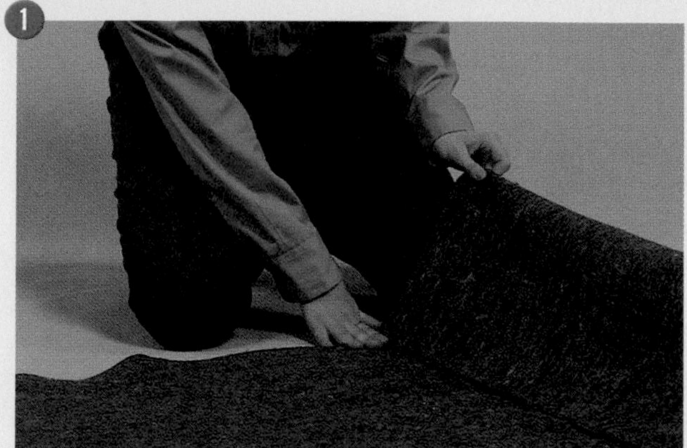

Fold blanket.

2

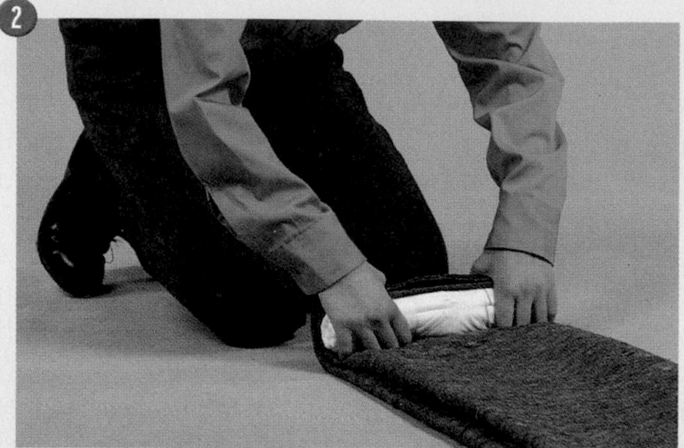

Insert rolled towel and roll from each end.

3

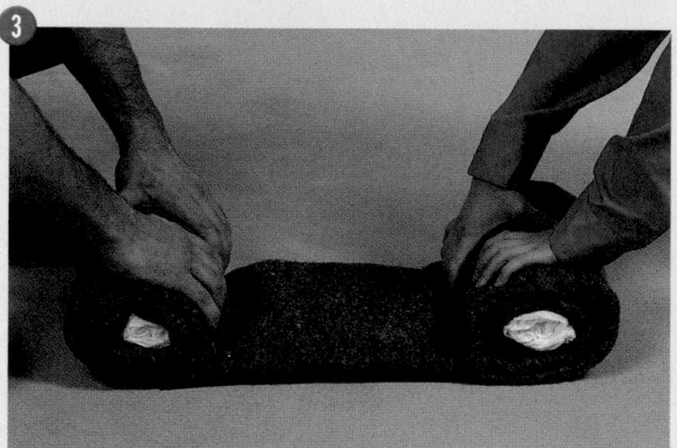

Roll the ends together.

4

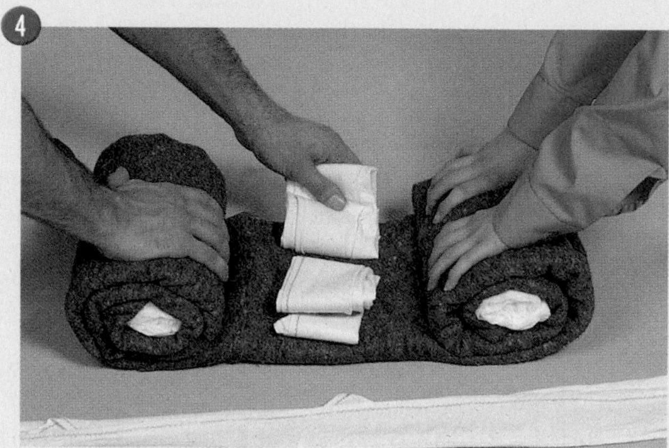

Place extra cravats inside.

5

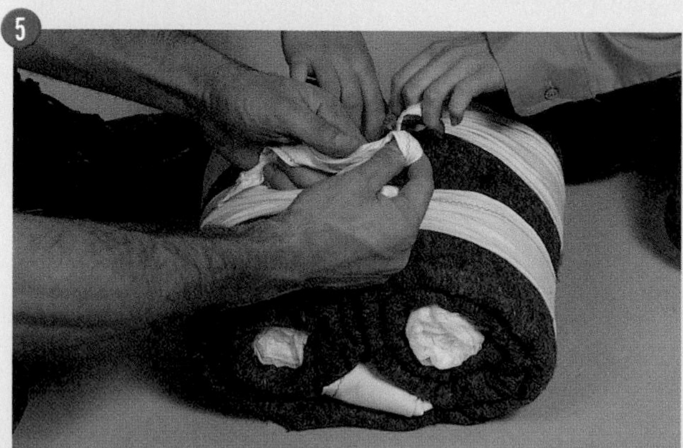

Tie with two cravats.

6

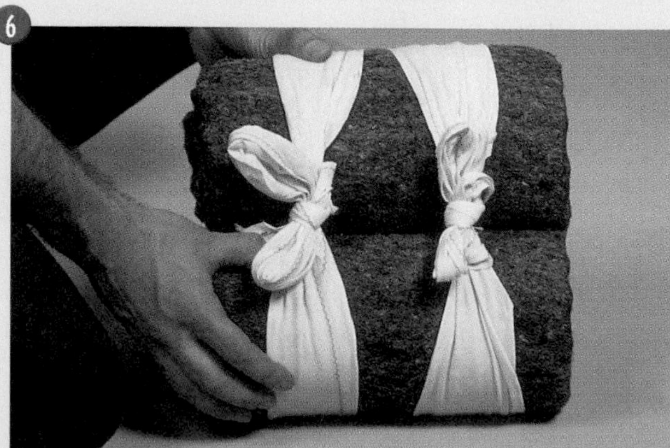

The finished blanket roll.

Skill Drill

Figure 5.33 Applying the Blanket Roll to Stabilize the Patient's Head and Neck

1

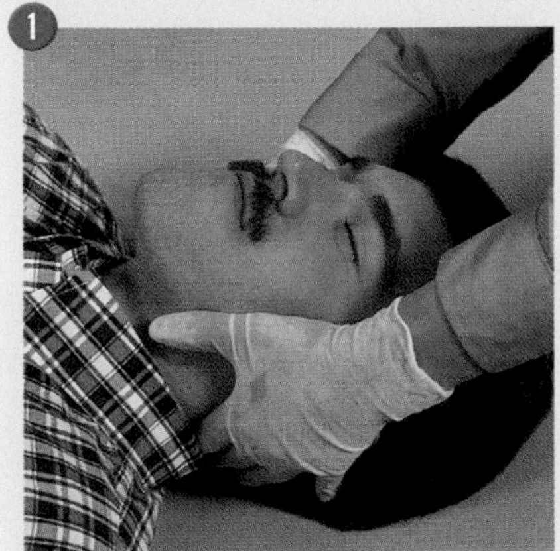

Stabilize the head.

2

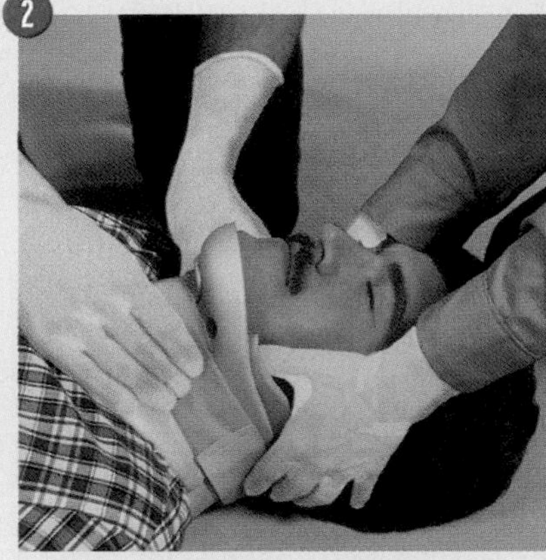

Apply a cervical collar.

3

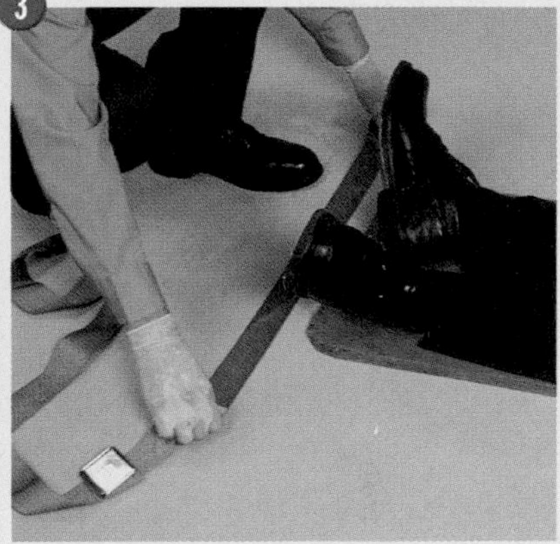

Place straps around backboard and patient.

4

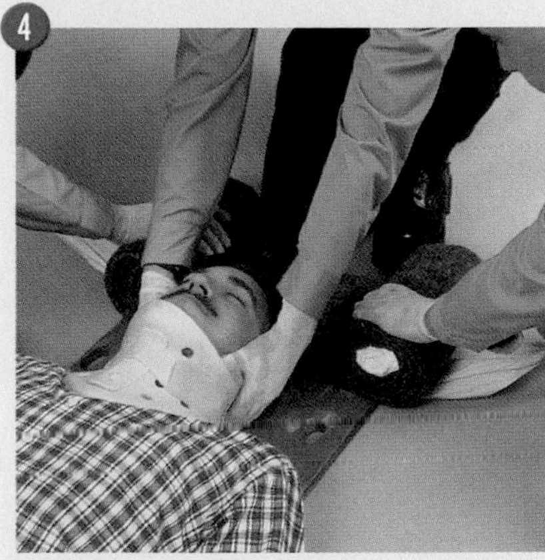

Insert the blanket roll.

5

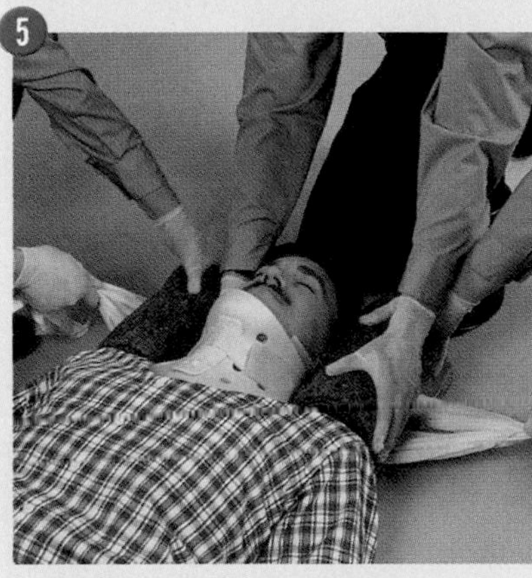

Roll blanket snugly against the neck and shoulders.

6

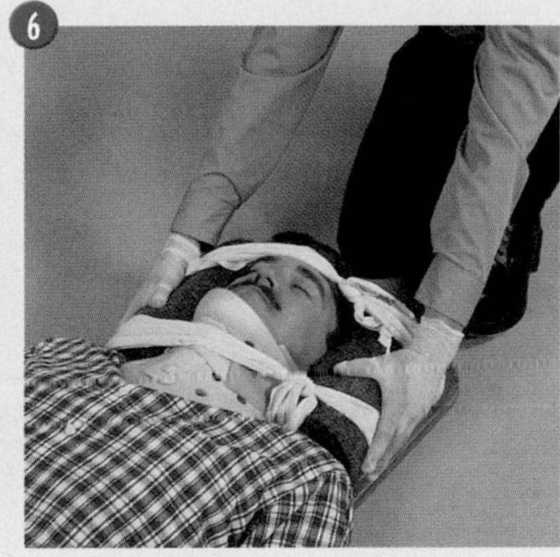

Tie two cravats around the blanket roll and patient's head.

7

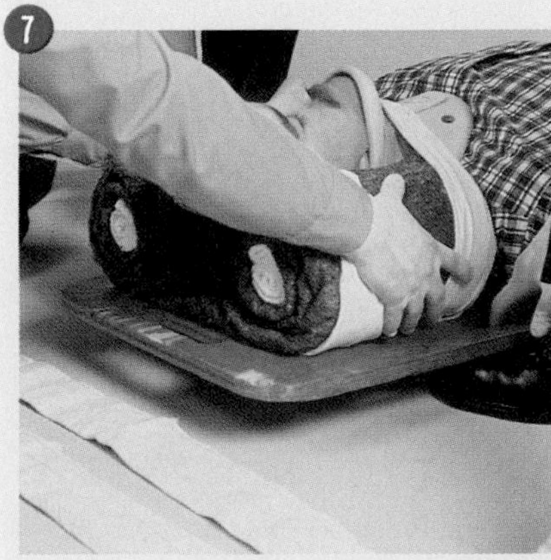

Continue to stabilize the patient's head.

8

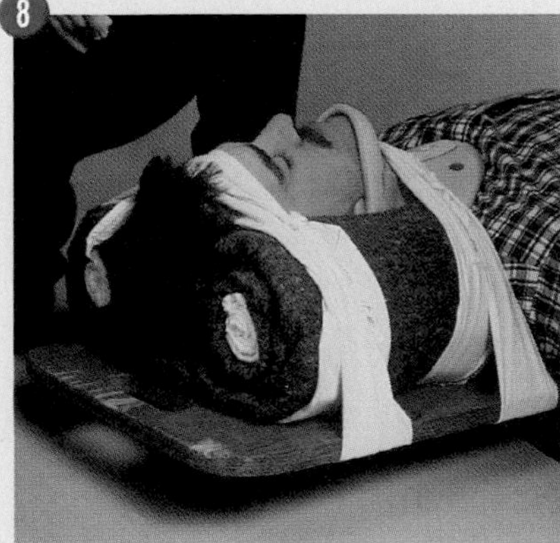

Tie two cravats around backboard.

9

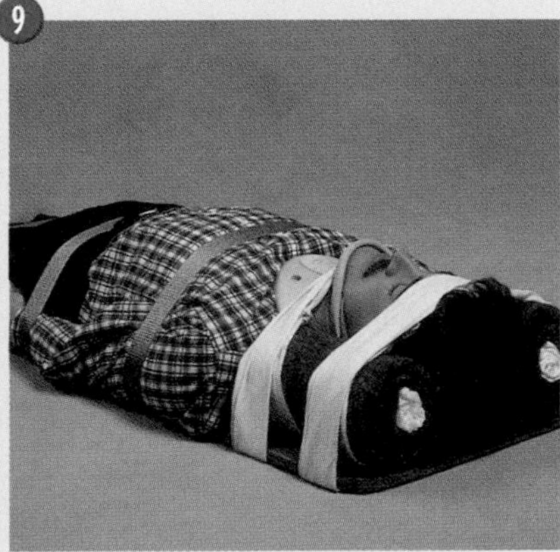

A secured patient.

Remember

Carefully monitor all immobilized patients for airway problems.

In an extreme emergency where a patient must be moved from a dangerous environment and a commercially prepared backboard is not available, you should improvise. Make sure that the improvised backboard is strong enough to carry the patient without breaking.

Improvised devices should be used only when a patient must be moved to prevent further injury or death and when a commercially prepared backboard is not available.

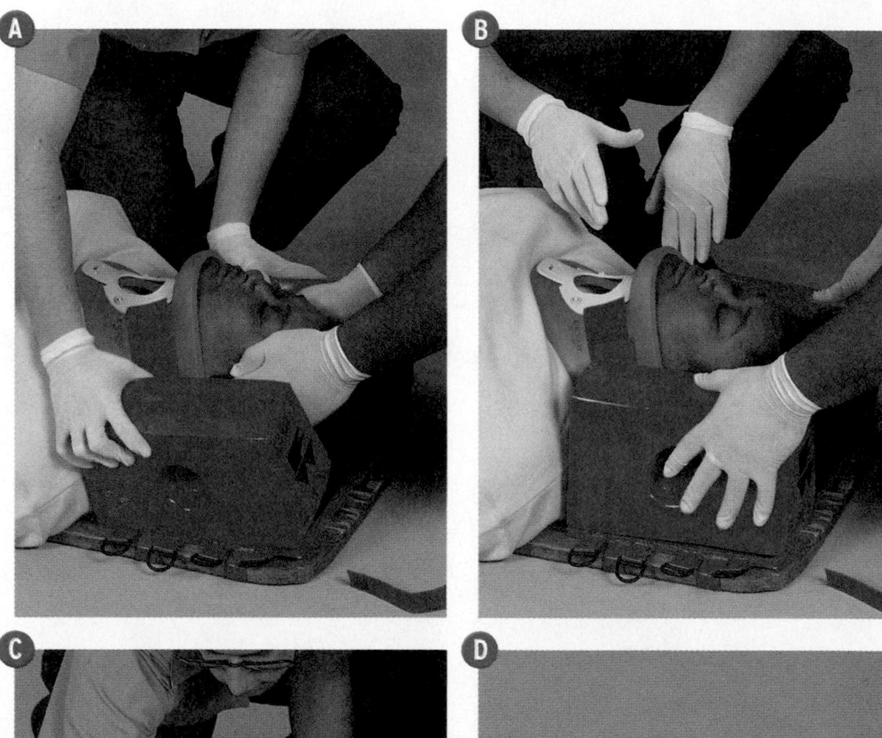

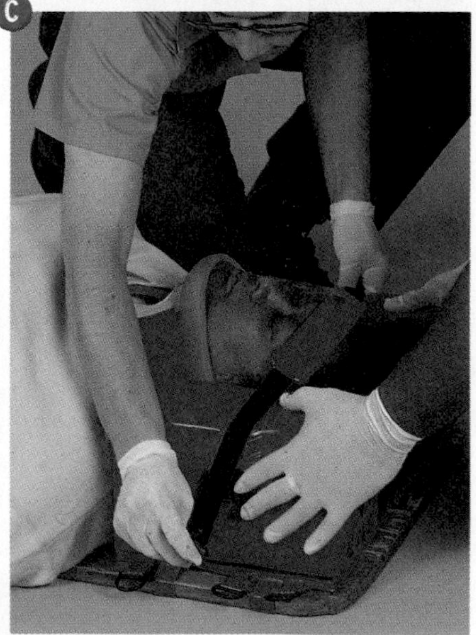

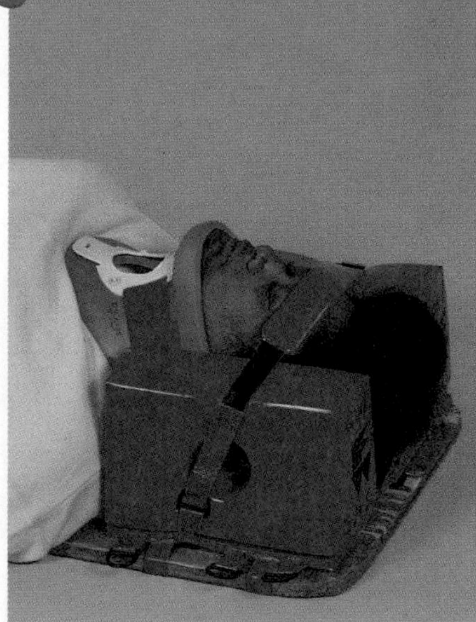

Figure 5.34 Application of a commercial device to stabilize a patient's head and neck. **A.** Apply the head blocks. **B.** Secure the device. **C.** Apply the immobilization straps. **D.** The head is immobilized.

Improvise

Some devices that you can use as backboards include:

- wide, sturdy planks
- doors
- ironing boards
- sturdy folding tables
- full-length lawn chair recliners

5

Prep Kit

Ready for Review

Ready for Review thoroughly summarizes the chapter.

As a first responder, you may sometimes have to move patients by yourself, particularly if the patient is in a dangerous environment or must be moved in order to receive CPR. This chapter covered six emergency patient drags. These drags enable you to move a patient out of an unsafe environment quickly and without equipment. They are useful even when the patient is heavier than the rescuer. Seven carries for nonambulatory patients were also presented. These carries enable two people to carry a patient with little equipment. Two walking assists were presented that allow you to help a patient who cannot walk without some help.

You should be familiar with certain equipment that your local ambulances carry. You may be asked to assist your EMS provider in lifting or moving patients. By learning how to assist with these devices, you can become a more valuable part of the EMS team. You should practice these skills with your local EMS provider. You must also know how to help move patients with spinal injuries. Stabilization and immobilization of trauma patients prevent further injury. Placing the patient on a backboard also makes moving easier. Because you will be called upon to help move patients onto backboards, it is important that you practice the skills involved with treating these patients.

Vital Vocabulary

The Vital Vocabulary are the key terms for this chapter.

arm-to-arm drag—*page 71*
blanket drag—*page 71*
cervical collar—*page 84*
clothes drag—*page 70*
cradle-in-arms carry—*page 74*
extremities—*page 74*
firefighter drag—*page 72*
logrolling—*page 87*
one-person walking assist—*page 80*
pack-strap carry—*page 75*
portable stretcher—*page 81*
recovery position—*page 69*
scoop stretcher—*page 83*
stair chair—*page 81*
straddle lift—*page 87*
straddle slide—*page 88*
two-person chair carry—*page 75*
two-person extremity carry—*page 74*
two-person seat carry—*page 74*
two-person walking assist—*page 80*

Skill Drills

The Skill Drills provide a visual summary of some of the more complex skills from the skills objectives.

Practice Points

The Practice Points are the key skills you need to know.

1. Placing a patient in the "recovery position."

2. Lifting and moving patients using good body mechanics.

3. Performing the following emergency patient drags:

A. Clothes drag

B. Blanket drag

C. Arm-to-arm drag

D. Firefighter drag

E. Emergency drag from a vehicle

4. Performing the following patient carries:

A. Two-person extremity carry

B. Two-person seat carry

C. Cradle-in-arms carry

D. Two-person chair carry

E. Pack-strap carry

F. Direct ground lift

G. Transfer from a bed to a stretcher

5. Performing the following walking assists for ambulatory patients:

A. One-person assist

B. Two-person assist

6. Assisting other EMS providers with the following devices:

A. Wheeled ambulance stretcher

B. Portable stretcher

C. Stair chair

D. Long backboard

E. Short backboard

F. Scoop stretcher

7. Assisting other EMS providers with the following procedures for patients with suspected spinal injuries:

A. Applying a cervical collar

B. Moving patients using backboards

C. Applying short backboard devices

D. Logrolling onto a long backboard

E. Straddle lifting onto a long backboard

F. Straddle sliding onto a long backboard

G. Strapping a patient onto a long backboard

H. Immobilizing a patient's head to a long backboard

Ready to Respond

Ready to Respond presents a fictitious scenario to help you review what you learned in this chapter.

You and your partner have been called to a senior citizens center to help evacuate patients because floodwaters may cut off the access road to the facility. The officer in charge assigns you and your partner to one wing that has four patients and asks that you bring the patients to the front lobby where they will be assigned to vehicles for evacuation.

1. The first gentleman tells you he can walk slowly, but he is weak. What technique could you use to to help this man?
   A. Straddle slide
   B. One-person walking assist
   C. Two-person extremity carry
   D. Pack-strap carry

2. The second room is occupied by a woman who has a brace on her ankle. She is not supposed to put weight on her sprained ankle. Which of the following carries would you consider using for this patient?
   A. Two-person extremity carry
   B. Pack-strap carry
   C. Two-person seat carry
   D. Direct ground lift

3. In the third room is an 82-year-old woman who says she has a heart condition and gets short of breath if she walks very far. How would you move this person?
   A. One-person walking assist
   B. Two-person extremity carry
   C. Pack-strap carry
   D. Two-person chair carry

4. The fourth person is confined to bed because she suffered a stroke two years ago. A nurse asks you to transfer this woman to a stretcher she furnishes for you. How would you move this woman to the stretcher?
   A. Direct ground lift
   B. Logroll
   C. Clothes drag
   D. Patient transfer technique

The following questions do not relate to the above scenario but test general knowledge.

5. The most commonly used technique for placing a patient on a backboard is:
   A. Straddle slide
   B. Logroll
   C. Straddle lift
   D. Direct ground lift

6. If you need to move a heavy unconscious person from a life threatening emergency, which of the following would you use?
   A. Straddle slide
   B. Straddle lift
   C. Firefighter drag
   D Clothes drag

7. Which is the correct order of steps to secure a patient with a possible head and neck injury to a backboard?
   1. Immobilize the head to the backboard
   2. Manually stabilize the head
   3. Immobilize the torso and legs
   4. Apply a cervical collar

   A. 4,2,1,3
   B. 2,4,3,1
   C. 3,2,4,1
   D. 2,4,1,3

MODULE 1 Quick Quiz

Preparatory

1. Place the sequence of events in the order in which they occur in an emergency.

A EMS response

B. Hospital care

C. Dispatch

D. Reporting

E. First response

2. The overall leader of the emergency medical services system is the physician.

A. True

B. False

3. First responders are a critical component of an emergency medical services system because they are.

A. Responsible for reporting such emergencies.

B. The first medically trained personnel to arrive on the scene.

C. Able to provide both basic and advanced life support.

D. Trained in traffic control.

4. Place the five stages of the normal reactions to stress in the order in which they usually occur.

A. Bargaining

B. Anger

C. Depression

D. Denial

E. Acceptance

5. List eight signs and symptoms of stress.

6. Universal precautions include all but which of the following?

A. Washing your hands after patient contact

B. Proper handling of used needles

C. Wearing eye protection during all patient contacts

D. Wearing medical gloves when handling patients

E. Avoiding mouth-to-mouth rescue breathing whenever possible

7. The manner in which an individual must act or behave when giving care is.
   A. Duty to act
   B. Standard of care
   C. Competency
   D. Negligence
   E. Implied care

8. Which of the following is not a condition of negligence?
   A. Breech of duty
   B. Abandonment
   C. Duty to act
   D. Resulting injuries
   E. Proximal cause

9. Which of the following describes any patient who does not refuse emergency care?
   A. Implied consent
   B. Expressed consent
   C. Consent for a minor
   D. Patient refusal

10. Match the following terms:

A. Superior	1. Toward the midline of the body
B. Distal	2. The back surface of the body
C. Proximal	3. Toward the head
D. Lateral	4. A structure that is nearer to the free end of an extremity
E. Medial	5. Describing structures that are closer to the trunk
F. Posterior	6. Away from the midline of the body

11. Oxygen is transported throughout the body by means of the
   A. Plasma
   B. White blood cells
   C. Platelets
   D. Red blood cells

MODULE 1 QuickQuiz *Continued*

Preparatory

12. Which of the following structures is not part of the digestive system?

A. Pharynx

B. Esophagus

C. Stomach

D. Kidney

E. Gall bladder

13. Which of the following situations does not require an emergency movement of a patient?

A. Hazardous materials are present

B. The accident scene cannot be protected

C. The patient has suffered cardiac arrest and must be moved to perform CPR

D. Danger of fire, explosion, or structural collapse

E. Bad weather conditions

14. Unconscious patients who are breathing adequately should be placed in the ____________ position.

A. recovery

B. unconscious

C. side lying

D. prone

15. A patient who has fallen from a tree should be moved using a ____________.

A. wheeled ambulance stretcher

B. portable stretcher

C. stair chair

D. long backboard

E. short backboard

1. D, C, E, A, B **2.** A **3.** B **4.** D, B, A, C, E **5.** (1) irritability, (2) inability to concentrate, (3) change in normal disposition, (4) difficulty in sleeping, (5) anxiety, (6) indecisiveness, (7) guilt, (8) loss of appetite, (9) loss of interest in sex, (12) loss of interest in work, (11) isolation **6.** C **7.** B **8.** B **9.** A **10.** A=3, B=4, C=5, D=6, E=1, F=2) **11.** D **12.** D **13.** E **14.** A **15.** D

Airway

MODULE 2

Module CONTENTS

Chapter 6

Airway Care and Rescue Breathing

TECHNOLOGY

- Online Chapter Pretest
- Web Links
- Online Glossary
- Anatomy Review
- Online Review Manual
- CyberClass

www.FirstResponderTraining.com

- Interactive First Responder

Chapter FEATURES

- Skill Drills
- Vital Vocabulary
- Voices of Experience
- Signs and Symptoms
- FYI
- Special Needs
- Safety Tips
- BSI Tips
- Caution
- Check Point
- Prep Kit

Objectives

Knowledge and Attitude Objectives

After studying this chapter, you will be expected to:

1. Identify the anatomic structures of the respiratory system and state the function of each structure.
2. State the differences in the respiratory systems of infants, adults, and children.
3. Describe the process used to check a patient's responsiveness.
4. Describe the steps in the head tilt–chin lift technique.
5. Describe the steps in the jaw-thrust technique.
6. Describe how to check for fluids, solids, and dentures in a patient's mouth.
7. State the steps needed to clear a patient's airway using finger sweeps and suction.
8. Describe the steps required to maintain a patient's airway using the recovery position, oral airways, and nasal airways.
9. Describe the signs of adequate breathing, the signs of inadequate breathing, the causes of respiratory arrest, and the major signs of respiratory arrest.

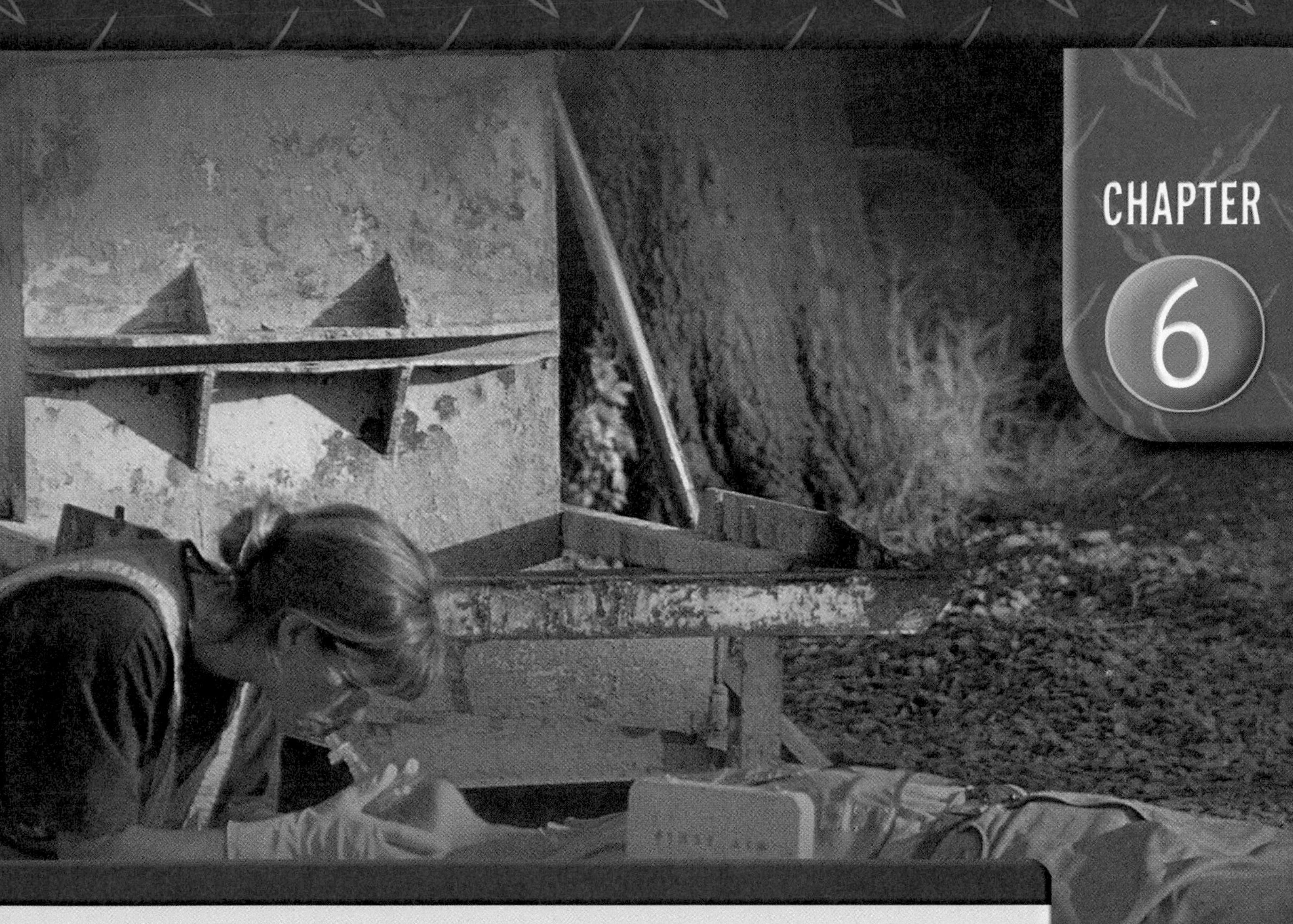

10. Describe how to check a patient for the presence of breathing.
11. Describe how to perform rescue breathing using a mouth-to-mask device, a mouth-to-barrier device, and mouth-to-mouth techniques.
12. Describe, in order, the steps for recognizing respiratory arrest and performing rescue breathing in adults, children, and infants.
13. Describe the differences between the signs and symptoms of partial airway obstruction and those of complete airway obstruction.
14. List the steps in managing a foreign body airway obstruction in conscious and unconscious adults, in conscious and unconscious children, and in conscious and unconscious infants.
15. List the special considerations needed to perform rescue breathing in patients with stomas.
16. Describe the special considerations of airway care and rescue breathing in children and infants.
17. Describe the hazards dental appliances present during the performance of airway skills.
18. Describe the steps in providing airway care to a patient in a vehicle.

Skill Objectives

As a first responder, you should be able to:

1. Demonstrate the head tilt–chin lift and jaw-thrust techniques for opening blocked airways.
2. Check for fluids, solids, and dentures in a patient's airway.
3. Correct a blocked airway using finger sweeps and suction.
4. Place a patient in the recovery position.
5. Insert oral and nasal airways.
6. Check for the presence of breathing.
7. Perform rescue breathing using a mouth-to-mask device, a mouth-to-barrier device, and mouth-to-mouth techniques.
8. Demonstrate the steps in recognizing respiratory arrest and performing rescue breathing on an adult patient, a child, and an infant.
9. Perform the steps needed to remove a foreign body airway obstruction in an adult patient, a child, and an infant.
10. Demonstrate rescue breathing on a patient with a stoma.
11. Perform airway management on a patient in a vehicle.

This chapter introduces the two most important lifesaving skills, airway care and rescue breathing. Patients must have an open airway passage and must maintain adequate breathing to survive. By learning and practicing the simple skills in this chapter, you can often make the difference between life and death for a patient.

A review of the major structures of the respiratory system is needed before you practice airway and rescue breathing skills. Once you learn the functions of these structures, you will be a long way down the road to becoming proficient in performing these skills.

The skills of airway care and rescue breathing are as easy as A and B—the "A" stands for airway, and the "B" stands for breathing. Because you must assess and correct the airway before you turn your attention to the patient's breathing status, it is helpful to remember the AB sequence. In Chapter 8, "C" will be added for the assessment and correction of the patient's circulation. As you learn the skills presented in this chapter and in Chapter 8, remember the ABC sequence. A second mnemonic that will be used throughout both this chapter and Chapter 8 is "check and correct." By using this two-step sequence for each of the ABCs, you will be able to remember the steps needed to check and correct problems involving the patient's airway, breathing, and circulation.

The "A" or airway section presents airway skills, including how to check the level of consciousness and manually correct a blocked airway by using the head tilt–chin lift and jaw-thrust techniques. You must check the patient's airway for foreign objects. If you find foreign objects, you must correct the problem and remove the objects by using either a manual technique or a suction device. You will learn when and how to use oral and nasal airways to keep the patient's airway open.

The "B" or breathing section describes how to check patients to determine whether or not they are breathing adequately. You will learn how to correct breathing problems by using three rescue breathing techniques: mouth-to-mask, mouth-to-barrier device, and mouth-to-mouth.

Finally, you will learn how to check patients to determine if they have an airway obstruction that can cause death in a few minutes. You will learn how to correct this condition using manual techniques that require no special equipment.

As you study this chapter, remember the check-and-correct process for both airway and breathing skills. Do not forget that the A and B skills presented in this chapter will be followed by C (for circulation) skills in Chapter 8. After you have learned the Airway, Breathing, and Circulation skills (the ABCs), you will be able to perform **cardiopulmonary resuscitation (CPR)**. CPR is used to save the lives of people suffering cardiac arrest.*

cardiopulmonary resuscitation (CPR) The artificial circulation of the blood and movement of air into and out of the lungs in a pulseless, nonbreathing patient.

Anatomy and Function of the Respiratory System

To maintain life, all organisms must receive a constant supply of certain substances. In human beings, these basic life-sustaining substances are food, water, and **oxygen**. A person can live several weeks without food because the body can use nutrients it has stored. Although the body does not store as much water, it is possible to live several days without fluid intake. But lack of oxygen, even for a few minutes, can result in irreversible damage and death.

The most sensitive cells in the human body are in the brain. If brain cells are deprived of oxygen and nutrients for four to six minutes, they begin to die. Brain death is followed by the death of the entire body. Once brain cells have been destroyed, they cannot be replaced. This is why it is important to understand the anatomy and function of the respiratory system.

The main purpose of the respiratory system is to provide oxygen and to remove carbon dioxide from the red blood cells as they pass through the lungs. This action forms the basis for your study of the lifesaving skill of CPR.

The parts of the body used in breathing are shown in **Figure 6.1** and include the mouth (**oropharynx**), the nose (**nasopharynx**), the throat, the **trachea** (windpipe), the lungs, the diaphragm (the dome-shaped muscle between the chest and the abdomen), and numerous chest

oxygen (O_2) A colorless, odorless gas that is essential for life.

oropharynx The posterior part of the mouth.

nasopharynx The posterior part of the nose.

trachea The windpipe.

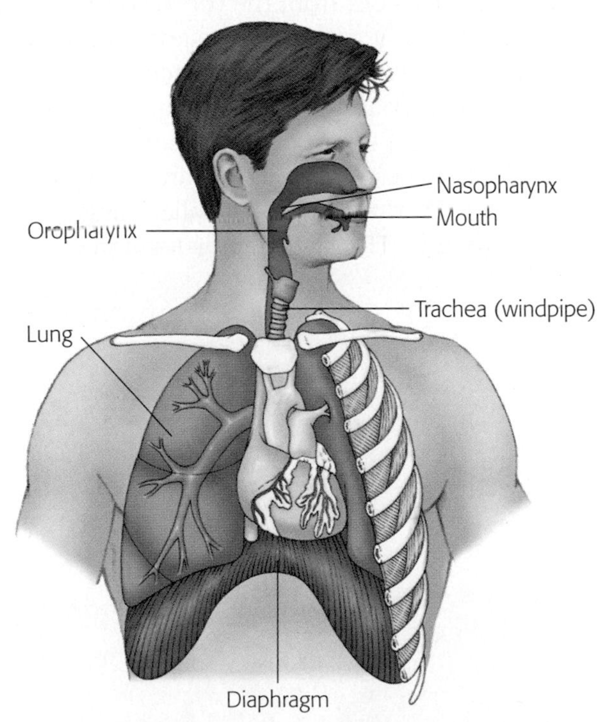

Figure 6.1 The respiratory system.

* The material presented in this book concerning CPR is intended to follow the CPR guidelines of the American Heart Association (AHA). Although the information presented here follows AHA guidelines at the time of publication, these guidelines are subject to periodic revision and updating. You should follow the AHA's most current CPR guidelines.

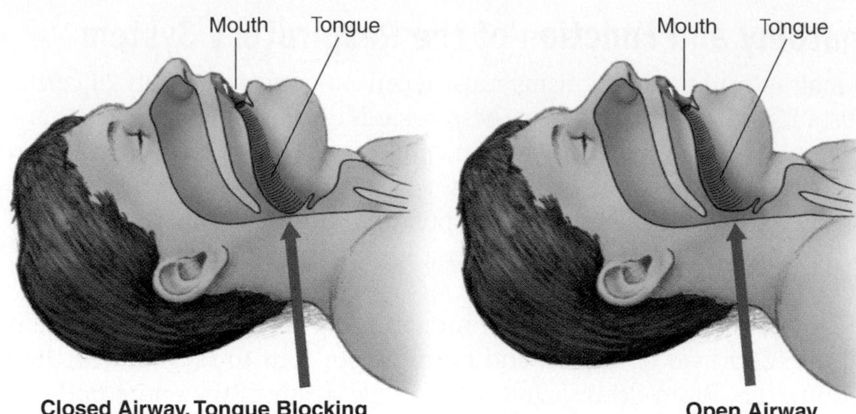

Figure 6.2 In an unconscious patient, the airway may be blocked by the tongue (left). Open airway (right).

mandible The lower jaw.

esophagus The tube through which food passes. It starts at the throat and ends at the stomach.

airway The passages from the openings of the mouth and nose to the air sacs in the lungs through which air enters and leaves the lungs.

bronchi The two main branches of the windpipe that lead into the right and left lungs. Within the lungs, they branch into smaller airways.

lungs The organs that supply the body with oxygen and eliminate carbon dioxide from the blood.

alveoli The air sacs of the lungs where the exchange of oxygen and carbon dioxide takes place.

capillaries The smallest blood vessels that connect small arteries and small veins. Capillary walls serve as the membrane to exchange oxygen and carbon dioxide.

muscles. Air enters the body through the nose and mouth. In an unconscious patient lying on his or her back, the passage of air through both nose and mouth may be blocked by the tongue (**Figure 6.2**). The tongue is attached to the lower jaw (**mandible**). When a person loses consciousness, the jaw relaxes and the tongue falls backward into the rear of the mouth, effectively blocking the passage of air from both nose and mouth to the lungs. A partially blocked airway often produces a snoring sound. At the bottom of the throat are two passages, the **esophagus** (the food tube) and the trachea. The epiglottis is a thin flapper valve that allows air to enter the trachea but prevents food or water from doing so. Air passes from the throat to the larynx (voice box), which can be seen externally as the Adam's apple in the neck. Below the trachea, the **airway** divides into the **bronchi** (two large tubes). The bronchi branch into smaller and smaller airways in the **lungs**. The lungs are located on either side of the heart and are protected by the sternum at the front and by the rib cage at the sides and back (**Figure 6.3**).

The airways branch into smaller and smaller passages, which end as tiny air sacs called **alveoli**. The alveoli are surrounded by very small

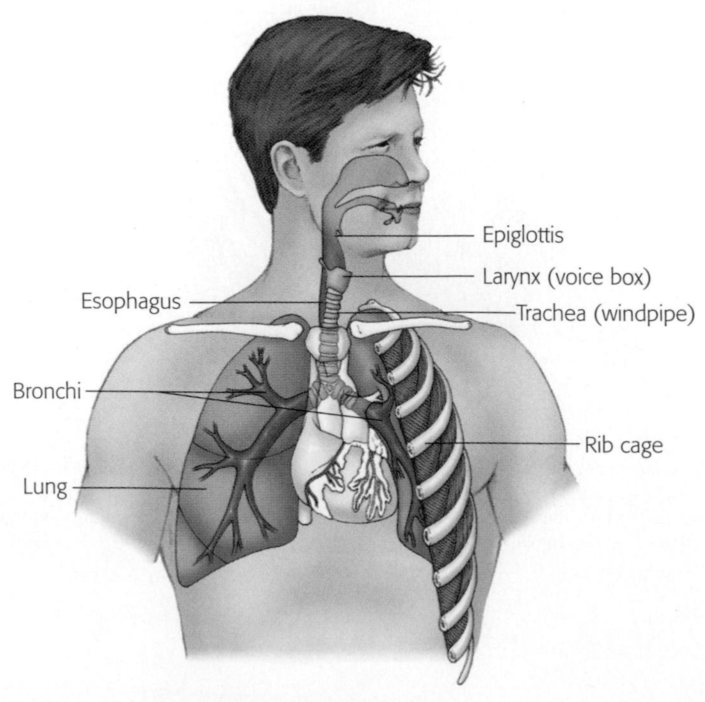

Figure 6.3 Anatomy of the respiratory system.

blood vessels, the **capillaries**. The actual exchange of gases takes place across a thin membrane that separates the capillaries of the circulatory system from the alveoli of the lungs (**Figure 6.4**). The incoming oxygen passes from the alveoli into the blood, and the outgoing carbon dioxide passes from the blood into the alveoli.

The lungs consist of soft, spongy tissue with no muscles. Therefore, movement of air into the lungs depends on movement of the rib cage and the diaphragm. As the rib cage expands, air is drawn into the lungs through the trachea. The diaphragm, a muscle that separates the abdominal cavity from the chest, is dome-shaped when it is relaxed. When the diaphragm contracts, it flattens and moves downward. This action increases the size of the chest cavity and draws air into the lungs through the trachea. In normal breathing, the combined actions of the diaphragm and the rib cage automatically produce adequate inhalation and exhalation (**Figure 6.5**).

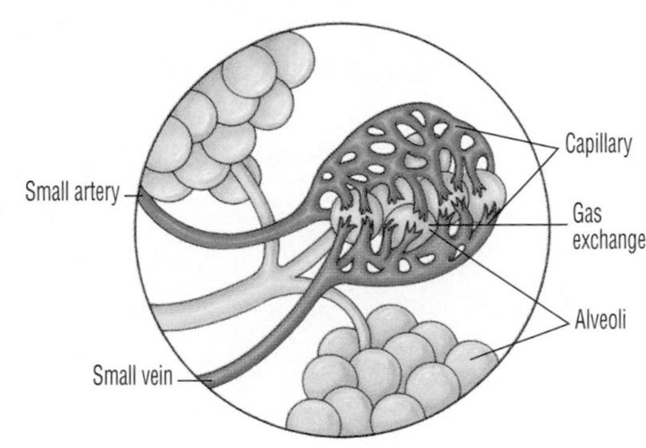

Figure 6.4 The exchange of gases occurs in the alveoli of the lungs.

Checkpoint

- What are the major structures of the respiratory system?
- What is the function of each structure?
- How are these functions interrelated?

"A" Is for Airway

The patient's airway is the pipeline that transports life-giving oxygen from the air to the lungs and transports the waste product, carbon dioxide, from the lungs to the air. In healthy individuals, the airway automatically stays open. An injured or seriously ill person, however, may not be able to protect the airway, and it may become blocked. If a patient cannot protect his or her airway, you, as a first responder, must take certain steps to check the condition of the patient's airway and correct the problem to keep the patient alive.

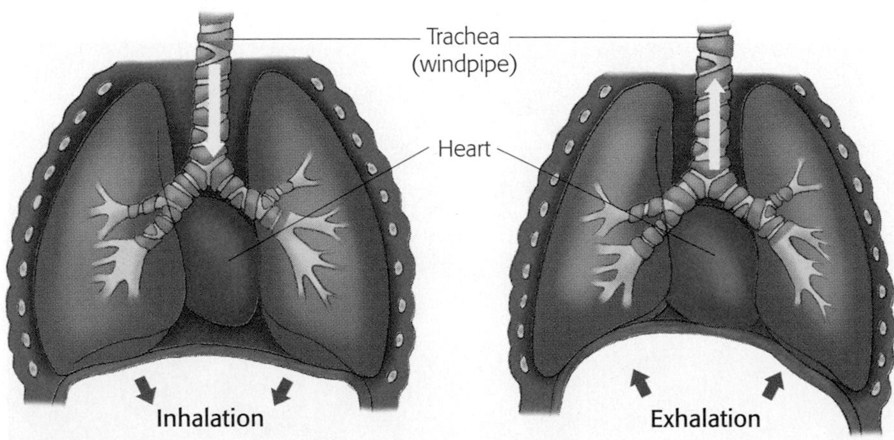

Figure 6.5 Normal mechanical act of breathing.

Special Needs

INFANTS AND CHILDREN

- The structures of the respiratory systems in children and infants are smaller than they are in adults. Thus the air passages of children and infants may be more easily blocked by secretions or by foreign objects.
- In children and infants, the tongue is proportionally larger than it is in adults. Thus the tongue of these smaller patients is more likely to block their airway than it would in an adult patient.
- Because the trachea of an infant or child is more flexible than that of an adult, it is more likely to become narrowed or blocked than that of an adult.
- The head of a child or an infant is proportionally larger than the head of an adult. You will have to learn slightly different techniques for opening the airway of children.
- Children and infants have smaller lungs than adults. You need to give them smaller breaths when you perform rescue breathing.
- Most children and infants have healthy hearts. When a child or infant suffers cardiac arrest (stoppage of the heart), it is usually because the patient has a blocked airway or has stopped breathing, not because there is a problem with the heart.

AIRWAY ASSESSMENT

- *Check*
- *Correct*
- *Check*
- *Correct*
- *Maintain*

Check for Responsiveness

The first step in assessing a patient's airway is to check the patient's level of responsiveness. When you first approach a patient, you can immediately find out whether the patient is conscious or unconscious by asking, "Are you okay? Can you hear me?" (**Figure 6.6**) If you get a response, you can assume that the patient is conscious and has an open airway. If there is no response, grasp the patient's shoulder and gently shake the patient. Then repeat your question. If the patient still does not respond, you can assume the patient is unconscious and that you will need more help. Before doing anything for the patient, call 9-1-1 ("phone first") if the EMS system has not already been activated, especially if you are the only rescuer. Position the patient by supporting the patient's head and neck and placing the patient on his or her back.

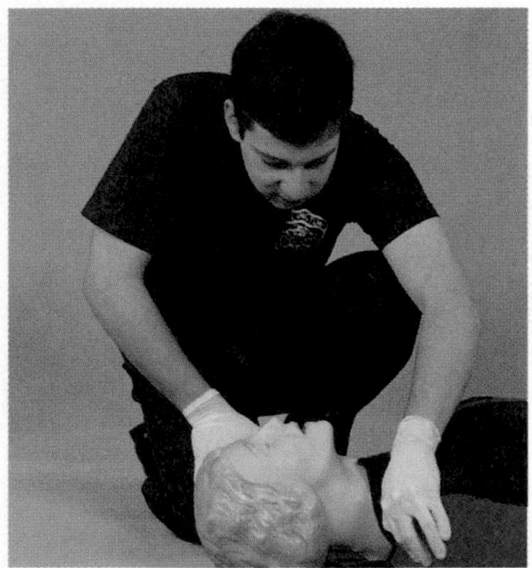

Figure 6.6 Establish the level of consciousness.

Correct the Blocked Airway

An unconscious patient's airway is often blocked (occluded) because the tongue has dropped back and is obstructing it. In this case, simply opening the airway may enable the patient to breathe spontaneously.

Head Tilt-Chin Lift Technique

To open the airway, place one hand on the forehead and place the fingers of the other hand under the bony part of the lower jaw near the chin. Push down on the forehead and lift up and forward on the chin. Be certain you are not merely pushing the mouth closed when you use this technique. This method of opening the airway is called the **head tilt–chin lift technique** (**Figure 6.7**).

head tilt–chin lift Opening the airway by tilting the patient's head backward and lifting the chin forward, bringing the entire lower jaw with it.

Follow these steps to perform the head tilt–chin lift technique:

1. Place the patient on his or her back and kneel beside the patient.
2. Place one hand on the patient's forehead and apply firm pressure backward with your palm. Move the patient's head back as far as possible.
3. Place the tips of the fingers of your other hand under the bony part of the lower jaw near the chin.
4. Lift the chin forward to help tilt the head back.

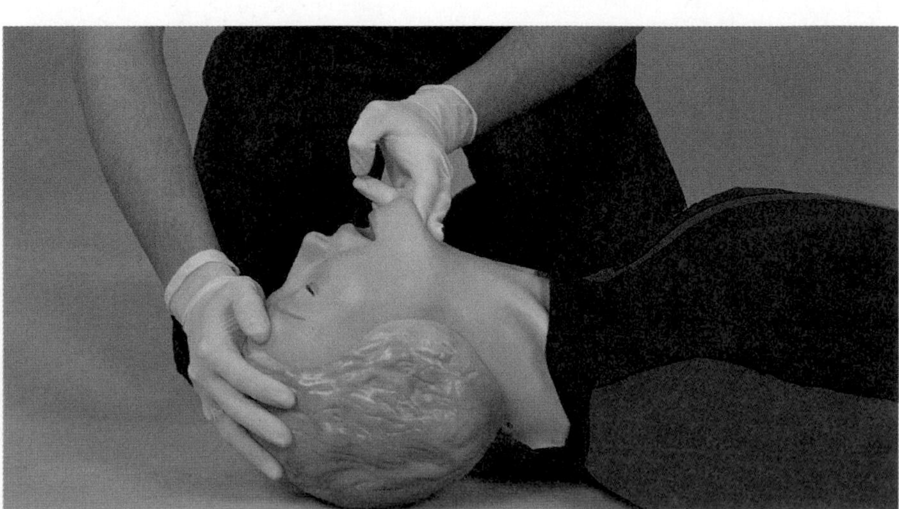

Figure 6.7 Open the patient's airway using the head tilt-chin lift technique.

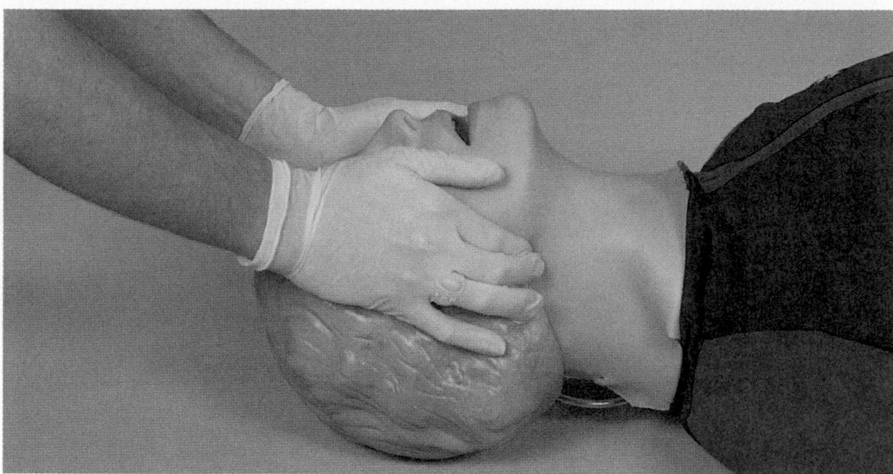

Figure 6.8 The jaw-thrust technique should open the patient's airway without extending the neck.

Jaw-Thrust Technique

The **jaw-thrust technique** or maneuver is another way to open a patient's airway. If the patient was injured in a fall, diving mishap, or automobile accident, do not tilt the head to open the airway. If the patient has a neck injury, tilting the head may cause permanent paralysis. If you suspect a neck injury, use the jaw-thrust technique. Open the airway by placing your fingers under the angles of the jaw and pushing upward. At the same time, use your thumbs to open the mouth slightly. The jaw-thrust technique should open the airway without extending the neck (**Figure 6.8**).

jaw-thrust technique Opening the airway by bringing the patient's jaw forward without extending the neck.

Follow these steps to perform the jaw-thrust technique:

1. Place the patient on his or her back and kneel at the top of the patient's head. Place your fingers behind the angles of the patient's lower jaw and move the jaw forward with firm pressure.
2. Tilt the head backward to a neutral or slight sniffing position. Do not extend the cervical spine in a patient who has suffered an injury to the head or neck.
3. Use your thumbs to pull the patient's lower jaw down, opening the mouth enough to allow breathing through the mouth and nose.

BSI Tip

Use body substance isolation (BSI) techniques whenever you may be in contact with body secretions that might contain blood.

Check for Fluids, Foreign Bodies, or Dentures

After you have opened the patient's airway by using either the head tilt–chin lift or the jaw-thrust technique, look in the patient's mouth to see if anything is blocking the patient's airway. Potential blocks include secretions, such as vomitus, mucus, or blood; foreign objects, such as candy, food, or dirt; and dentures or false teeth that may have become dislodged and are blocking the patient's airway (**Figure 6.9**). If you find anything in the patient's mouth, remove it by using one of the following techniques. If the patient's mouth is clear, consider using one of the devices described in the section on airway devices.

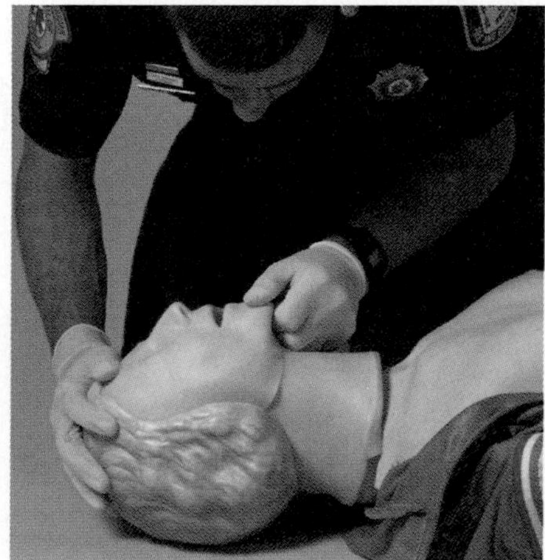

Figure 6.9 Check for fluids, foreign bodies, and dentures.

Correct the Airway Using Finger Sweeps or Suction

Vomitus, mucus, blood, and foreign objects must be cleared from the patient's airway. This can be done by using finger sweeps, suctioning, or the recovery position.

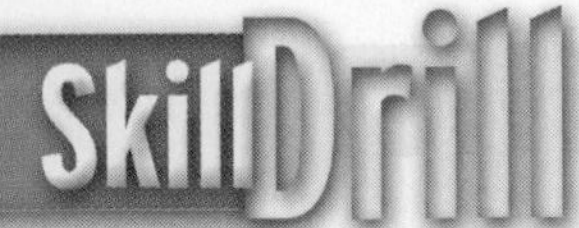

Figure 6.10 Clearing the Airway Using Finger Sweeps

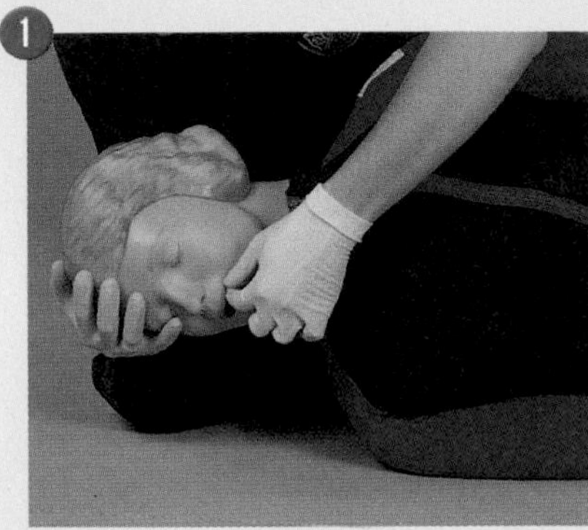

1. Turn the patient onto his or her side.

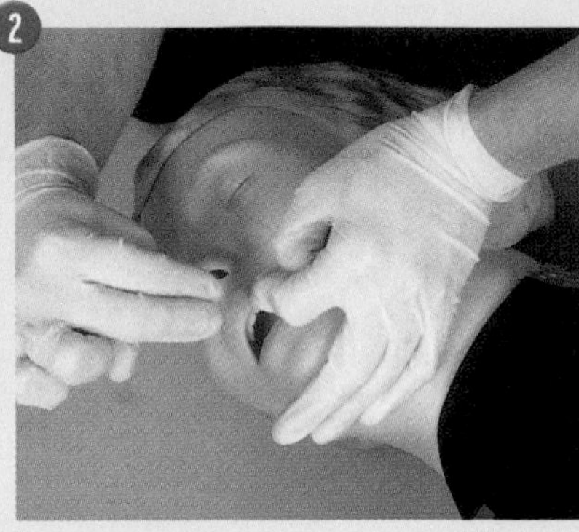

2. Insert your finger into the patient's mouth.

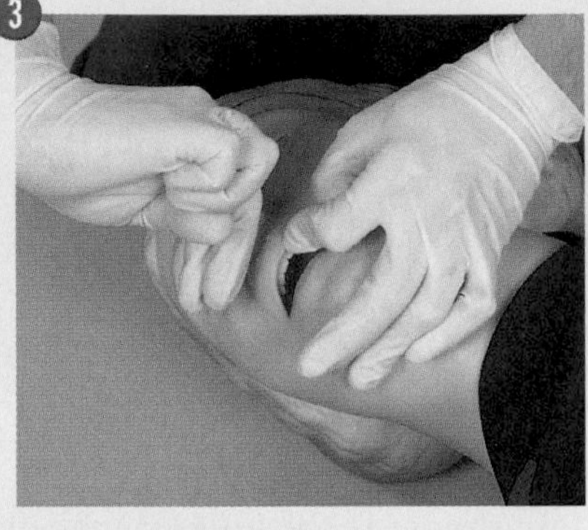

3. Curve your finger into a C-shape and sweep it from one side of the back of the mouth to the other.

Finger Sweeps

Finger sweeps can be done quickly and require no special equipment except a set of medical gloves. To perform a finger sweep, turn the patient's head to one side and use your gloved index and middle fingers to scoop out as much of the material as possible (**Figure 6.10**). A gauze pad wrapped around your gloved fingers may help remove the obstructing materials. Repeat the finger sweeps until you have removed all the foreign material in the patient's mouth. Finger sweeps should be your first attempt at clearing the airway even if suction equipment is available.

CAUTION

If the possibility of a spinal cord injury exists, be sure to logroll the patient onto his or her side and keep the head and neck in a neutral position. Open the mouth and use your gloved fingers in the same manner to clean out the mouth.

manual suction device A hand-powered device used for clearing the upper airway of mucus, blood, or vomitus.

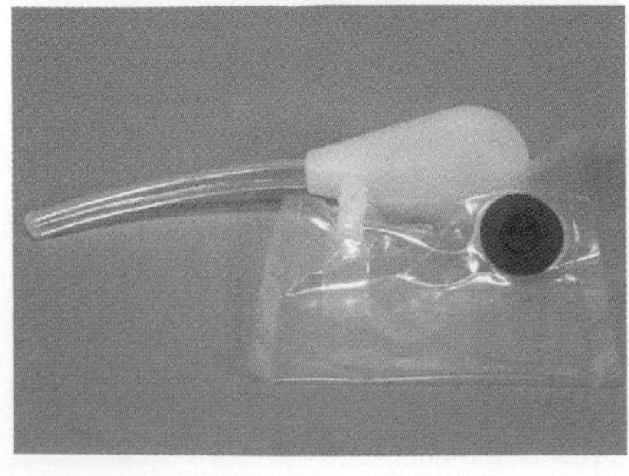

Figure 6.11 Manual suction devices.

Suctioning

Sometimes just sweeping out the mouth is not enough to clear the materials completely from the mouth and upper airway. Suction machines can be helpful in removing secretions such as vomitus, blood, and mucus from the patient's mouth. Two types of suction devices are available—manual and mechanical.

Manual Suction Devices Several **manual suction devices** are available to first responders (**Figure 6.11**). These devices are relatively inexpensive and are compact enough to fit into first responder life support kits. With most manual suction devices, you insert the end of the suction tip into the patient's mouth and squeeze or pump the hand-powered pump. Be sure that you do not insert the tip of the suction farther than you can see. Manual suction devices are used in the same way as the mechanical suction devices described in the following section. The only difference is the power source. Be sure to follow local medical protocols on first responders' authorization to use suction devices in the field.

Mechanical Suction Devices A **mechanical suction device** uses either a battery-powered pump or an oxygen-powered **aspirator** to create a vacuum that will draw the obstructing materials from the patient's airway (**Figure 6.12**). Usually, both a rigid suction tip and a flexible whistle tip catheter can be used with mechanical suction devices. To use this type of suction machine, you must first learn how to operate the device and control the force of the suction.

When using mechanical suction, first clear the mouth of large pieces of material with your gloved fingers. After the mouth is clear, turn the suction device on and use the rigid tip to remove most of the remaining material. Do not suction for more than 15 seconds at a time because the suction draws air out of the patient's airway, as well as any obstructing material.

If the rigid tip has a suction control port (a small hole located close to the tip's handle), you must place a finger over the hole to create the suction (**Figure 6.13**). Do not keep your finger over this control port for longer than 15 seconds at a time because you may rob the patient of oxygen.

After you have cleared most of the obstructing material out of the patient's mouth and upper airway with the rigid tip, change to the flexible tip and clear out material from the deeper parts of the patient's throat (**Figure 6.14**).

Flexible whistle tip catheters also have suction control ports, which are located close to the end of the catheter that attaches to the suction machine. Again, place a finger over the control port to achieve suction.

Suctioning the airway (either manually or mechanically) is a lifesaving technique. Although a gauze pad and your gloved fingers can do most of the work, the use of supplementary suction devices enables you to remove much more obstructing material from the patient's airway.

Maintain the Airway

If a patient is unable to keep the airway open, you must open the airway manually. You have learned how to do this by using the head tilt–chin lift or jaw-thrust techniques to open the airway.

Remember

Do not suction any deeper than you can see.

mechanical suction device An electrically or battery powered device used for clearing the upper airway of mucus, blood, or vomitus.

aspirator A suction device.

Special Needs

INFANTS AND CHILDREN

- When suctioning a child's airway, suction for no more than 10 seconds at a time.
- When suctioning an infant's airway, suction for no more than 5 seconds at a time.

Remember

Do not forget to ventilate all patients who are not breathing.

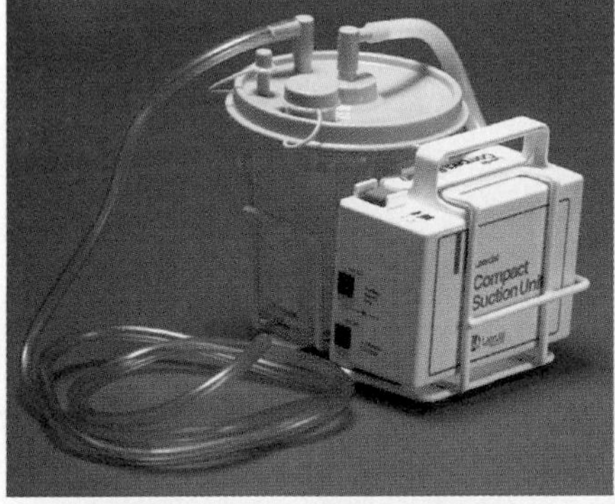

Figure 6.12 Battery-powered suction device.

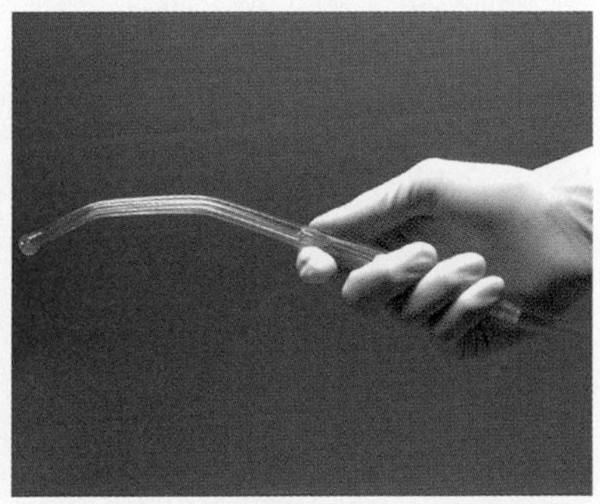

Figure 6.13 Rigid suction tip.

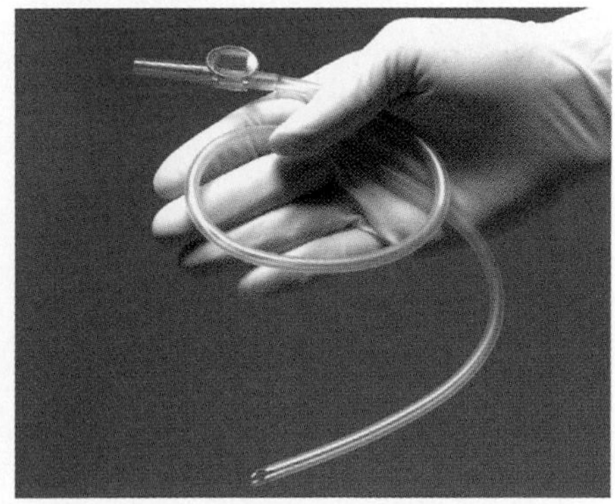

Figure 6.14 Flexible suction catheter.

BSI Tip

Use body substance isolation (BSI) techniques when clearing the patient's airway.

Unconscious patients will not be able to keep their airway open. You can continue to keep their airway open by using the head tilt–chin lift or jaw-thrust technique. To do this, you must continue holding the patient's head to maintain the head tilt or the jaw-thrust position.

If the patient is breathing adequately, you can keep the airway open by placing the patient in the recovery position. You can also insert an oral or nasal airway to keep the patient's airway open. These two mechanical airway devices will maintain the patient's airway after you have opened it manually.

Recovery Position

If an unconscious patient is breathing and the patient has not suffered trauma, one way to keep the airway open is to place the patient in the recovery position. The recovery position helps keep the patient's airway open by allowing secretions to drain out of the mouth instead of draining into the trachea. It also uses gravity to help keep the patient's tongue and lower jaw from blocking the airway.

To place a patient in the recovery position, carefully roll the patient onto one side as you support the patient's head. Roll the patient as a unit without twisting the body. You can use the patient's hand to help hold his or her head in a good position. Place the patient's face on its side so any secretions drain out of the mouth. The head should be in a position similar to the tilted back position of the head tilt–chin lift technique. See **Figure 6.15** for a demonstration of the recovery position.

Oral Airway

An **oral airway** has two primary purposes. It is used to maintain the patient's airway after you have manually opened the airway. It also functions as a pathway through which you can suction the patient. Oral airways can be used for unconscious patients who are breathing or who are in **respiratory arrest**. An oral airway can be used in any unconscious patient who does not have a **gag reflex**. Oral airways cannot be used in conscious patients because they have a gag reflex. These airways can be used with mechanical breathing devices such as the **pocket mask**.

oral airway An airway adjunct that is inserted into the mouth to keep the tongue from blocking the upper airway. It is also called an oropharyngeal or nasopharyngeal airway.

gag reflex A strong involuntary effort to vomit caused by something being placed or caught in the throat.

respiratory arrest Sudden stoppage of breathing.

pocket mask A mechanical breathing device used to administer mouth-to-mask rescue breathing.

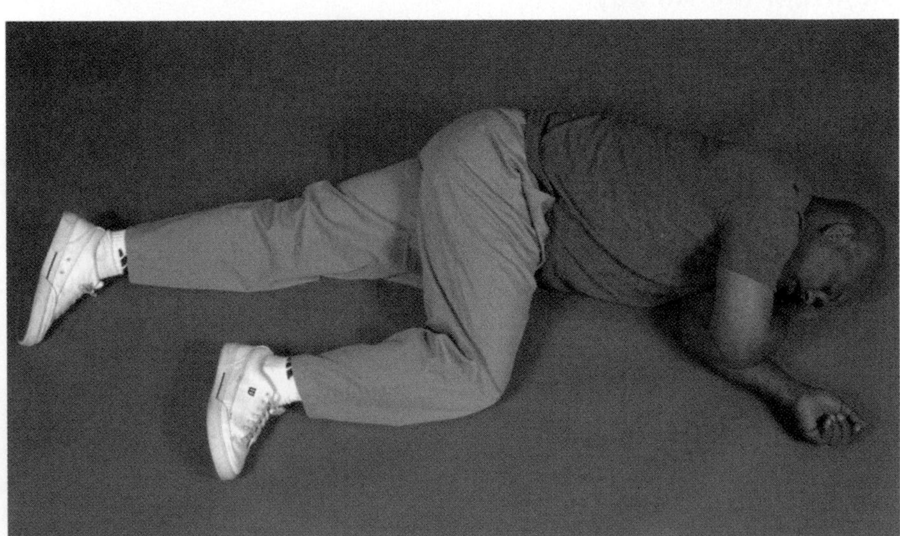

Figure 6.15 Recovery position for an unconscious patient.

There are two styles of oral airways. One has an opening down the center, and the other has a slot along each side. The opening or slot permits the free flow of air and allows you to suction through the airway (**Figure 6.16**). Before you insert the oral airway, you need to select the proper size. Choose the proper size by measuring from the earlobe to the corner of the patient's mouth. When properly inserted, the airway will rest inside the mouth. The curve of the airway should follow the contour of the tongue. The flange should rest against the lips. The other end should be resting in the back of the throat.

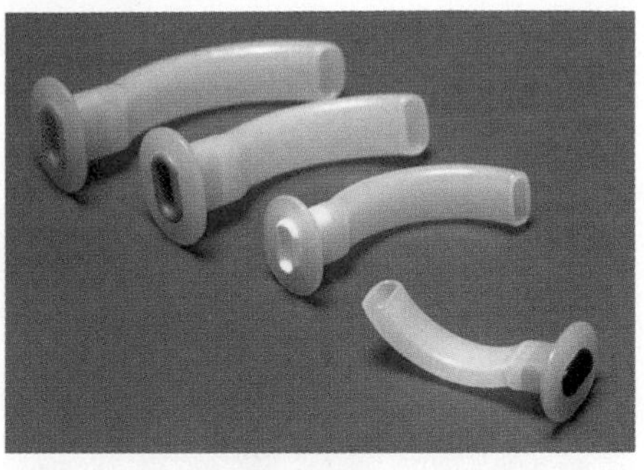

Figure 6.16 Oral airways.

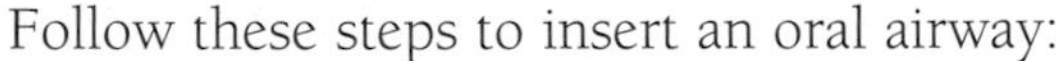

Follow these steps to insert an oral airway:

1. Select the proper sized airway by measuring from the patient's earlobe to the corner of the mouth (**Figure 6.17, step 1**).
2. Open the patient's mouth with one hand after manually opening the patient's airway with a head tilt–chin lift or jaw-thrust technique.
3. Hold the airway upside down with your other hand. Insert the airway into the patient's mouth and guide the tip of the airway along the roof of the patient's mouth, advancing it until you feel resistance (**Figure 6.17, step 2**).
4. Rotate the airway 180° until the flange comes to rest on the patient's teeth or lips (**Figure 6.17, step 3**).

Be especially careful when you insert the airway. You could injure the roof of the patient's mouth by the rough insertion of an oral airway. Remember that an oral airway does not open the patient's airway. It will maintain the open airway after you have opened it with a manual technique.

Skill Drill

Figure 6.17 Inserting an Oral Airway

1

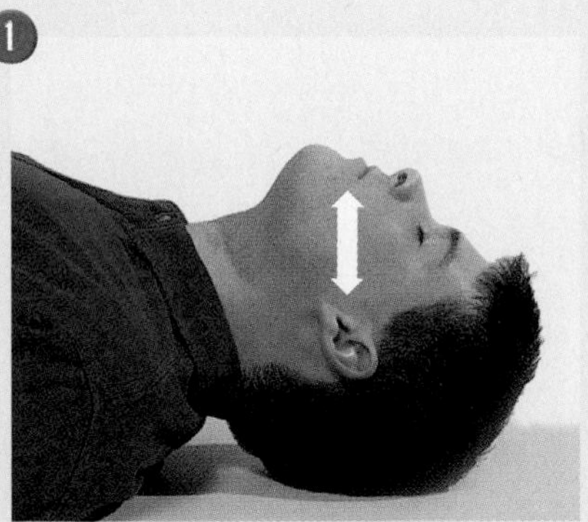

Proper sizing of an oral airway.

2

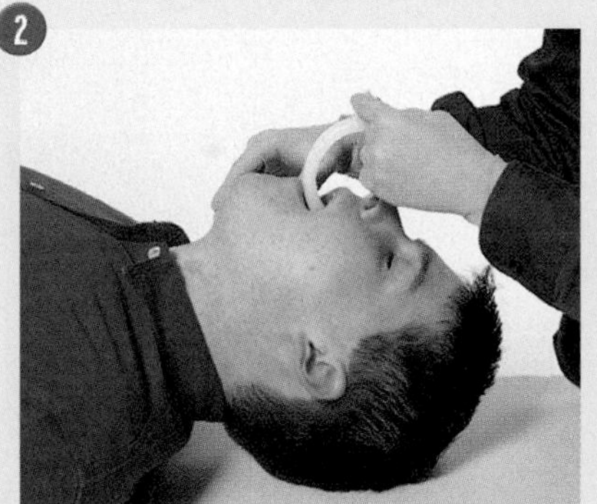

Inserting the oral airway.

3

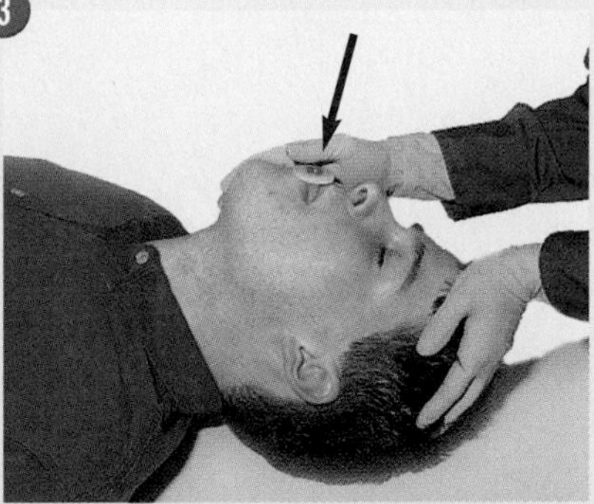

Proper position of flange after insertion.

nasal airway An airway adjunct that is inserted into the nostril of a patient who is not able to maintain a natural airway. It is also called a nasopharyngeal airway.

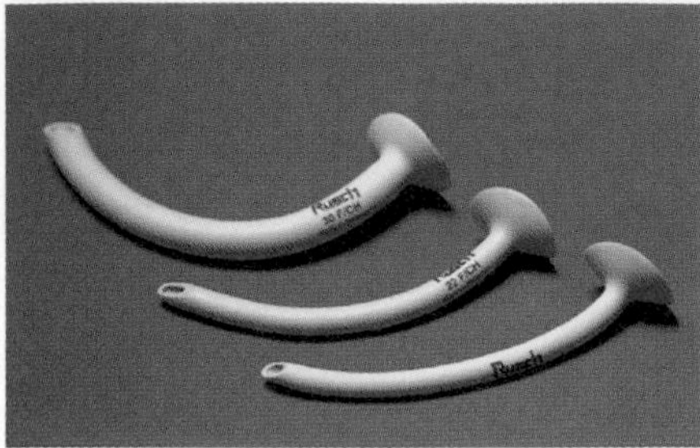

Figure 6.18 Nasal airways.

Nasal Airway

A second type of device you can use to keep the patient's airway open is a **nasal airway** (**Figure 6.18**). This device is inserted into the patient's nose. Nasal airways can be used in both unconscious and conscious patients who are not able to maintain an open airway. Usually a patient will tolerate a nasal airway better than an oral airway. It is not as likely to cause vomiting. One disadvantage of a nasal airway is that you cannot suction through it if the inside diameter of the airway is too small for a whistle tip suction catheter.

You will have to select the proper size nasal airway for the patient. Measure from the tip of the patient's nose to the bottom of the ear. Coat the airway with a water-soluble lubricant before inserting it. This makes it easier for you to insert the airway and reduces the chance of trauma to the patient's airway.

Insert the airway in the larger nostril. As you insert the airway, follow the curvature of the floor of the nose. The airway is fully inserted when the flange or trumpet rests against the patient's nostril. At this point, the other end of the airway will reach the back of the patient's throat and an open airway for the patient can be maintained.

Follow these steps to insert a nasal airway:

1. Select the proper sized airway by measuring from the tip of the patient's nose to the earlobe (**Figure 6.19, step 1**).
2. Coat the airway with a water-soluble lubricant.
3. Select the larger nostril.
4. Gently stretch the nostril open by using your thumb.
5. Gently insert the airway until the flange rests against the nose (**Figure 6.19, steps 2 and 3**). Do not force the airway. If you feel any resistance, remove the airway and try to insert it in the other nostril.

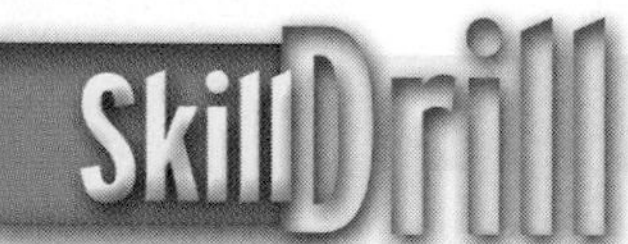

Figure 6.19 Inserting a Nasal Airway

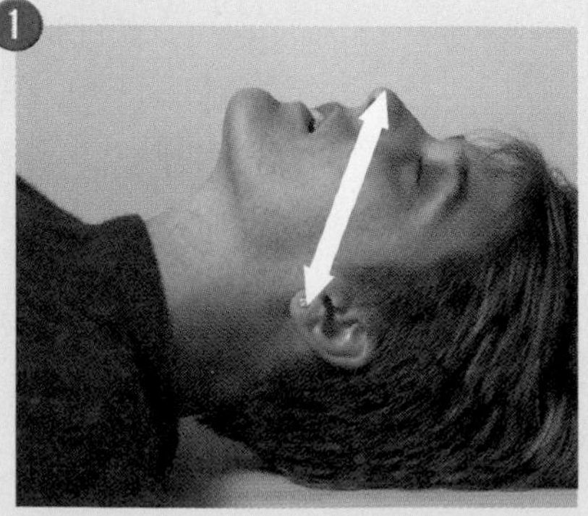

1 Proper sizing of a nasal airway.

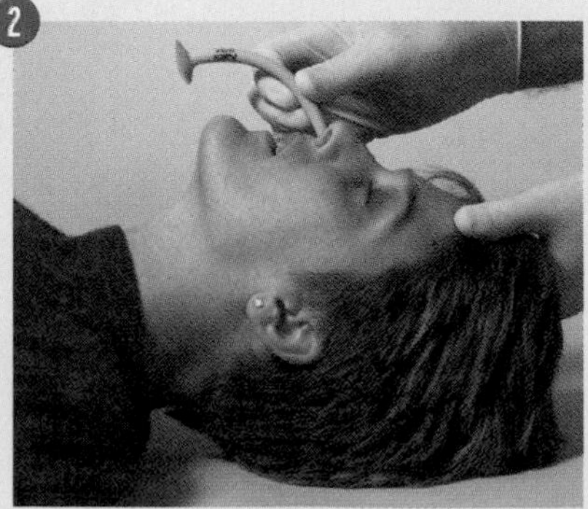

2 Inserting a nasal airway.

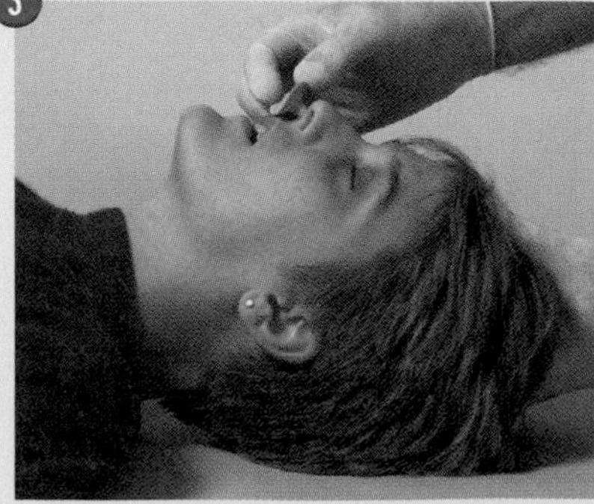

3 Proper position of flange after insertion.

Practice selecting the proper size and inserting the airway until you can do it quickly and smoothly.

CAUTION

If a patient has suffered severe head trauma, there is some chance that a nasal airway may further damage the brain. You should check with your local medical control to determine the protocol for using a nasal airway in these patients.

Check✓point

Fill in the following blanks:

- ◯ First, check the patient for ______________________________
- ◯ Correct the blocked airway by 1. ______________________________ or
  2. ______________________________
- ◯ Check for 1. ______________________________
  2. ______________________________ or
  3. ______________________________
- ◯ Correct the airway using 1. ______________________________ or
  2. ______________________________
- ◯ Maintain the airway by 1. ______________________________
  2. ______________________________ or
  3. ______________________________

"B" Is for Breathing

After you have checked and corrected the patient's airway, you should move on to check and correct the patient's breathing. To do this, you must understand the signs of adequate breathing, the signs of inadequate breathing, and the signs and causes of respiratory arrest.

Remember

To *open* the patient's airway:

1. Perform the head tilt-chin lift technique, or
2. Perform the jaw-thrust technique.

To *maintain* the patient's airway,

1. Continue to apply the head tilt-chin lift technique, or
2. Continue to apply the jaw-thrust technique, or
3. Insert an oral airway, or
4. Insert a nasal airway, or
5. Place the patient in the recovery position.

After you open and maintain the patient's airway, you need to continue to monitor the status of the patient's breathing.

Special Needs

CHILDREN

The roof of a child's mouth is much more fragile than that of an adult. This means you must be especially careful to avoid injuring it as you insert the oral airway. The technique for inserting an oral airway in a child is almost the same as for an adult patient. However, to make it easier to insert the airway, use two or three stacked tongue blades and depress the tongue. This will press the tongue forward and away from the roof of the mouth so you can insert the airway.

Signs & Symptoms

RESPIRATORY ARREST

- No chest movement
- No breath sounds
- No air movement
- Blue skin (cyanosis), especially around the lips

Signs of Adequate Breathing

To check for adequate breathing, you must look, listen, and feel at the same time. If a patient is breathing adequately, you can look for the rise and fall of the patient's chest, you can listen for the sounds of air passing into or out of the patient's nose and mouth, and you can feel the air moving on the side of your face. Place the side of your face close to the patient's nose and mouth and watch the patient's chest. In this way, you can look for chest movements, listen for the sounds of air moving, and feel the air as it moves in and out of the patient's nose and mouth. A normal adult has a resting breathing rate of approximately 12 to 20 breaths per minute. Remember that one breath includes both an inhalation and an exhalation.

Signs of Inadequate Breathing

If a patient is breathing inadequately, you will detect signs of abnormal respirations. Noisy respirations, wheezing, or gurgling indicate partial blockage or constriction somewhere along the respiratory tract. Rapid or gasping respirations may indicate that the patient is not receiving an adequate amount of oxygen due to illness or injury. The patient's skin may be pale or even blue, especially around the lips or fingernail beds.

The most critical sign of inadequate breathing is respiratory arrest (total lack of respirations). This critical state is characterized by no chest movements, no breath sounds, and no air against the side of your face. In patients with severe hypothermia, respirations can be slowed (and/or shallow) to the point that the patient appears clinically dead.

There are many causes of respiratory arrest. By far the most common cause is heart attack, which claims more than 500,000 lives each year. Other major causes of respiratory arrest include:

- Mechanical blockage or obstruction caused by the tongue
- Vomitus, particularly in a patient weakened by an illness such as a stroke
- Foreign objects: teeth, dentures, balloons, marbles, pieces of food, or pieces of hard candy (especially in small children)
- Illness or disease such as heart attack or severe stroke
- Drug overdose
- Poisoning
- Severe loss of blood
- Electrocution by electrical current or lightning

Check for the Presence of Breathing

After establishing the loss of consciousness and opening the airway of the unconscious patient, check for breathing by looking, listening, and feeling (**Figure 6.20**):

- Look for the rising and falling of the patient's chest.
- Listen for the sound of air moving in and out of the patient's nose and mouth.
- Feel for the movement of air on the side of your face and ear.

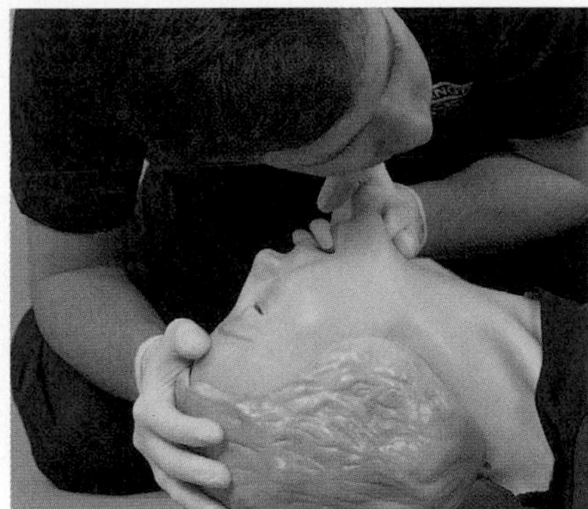

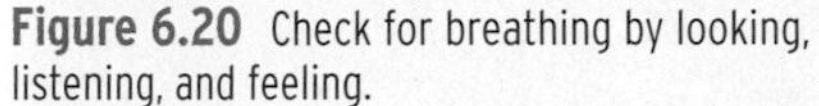

Figure 6.20 Check for breathing by looking, listening, and feeling.

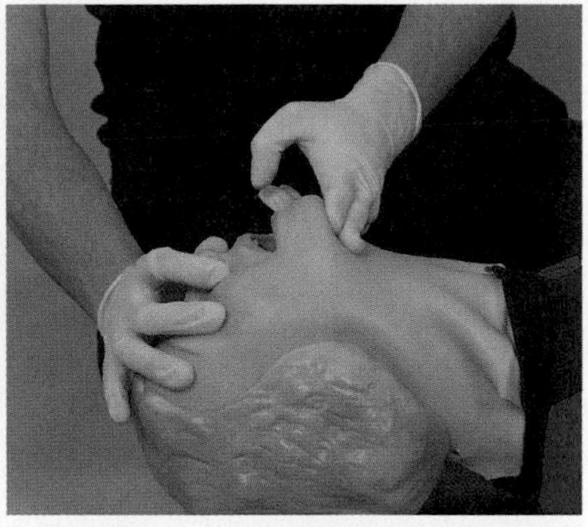

Figure 6.21 To perform resuce breathing, pinch the patient's nose with your thumb and forefinger.

Continue to look, listen, and feel for at least 3 to 5 seconds; if you do not, you risk checking the patient between breaths and missing any signs of breathing that are present. Your breathing check should take no more than 10 seconds. If there are no signs of breathing, proceed to the next step and correct the lack of breathing by beginning rescue breathing. If the patient is breathing adequately (about 12 to 20 times a minute), you can continue to maintain the airway and monitor the rate and depth of respirations to ensure adequate breathing continues.

Correct the Breathing

You must breathe for any patient who is not breathing. As you perform **rescue breathing**, keep the patient's airway open by using the head tilt–chin lift method (or the jaw-thrust method for patients with head or neck injuries). To perform rescue breathing, blow your air into the patient's mouth. Pinch the patient's nose with your thumb and forefinger, take a deep breath, and blow slowly for 2 seconds (**Figure 6.21**).

Use slow, gentle, sustained breathing and just enough breath to make the patient's chest rise. This minimizes the amount of air blown into the stomach. Remove your mouth and allow the lungs to deflate. Breathe for the patient a second time. After these first two breaths, breathe once into the patient's mouth every 4 to 5 seconds. The rate of breaths should be 10 to 12 per minute for an adult.

Rescue breathing can be done by using a mouth-to-mask device, a barrier device, or just your mouth. The mouth-to-mask and barrier devices prevent you from putting your mouth directly on the patient's mouth. These devices should be available to you as a first responder.

If a rescue breathing device is not available, you must weigh the potential good to the patient against the limited chance that you will contract an infectious disease if you perform mouth-to-mouth rescue breathing.

rescue breathing Artificial means of breathing for a patient.

mouth-to-mask ventilation device A piece of equipment that consists of a mask, a one-way valve, and a mouthpiece. Rescue breathing is performed by breathing into the mouthpiece after placing the mask over the patient's mouth and nose.

Mouth-to-Mask Rescue Breathing

Your first responder life support kit should contain an artificial ventilation device that enables you to perform rescue breathing without mouth-to-mouth contact with the patient. This simple piece of equipment is called a **mouth-to-mask ventilation device**. A mouth-to-mask ventilation device consists of a mask that fits over the patient's face, a one-way

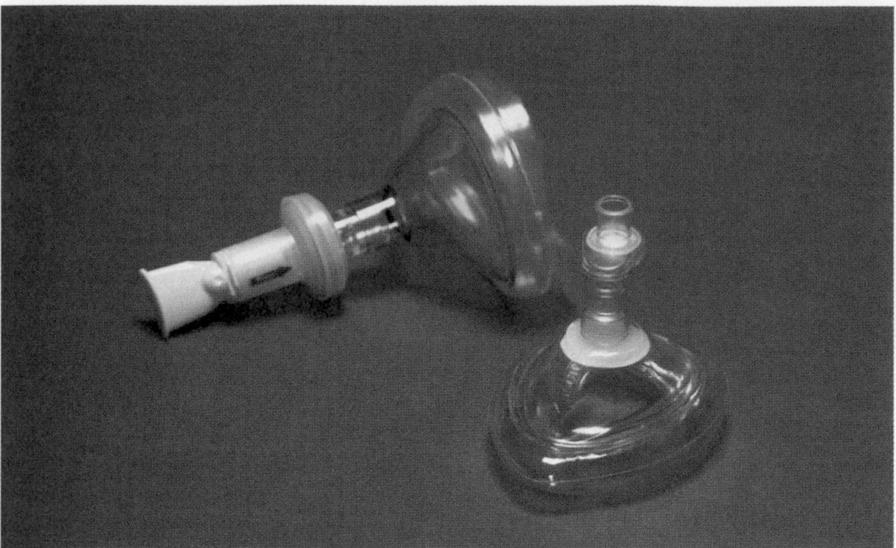

Figure 6.22 Types of mouth-to-mask ventilation devices.

valve, and a mouthpiece through which the rescuer breathes. It may also have an inlet port for supplemental oxygen and a tube between the mouthpiece and the mask. These devices are shown in **Figure 6.22**. Because mouth-to-mask devices prevent direct contact between you and the patient, they reduce the risk of transmitting infectious diseases.

To use a mouth-to-mask ventilation device for rescue breathing, follow these steps:

1. Position yourself at the patient's head.
2. Use the head tilt–chin lift or jaw-thrust technique to open the patient's airway (**Figure 6.23, steps 1 and 2**).
3. Place the mask over the patient's mouth and nose. Make sure that the mask's nose notch is on the nose and not the chin.
4. Grasp the mask and the patient's jaw, using both hands. Use the thumb and forefinger of each hand to hold the mask tightly against the face. Hook the other three fingers of each hand under the patient's jaw and lift up to seal the mask tightly against the patient's face (**Figure 6.23, step 3**).
5. Maintain an airtight seal as you pull up on the jaw to maintain the proper head position.
6. Take a deep breath, then seal your mouth over the mouthpiece.
7. Breathe slowly into the mouthpiece for 2 seconds (**Figure 6.23, step 4**). Breathe until the patient's chest rises.
8. Monitor the patient for proper head position, air exchange, and vomiting.

Practice this technique frequently on a manikin until you can do it well.

Skill Drill

Figure 6.23 Performing Mouth-to-Mask Rescue Breathing

1

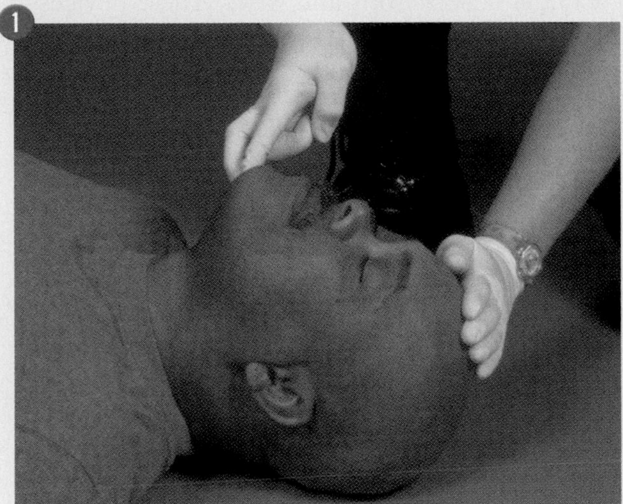

Open the airway using the head tilt-chin lift technique.

2

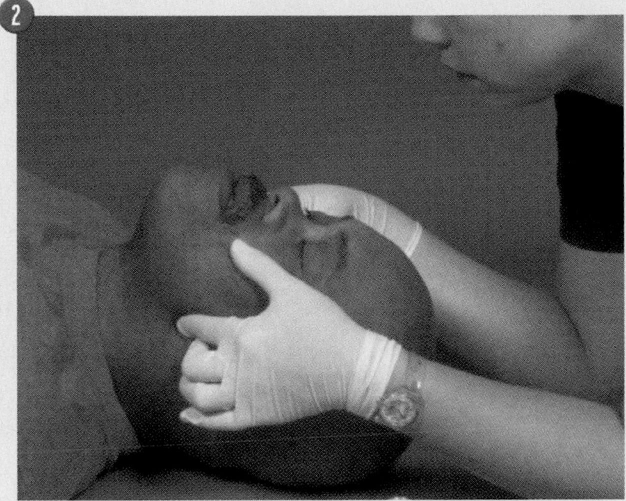

Or, open the airway using the jaw-thrust technique.

3

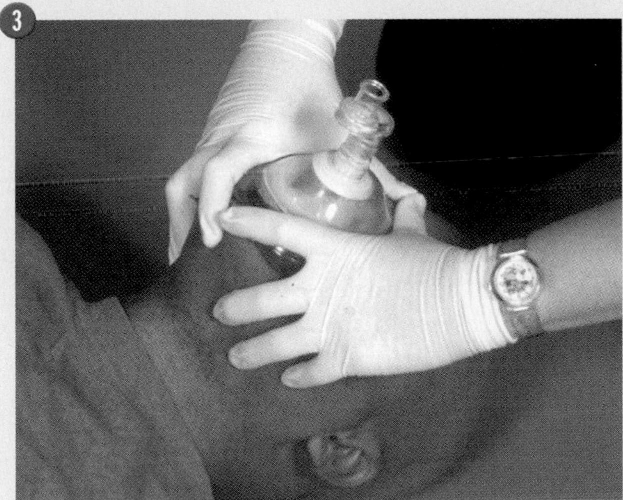

Seal the mask against the patient's face.

4

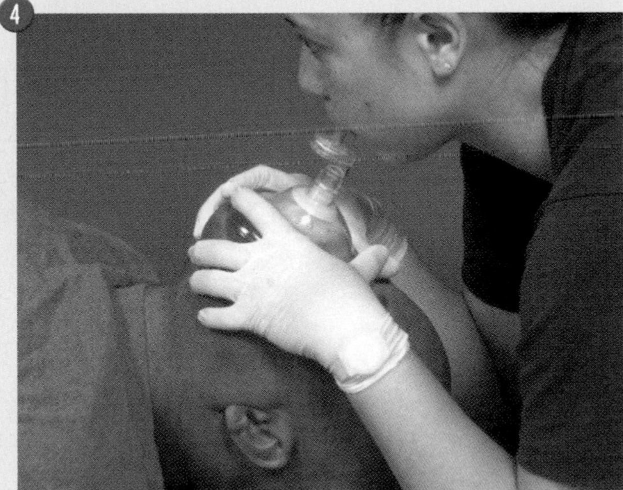

Breathe through the mouthpiece.

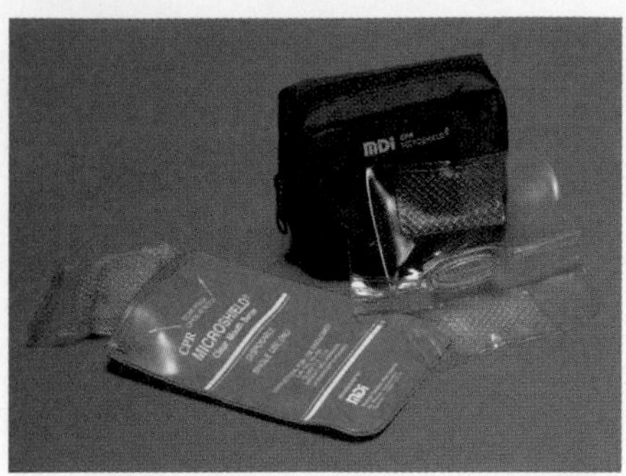

Figure 6.24 Barrier devices.

Mouth-to-Barrier Rescue Breathing

Mouth-to-barrier devices also provide a barrier between the rescuer and the patient (**Figure 6.24**). Some of these devices are small enough to carry in your pocket. Although a wide variety of devices is available, most of them consist of a port or hole that you breathe into and a mask or plastic film that covers the patient's face. Some also have a one-way valve that prevents backflow of secretions and gases. These devices provide variable degrees of infection control.

To perform mouth-to-mouth rescue breathing with a barrier device, follow these steps (**Figure 6.25**):

1. Open the airway with the head tilt–chin lift technique.
2. Press on the forehead to maintain the backward tilt of the head.
3. Pinch the patient's nostrils together with your thumb and forefinger.
4. Keep the patient's mouth open with the thumb of whichever hand you are using to lift the patient's chin.
5. Place the barrier device over the patient's mouth.
6. Take a deep breath, then make a tight seal by placing your mouth on the barrier device around the patient's mouth.
7. Breathe slowly into the patient's mouth for 2 seconds. Breathe until the patient's chest rises.
8. Remove your mouth and allow the patient to exhale passively. Check to see that the patient's chest falls after each exhalation.
9. Repeat this rescue breathing sequence 10 to 12 times per minute (one breath every 4 to 5 seconds) for an adult.

Mouth-to-Mouth Rescue Breathing

Mouth-to-mouth rescue breathing is an effective way of providing artificial ventilation for nonbreathing patients. It requires no equipment except you. However, because there is a somewhat higher risk of contracting a disease when using this method, you should use a mask or barrier breathing device if available. If a rescue breathing device is not available, you must weigh the potential good to the patient against the limited chance that you will contract an infectious disease from mouth-to-mouth breathing.

To perform mouth-to-mouth rescue breathing, follow these steps:

1. Open the airway with the head tilt–chin lift technique.
2. Press on the forehead to maintain the backward tilt of the head.
3. Pinch the patient's nostrils together with your thumb and forefinger.
4. Keep the patient's mouth open with the thumb of whichever hand you are using to lift the patient's chin.
5. Take a deep breath, then make a tight seal by placing your mouth over the patient's mouth.
6. Breathe slowly into the patient's mouth for 2 seconds. Breathe until the patient's chest rises.
7. Remove your mouth and allow the patient to exhale passively. Check to see that the patient's chest falls after each exhalation.
8. Repeat this rescue breathing sequence 10 to 12 times per minute for adult patients and about 20 times per minute for children and infants.

Remember

The three methods for performing rescue breathing are all potentially lifesaving. You should use a mouth-to-mask or mouth-to-barrier breathing device whenever possible. If a rescue breathing device is not available, you must weigh the potential good to the patient against the limited chance that you will contract an infectious disease from mouth-to-mouth breathing.

Skill Drill

Figure 6.25 Performing Mouth-to-Barrier Rescue Breathing

1

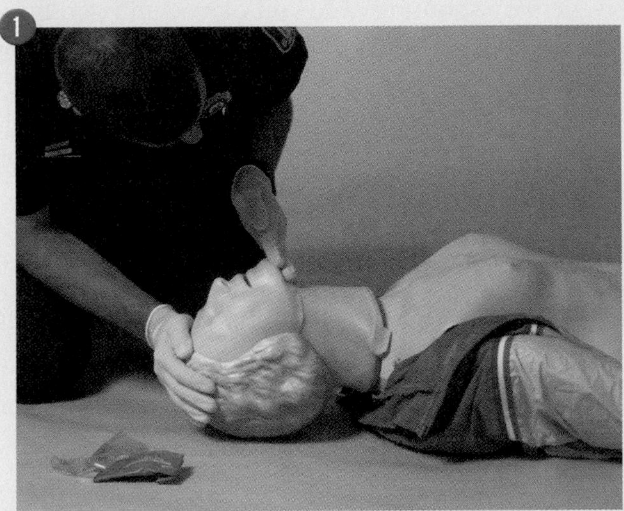

Open the airway using the head tilt-chin lift technique.

2

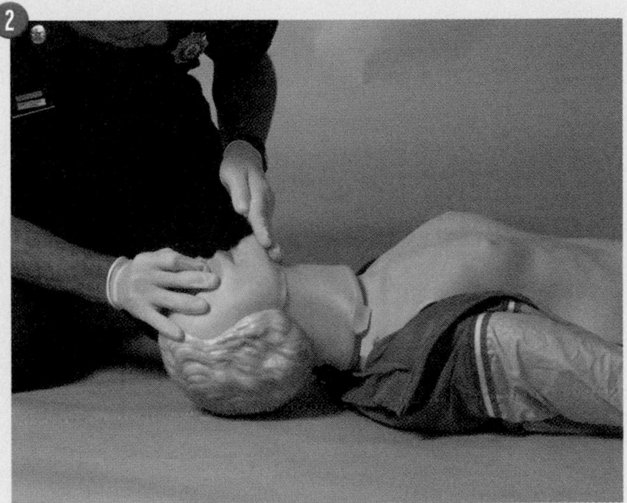

Pinch the patient's nostrils together.

3

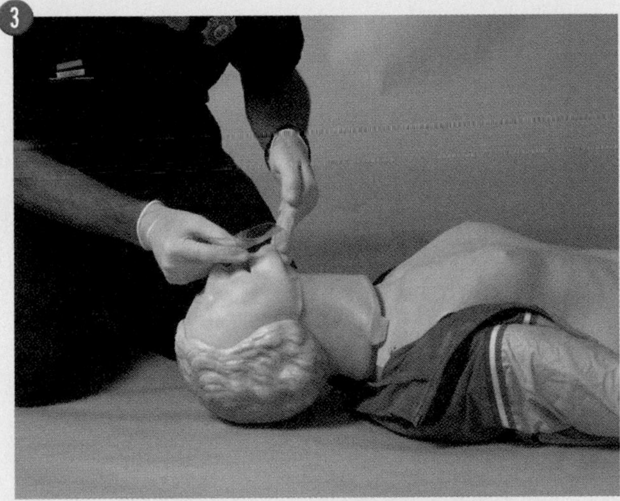

Place the barrier device over the patient's mouth.

4

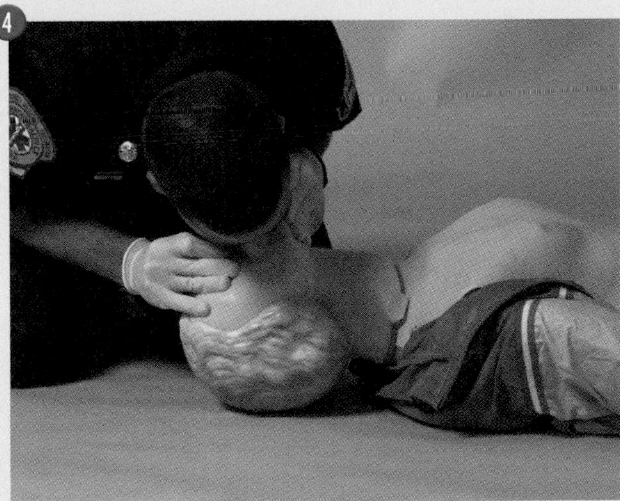

Perform rescue breathing.

Airway and Breathing Review

Assume that all patients may be in respiratory arrest until you can assess them and determine whether they are breathing adequately. A summary of the steps required to recognize respiratory arrest and perform rescue breathing in adults follows.

Airway

1. *Check* for responsiveness by shouting "Are you okay?" and gently shaking the patient's shoulder. If the patient is unresponsive and the EMS system has not been notified, activate the EMS system. Place the patient on his or her back.
2. *Correct* a closed airway by using the head tilt–chin lift technique or, if the patient has suffered any injury to the head or neck, the jaw-thrust technique.
3. *Check* the mouth for secretions, vomitus, or solid objects.
4. *Correct* a blocked airway, if needed, by using finger sweeps or suction to remove foreign substances.
5. *Maintain* the airway by manually holding it open or by using an oral or nasal airway.

Breathing

1. *Check* for the presence of breathing:
   - *Look* for the rising and falling of the patient's chest.
   - *Listen* for the sound of air moving in and out of the patient's nose and mouth.
   - *Feel* for air moving on the side of your face and ear.

Continue to look, listen, and feel for at least 3 to 5 seconds. If the patient is breathing adequately, place him or her in the recovery position. If the patient is not breathing, go to step 2.

2. *Correct* the lack of breathing by performing rescue breathing using a mouth-to-mask or mouth-to-barrier device, if available. Blow slowly into the patient's mouth for 2 seconds, using slow, gentle, sustained breaths with enough force to make the chest rise. Remove your mouth and allow the lungs to deflate. Breathe for the patient a second time. After these first two breaths, breathe once into the patient's mouth about every 4 to 5 seconds.

Generally, when mouth-to-mouth rescue breathing is necessary, **external cardiac compressions** are also required. External cardiac compressions, the "C" part of the ABCs, are explained in Chapter 8. A skill performance sheet titled "Adult One-Rescuer CPR" is shown in **Figure 6.26** for your review and practice.

external cardiac compressions A means of applying artificial circulation by applying rhythmic pressure and relaxation on the lower half of the sternum.

Performing Rescue Breathing on Children and Infants

The "A" steps required to check and correct the patient's airway and the "B" steps needed to check and correct the patient's breathing are similar for adults, children, and infants. However, there are some differences. You must learn and practice the different airway and breathing sequences for children and infants.

Figure 6.26 Skill Performance Sheet

Adult One-Rescuer CPR

Steps	Adequately Performed
1. Establish unresponsiveness. Activate the EMS system.	
2. Open airway using head tilt-chin lift. (If trauma is present use jaw-thrust.) Check breathing (look, listen, and feel).*	
3. Give two slow breaths at 2 seconds per breath. If airway is obstructed, reposition head and try to ventilate again.† Watch chest rise, allow for exhalation between breaths.	
4. Check for signs of circulation. Check carotid pulse and look for signs of coughing and movement. If breathing is absent but pulse is present, provide rescue breathing (1 breath every 4 to 5 seconds, about 10 to 12 breaths per minute).	
5. If no pulse, give cycles of 15 chest compressions (rate, 100 compressions per minute) followed by 2 slow breaths.	
6. After 4 cycles of 15 to 2 (about 1 minute), check pulse. *If no pulse, continue 15 to 2 cycle beginning with chest compressions.	

* *If victim is unresponsive but breathing, place in recovery position.* ***Based on the latest CPR guidelines.***

† *If still unsuccessful, begin the unresponsive Foreign Body Airway Obstruction (FBAO) sequence.*

Rescue Breathing for Children

For purposes of performing rescue breathing, a child is a person between one and eight years of age. The steps for determining responsiveness, checking and correcting airways, and checking and correcting a child's breathing are essentially the same as for an adult patient, but you should keep the following differences in mind:

1. Children are smaller, and you will not have to use as much force to open their airways and tilt their heads.
2. You should perform rescue breathing for 1 minute before activating the EMS system ("phone fast") if you are on the scene by yourself and EMS has not been notified.
3. Each rescue breath should be slightly shorter for a child, given over a period of 1 to 1½ seconds instead of over a period of 2 seconds for an adult patient.
4. The rate of rescue breathing is slightly faster for children. Give 1 rescue breath every 3 seconds (about 20 rescue breaths per minute), instead of the adult rate of one rescue breath every 4 to 5 seconds (about 12 rescue breaths per minute).

Figure 6.27 Skill Performance Sheet

Child One-Rescuer CPR

Steps	Adequately Performed
1. Establish unresponsiveness. If second rescuer is available, have him or her activate the EMS system.	
2. Open airway using head tilt-chin lift. (If trauma is present, use jaw-thrust.) Check breathing (look, listen, and feel).*	
3. Give two effective breaths (1 to 1½ seconds per breath); if airway is obstructed, reposition head and try to ventilate again.† Watch chest rise, allow for exhalation between breaths.	
4. Check for signs of circulation. Check carotid pulse and look for signs of coughing or movement. If breathing is absent but pulse is present, provide rescue breathing (1 breath every 3 seconds, about 20 breaths per minute).	
5. If no pulse, give 5 chest compressions (rate 100 compressions per minute), followed by one slow breath.	
6. After about 1 minute of rescue support, check pulse.* If rescuer is alone, activate the EMS system. If no pulse, continue 5:1 cycles.	

* *If victim is unresponsive but breathing, place in recovery position.* *Based on the latest CPR guidelines.*

† *If still unsuccessful, begin the unresponsive Foreign Body Airway Obstruction (FBAO) sequence.*

A skill performance sheet titled "Child One-Rescuer CPR" is shown in **Figure 6.27** for your review and practice.

Rescue Breathing for Infants

If the patient is an infant (under one year of age), you must vary rescue breathing techniques slightly. Keep in mind that an infant is tiny and must be treated very gently. The steps in rescue breathing for an infant are as follows:

Airway

1. *Check* for responsiveness by gently shaking the infant's shoulder or tapping the bottom of the foot (**Figure 6.28, step 1**). If the infant is unresponsive, place the infant on his or her back and proceed to step 2.
2. *Correct* the airway, if it is closed, by using the head tilt–chin lift technique (**Figure 6.28, step 2**). Do not tip the infant's head back too far because this may block the infant's airway. Tilt it only enough to open the airway.
3. *Check* for any visible secretions or foreign objects.
4. *Correct* any airway problems. Use finger sweeps only if there is a foreign object visible. If suction is needed, use it gently.
5. *Maintain* the airway by continuing to use the head tilt–chin lift technique.

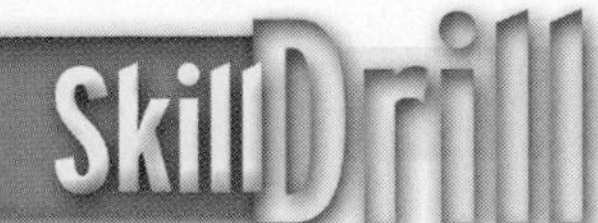

Figure 6.28 Infant Rescue Breathing

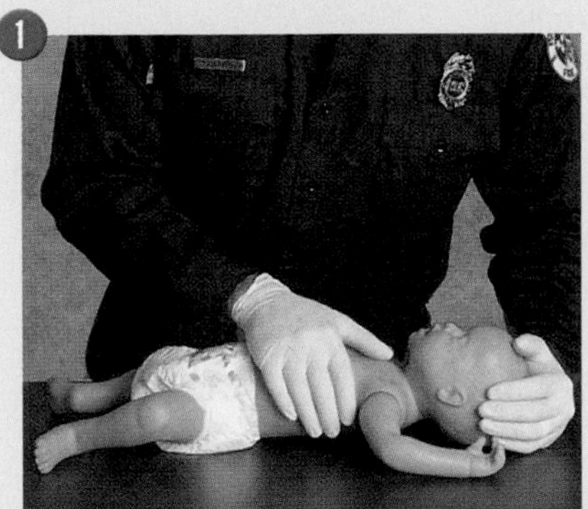

1 Establish the patient's level of responsiveness.

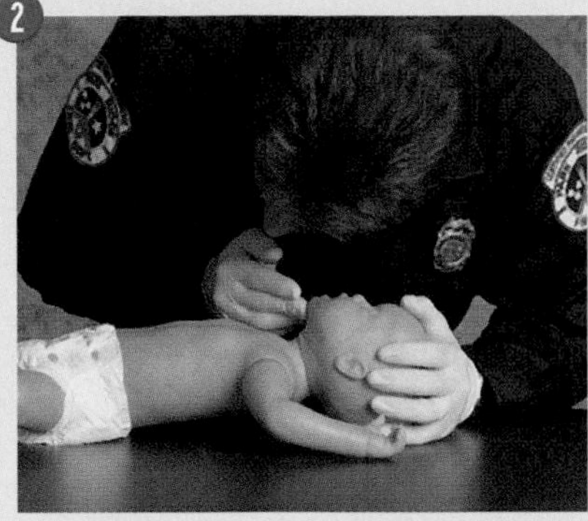

2 Open the infant's airway using the head tilt-chin lift technique and check for breathing by looking, listening, and feeling.

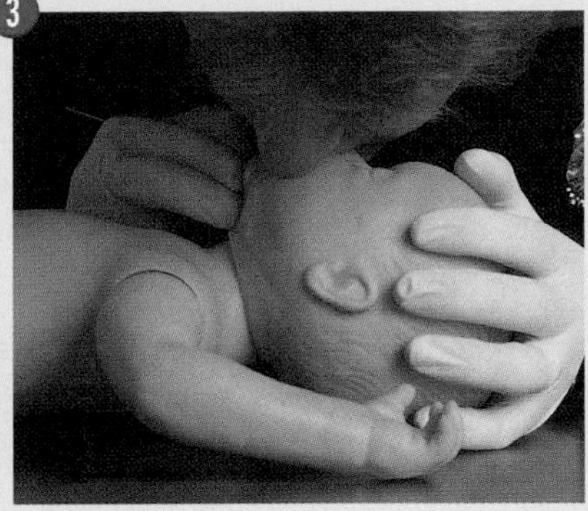

3 Perform infant rescue breathing.

Breathing

1. *Check* for the presence of breathing:
   - *Look* for the rising and falling of the infant's chest.
   - *Listen* for the sound of air moving in and out of the infant's mouth and nose.
   - *Feel* for the movement of air on the side of your face and ear (**Figure 6.28, step 2**).

Continue to look, listen, and feel for at least 3 to 5 seconds. If there is adequate breathing, place the patient in the recovery position. If there is no breathing, go to step 2.

2. *Correct* the lack of breathing by performing rescue breathing (**Figure 6.28, step 3**). Cover the infant's mouth and nose with your mouth. Blow gently into the infant's mouth and nose for 1 to $1\frac{1}{2}$ seconds. Watch the chest rise with each breath. Remove your mouth and allow the lungs to deflate. Breathe for the infant a second time. After these first two breaths, breathe into the infant's mouth and nose every 3 seconds (20 rescue breaths per minute).

Often when mouth-to-mouth rescue breathing is necessary, external cardiac compressions are also required. External cardiac compressions, the "C" part of the ABCs, are explained in Chapter 8. A skill performance sheet titled "Infant One-Rescuer CPR" is shown in **Figure 6.29**, page 124 for your review and practice.

Foreign Body Airway Obstruction

Causes of Airway Obstruction

Your attempt to perform rescue breathing may not be effective because of an airway obstruction. The most common airway obstruction is the

airway obstruction Partial or complete obstruction of the respiratory passages resulting from blockage by food, small objects, or vomitus.

Figure 6.29 Skill Performance Sheet

Infant One-Rescuer CPR

Steps	Adequately Performed
1. Establish unresponsiveness. If second rescuer is available, have him or her activate the EMS system.	
2. Open airway using the head tilt-chin lift. (If trauma is present, use jaw-thrust.) Check breathing (look, listen, and feel).*	
3. Give two effective breaths (1 to 1½ seconds per breath); if airway is obstructed, reposition head and try to ventilate again.† Watch chest rise, allow for exhalation between breaths.	
4. Check for signs of circulation. Check brachial pulse and look for signs of coughing or movement. If breathing is absent but pulse is present, provide rescue breathing (1 breath every 3 seconds, about 20 breaths per minute).	
5. If no pulse, give 5 chest compressions (rate at least 100 compressions per minute), followed by one slow breath.	
6. After about 1 minute of rescue support, check pulse.* If rescuer is alone, activate the EMS system. If no pulse, continue 5:1 cycles.	

* *If victim is unresponsive but breathing, place in recovery position.*

Based on the latest CPR guidelines.

† *If still unsuccessful, begin the unresponsive Foreign Body Airway Obstruction (FBAO) sequence.*

Checkpoint

- What are the signs of adequate breathing?
- What are the signs of inadequate breathing?
- What are the causes of respiratory arrest?
- What are the major signs of respiratory arrest?
- What are three ways to check for the presence of breathing?
- What are the steps for performing rescue breathing using each of the following methods:
  - Mouth-to-mask device?
  - Mouth-to-barrier device?
  - Mouth-to-mouth?

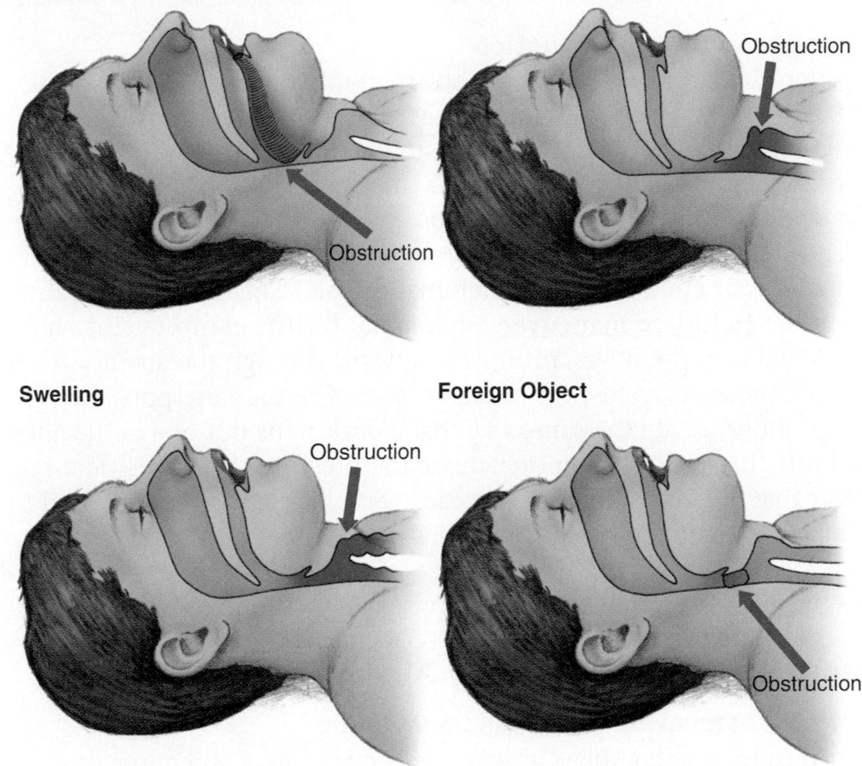

Figure 6.30 Common causes of airway obstruction.

tongue. If the tongue is blocking the airway, the head tilt–chin lift technique or the jaw-thrust technique should open the airway. However, if a foreign body is lodged in the air passages, you must use other techniques.

Food is the most common foreign object that causes an airway obstruction. An adult may choke on a large piece of meat; a child may inhale candy, a peanut, or a piece of a hot dog. Children may put small objects in their mouths and inhale such things as toys or balloons. Vomitus may obstruct the airway of a child or an adult (**Figure 6.30**).

Types of Airway Obstruction

Airway obstruction may be partial or complete. The first step in caring for a conscious person who may have an obstructed airway is to ask, "Are you choking?" If the patient can reply to your question, the airway is not completely blocked. If the patient is unable to speak or cough, the airway is completely blocked.

Partial Airway Obstruction

In partial airway obstruction, the patient coughs and gags. This indicates that some air is passing around the obstruction. The patient may even be able to speak, although with difficulty.

To treat a partially obstructed airway, encourage the patient to cough. Coughing is the most effective way of expelling a foreign object. If the patient is unable to expel the object by coughing (if, for example, a bone is stuck in the throat), you should arrange for the patient's T ***prompt transport*** to an appropriate medical facility. Such a patient must be monitored carefully while awaiting transport and during transport because a partial obstruction can become a complete obstruction at any moment.

Complete Airway Obstruction

A patient with a complete airway obstruction will have different signs and symptoms. The body quickly uses all the oxygen breathed in with the last breath. The patient is unable to breathe in or out and, because he or she cannot exhale air, speech is impossible. If the airway is completely obstructed, the patient will lose consciousness in 3 to 4 minutes.

The currently accepted treatment for a completely obstructed airway in an adult or child involves abdominal thrusts. This technique is also called the **Heimlich maneuver**. Abdominal thrusts compress the air that remains in the lungs, pushing it upward through the airway so that it exerts pressure against the foreign object. The pressure pops the object out, in much the same way that a cork pops out of a bottle after the bottle has been shaken to increase the pressure. Many rescuers report that abdominal thrusts can cause an obstructing piece of food to fly across the room. A person who has had an obstruction removed from their airway by the Heimlich maneuver should be T ***transported*** to a hospital for examination by a physician.

Heimlich maneuver A series of manual thrusts to the abdomen to relieve upper airway obstruction.

Management of Foreign Body Airway Obstructions

Airway Obstruction in a Conscious Adult

The steps to treat complete airway obstruction vary, depending on whether the patient is conscious or unconscious. If the patient is conscious, stand behind the patient and perform the abdominal thrusts while the patient is standing or seated in a chair.

Locate the xiphoid process (the bottom of the sternum) and the navel. Place one fist above the navel and well below the xiphoid process, thumb side against the patient's abdomen. Grasp your fist with your other hand. Then apply abdominal thrusts sharply and firmly, bringing your fist in and slightly upward. Do not give the patient a bear hug; rather, apply pressure at the point where your fist contacts the patient's abdomen. Each thrust should be distinct and forceful. Repeat these abdominal thrusts until the foreign object is expelled or until the patient becomes unconscious (**Figure 6.31**).

Review the following sequence until you can carry it out automatically. To assist a conscious patient with a complete airway obstruction, you must:

1. Ask, "Are you choking? Can you speak?" If there is no response, assume that the airway obstruction is complete.
2. Stand behind the patient and deliver an abdominal thrust (position the thumb side of your fist above the patient's navel and well below the xiphoid process). Press into the patient's abdomen with a quick upward thrust.
3. Repeat the abdominal thrusts until either the foreign body is expelled or the patient becomes unconscious.
4. If the patient is obese or in the late stages of pregnancy, use chest thrusts instead of abdominal thrusts. Chest thrusts are done by standing behind the patient and placing your arms under the patient's armpits to encircle the patient's chest. Press with quick backward thrusts.

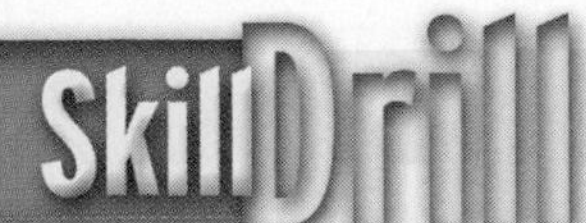

Figure 6.31 Airway Obstruction in a Conscious Patient

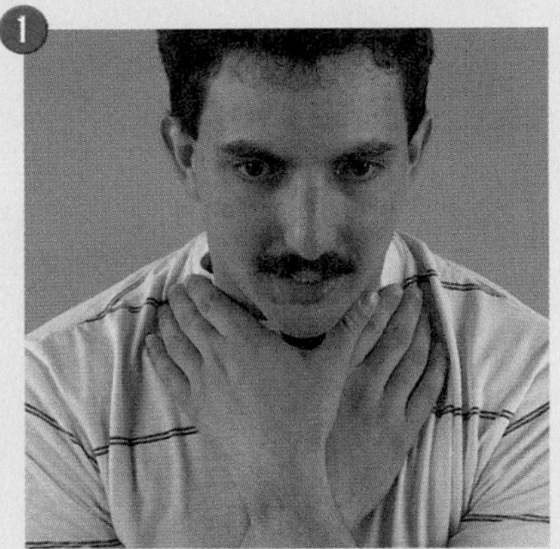

1 Look for a sign of choking.

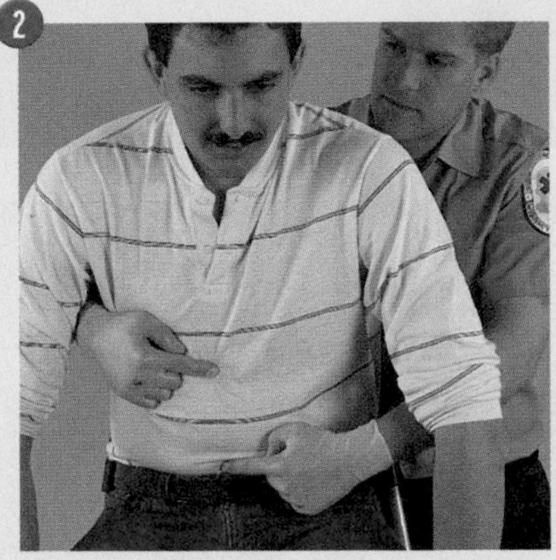

2 Locate the xiphoid process and the navel.

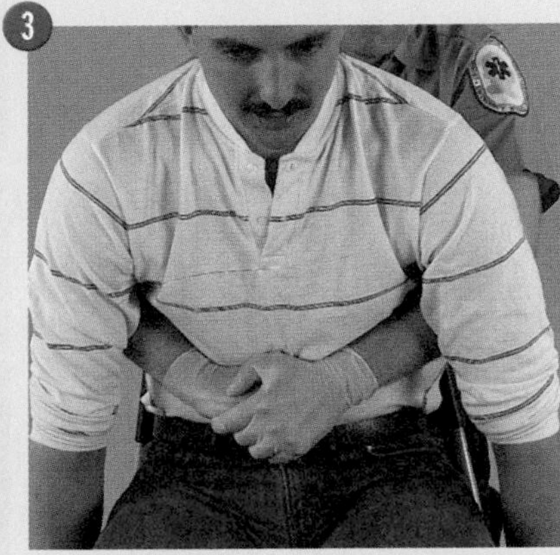

3 Apply abdominal thrusts.

A skill performance sheet titled "Conscious Adult—Foreign Body Airway Obstruction" is shown in **Figure 6.32** for your review and practice.

Figure 6.32 Skill Performance Sheet

Conscious Adult–Foreign Body Airway Obstruction

Steps	Adequately Performed
1. Ask "Are you choking?"	
2. Give abdominal thrusts (chest thrusts for pregnant or obese victim).	
3. Repeat thrusts until effective or victim becomes unconscious.	
Adult Foreign Body Airway Obstruction–Victim Becomes Unconscious.	
4. Activate the EMS system.	
5. Perform a tongue-jaw lift followed by a finger sweep to remove the object.	
6. Open airway and try to ventilate; if obstructed, reposition head and try to ventilate again.	
7. Give up to five abdominal thrusts.	
8. Repeat steps 5 through 7 until effective.*	

* *If victim is unresponsive but breathing, place in recovery position.*

Based on the latest CPR guidelines.

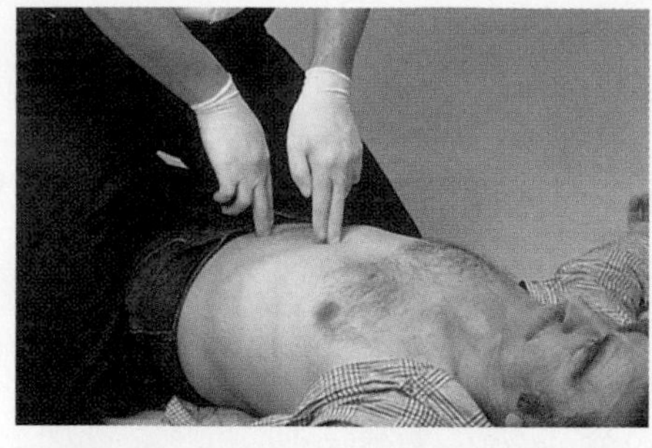
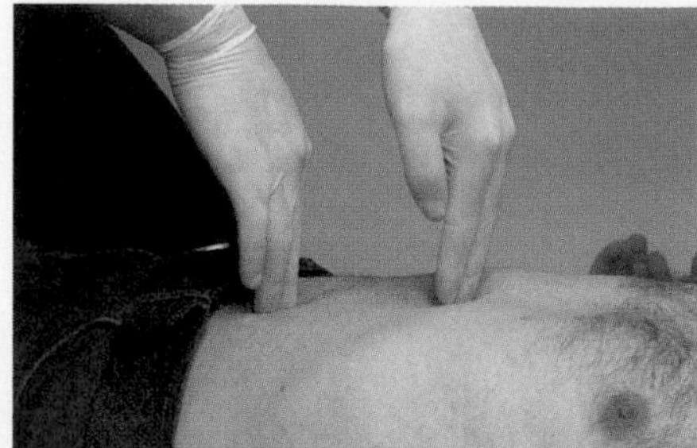

Figure 6.33 Locating the xiphoid process and the navel in an unconscious patient.

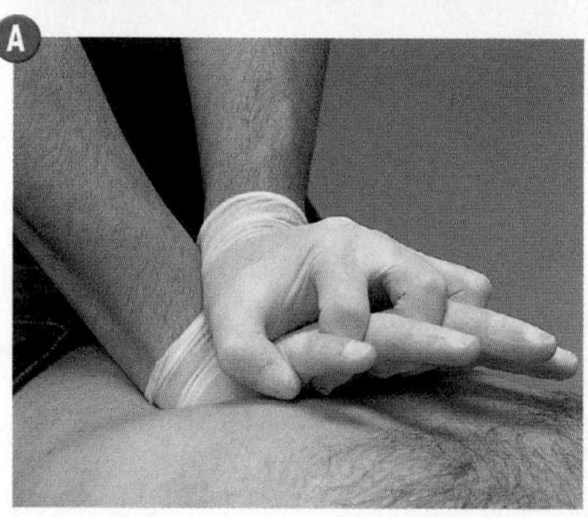
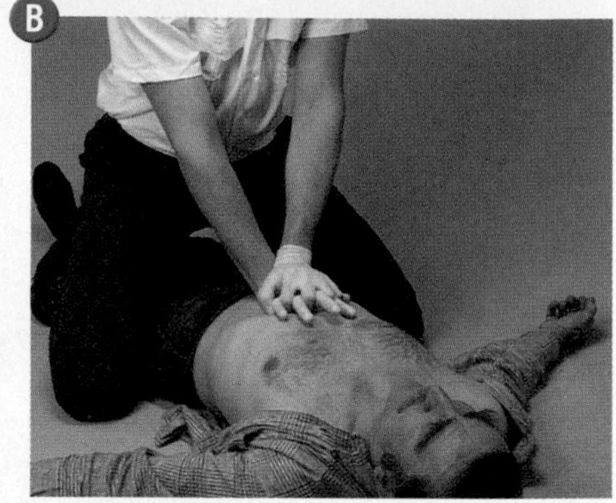

Figure 6.34 Performing an abdominal thrust on an unconscious adult. **A.** Place one hand above the navel and below the xiphoid process and the other hand on top of your first hand. **B.** Thrust inward and slightly upward.

Airway Obstruction in an Unconscious Adult

You can perform abdominal thrusts on patients who are unconscious or so large that you cannot encircle them with your arms by placing the patient flat on his or her back. Straddle the patient. Locate the xiphoid process and the navel (**Figure 6.33**). Place the heel of one hand slightly above the navel and well below the xiphoid process. Place your other hand directly on top of the first hand. Lean your shoulders forward and quickly press in and slightly upward (**Figure 6.34**). The force of the thrust should come from your shoulders and be delivered in the midline of the abdomen, not to either side.

Review the following sequence until you can carry it out automatically. To assist an unconscious patient with a complete airway obstruction, you must:

1. Verify unconsciousness. Ask the patient, "Are you okay?" Tap or gently shake the patient's shoulder. If the patient is unresponsive, call 9-1-1 immediately ("phone first") to activate the EMS system if this has not been done.
2. Support the patient's head and neck as you place the patient on his or her back.
3. Open the airway by using the head tilt–chin lift technique. If trauma to the head or neck is suspected, use the jaw-thrust technique.
4. Check for breathing for at least 3 to 5 seconds. If breathing is absent, proceed with step 5.
5. Attempt rescue breathing. If there is an obstruction, air will not move into or out of the patient. Proceed with step 6.
6. Reposition the head to improve the likelihood of opening the airway. Repeat the head tilt–chin lift or jaw-thrust technique to open the airway.
7. Attempt rescue breathing again. If there is still no air movement, assume the presence of complete obstruction and proceed with steps 8 through 11.

Figure 6.35 Skill Performance Sheet

Unconscious Adult–Foreign Body Airway Obstruction

Steps	Adequately Performed
1. Establish unresponsiveness. Activate the EMS system.	
2. Open airway, check breathing (look, listen, and feel), try to ventilate; if obstructed, reposition head and try to ventilate again.	
3. Give up to five abdominal thrusts.	
4. Perform a tongue-jaw lift followed by a finger sweep to remove the object.	
5. Try to ventilate; if still obstructed, reposition the head and try to ventilate again.	
6. Repeat steps 3 through 5 until effective.*	

* *If victim is unresponsive but breathing, place in recovery position.* ***Based on the latest CPR guidelines.***

8. Deliver an abdominal thrust. Straddle the patient and place the heel of your hand slightly above the navel and well below the xiphoid process. Place your other hand on top of the first hand and press into the abdomen with a quick thrust inward and slightly upward. If the foreign body is not expelled, repeat the abdominal thrust four times. If this does not work, proceed to step 9.
9. Use the tongue-jaw lift to open the patient's mouth so you can check for obstructions. Grasp the lower jaw, placing your thumb on the tongue, and wrap your gloved fingers around the chin. Lift the jaw to open the mouth. Holding the patient's tongue down against the lower jaw with your thumb may offer better access to sweep an object from the throat.
10. Use your finger to sweep the mouth clear. Curve your finger into a C-shape and sweep it from one side of the back of the mouth to the other.
11. Attempt rescue breathing again. If there is still an obstruction, proceed with step 12.
12. Repeat abdominal thrusts, finger sweeps, and breathing attempts until the airway is cleared.

A skill performance sheet titled "Unconscious Adult—Foreign Body Airway Obstruction" is shown in **Figure 6.35** for your review and practice.

Airway Obstruction in a Conscious Child

The steps for relieving an airway obstruction in a conscious child (one to eight years old) are the same as for an adult patient. The anatomic differences between adults and children/infants require that you make some adjustments in your technique. When opening the airway of a child or infant, tilt the head back just past the neutral position. Tilting the head too far back (hyperextending the neck) can actually obstruct the airway of a child or infant.

Figure 6.36 Skill Performance Sheet

Conscious Child–Foreign Body Airway Obstruction

Steps	Adequately Performed
1. Ask "Are you choking?"	
2. Give abdominal thrusts.	
3. Repeat thrusts until effective or victim becomes unconscious.	
Child Foreign Body Airway Obstruction–Victim Becomes Unconscious	
4. If second rescuer is available, have him or her activate the EMS system.	
5. Perform a tongue-jaw lift, and if you see the object, perform a finger sweep to remove it.	
6. Open airway and try to ventilate; if obstructed, reposition head and try to ventilate again.	
7. Give up to five abdominal thrusts.	
8. Repeat steps 5 through 7 until effective.*	
9. If airway obstruction is not relieved after about 1 minute, activate the EMS system.	

* *If victim is unresponsive but breathing, place in recovery position.*

Based on the latest CPR guidelines.

A skill performance sheet titled "Conscious Child—Foreign Body Airway Obstruction" is shown in **Figure 6.36**, for your review and practice.

Airway Obstruction in an Unconscious Child

The steps for relieving a complete airway obstruction in an unconscious child (one to eight years old) are almost the same as those for an unconscious adult. The only difference is that with a child you should perform a finger sweep only if you can see the object that is obstructing the airway. Because the child's airway is so much smaller than an adult's, it is important that you do not push the foreign object farther down into the child's airway. If you are alone, you should attempt to remove the foreign body obstruction for 1 minute before you stop to activate the EMS system.

A skill performance sheet titled "Unconscious Child—Foreign Body Airway Obstruction" is shown in **Figure 6.37** for your review and practice.

Airway Obstruction in a Conscious Infant

The steps for relieving an airway obstruction in a conscious infant (less than one year old) must take into consideration that an infant is very fragile. An infant's airway structures are very small, and they are more easily injured than those of an adult. If you suspect an airway obstruction, assess the infant to determine if there is any air exchange. If the infant is crying, the airway is not completely obstructed. Ask the person

Figure 6.37 Skill Performance Sheet

Unconscious Child–Foreign Body Airway Obstruction

Steps	Adequately Performed
1. Establish unresponsiveness. If second rescuer is available, have him or her activate the EMS system.	
2. Open airway, check breathing (look, listen, and feel), try to ventilate; if obstructed, reposition head and try to ventilate again.	
3. Give up to five abdominal thrusts.	
4. Perform a tongue-jaw lift and if you see the object, perform a finger sweep to remove it.	
5. Try to ventilate; if still obstructed, reposition the head and try to ventilate again.	
6. Repeat steps 3 through 5 until effective.*	
7. If airway obstruction is not relieved after about 1 minute, activate the EMS system.	

* *If victim is unresponsive but breathing, place in recovery position.*

Based on the latest CPR guidelines.

who was with the infant what was happening when the infant stopped breathing. This person may have seen the infant put a foreign body into his or her mouth.

If there is no movement of air from the infant's mouth and nose, suspect an airway obstruction. To relieve an airway obstruction in an infant, use a combination of back blows and chest thrusts. You must have a good grasp of the infant in order to alternate the back blows and the chest thrusts.

Review the following sequence until you can carry it out automatically. To assist a conscious infant with a complete airway obstruction, you must:

1. Assess the infant's airway and breathing status. Determine that there is no air exchange.
2. Place the infant in a face-down position over one arm so that you can deliver five back blows. Support the infant's head and neck with one hand, and place the infant face down with the head lower than the trunk. Rest the infant on your forearm and support your forearm on your thigh. Use the heel of your hand and deliver up to five back blows forcefully between the infant's shoulder blades.
3. Support the head and turn the infant face up by sandwiching the infant between your hands and arms. Rest the infant on his or her back with the head lower than the trunk.
4. Deliver up to five chest thrusts in the middle of the sternum. Use two fingers to deliver the chest thrusts in a firm manner.
5. Repeat the series of back blows and chest thrusts until the foreign object is expelled or until the infant becomes unconscious.

Figure 6.38 Skill Performance Sheet

Conscious Infant–Foreign Body Airway Obstruction

Steps	Adequately Performed
1. Confirm complete airway obstruction. Check for serious breathing difficulty, ineffective cough, no strong cry.	
2. Give up to five back blows and five chest thrusts.	
3. Repeat step 2 until effective or victim becomes unconscious.	
Infant Foreign Body Airway Obstruction–Victim Becomes Unconscious	
4. If second rescuer is available, have him or her activate the EMS system.	
5. Perform a tongue-jaw lift, and if you see the object, perform a finger sweep to remove it.	
6. Open airway and try to ventilate; if obstructed, reposition head and try to ventilate again.	
7. Give up to five back blows and up to five chest thrusts.	
8. Repeat steps 5 through 7 until effective.*	
9. If airway obstruction is not relieved after about 1 minute, activate the EMS system.	

* *If victim is unresponsive but breathing, place in recovery position.*

Based on the latest CPR guidelines.

A skill performance sheet titled "Conscious Infant-Foreign Body Airway Obstruction" is shown in **Figure 6.38** for your review and practice.

Airway Obstruction in an Unconscious Infant

Use the same sequence of back blows and chest thrusts steps for relieving an airway obstruction in an unconscious infant (less than one year old). However, the steps taken to determine unconsciousness and the presence of an airway obstruction are somewhat different.

Review the following sequence until you can carry it out automatically. To assist an unconscious infant with a complete airway obstruction, you must:

1. Determine unresponsiveness by gently shaking the shoulder or by gently tapping the bottom of the foot.
2. Position the infant on a firm, hard surface and support the head and neck.
3. Open the airway using the head tilt–chin lift technique. Be careful not to tilt the infant's head back too far.
4. Check for breathing by placing your ear close to the infant's mouth and nose. Listen and feel for the infant's breathing.
5. If the infant is not breathing, begin rescue breathing. If rescue breathing is unsuccessful, proceed to step 6.

Figure 6.39 Skill Performance Sheet

Unconscious Infant–Foreign Body Airway Obstruction

Steps	Adequately Performed
1. Establish unresponsiveness. If second rescuer is available, have him or her activate the EMS system.	
2. Open airway, check breathing (look, listen, and feel), try to ventilate; if obstructed, reposition head and try to ventilate again.	
3. Give up to 5 back blows and 5 chest thrusts.	
4. Perform a tongue-jaw lift, and if you see the object, perform a finger sweep to remove it.	
5. Try to ventilate; if still obstructed, reposition the head and try to ventilate again.	
6. Repeat steps 3 through 5 until effective.*	
7. If airway obstruction is not relieved after about 1 minute, activate the EMS system.	

* *If victim is unresponsive but breathing, place in recovery position.*

Based on the latest CPR guidelines.

6. Reposition the airway and reattempt rescue breathing.

Note: Up to this point, the steps are similar to those used for infant rescue breathing.

7. Deliver up to five back blows using the same technique as for a conscious infant.
8. Deliver up to five chest thrusts using the same technique as for a conscious infant.
9. Perform a tongue-jaw lift and remove any foreign object that you can see.
10. Repeat the sequence of back blows and chest thrusts until the foreign body is expelled.

A skill performance sheet titled "Unconscious Infant-Foreign Body Airway Obstruction" is shown in **Figure 6.39** for your review and practice.

Check✓point

- ◯ What are the signs and symptoms of a partial airway obstruction?
- ◯ How do you treat a partial airway obstruction?
- ◯ What are the signs and symptoms of a complete airway obstruction?
- ◯ What are the steps for treating a complete airway obstruction in a conscious adult? In an unconscious adult?
- ◯ How does the treatment of a complete airway obstruction differ for a child and an infant?

Remember

Though the sequences listed for relieving airway obstructions may seem complicated, keep in mind that they all contain the following steps:

1. Determine responsiveness or unresponsiveness.
2. Open the airway.
3. Determine if there is any air exchange.
4. If a complete obstruction is present, perform abdominal thrusts on adults and children or back blows and chest thrusts on infants.
5. Perform finger sweeps on adult patients, but do not perform finger sweeps on children and infants unless you can see the foreign object.

Voices of Experience

Efforts of Paramedic, Off-Duty Fire Captain Save Ejected Car Occupants

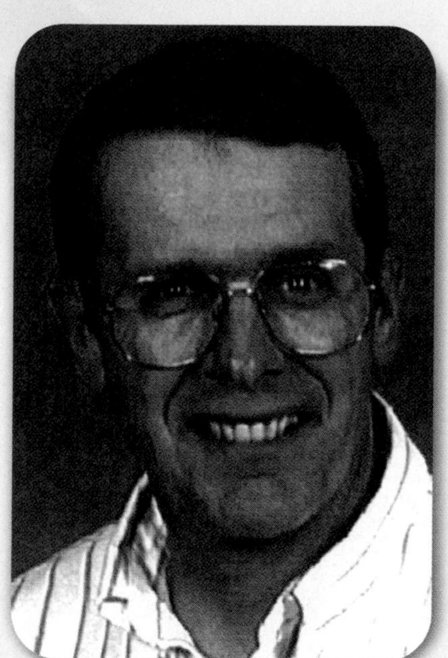

On the morning of September 2, 2000, three Arizona State college co-eds were driving to San Diego for the Labor Day weekend. Their sports utility vehicle left the roadway and rolled, end over end, ejecting the two women in the back seat.

As a full-time paramedic working for AMR in the Rural East County of San Diego, I arrived to find two major trauma patients and Rick Williams, an off-duty Santee Fire Department Captain/ Paramedic, attending to the injured victims. My initial triage indicated two "immediate" patients and one "delayed." Both "immediate" patients had airway problems that required aggressive treatment. A closer look at the most critical patient's chief complaint revealed that she had to be intubated. She was intubated and ventilated while en route to the trauma center, arriving approximately 47 minutes after our initial dispatch.

I have been a licensed full-time paramedic for over 25 years and have run on thousands of calls. There are occasions in EMS when everything seems to go right. When this happens, the patient benefits with a positive outcome. Such was the case on this call. Using his cell phone, Rick had called for an air ambulance after calling 9-1-1. He was instrumental in maintaining cervical spine immobilization on the combative patient and initially opening the airway of the unconscious patient.

“He was instrumental in maintaining cervical spine immobilization on the combative patient and initially opening the airway of the unconscious patient.”

It is most rewarding when patients call to personally thank you for saving their lives, as this young woman did. She could have very easily died from her injuries, had not everything fallen into place in just the right way. That day the EMS system performed perfectly, thanks to the heroic actions of one off-duty Fire Captain/Paramedic! ❖

Rick Foehr, BA, EMT-P
American Medical Response
San Diego, CA
Grossmont Rural EMS
Medic 17
Alpine, CA

Special Considerations

Rescue Breathing for Patients with Stomas

Some individuals have had surgery that removed part or all of the larynx (voice box). In these patients, the upper airway has been rerouted to open through a **stoma** in the neck. These patients are called **neck breathers**. Rescue breathing must therefore be given through the stoma (hole) in the patient's neck. The technique is called **mouth-to-stoma breathing**.

stoma An opening in the neck that connects the windpipe (trachea) to the skin.

neck breathers Patients who have a stoma and breathe through the opening in their neck.

mouth-to-stoma breathing Rescue breathing for patients who, because of surgical removal of the larynx, have a stoma.

The steps in performing mouth-to-stoma breathing are:

1. Check every patient for the presence of a stoma.
2. If you locate a stoma, keep the patient's neck straight; do not hyperextend the patient's head and neck.
3. Examine the stoma and clean away any mucus in it.
4. If there is a breathing tube in the opening, remove it to be sure it is clear. Clean it rapidly and replace it into the stoma. Moistening the tube will make it easier to insert the tube.
5. Place your mouth directly over the stoma and use the same procedures as in mouth-to-mouth breathing. It is not necessary to seal the mouth and nose of most neck breathers.
6. If the patient's chest does not rise, he or she may be a partial neck breather. In these patients, you must seal the mouth and nose with one hand and then breathe through the stoma (**Figure 6.40**).

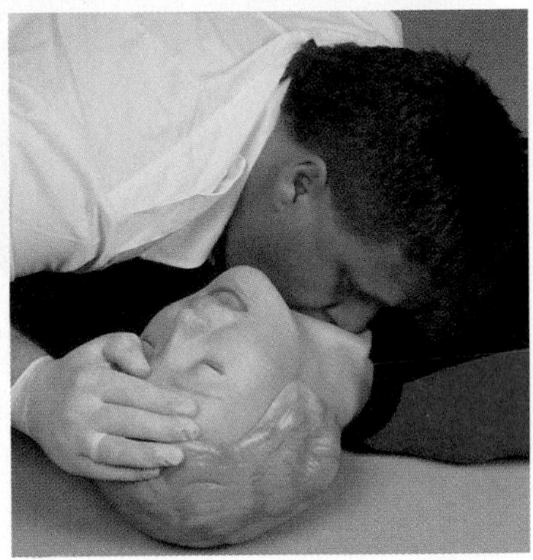

Figure 6.40 Perform mouth-to-stoma rescue breathing by using the same procedure as in mouth-to-mouth breathing, by breathing through the stoma.

Gastric Distention

Gastric distention occurs when air is forced into the stomach instead of the lungs. This makes it harder to get an adequate amount of air into the patient's lungs, and it increases the chance that the patient will vomit. Breath slowly into the patient's mouth just enough to make the chest rise. Remember that the lungs of children and infants are smaller, and require smaller breaths during rescue breathing. The excess air may enter the stomach and cause gastric distention. Preventing gastric distention is much better than trying to cure the results of it.

Dental Appliances

Do not remove dental appliances that are firmly attached. They may help keep the mouth fuller so you can make a better seal between the patient's mouth and your mouth or a breathing device. Loose dental appliances, however, may cause problems. Partial dentures may become dislodged during trauma or while you are performing airway care and rescue breathing. If you discover loose dental appliances during your examination of the patient's airway, remove the dentures to prevent them from occluding the airway. Try to put them in a safe place so they will not get damaged or lost.

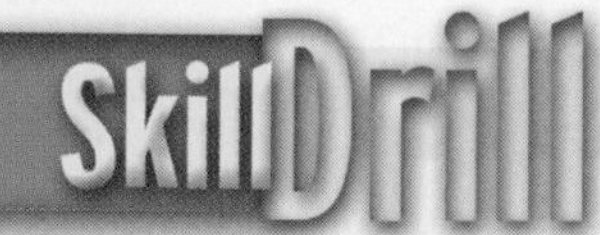

Figure 6.41 Airway Management in a Vehicle

1

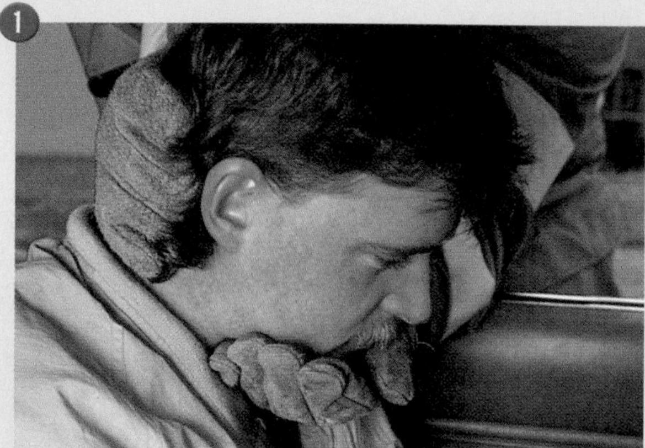

To open the airway, place one hand under the chin and the other hand on the back of the patient's head.

2

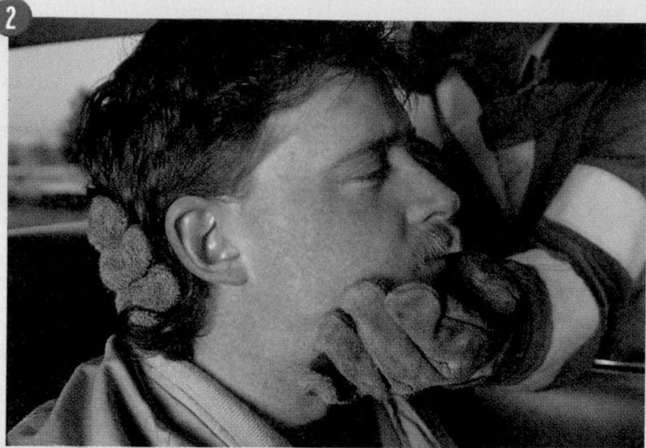

Raise the head to neutral position to open airway.

Airway Management in a Vehicle

FYI

If you arrive on the scene of an automobile accident and find that the patient has airway problems, how can you best assist the patient and maintain an open airway? If the patient is lying on the seat or floor of the car, you can apply the standard jaw-thrust technique. Use the jaw-thrust technique if there is any possibility that the accident could have caused a head or spinal injury.

When the patient is in a sitting or semireclining position, approach him or her from the side by leaning in through the window or across the front seat. Grasp the patient's head with both hands. Put one hand under the patient's chin and the other hand on the back of the patient's head just above the neck, as shown in **Figure 6.41**. Maintain slight upward pressure to support the head and cervical spine and to ensure that the airway remains open. This technique will often enable you to maintain an open airway without moving the patient. This technique has several advantages:

1. You do not have to enter the automobile.
2. You can easily monitor the patient's carotid pulse and breathing patterns by using your fingers.
3. It stabilizes the patient's cervical spine.
4. It opens the patient's airway.

Checkpoint

- ◯ How do you perform rescue breathing on a neck breather?
- ◯ What are the steps in maintaining the airway of a patient in a vehicle?

6

Prep Kit

Ready for Review

Ready for Review thoroughly summarizes the chapter.

In this chapter, you have learned the anatomy and physiology of the respiratory system and the procedure for performing rescue breathing. When a patient experiences possible respiratory arrest, you should: check for responsiveness; correct the blocked airway using the head tilt–chin lift or jaw-thrust technique; check for fluids, solids, or dentures in the mouth; and correct the airway, if needed, using finger sweeps or suction. Maintain the airway by continuing to manually hold the airway open, by placing the patient in the recovery position, or by inserting an oral or a nasal airway. Check for breathing by looking, listening, and feeling for air movement, and correct any problems by using a mouth-to-mask or a mouth-to-barrier device or by performing mouth-to-mouth rescue breathing. It is important to learn the sequences for adults, children, and infants.

If the patient's airway is obstructed, you must perform abdominal or chest thrusts. Use back blows and chest thrusts for infants with airway obstructions. You should also know how to perform rescue breathing on a patient with a stoma. A simple technique enables you to manage the airway of a patient who is in a vehicle.

You should learn these lifesaving skills thoroughly. Practice them until they become almost automatic for you. In Chapter 8, these skills will be combined with circulation skills so that you can learn and perform CPR. To keep your skills up-to-date, maintain current certification through an agency that uses the American Heart Association standards.

Vital Vocabulary

The Vital Vocabulary are the key terms for this chapter.

airway—*page 104*
airway obstruction—*page 123*
alveoli—*page 104*
aspirator—*page 109*
bronchi—*page 104*
capillaries—*page 104*
cardiopulmonary resuscitation (CPR)—*page 102*
esophagus—*page 104*
external cardiac compressions—*page 120*
gag reflex—*page 110*
head tilt–chin lift—*page 106*
Heimlich maneuver—*page 126*
jaw-thrust technique—*page 107*
lungs—*page 104*
mandible—*page 104*
manual suction device—*page 108*
mechanical suction device—*page 109*
mouth-to-mask ventilation device—*page 115*
mouth-to-stoma breathing—*page 135*
nasal airway—*page 112*
nasopharynx—*page 103*
neck breathers—*page 135*
oral airway—*page 110*
oropharynx—*page 103*
oxygen (O_2)—*page 103*
pocket mask—*page 110*
rescue breathing—*page 115*
respiratory arrest—*page 110*
stoma—*page 135*
trachea—*page 103*

Skill Drills

The Skill Drills provide a visual summary of some of the more complex skills from the skills objectives.

Practice Points

The Practice Points are the key skills you need to know.

1. Performing the head tilt–chin lift and jaw-thrust techniques for opening blocked airways.
2. Checking for fluids, solids, and dentures in a patient's airway.
3. Correcting a blocked airway using finger sweeps and suction.
4. Placing a patient in the recovery position.
5. Inserting oral and nasal airways.
6. Checking for the presence of breathing.
7. Performing rescue breathing using a mouth-to-mask device, a mouth-to-barrier device, and mouth-to-mouth techniques.
8. Demonstrating the steps in recognizing respiratory arrest and performing rescue breathing on an adult patient, a child, and an infant.
9. Performing the steps needed to remove a foreign body airway obstruction in an adult patient, a child, and an infant.
10. Demonstrating rescue breathing on a patient with a stoma.
11. Performing airway management on a patient in a vehicle.

Ready to Respond

Ready to Respond presents a fictitious scenario to help you review what you learned in this chapter.

Questions 1 – 5 are based on this scenario. You are called to a day care center for the report of a child choking. The day care worker tells you that a four-year-old child may have put something in his mouth. The child does not respond to your verbal stimuli or your touch on the shoulder.

1. Your next step should be
  A. Perform rescue breathing
  B. Open the airway
  C. Check for foreign bodies
  D. Place the child in the recovery position

2. If you need to open the airway you should use the
  A. Jaw-thrust technique
  B. Cross finger technique
  C. Head tilt–chin lift technique
  D. Mouth-to-nose technique

3. If the airway is obstructed, how should you remove the obstruction?
  A. Back blows only
  B. Abdominal thrusts only
  C. Back blows and abdominal thrusts
  D. Tongue-jaw lift

4. You should perform a finger sweep
  A. After the abdominal thrusts
  B. In all patients
  C. Only when you can see the obstruction
  D. Only when the abdominal thrusts do not work

5. If you are not able to ventilate this patient, you should
  A. Use the jaw-thrust technique and ventilate
  B. Reposition the head and try to ventilate again
  C. Give a bigger rescue breath
  D. Give abdominal thrusts

Questions 6 – 9 are based on this scenario. You are called to a city park for a reported accident. You find a 25-year-old woman who has hit a tree while inline skating.

6. Your first step in assessing this patient should be
  A. Shake her shoulder
  B. Check her pulse
  C. Check for breathing
  D. Establish her level of responsiveness

7. To open the airway, you should use
  A. Head tilt–chin lift technique
  B. Tongue-jaw lift technique
  C. Jaw-thrust technique
  D. An oral airway

8. As you open this patient's airway, you should also
  A. Check the carotid pulse
  B. Stabilize the patient's neck
  C. Check the patient's level of responsiveness
  D. Perform rescue breathing

9. In performing rescue breathing you should give____ slow breath(s) at ___ second(s) per breath
  A. 1, 2
  B. 2, 1
  C. 1, 3
  D. 2, 2

MODULE 2 QuickQuiz

Airway

1. In an unconscious patient, a blocked airway is most likely caused by
   A. Foreign object
   B. The tongue
   C. The epiglottis
   D. The larynx

2. Your first effort to ensure that the patient's airway is open should be
   A. Shake the patient to determine responsiveness
   B. Attempt to give rescue breaths
   C. Position the head properly
   D. Clear foreign matter from the throat

3. To open the airway in an unconscious adult with no suspected spinal injury, you should use the
   A. Jaw-thrust technique
   B. Manual suction device
   C. Head lift–chin tilt technique
   D. Tongue-jaw lift technique

4. If a patient is coughing forcefully with something caught in the throat
   A. Give abdominal thrusts
   B. Sweep out the mouth
   C. Check the pulse
   D. Encourage the patient to cough

5. If gastric distention occurs while you are doing CPR, it is probably caused by
   A. Rescue breaths that are too small
   B. Too much force while doing chest compressions
   C. Air entering the patient's stomach
   D. Too much fluid in the patient's stomach

1.B 2.C 3.B 4.D 5.C

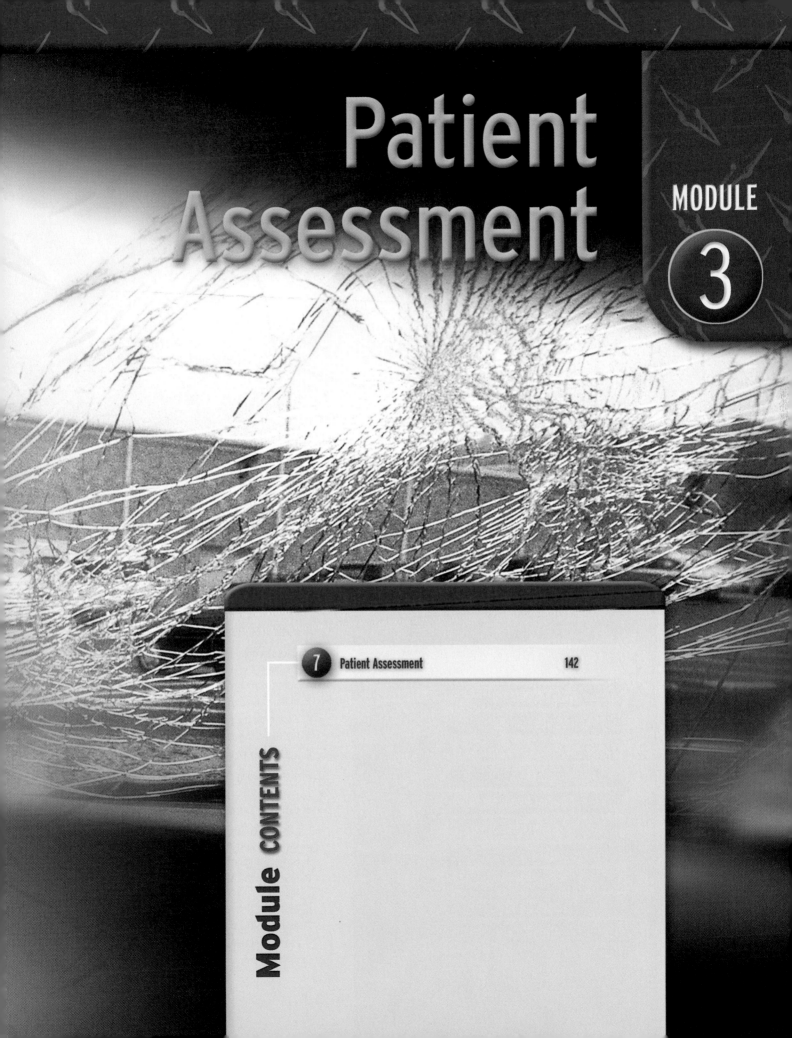

Patient Assessment

MODULE 3

Module CONTENTS

Chapter 7

Patient Assessment

TECHNOLOGY

- Online Chapter Pretest
- Web Links
- Online Glossary
- Anatomy Review
- Online Review Manual
- CyberClass

www.FirstResponderTraining.com

- Interactive First Responder

Chapter FEATURES

- Skill Drills
- Vital Vocabulary
- Voices of Experience
- Signs and Symptoms
- FYI
- Special Needs
- Safety Tips
- BSI Tips
- Caution
- Check Point
- Prep Kit

Objectives

Knowledge and Attitude Objectives

After studying this chapter, you will be expected to:

1. Discuss the importance of each of the following steps in the patient assessment sequence:
   - A. Scene size-up
   - B. Initial patient assessment
   - C. Examining the patient from head to toe
   - D. Obtaining the patient's medical history
   - E. Performing an on-going assessment
2. Discuss the components of a scene size-up.
3. Describe why it is important to get an idea of the number of patients at an emergency scene as soon as possible.
4. List and describe the importance of the following steps of the initial patient assessment:
   - A. Forming a general impression of the patient
   - B. Assessing the patient's responsiveness and stabilizing the spine if necessary
   - C. Assessing the patient's airway
   - D. Assessing the patient's breathing
   - E. Assessing the patient's circulation
   - F. Updating responding EMS units

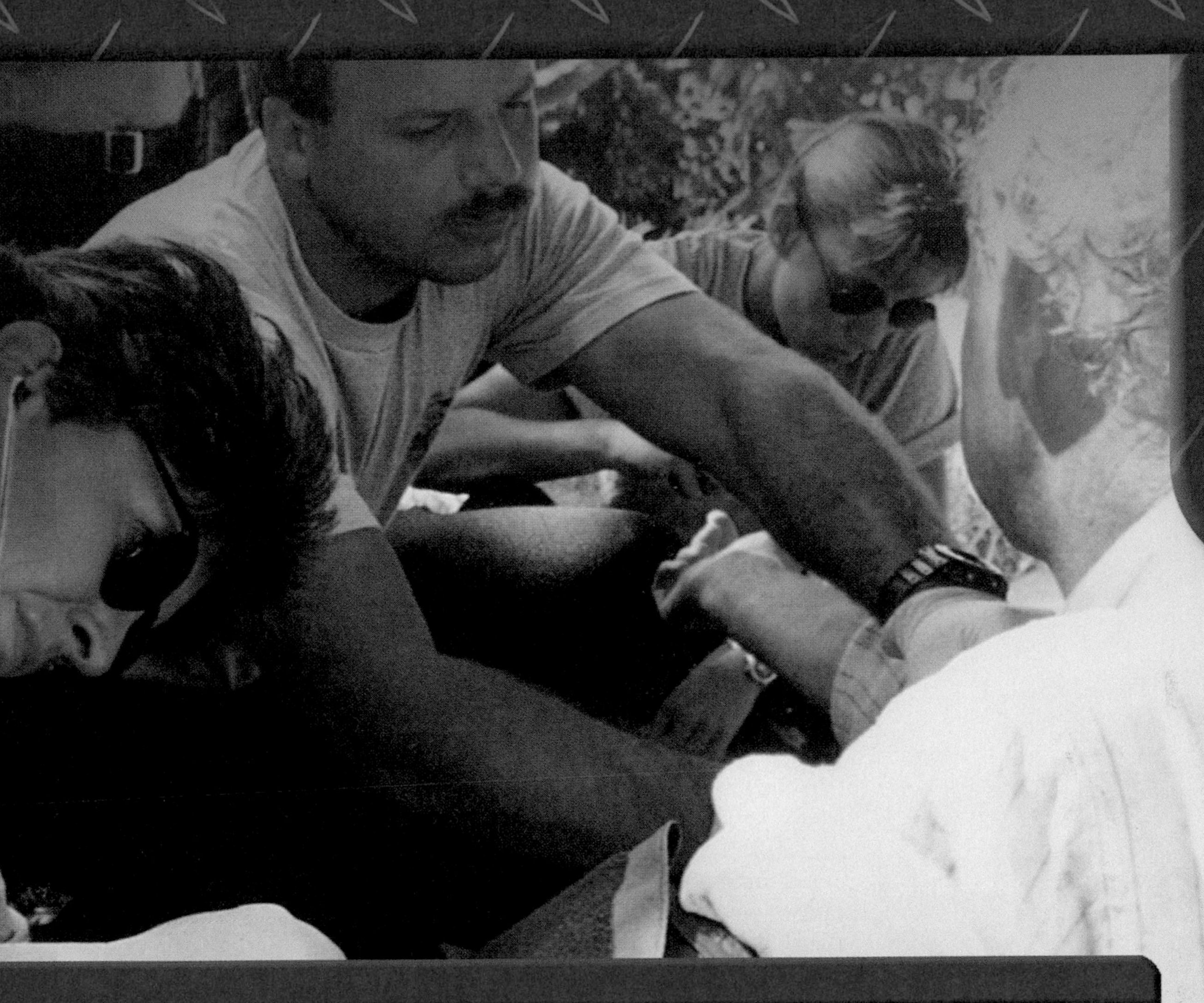

CHAPTER

7

5. Describe the differences in checking airway, breathing, and circulation when the patient is an adult, a child, or an infant.

6. Explain the significance of the following signs: respiration, circulation, skin condition, pupil size and reactivity, level of consciousness.

7. Describe the sequence used to perform a head-to-toe physical examination.

8. State the areas of the body that you should examine during a physical examination.

9. Describe the importance of obtaining the patient's medical history.

10. State the information that you should obtain when taking a patient's medical history.

11. List the information that should be addressed in your hand-off report about the patient's condition.

12. List the differences between performing a patient assessment on a trauma patient and performing one on a medical patient.

13. Describe the components of the on-going assessment.

Skill Objectives

As a first responder, you should be able to:

1. Perform the following five steps of the patient assessment sequence given a real or simulated incident:
   A. Scene size-up
   B. Initial patient assessment, including:
      (1) Forming a general impression of the patient
      (2) Assessing the patient's responsiveness and stabilizing the patient's spine if necessary
      (3) Assessing the patient's airway
      (4) Assessing the patient's breathing
      (5) Assessing the patient's circulation (including severe bleeding) and stabilizing those functions if necessary
      (6) Updating responding EMS units
   C. Examination of the patient from head to toe
   D. Obtaining the patient's medical history using the SAMPLE format
   E. Performing an on-going assessment
2. Identify and measure the following signs on adult, child, and infant patients: respiration, pulse, capillary refill, skin color, skin temperature, skin moisture, pupil size and reactivity, level of consciousness.

As a first responder, you will be the first trained EMS person on many emergency scenes. Your initial actions will affect not only you, but also the patient and other responders. Your assessment of the scene and the patient will affect the level of care requested for the patient.

It is important that you are able to perform a systematic patient assessment to determine what injuries or illness the patient has suffered. The patient assessment sequence consists of the following steps:

1. Perform a scene size-up.
2. Perform an initial patient assessment to identify immediate threats to life.
3. Examine the patient from head to toe.
4. Obtain the patient's medical history.
5. Perform an on-going assessment.

By performing these five steps, you can systematically gather the information you need. After you have learned these steps, you will discover that you can modify them to gather needed information about a patient who is suffering from a medical problem instead of a patient who is suffering from trauma.

FYI

The skills and knowledge presented in this chapter follow an **assessment-based care** model. With assessment-based care, the treatment rendered is based on the patient's symptoms.

Assessment-based care requires a careful and thorough evaluation of the patient to provide appropriate care. If a given condition has already been diagnosed by a physician and is known to the patient, you will sometimes know the patient's diagnosis. Other times, you will have to respond to the signs and symptoms you find during the assessment process. Throughout this text, you will find signs and symptoms of certain medical conditions.

Careful and thorough study of the skills and knowledge related to patient assessment will go a long way in helping you perform as a valuable member of the EMS team in your community.

assessment-based care A system of patient evaluation in which the chief complaint of the patient and other signs and symptoms are gathered. The care given is based on this information rather than on a formal diagnosis.

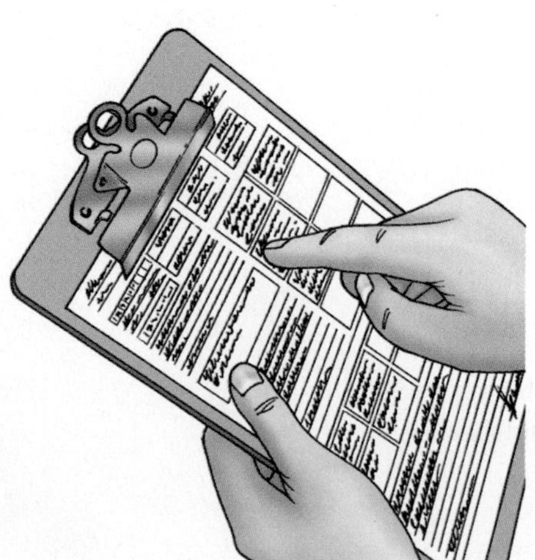

Figure 7.1 Review dispatch information.

Patient Assessment Sequence

The patient assessment sequence is designed to give you a framework so you can safely approach an emergency scene, determine the need for additional help, examine the patient to determine if injuries or illnesses are present, obtain the patient's medical history, and report the results of your assessment to other EMS personnel. A complete patient assessment consists of five steps.

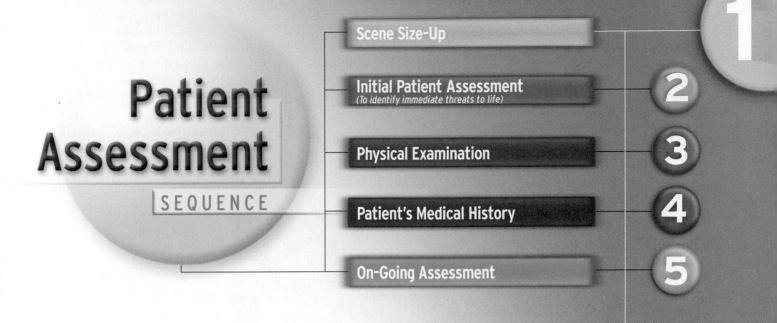

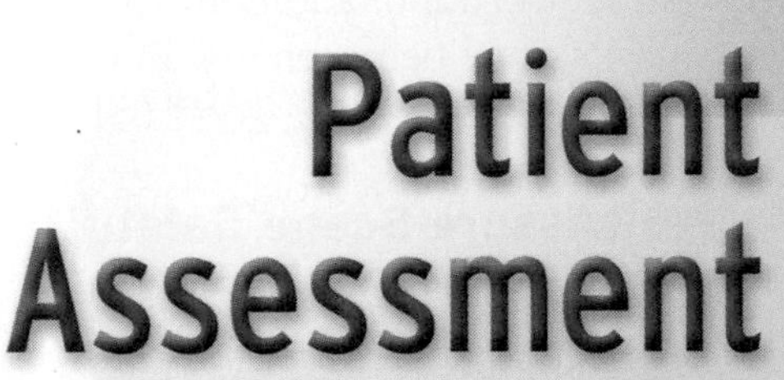

Scene Size-Up
Initial Patient Assessment
(To identify immediate threats to life)
Physical Examination
Patient's Medical History
On-Going Assessment

1 2 3 4 5

Scene Size-Up

- Review Dispatch Information FYI
- Observe Body Substance Isolation Procedures
- Assure Scene Safety
- Determine the Mechanism of Injury or Nature of the Illness
- Determine the Need for Additional Resources

Perform a Scene Size-Up

The scene size-up is a general overview of the incident and its surroundings. Based on this information, you can make decisions about the safety of the scene, what type of incident is present, any mechanism of injury, and the need for additional resources.

Review Dispatch Information

FYI

Your scene size-up begins before you arrive at the actual scene of the emergency. You can anticipate possible conditions by reviewing and understanding dispatch information. Your dispatcher should have obtained the following information: the location of the incident, the main problem or type of incident, the number of people involved, and the safety level of the scene. As you receive the dispatcher's information, you should begin to assess it (**Figure 7.1**).

In addition to the information you obtain from the dispatcher, other factors could affect your actions. Consider, for example, the time of day, the day of the week, and weather conditions. A call from a school during school hours may require a different response than a call during the weekend. Finally, think about the resources that may be needed and mentally prepare for other situations you may find when you arrive on the scene.

If you happen on a medical emergency, notify the emergency medical dispatch center by using your two-way radio. If you do not have a two-way radio, send someone to call for help. Relay the following information: the location of the incident, the main problem or type of incident, the number of people involved, and the safety of the scene.

Observe Body Substance Isolation

Before you arrive at the scene, you should prepare by anticipating the types of body substance isolation (BSI) that may be required. You should always have gloves readily available. Consider whether the use of additional protection, such as eye protection, gowns, or masks, may be necessary. In other words, try to anticipate your needs for equipment to ensure good BSI.

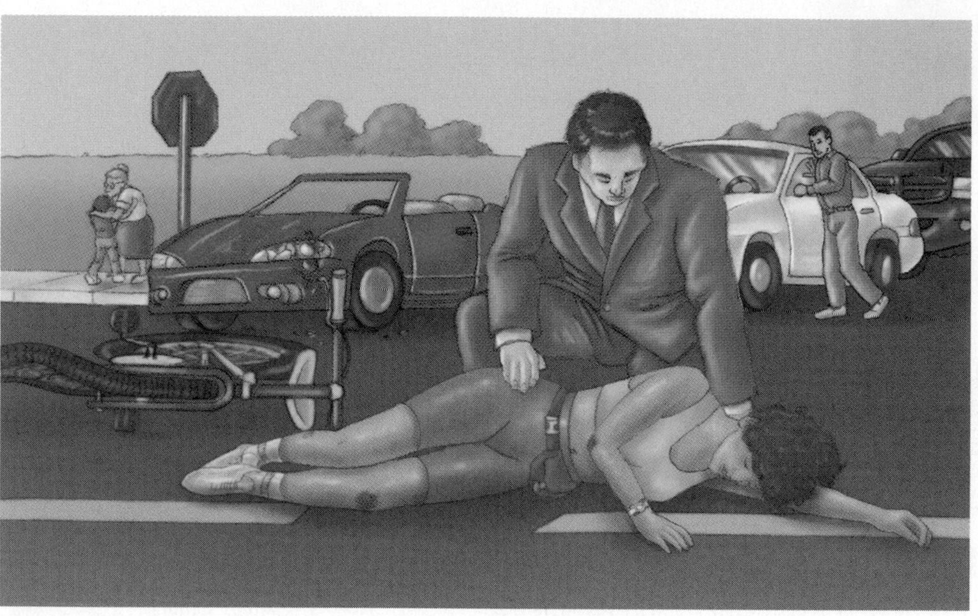

Figure 7.2 Perform a scene size-up.

Assure Scene Safety

When you arrive at the scene, remember to park your vehicle so that it helps secure the scene and minimizes traffic blockage.
As you approach the scene, scan the area to determine the extent of the incident, the possible number of people injured, and the presence of possible hazards (**Figure 7.2**). It is important to scan the scene to ensure that you are not putting yourself in danger.

Hazards can be visible or invisible. Visible hazards include such things as the scene of a crash, fallen electrical wires, traffic, spilled gasoline, unstable buildings, a crime scene, and crowds. Unstable surfaces such as slopes, ice, and water pose potential hazards. Invisible hazards include electricity, hazardous materials, and poisonous fumes. Downed electrical wires or broken poles may indicate an electrical hazard. Never assume a downed electrical wire is safe. Confined spaces such as farm silos, industrial tanks, and below-ground pits often contain poisonous gases or lack enough oxygen to support life. Hazardous materials placards may indicate the presence of a chemical hazard.

Note the hazards, consider your ability to manage them and decide whether to call for assistance. This assistance may include the fire department, additional EMS units, law enforcement officers, heavy rescue equipment, hazardous materials teams, electric or gas company personnel, or other special resources. If a hazardous condition exists, make every effort to ensure that bystanders, rescuers, and patients are not exposed to it unnecessarily. If possible, see to it that any hazardous conditions are corrected or minimized as soon as possible. Noting such conditions early keeps them from becoming part of the problem later.

Some emergency scenes will not be safe for you to enter. These scenes will require personnel with special training and equipment. If a scene is unsafe, keep people away until specially trained teams arrive. It is also important to identify potential exit routes from the scene in case a hazard becomes life threatening to you or your patients.

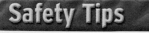

> **Safety Tips**
>
> Never enter an enclosed space unless you have received proper training and are equipped with self-contained breathing apparatus (SCBA).

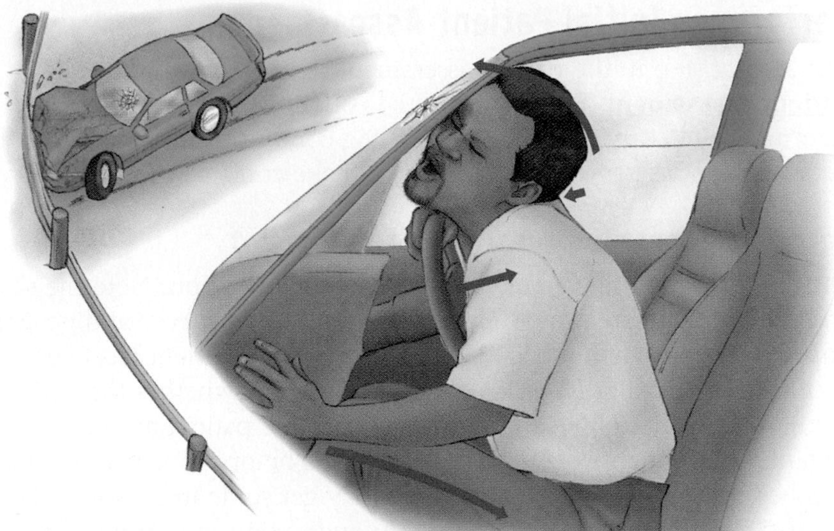

Figure 7.3 Determine the mechanism of injury.

Mechanism of Injury or Nature of Illness

As you approach the scene, look for clues that may indicate how the accident happened (**Figure 7.3**). This is called the mechanism of injury. If you can determine the mechanism of injury or the nature of the illness, you can sometimes predict the patient's injuries. For example, a ladder lying on the ground next to a spilled paint bucket probably indicates that the patient fell from the ladder and may have broken bones. If the incident is an automobile accident, knowing what type of accident occurred makes it possible to anticipate the types of injuries that may be present. For example, a rollover accident results in different injuries than a car-tree collision. It is also possible to anticipate injuries by examining the extent of damage to an automobile. If the windshield is broken, look for head and spine injuries; if the steering wheel is bent, check for a chest injury. (See Chapter 13 for more information on mechanisms of injury that result in musculoskeletal injuries.) Ask the patient (if conscious) or family members or bystanders for additional information about the mechanism of injury. The same type of overview that gives you information at the scene of an accident can also help provide information about a patient's condition. Again, ask the patient, family, or bystanders why you were called.

You should not, however, rule out any injury without conducting a head-to-toe physical examination of the patient. The mechanism of the accident may provide clues, but it cannot be used to determine what injuries are present in a particular patient. In the previous example, the painter may have had a heart attack before beginning to climb the ladder.

Determine Need for Additional Resources

If there is more than one patient, count the total number of patients. Call for additional assistance if you think you will need help. It may be necessary to sort patients into groups according to the severity of their injuries to determine which patients should be treated and transported first. The topic of "triage," or patient sorting, is covered more thoroughly in Chapter 16.

Note: Call for additional assistance before beginning to treat the patient(s). It will take time for more help to arrive, so the sooner you request aid, the better. In addition, you are less likely to call for help if you first become involved in patient care, and this can be detrimental to the patient's chances for recovery.

Perform an Initial Patient Assessment

The second step in the patient assessment sequence is the **initial patient assessment**. During the initial patient assessment, you can determine and correct any life-threatening conditions. Do all steps in the initial patient assessment quickly as you make contact with the patient.

2

Initial Patient Assessment
(To identify immediate threats to life)

- Form a General Impression of the Patient
- Assess Responsiveness (AVPU)
- Check the Patient's Airway
- Check the Patient's Breathing
- Check the Patient's Circulation (including severe bleeding)
- Acknowledge the Patient's Primary Complaint
- Update Responding EMS Units

Form a General Impression of the Patient

As you approach the patient, form a general impression. Note the sex and the approximate age of the patient. Your scene survey and general impressions may help you determine whether the patient has experienced trauma or illness. (If you cannot determine whether the patient is suffering from an illness or an injury, treat the patient as a trauma patient.) The patient's position or the sounds he or she is making may also be indicators of the problem. You may get some impression of the patient's level of consciousness. Although your first impression is valuable, do not let it block out later information that may lead you in another direction.

Assess Responsiveness

The first part of determining the patient's responsiveness is to introduce yourself. Many patients will be conscious and able to interact with you. As you approach the patient, tell the patient your name and function (**Figure 7.4**). For example, "I'm Jill Smith from the Sheriff's Department, and I'm here to help you." This simple introduction helps establish:

- Your reason for being at the accident
- The fact that you will be helping the patient
- The level of consciousness of the patient

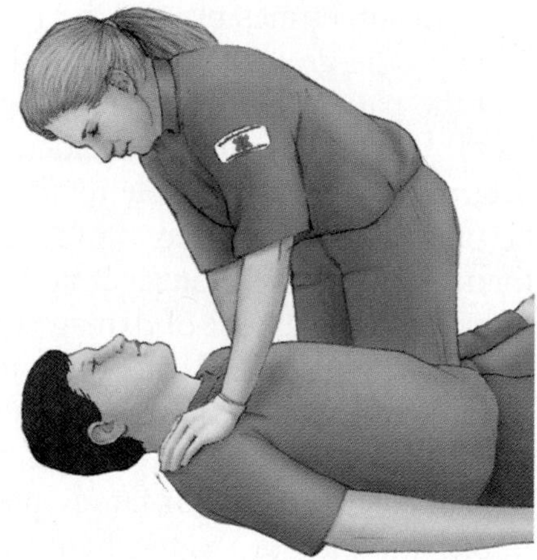

Figure 7.4 As you approach the patient, introduce yourself. If a patient appears unconscious, gently touch or shake the patient's shoulder to get a response.

The introduction is your first contact with the patient. It should put the patient at ease by conveying the fact that you are a trained person ready to help.

Next, ask the patient's name, and then use it when talking with the patient, family, or friends. The patient's response helps you determine the patient's level of consciousness. Avoid telling the patient that everything will be all right.

Even if the patient appears to be unconscious, introduce yourself and talk with the patient as you conduct the rest of the patient assessment. Many patients who appear to be unconscious can hear your voice and need the reassurance it carries. Do not say anything you do not want the patient to hear!

initial patient assessment The first actions taken to form an impression of the patient's condition; to determine the patient's responsiveness and introduce yourself to the patient; to check the patient's airway, breathing, and circulation; and to acknowledge the patient's chief complaint.

If a patient appears to be unconscious, call to the patient in a tone of voice that is loud enough for the patient to hear. If the patient does not respond to the sound of your voice, gently touch the patient or shake the patient's shoulder.

The patient's level of consciousness can range from fully conscious to unconscious. Describe the patient's level of consciousness using the four-level **AVPU scale**:

A *Alert.* An alert patient is able to answer the following questions accurately and appropriately: What is your name? Where are you? What is today's date? A patient who can answer these questions is said to be "alert and oriented."

V *Verbal.* A patient is said to be "responsive to verbal stimulus" even if the patient only reacts to loud sounds.

P *Pain.* A patient who is responsive to pain will not respond to a verbal stimulus but will move or cry out in response to pain. Response to pain is tested by pinching the patient's earlobe or pinching the patient's skin over the collarbone. If the patient withdraws from the painful stimulus, he or she is said to be "responsive to painful stimuli."

U *Unresponsive.* An unresponsive patient will not respond to either a verbal or a painful stimulus. This patient's condition is described as "unresponsive."

AVPU scale A scale to measure a patient's level of consciousness. The letters stand for Alert, Verbal, Pain, and Unresponsive.

If the patient has suffered any type of major trauma, you should provide manual stabilization of the patient's neck as soon as possible. This will prevent any further injury to the neck and spinal column.

BSI Tip

Remember that performing a patient assessment may bring you in contact with the patient's blood, body fluids, waste products, and mucous membranes. You need to wear approved gloves and take other precautions to ensure that you maintain body substance isolation (BSI) to prevent any exposure to infected body fluids. Follow the latest standards from the CDC and OSHA.

Check the Patient's Airway

The third part of the initial assessment is to check the patient's airway. If the patient is alert and able to answer questions without difficulty, then the airway is open. If the patient is not responsive to verbal stimuli, then you must assume that the airway may be closed. In the case of an unconscious patient, open the airway by using the head tilt–chin lift technique for patients with medical problems, and the jaw-thrust technique (without tilting the patient's head) for patients who have suffered trauma. After the airway is open, inspect it for foreign bodies or secretions. Clear the airway as needed. You may need to insert an airway adjunct to keep the airway open. (See Chapter 6 for information about airway adjuncts.)

Special Needs

CHILDREN

Infants and children may not have the verbal skills to answer the questions used to assess responsiveness in adults. Therefore, you should assess the interaction of children and infants with their environment and with their parents.

Check the Patient's Breathing

If the patient is conscious, assess the rate and quality of the patient's breathing. Does the chest rise and fall with each breath? Or does the patient appear to be short of breath? If the patient is unconscious, check for breathing by placing the side of your face next to the patient's nose and mouth. You should be able to hear the sounds of breathing, see the chest rise and fall, and even feel the movement of air on your

Remember

A is for Airway
B is for Breathing
C is for Circulation

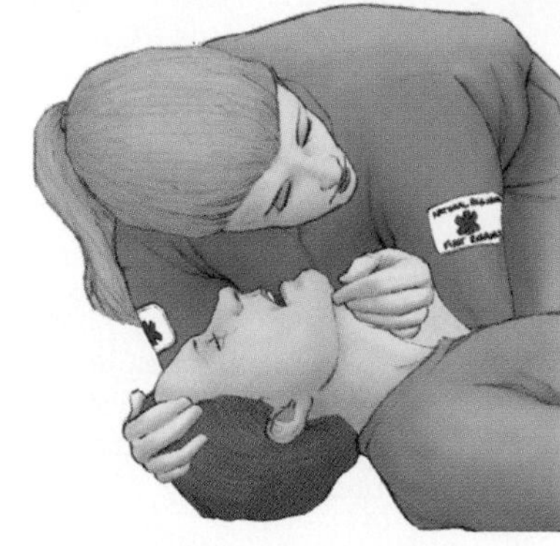

Figure 7.5 Check the patient's breathing.

cheek (**Figure 7.5**). If breathing is difficult, or if you hear unusual sounds, you may have to remove an object from the patient's mouth, such as food, vomitus, dentures, gum, chewing tobacco, or broken teeth.

If you cannot detect any movement of the chest and no sounds of air are coming from the nose and mouth, breathing is absent. Take immediate steps to open the patient's airway and perform rescue breathing. If trauma is suspected protect the cervical spine by keeping the patient's head in a neutral position and using the jaw-thrust technique to open the airway. Maintain cervical stabilization until the head and neck are immobilized (these procedures are covered in Chapter 6).

Check the Patient's Circulation

Next, check the patient's circulation (heartbeat). If the patient is unconscious, take the carotid pulse (**Figure 7.6**). Place your index and middle fingers together and touch the larynx (Adam's apple) in the patient's neck. Then slide your two fingers off the larynx toward the patient's ear until you feel a slight notch. Practice this maneuver until you are able to find a carotid pulse within 5 seconds of touching the patient's larynx. If you cannot feel a pulse with your fingers in 5 to 10 seconds, begin cardiopulmonary resuscitation (CPR), which is covered in Chapter 8.

If the patient is conscious, assess the radial pulse rather than the carotid pulse. Place your index and middle fingers on the patient's wrist at the thumb side. You should practice taking the radial pulse often to develop this skill (**Figure 7.7**).

Next, quickly check the patient for severe bleeding. If you discover severe bleeding, you must take immediate action to control it by applying direct pressure over the wound. These procedures are covered in Chapter 12. Quickly assess the patient's skin color and temperature. This assessment will give you an idea of whether the patient is suffering from internal bleeding and shock. It is important to check the color of the patient's skin when you arrive on the scene so that you can tell if the color changes as time goes on.

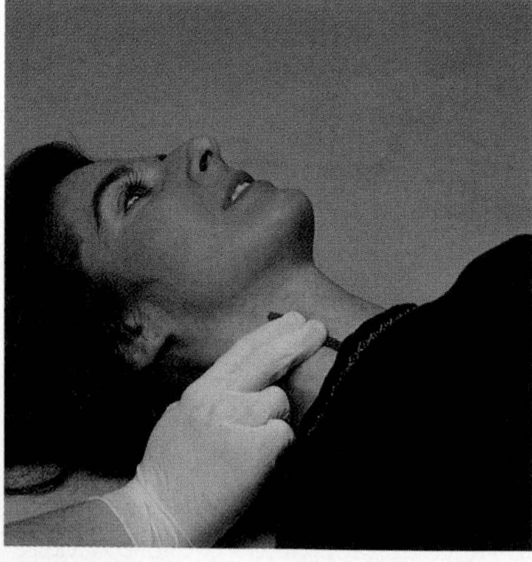

Figure 7.6 Check an unconscious patient's circulation by taking the carotid pulse.

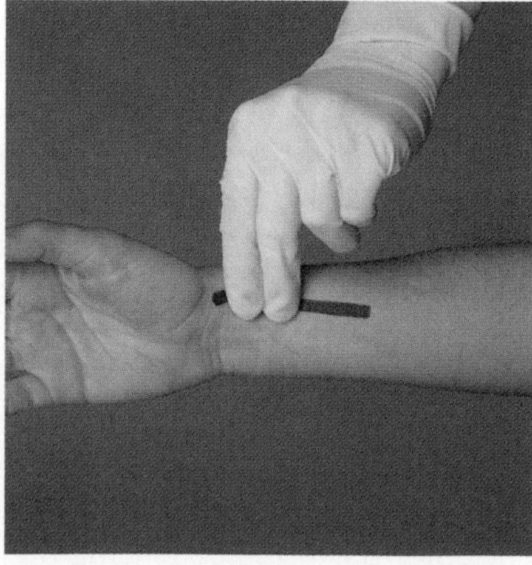

Figure 7.7 Take the radial pulse if the patient is conscious.

Special Needs

CHILDREN

To assess circulation in an infant, check the brachial pulse, located on the inside of the upper arm. You can feel the brachial pulse by placing your index and middle fingers on the inside of the infant's arm halfway between the shoulder and the elbow (**Figure 7.8**). Check for 5 to 10 seconds.

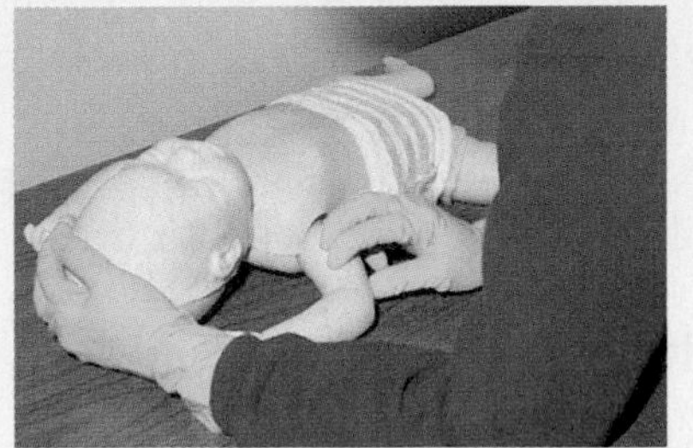

Figure 7.8 Take the brachial pulse if the patient is an infant.

Skin color is described as:

- Pale (whitish, indicating decreased circulation to that part of the body or to all of the body)
- Flushed (reddish, indicating excess circulation to that part of the body)
- Blue (also called **cyanosis**, indicating lack of oxygen and possible airway problems)
- Yellow (indicating liver problems)
- Normal

cyanosis Bluish coloration of the skin resulting from poor oxygenation of the circulating blood.

chief complaint The patient's response to a question such as "What happened?" or "What's wrong?"

Patients with deeply pigmented skin may show color changes in the fingernail beds, in the whites of the eyes, or inside the mouth.

Acknowledge the Patient's Chief Complaint

As you perform the initial patient assessment, you will often form an impression of the patient's **chief complaint**. It is important to acknowledge the patient's chief complaint and provide reassurance. A conscious patient will often complain of an injury that causes great pain or results in obvious bleeding. However, the injury that the patient complains of may not be the most serious injury (**Figure 7.9**). Do not allow a conscious patient's comments to distract you from completing the patient assessment sequence. You can acknowledge the patient's chief complaint by saying something like, "Yes, I can see that your arm appears to be broken, but let me finish checking you completely in case there are any other injuries. I will then treat your injured arm." In an unconscious patient, the primary "complaint" is unconsciousness.

BSI Tip

Remember to wear gloves to avoid contact with body fluids that may contain blood.

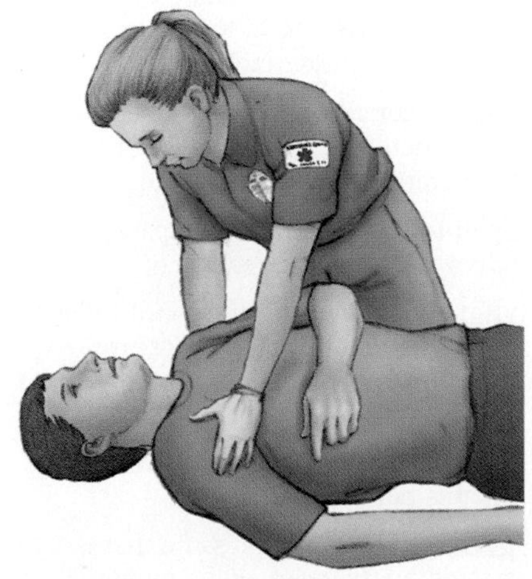

Figure 7.9 Acknowledge the patient's chief complaints.

Update Responding EMS Units

In some EMS systems you will be expected to update responding EMS units about the condition of your patient. This report should include age and sex of the patient, the chief complaint, level of responsiveness, and status of airway, breathing, and circulation. This update helps them know what to expect when they arrive on the scene.

Perform a Physical Examination

The **physical examination** of the patient from head to toe is done to assess non-life-threatening conditions after you have completed the initial assessment and stabilized life-threatening conditions. This exam helps you locate and begin initial management of the signs and symptoms of illness or injury. After you complete the physical examination, review any positive signs and symptoms of injury or illness. This review will help you to get a better picture of the patient's overall condition.

Signs and Symptoms

In a careful and systematic patient assessment, you need to understand the difference between a **sign** and a **symptom**. You need to be able to assess selected signs and report them systematically. You also need to be able to understand and report the symptoms that the patient reports.

Simply put, a sign is something about the patient you can see or feel for yourself. A symptom is something the patient tells you about his or her condition, such as "My back hurts" or "I think I am going to vomit."

The first step of the physical examination is to determine the patient's **vital signs**. These consist of respiration, pulse, and temperature. (Blood pressure, a fourth vital sign, is not routinely taken by first responders; however, your EMS service may include it as an optional skill. It is covered in Chapter 19.)

Respiration

The **respiratory rate** is a vital sign that indicates how fast the patient is breathing. It is measured as breaths per minute. In a normal adult, the resting respiratory rate is between 12 and 20 breaths per minute. One cycle of inhaling (breathing in) and exhaling (breathing out) is counted as one breath (respiration). Count the patient's breaths for one minute to determine the respiratory rate.

Respirations may be rapid and shallow (characteristic of shock) or slow (characteristic of a stroke or drug overdose). Respirations may also be described as deep, wheezing, gasping, panting, snoring, noisy, or labored. If the patient is not breathing, respiration is described as "absent," a condition that would have been addressed during the initial assessment.

When you are checking the rate or noting the quality of respirations, make sure that your face or hand is close enough to the patient's face to feel the exhaled air on your skin. Also watch for the rise and fall of the chest. When counting respirations in a conscious patient, try not to let the patient know that you are counting. If the patient knows you are counting respirations, you may not get an accurate count.

Pulse

The second vital sign is the **pulse**, which indicates the speed and force of the heartbeat. A pulse can be felt anywhere on the body where an artery passes over a hard structure such as a bone. Although there are many such places on the body, the four most common pulse points are the radial (wrist), the carotid (neck), the brachial (arm), and the posterior tibial (ankle).

3

Physical Examination

- Determine the Patient's Vital Signs
- Inspect for Signs of Injury
- Examine the Patient from Head to Toe

physical examination The step in the patient assessment sequence in which the first responder carefully examines the patient from head to toe, looking for additional injuries and other problems.

sign A condition that you observe in a patient, such as bleeding or the temperature of a patient's skin.

symptom A condition the patient tells you, such as "I feel dizzy."

vital signs Signs of life, specifically pulse, respiration, blood pressure, and temperature.

respiratory rate The speed at which a person is breathing (measured in breaths per minute).

pulse The wave of pressure that is created by the heart as it contracts and forces blood out of the heart and into the major arteries.

The most commonly taken pulse is the **radial pulse**, located at the wrist where the radial artery passes over one of the forearm bones, the radius (see Figure 7.7 on page 150). The carotid pulse is taken over a **carotid artery**, located on either side of the patient's neck just under the jawbone (see Figure 7.6 on page 150). The **brachial pulse** is taken on the inside of the arm, halfway between the shoulder and the elbow (see Figure 7.8 on page 151). The **posterior tibial pulse** is located on the inner aspect of the ankle just behind the ankle bone (**Figure 7.10**).

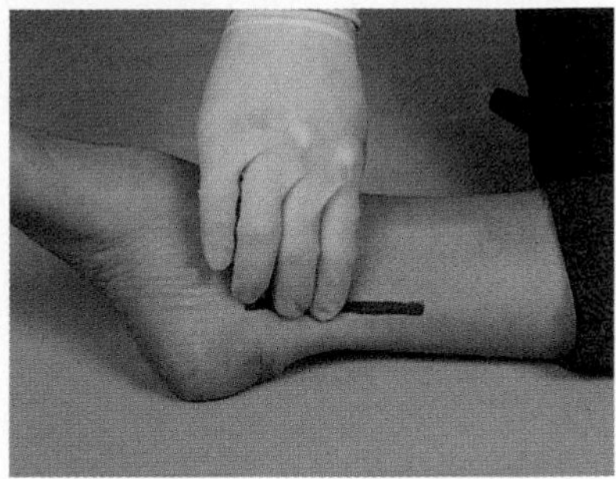

Figure 7.10 Taking the ankle pulse.

In general, you should take the radial pulse of a conscious patient and the carotid pulse of an unconscious patient. When examining an infant, use the brachial pulse. The posterior tibial pulse is used to assess the circulatory status of a leg.

To check a patient's pulse, you need to determine three things: rate, rhythm, and quality.

To determine the pulse rate (heartbeats per minute), find the patient's pulse with your fingers, count the beats for 30 seconds, and multiply by 2. In a normal adult, the resting pulse rate is about 60 to 80 beats per minute, although in a physically fit person (such as a jogger) the resting rate may be lower (about 40 to 60 beats per minute). In children, the pulse rate is normally faster (about 80 to 100 beats per minute). (See Chapter 15.)

A very slow pulse (fewer than 40 beats per minute) can be the result of a serious illness, whereas a very fast pulse (more than 120 beats per minute) can indicate that the patient is in shock. Remember, however, that a person who is in excellent physical condition may have a pulse rate of less than 50 beats per minute, and a person who is simply anxious or worried could have a fast pulse rate (more than 110 beats per minute).

You should also be able to determine the rhythm and describe the quality of the pulse. Note whether the pulse is regular or irregular. A strong pulse is often referred to as a **bounding pulse**. This is similar to the heart rate that follows physical exertion such as running or lifting heavy objects. The beats are very strong and well defined. A weak pulse is often called a **thready pulse**. The pulse is present, but the beats are not easily detected. A thready pulse is a more dangerous sign than a bounding pulse. A bounding pulse can be dangerous if the patient has high blood pressure and is at risk for a stroke.

Capillary Refill

Capillary refill is the ability of the circulatory system to return blood to the capillary vessels after the blood has been squeezed out. The capillary refill test is done on the patient's fingernails or toenails. To perform this test, squeeze the patient's nail bed firmly between your thumb and forefinger (**Figure 7.11**, page 154). The patient's nail bed will look pale. Release the pressure. Count two seconds by saying "capillary refill." The patient's nail bed should become pink. This indicates a normal capillary refill time.

If the patient has lost a lot of blood and is in shock, or if the blood vessels supplying that limb have been damaged, the capillary refill will

radial pulse Wrist pulse.

carotid pulse A pulse that can be felt on each side of the neck where the carotid artery is close to the skin.

carotid arteries The principle arteries of the neck. They supply blood to the face, head, and brain.

brachial pulse Pulse located in the arm between the elbow and shoulder; used for checking pulse in infants.

posterior tibial pulse Ankle pulse.

bounding pulse A strong pulse (similar to the pulse that follows physical exertion like running or lifting heavy objects).

thready pulse A weak pulse.

capillary refill The ability of the circulatory system to restore blood to the capillary blood vessels after it has been squeezed out by the examiner.

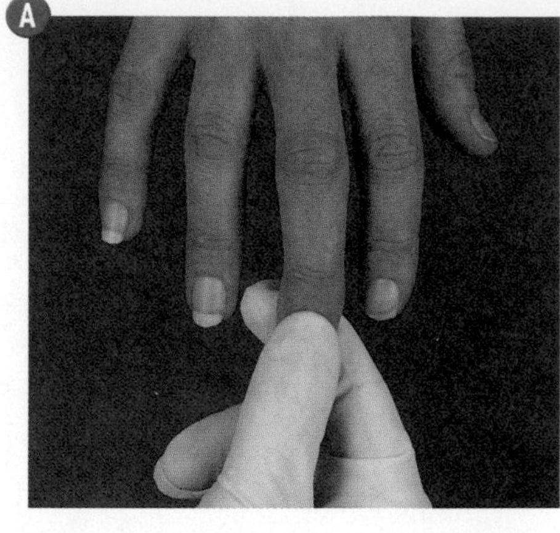
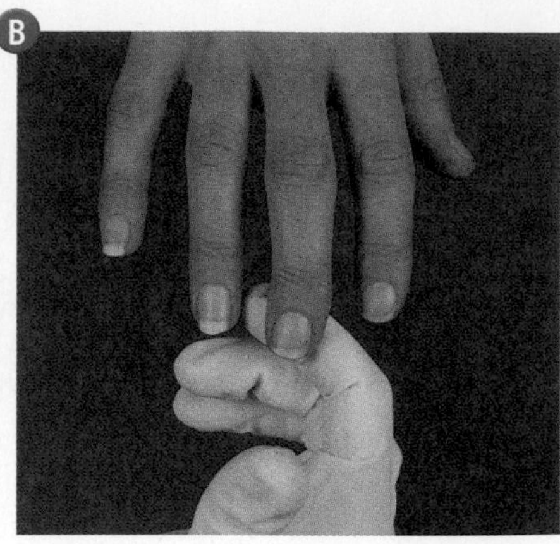

Figure 7.11 Checking capillary refill time. **A.** Squeeze the nail bed between your thumb and forefinger. **B.** Release the pressure.

be delayed or entirely absent. Capillary refill will be delayed in a cold environment and should not be used as the sole means for assessing the circulatory status of an extremity. Check with your medical director to determine if you should use the capillary refill test.

Skin Condition

The patient's skin should be checked for color and moisture. For information on checking skin color, see **Table 7.2** on page 158.

Normal body temperature is about 98.6°F, or 37°C. Precise body temperature is taken with a thermometer, but you can estimate a patient's body temperature by placing the back of your hand on the patient's forehead. The patient's skin temperature is judged, in relation to your skin temperature, as hot or cold.

Some illnesses can cause the skin to become excessively moist or excessively dry. Therefore, together with its relative temperature, the patient's skin might be described as hot and dry, hot and moist, cold and dry, or cold and moist.

After you have determined the patient's vital signs, you should also be able to identify and measure these other important signs: pupil size and reactivity, and level of consciousness.

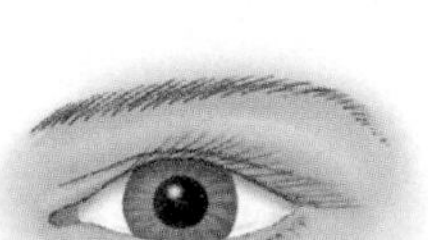

Normal pupil

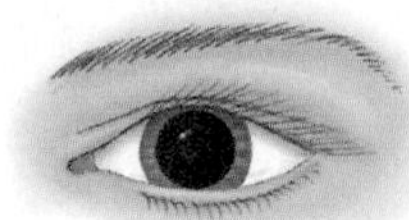

Dilated pupil

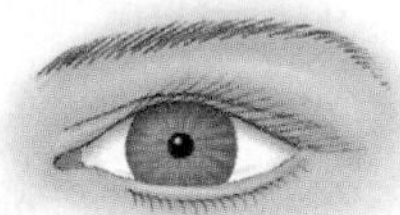

Constricted pupil

Figure 7.12 Normal, dilated, and constricted pupils.

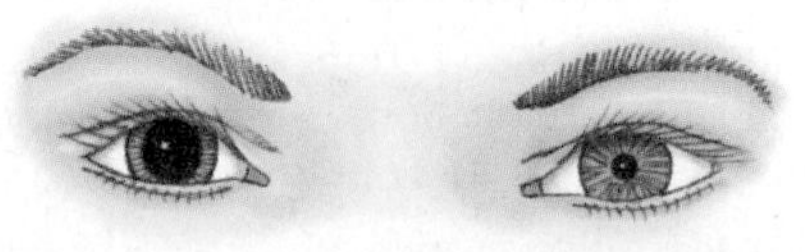

Figure 7.13 Unequal pupils may indicate a stroke or injury to the brain.

pupil The circular opening in the middle of the eye.

Pupil Size and Reactivity

FYI

It is important to examine each eye to detect signs of head injury, stroke, or drug overdose. Look to see whether the **pupils** are of equal size and whether they both react (contract) when light is shone into them (**Figure 7.12**). The following findings are abnormal:

- ***Pupils of unequal size***. Unequal pupils can indicate a stroke or injury to the brain (**Figure 7.13**). A small percentage of people normally have unequal pupils, but unequal pupils are usually a valuable diagnostic sign in an injured or ill patient.
- ***Pupils that remain constricted***. Constricted pupils are often present in a person who is taking narcotics. They are also a sign of certain central nervous system diseases.
- ***Pupils that remain dilated (enlarged)***. Dilated pupils indicate a relaxed or unconscious state. Pupils will dilate within 30 to 60 seconds of cardiac arrest. Head injuries and the use of certain drugs such as barbiturates can also cause dilated pupils.

Level of Consciousness

You will usually assess the patient's level of consciousness as part of your initial assessment. However, it is important to observe and note any changes that occur between the time of your arrival and the time you turn over the patient's care to personnel at the next level of the EMS system. Report any changes from one level of consciousness to another, using the AVPU scale (see page 149).

Signs Review

Signs are indicators of illness or injury that a first responder can observe in a patient. They help you to determine what is wrong with the patient and the severity of the patient's condition. Vital signs include the patient's respirations (respiratory status), pulse (circulatory status), skin condition, and temperature. Other signs include pupil size and reaction, and level of consciousness.

To assess a patient's respiratory status, determine the patient's breathing rate and whether breaths are rapid or slow, shallow or deep, noisy or quiet. In assessing a patient's circulatory status, you determine the rate, rhythm, and quality of the victim's pulse. You can also determine if the patient's capillary refill is normal, slow, or absent. Although you may not be able to determine the patient's exact temperature, you will be able to state whether the patient is hot or cold. Skin condition is measured by color and moisture, and can be described as pale, flushed, blue, yellow, normal, dry, or moist. To assess the patient's pupils, check to see whether the pupils are equal or unequal in size and whether they remain constricted or dilated. Use the AVPU scale to assess the patient's level of consciousness: alert, responsive to verbal stimuli, responsive to pain, or unresponsive.

Check✓point

Describe the importance of the following signs:

- ○ Respirations
- ○ Pulse
- ○ Temperature
- ○ Skin color and moisture
- ○ Capillary refill
- ○ Pupil size and reactivity
- ○ Level of consciousness

Inspect for Signs of Injury

As you perform the patient examination, look and feel for the following signs of injury: deformities, open injuries, tenderness, and swelling. Use the acronym DOTS to remember these signs (**Table 7.1**).

Table 7.1

Signs of Injury

D	Deformities
O	Open Injuries
T	Tenderness
S	Swelling

Examine the Patient from Head to Toe

Conduct a thorough, hands-on, head-to-toe examination in a logical, systematic manner. It is important to conduct the examination the same way each time to be sure you search all areas of the body for injuries. Use a clear, concise format to communicate your findings to other medical personnel.

The head-to-toe examination can be done whether the patient is conscious or unconscious. Watch the reactions of a conscious patient to your examination. You may want to ask what the patient is feeling as you proceed with your examination. Remember that your examination is the main focus of this part of the assessment. Do not ask the patient so many questions that you are not doing a thorough physical examination.

If the patient is unconscious, it is vitally important that you assess the airway, breathing, and circulation during the initial assessment. After you have established breathing and pulse, begin a head-to-toe examination of the unconscious patient. Examining an unconscious patient is difficult because the patient cannot cooperate or tell you where something hurts. Your examination often will elicit grimaces or moans from an unconscious patient.

Assume that all unconscious, injured patients have spine injuries. Stabilize the head and spine to minimize movement during the patient examination. It is essential to fully immobilize all injured, unconscious patients on a **backboard** before transporting them. (See Chapter 5.) You should also be cautious when treating a patient who is unconscious because of illness.

backboard A straight board used for splinting, extricating, and transporting patients with suspected spine injuries.

Examine the Head

Use both hands to examine thoroughly all areas of the scalp (**Figure 7.14**). Do not move the patient's head! This is especially important if the patient is unconscious or has suffered a spine injury. Injuries to the head bleed a lot. Be sure to find the actual wound; do not be fooled by globs of matted, bloody hair.

If necessary, remove the patient's eyeglasses and put them in a safe place. Many patients who need glasses become upset if their glasses are taken away. Use your judgment in each case. Be considerate of the patient.

If the patient is wearing a wig, it may be necessary to remove the hairpiece to complete the head examination. Be sure to check the entire head for bumps, areas of tenderness, and bleeding.

Examine the Eyes

Cover one eye for five seconds. Then quickly open the eyelid and watch the pupil, the dark part at the center of the eye. The normal reaction of the pupil is to contract (get smaller). This should happen in about one second. If you are examining a patient's eyes at night or in the dark, use a flashlight and aim the light at the closed eye (**Figure 7.15**).

A pupil that fails to react to light or pupils that are unequal in size may be important diagnostic signs and should be reported to personnel at the next level of medical care.

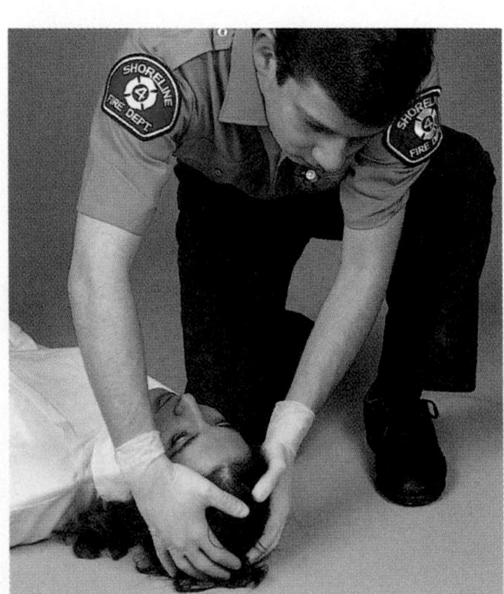

Figure 7.14 Use both hands to examine the head.

Examine the Nose

Examine the nose for tenderness or deformity, which may indicate a broken nose. Check to see if there is any blood or fluid coming from the nose.

Examine the Mouth

Your first examination of the mouth should have taken place when you checked to see whether the patient was breathing. Now recheck the mouth for foreign objects such as food, vomitus, dentures, gum, chewing tobacco, and loose teeth. Be sure to carefully clear away any material

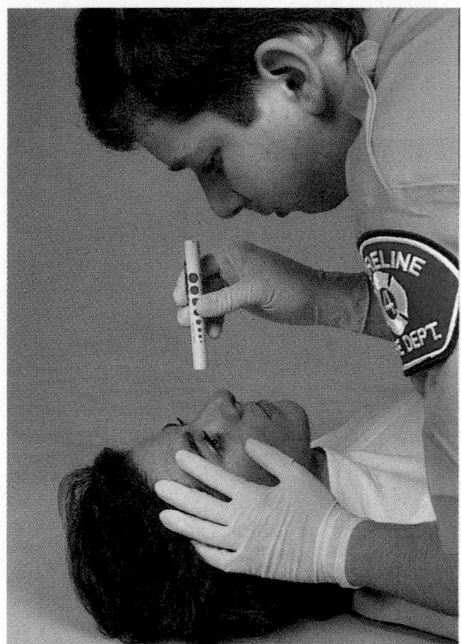

Figure 7.15 Examine the patient's eyes.

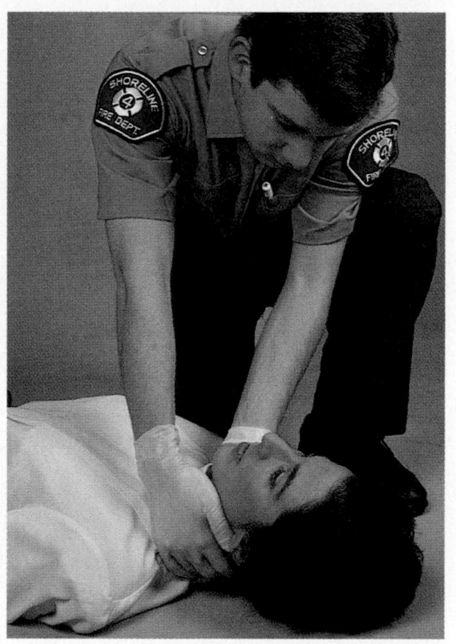

Figure 7.16 Use both hands to examine the patient's neck.

that obstructs the patient's breathing. In addition, you should be ready to deal with vomiting. It is important to prevent **aspiration** (inhalation) of vomitus into the lungs.

Use your sense of smell to determine whether any unusual odors are present. A patient who is sick with diabetes may have a fruity breath odor. Do not allow the presence of alcohol on the patient's breath to change the way you treat the patient. In fact, if you detect alcohol, you should conduct an especially careful physical examination, particularly if the patient appears to be severely injured. Remember to place any unconscious patient who has not suffered trauma in the recovery position. This helps keep the patient's airway open and prevents aspiration of vomitus into the airway or lungs.

aspiration Breathing in foreign matter such as food, drink, or vomitus into the airway or lungs.

stoma An opening.

Examine the Neck

Examine the neck carefully using both hands, one on each side of the patient's neck. Be sure to touch the vertebrae (the bony part of the back of the neck) to see whether gentle pressure produces pain (**Figure 7.16**).

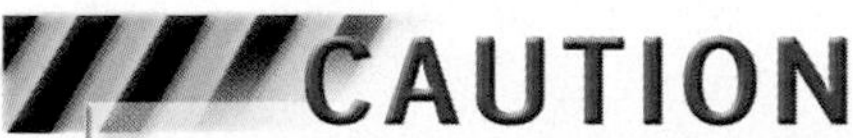

CAUTION

Be careful not to move the neck or head!

Check the neck veins. Swollen (distended) neck veins may indicate heart problems or major trauma to the chest.

Examine the neck for a **stoma** (opening), which indicates that the patient is a "neck breather." A neck breather is a person who has undergone major surgery in which the airway above the stoma has been removed. The stoma may be the patient's only means of breathing, and the patient may not be able to speak normally. The stoma is usually concealed behind an article of clothing or a bib.

As your hands move down the patient's scalp and onto the neck, check for the presence of an emergency medical identification neck chain. Any chain around a patient's neck should be examined for medical information. The internationally recognized symbol shown in **Figure 7.17** is found on necklaces, arm bracelets, ankle bracelets, and wallet cards and is carried by people who have a medical condition that warrants special attention if they become ill or injured. If you find such a warning on a patient, it is your responsibility to give this information to the next person in the EMS system.

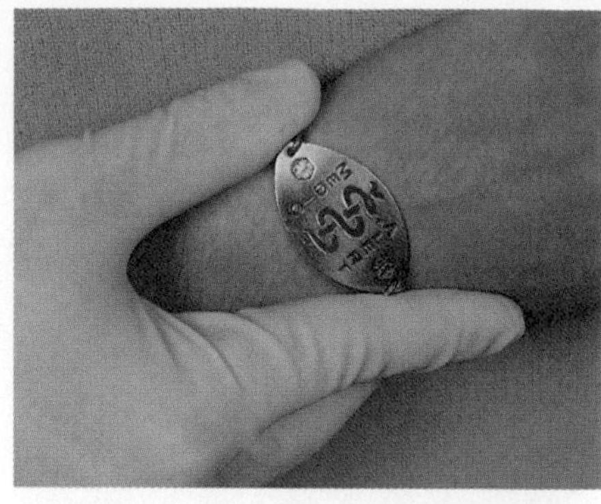

Figure 7.17 Medical identification is found on wrist and ankle bracelets, necklaces, and wallet cards.

Examine the Face

While you are performing the hands-on examination of the head and neck, be sure to note the color of the facial skin, its temperature, and whether it is moist or dry (**Table 7.2**).

After you have completed the head examination, be sure to note any bumps, bruises, cuts, or other abnormalities.

Examine the Chest

If the patient is conscious, ask him or her to take a deep breath and tell you whether there is any pain on **inhalation** or **exhalation**. Note whether the patient breathes with difficulty. Look and listen for signs of difficult breathing such as coughing, wheezing, or foaming at the mouth.

It is important to look at both sides of the chest completely, noting any injuries, bleeding, or sections of the chest that move abnormally, unequally, or painfully. Unequal motion of one side or section may be a sign of a serious condition, called a **flail chest**, that can result from multiple rib fractures. Be sure to run your hands over all parts of the chest. Like the head and neck examinations, this must be accomplished with minimal patient movement (**Figure 7.18**).

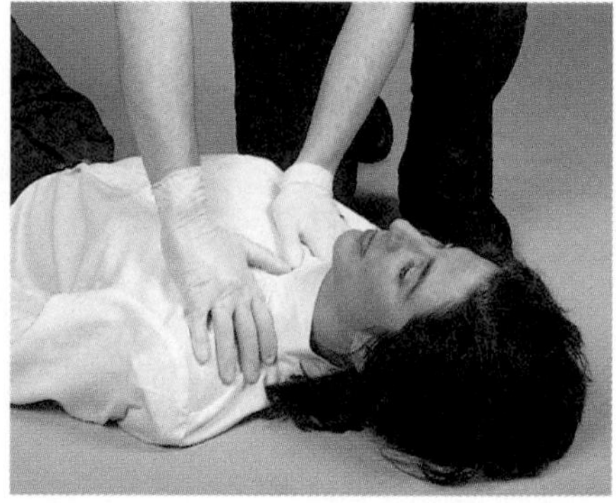

Figure 7.18 Examine the patient's chest.

Apply firm but gentle pressure to the collarbone (**clavicle**) to check for **fractures**. Check the chest for fractured ribs by placing your hands

inhalation Breathing in.

exhalation Breathing out.

flail chest A condition that occurs when three or more ribs are broken each in two places, and the chest wall lying between the fractures becomes a free-floating segment.

clavicle The collarbone.

fracture Any break in a bone.

Table 7.2

Skin Color

Color	Term	Sign of
Red	Flushed	Fever or sunburn
White	Pale	Shock
Blue	Cyanotic	Airway obstruction
Yellow	Jaundiced	Liver disease

on the chest and pushing down gently but firmly. Then put your hands on each side of the chest and push inward, squeezing the chest.

abdomen The body cavity, lying between the thorax and the pelvis that contains the major organs of digestion and excretion.

Examine the Abdomen

Continue your examination downward to the **abdomen** (stomach and groin). Look for any signs of external bleeding, penetrating injuries, or protruding parts, such as intestines (**Figure 7.19**).

Ask the patient to relax the stomach muscles and observe whether the stomach remains rigid. Rigidity is often a sign of abdominal injury. Swelling is also a sign of abdominal injury.

Note whether the clothing has been soiled with urine or feces. This may be an important diagnostic sign for certain illnesses or injuries, such as stroke. Make sure you check the genital area for external injuries. Although both the patient and you may be socially uncomfortable during this examination, it must be done if there is any suspicion of injury.

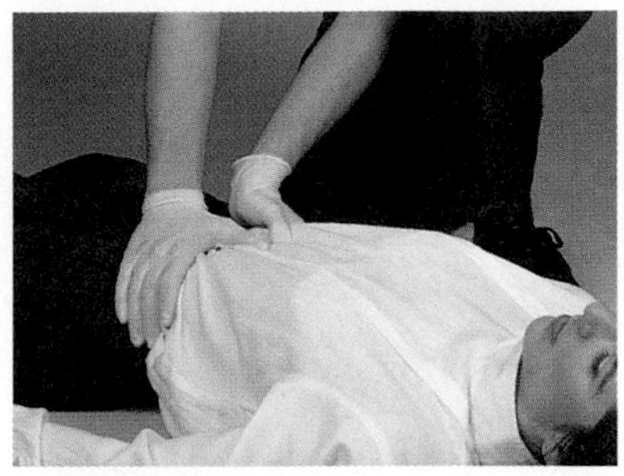

Figure 7.19 Examine the patient's abdomen.

Remember

Continue talking to the patient throughout the entire patient assessment. Tell the patient what you are doing and why.

Examine the Pelvis

Next check for fractures of the pelvis. First check for signs of obvious bruising, bleeding, or swelling. If no pain is reported by the patient, then gently press on the pelvic bones. If the patient reports pain or tenderness or if you note any movement, a severe injury may be present in this region (**Figure 7.20**).

Examine the Back

FYI

The patient's back should be checked one side of the back at a time, using one hand to gently lift the patient's shoulder and the other to slide downward in the examination (**Figure 7.21**). In cases where a patient has been injured, stabilize the head and neck to prevent movement while you examine the patient.

As you check each side of the back, be sure that your hands go all the way to the midline of the patient's body so you can feel the spinal column. Check half the back from one side; then switch and check the other side in the same manner. This ensures that no part of the back is missed during the examination. If the patient is lying on his or her side or stomach, it will be much easier to examine the patient's back. If the patient must be rolled on a backboard, you can examine the patient's back while the patient is on his or her side. Do not wait for a backboard if this will delay your examination of the patient.

A

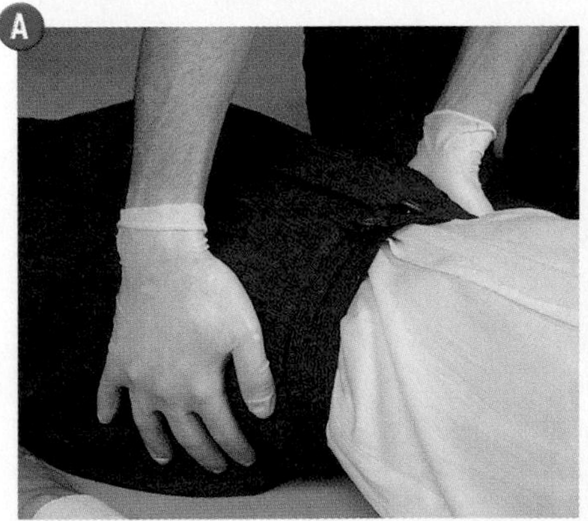

B

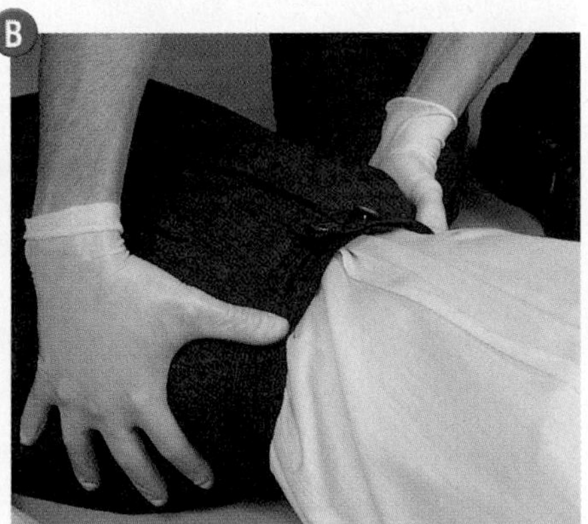

Figure 7.20 Examine the patient's pelvis by gently pressing on the pelvic bones. **A.** Place your hands on both sides of the pelvis. **B.** Push downward and push inward.

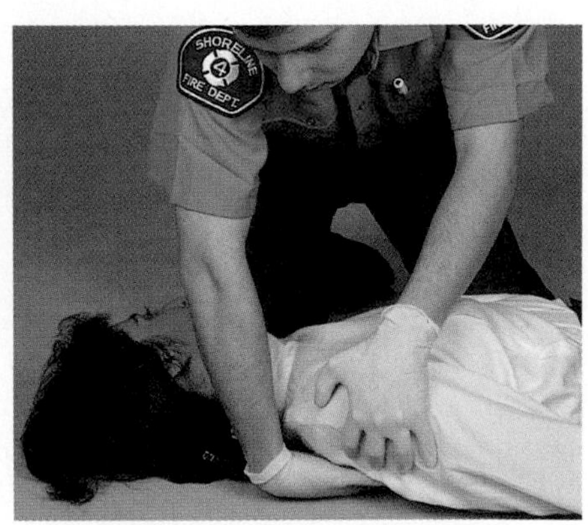

Figure 7.21 Examine the patient's back.

Examine the Extremities

Do a systematic examination of each extremity to determine if there are any injuries. This examination consists of the following five steps:

1. Observe the extremity to determine if there is any visible injury. Look for bleeding and deformity.
2. Examine for tenderness in each extremity by encircling it with both hands and gently, but firmly, squeezing each part of the limb. Watch the patient's face and listen to see if the patient shows any signs of pain.
3. Ask the patient to move the extremity. Check for normal movement. Determine if there is any pain when the patient moves the extremity.

CAUTION

Do not ask the patient to move an extremity if you find any deformity or tenderness during the first two steps.

4. Check for sensation by touching the bare skin of each extremity. See if the patient can feel your touch.
5. Assess the circulatory status of each extremity by checking for the presence of a pulse in that extremity and by checking for capillary refill.

arm Part of the upper extremity that extends from the shoulder to the elbow.

Each upper extremity consists of the **arm**, the forearm, the wrist, and the hand. The arm extends from the shoulder to the elbow; the forearm extends from the elbow to the wrist.

Examine one upper extremity at a time (**Figure 7.22**):

1. ***Observe the extremity***. Start by looking at its position. Is it in a normal or an abnormal position? Does it look broken (deformed) to you?
2. ***Examine for tenderness***. Encircle the upper extremity with your hands. Work from the shoulder downward to the hand. Firmly squeeze the limb to locate any possible fractures.

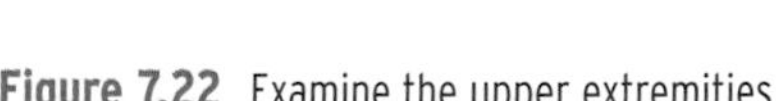

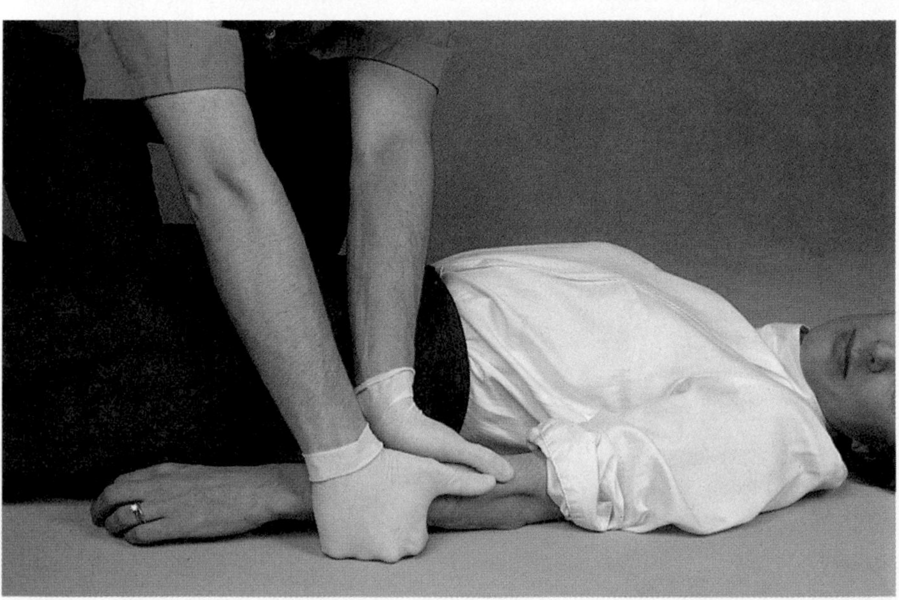

Figure 7.22 Examine the upper extremities one at a time.

3. ***Check for movement***. Take the patient's hand in yours and ask the patient to squeeze your hand. Squeezing is usually painful for the patient if there is a fracture or other injury. If a conscious patient cannot squeeze your hand, you should assume that the extremity is seriously injured or paralyzed.
4. ***Check for sensation***. Ask the patient if he or she feels any tingling or numbness in the extremity. Such tingling or numbness may be a sign of a spine injury. Check for sensation by touching the palm of the patient's hand. See if the patient can feel your touch.
5. ***Assess the circulatory status***. Check the patient's radial pulse. Absence of a radial pulse indicates blood vessel damage. Check the fingers for capillary refill. Check the color, temperature, and moisture of the hand.

Repeat this examination for the other upper extremity.

Each lower extremity consists of the thigh, the **leg**, the ankle, and the foot. The thigh extends from the hip to the knee. The leg extends from the knee to the ankle.

leg The lower extremity; specifically, the lower portion, from the knee to the ankle.

Examine one lower extremity at a time (**Figure 7.23**):

1. ***Observe the extremity***. Look at the position and shape of the lower extremity. Is it deformed? Is the foot rotated inward or outward?
2. ***Examine for tenderness***. Encircle the lower extremity with your hands, as you did with the upper extremities. Move from the groin to the foot. Be sure to make contact with all surfaces of the limb. Use firm but gentle pressure to identify tender (injured) areas. You are not handling eggs but are attempting to locate injuries.
3. ***Check for movement***. Ask the patient to move the limb only if you have found no signs of injury in the first two steps. If there is a significant injury, movement will probably be painful. If a conscious patient cannot move the foot or toes, the limb is seriously injured or paralyzed.
4. ***Check for sensation***. Ask the patient whether he or she can feel your touch as you examine the extremity. Tingling or numbness in a limb is a sign of spine injury.
5. ***Assess circulatory status***. Check the posterior tibial (ankle) pulse, located just behind the ankle bone on the medial (inner) side of the ankle. Absence of this pulse indicates blood vessel damage, which is sometimes caused by fractures. Check the toes for capillary refill. Check the skin color, temperature, and moisture of the extremity.

Repeat this examination for the other lower extremity.

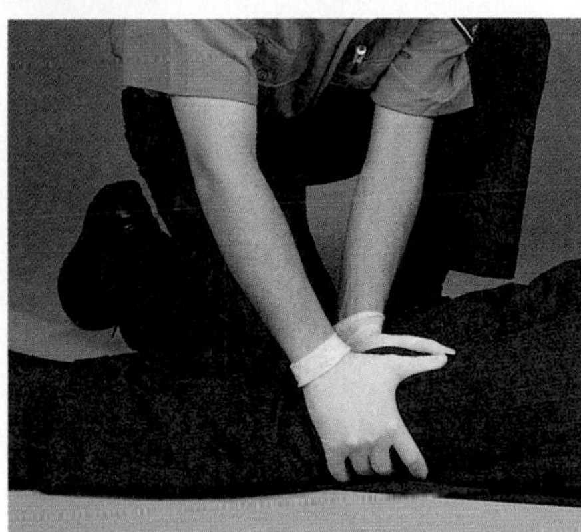

Figure 7.23 Examine the lower extremities one at a time.

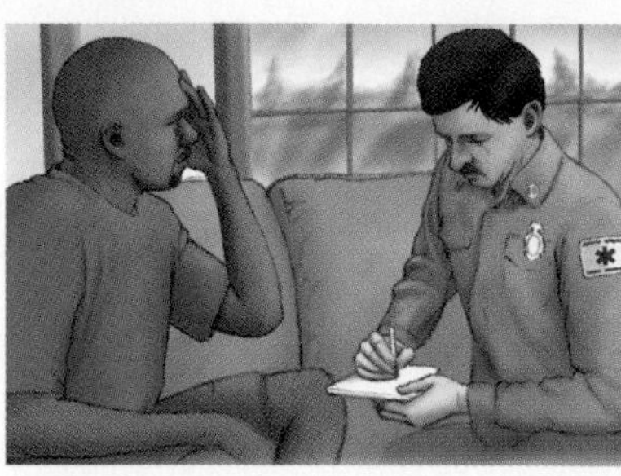

Figure 7.24 Obtain the patient's medical history (SAMPLE).

4 Patient's Medical History

- Check for Medical ID
- Obtain History from Patients/Relatives/Bystanders
- Obtain SAMPLE History

SAMPLE history A patient's medical history. S=signs/symptoms, A=allergies, M=medications, P=pertinent past history, L=last oral intake, E=events associated with the illness or injury.

Obtain the Patient's Medical History

Knowing the patient's health status prior to the incident can help medical personnel give proper treatment and avoid measures that might endanger the patient further. Therefore, you should attempt to gather important facts about the patient's general medical history (**Figure 7.24**). Important questions include:

- How old are you?
- Do you have any existing medical problems (such as a heart condition or diabetes)?
- Are you under the care of a physician at the present time?
- Do you have any allergies?

If the patient is unconscious, a family member, friend, or co-worker may be able to answer these questions. Important information can often be found on a medical identification necklace, bracelet, or card.

One of the most commonly used medical history formats is the SAMPLE history (**Table 7.3**). Each letter in the SAMPLE history stands for a different part of the medical history.

Table 7.3

SAMPLE Medical History

S	Signs and symptoms of the injury or illness that caused the patient to call for emergency medical services. Patients should describe signs and symptoms in their own words.
A	Allergies. Patients may be allergic to medicines, food, or airborne particles.
M	Medications. What medications is the patient taking? Ask about medications prescribed by the patient's physician and over-the-counter (nonprescription) medicines.
P	Pertinent past medical history. What events or symptoms might be related to the patient's current illness? For example, it would be important to know whether a patient experiencing severe chest pain had a previous heart attack.
L	Last oral intake. When was the last time the patient had anything to eat or drink? Find out what the patient last ate or drank and how much he or she consumed.
E	Events associated with or leading to this injury or illness. Knowing these events will help you put together the pieces of the medical history puzzle. Let patients describe these events in their own words.

These six areas of a patient's medical history give you important information about the problem. Pass this information on to other EMS and hospital personnel.

Provide On-Going Assessment

The patient assessment sequence helps you determine each patient's initial condition. Patients who appear stable can become unstable quickly. Therefore, it is essential that you watch all patients carefully for changes in status. As a general rule, you should monitor the patient's vital signs every 15 minutes. Continue to maintain an open airway, monitor breathing and pulse for rate and quality, and observe the skin color and temperature. If the patient is unstable, take the patient's vital signs every 5 minutes. If the patient's condition changes, repeat the physical examination. Check to see if the interventions you took were effective. Continue to talk with the patient. Tell the patient what you are doing and give reassurance.

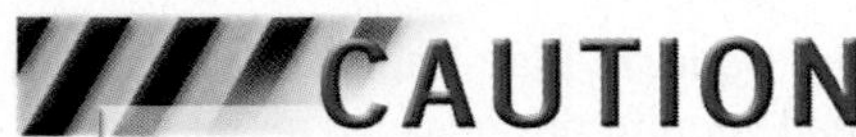

Serious changes can occur rapidly!

Providing a "Hand-off" Report

It is important that you describe your findings concisely and accurately to the emergency medical personnel who take over the care of your patients in a "hand-off" report (**Figure 7.25**, page 165).

The easiest way to report your patient assessment results is to use the same systematic approach you followed during the patient assessment:

1. Provide the age and sex of the patient.
2. Describe the history of the incident.
3. Describe the patient's chief complaint.
4. Describe the patient's level of responsiveness.
5. Report the status of the vital signs: airway, breathing, and circulation (including severe bleeding).
6. Describe the results of the physical examination.
7. Report any pertinent medical conditions using the SAMPLE format.
8. Report the interventions provided.

Working in a systematic manner will help ensure that you do not overlook any significant symptoms, signs, or injuries and will help to make the hand-off report complete and accurate. For example, a hand-off report on a 23-year-old man injured in an automobile accident might include the following information:

1. The patient is a 23-year-old man.
2. He was involved in a two-car, head-on collision.

5

On-Going Assessment

- Repeat Initial Assessment
- Repeat Physical Exam as Needed
- Check Effectivness of Treatment
- Calm Patient
- Provide Hand-off Report

Voices of Experience

Rescuers Free Trapped Canoeist from Rapids

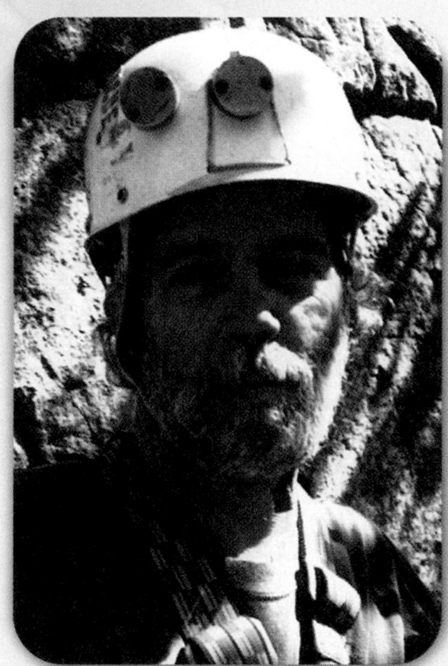

On August 10, 1994, while waiting to serve as Trip Leader to a commercial white water rafting trip on Tennessee's Ocoee River, a Tennessee Park Ranger drove up to me and asked me to collect my gear and come with him to lend my swiftwater rescue training to a critical situation.

En route to a section of the river known as "Squeeze Play Rapid" the ranger informed me of a swiftwater rescue that had been in progress for about one hour. Upon arrival, first responders told me that a canoeist was trapped in his boat, which had broached on a rock in the middle of the rapid. I could see the victim from the road. Wilderness first responders who had been on the river when the incident occurred were holding his head out of the water. There were many ropes tied to the canoe and attempts were being made to pull the boat free.

I was able to get to the victim with my rescue gear and the help of a kayaker. Once there, I quickly determined that if we were to free the canoe, the patient would be in more trouble because he was trapped in the canoe by a paddle that had bent around his legs. I cut all but one rope free, got out my rescue saw, and proceeded to cut the canoe in half just behind the patient. The entire time the patient was alert and oriented with his airway just out of the water and being maintained by first responders.

"A quick assessment of the patient showed mild hypothermia with a closed fracture of the right lower leg and two deep puncture wounds in the right thigh."

After cutting the canoe in half, I was able to relieve the pressure on his legs and move him to a raft that had been paddled out to us by other river guides. A quick assessment of the patient showed mild hypothermia with a closed fracture of the right lower leg and two deep puncture wounds in the right thigh. The patient was splinted and moved to the shore where an ALS unit was standing by. He was transported to a local hospital emergency room where his injuries were treated.

It is important to note that one should never attempt a swiftwater rescue unless trained and certified in this type of rescue. However, thanks to experienced swiftwater-trained first responders and a well-handled rescue, a tragedy was averted. The patient is still canoeing today, and I have a nice flower planter in my yard—the back half of the canoe. ❖

Russell L. Miller, Critical Care, Wilderness Paramedic
Director, Wilderness Safety Consultants
Program Director of EMS Education
Cleveland State Community College
Cleveland, Tennessee

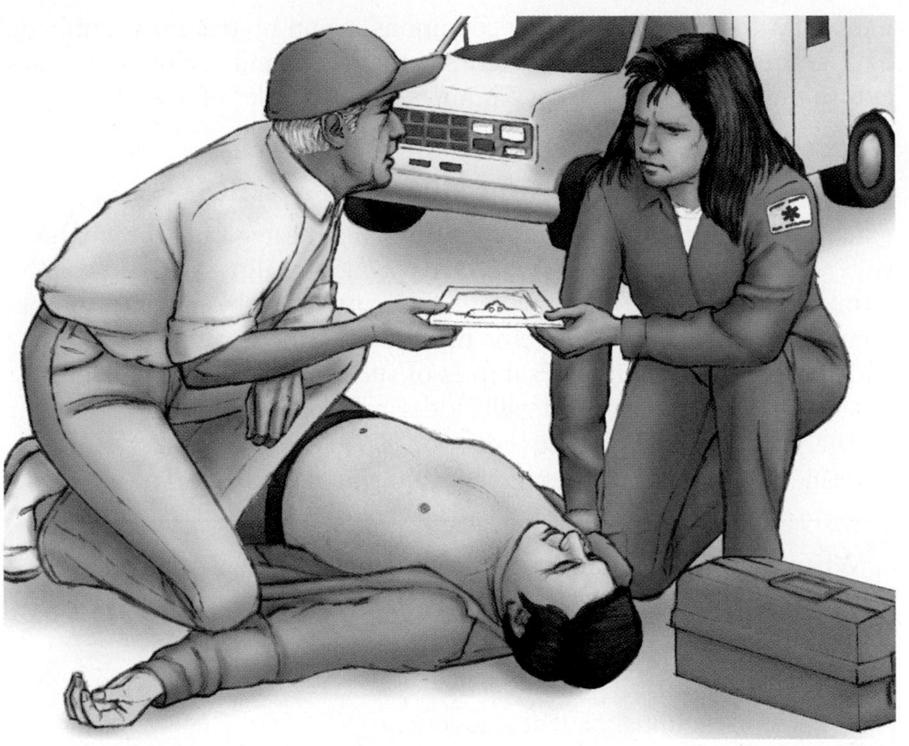

Figure 7.25 Report your findings in a hand-off report.

3. He is complaining of stomach pain and has a 2-inch cut on his forehead.
4. He is conscious and alert.
5. His pulse is 78 beats per minute and strong. His respirations are 16 breaths per minute and are regular and deep.
6. Examination revealed a 2-inch cut on his forehead, marks on his stomach, and moderate pain midway between his right knee and ankle.
7. He has no known medical conditions.
8. The patient is on his back, covered with a blanket to preserve his body heat. We have bandaged his laceration and immobilized his leg with an inflatable splint.

Remember that the purpose of the patient assessment sequence is to:

- Assist you in finding the patient's injuries so you can treat them.
- Obtain information about the patient's condition, which you provide to the EMS personnel at the next level of medical care.

With practice, you can complete the entire patient assessment sequence in about two minutes. This is not a complete medical examination but, as the name implies, is a patient assessment by first responders.

Examine every patient involved in an incident before you begin major treatment of any single patient. The exceptions to this rule are airway, breathing, and circulatory problems (severe bleeding or shock), which you must treat as you encounter them during patient assessment.

Except for these life-threatening conditions, begin no treatment until you have examined all patients to determine the extent and severity of injuries and to make sure that you treat injuries in their order of severity.

A Word about Trauma and Medical Patients

trauma A wound or injury.

illness Sickness.

Patients can generally be divided into two main categories: those who suffer from **trauma** and those who have a sudden **illness**. Trauma is the term used for an injury to a patient. The injury may be major or minor. Some incidents that cause trauma include falls, motor vehicle crashes, and sports-related injuries. Examples of sudden illnesses include heart attacks, strokes, asthma, and gallbladder problems.

The patient assessment sequence you have learned can be used to examine patients who have suffered from trauma, illnesses, or both.

When examining trauma patients, follow the sequence as you learned it:

1. Size up the scene.
2. Perform an initial patient assessment:
   a. Form a general impression of the patient.
   b. Assess the patient's responsiveness and stabilize the patient's spine if necessary.
   c. Assess the patient's airway.
   d. Assess the patient's breathing.
   e. Assess the patient's circulation (including severe bleeding) and stabilize if necessary.
   f. Update the responding EMS units.
3. Examine the patient from head to toe.
4. Obtain the patient's medical history using the SAMPLE format.
5. Provide on-going assessment.

This sequence gives you the information about the trauma patient in a logical order. It allows you to assess the most critical factors first. Although you may have to vary the order of the steps somewhat for certain patients, you should try to generally follow this order.

When dealing with a patient with a sudden illness, you can modify the preceding sequence slightly. The first two steps of the patient assessment sequence are the same for both illness and injury. However, when dealing with an illness, change the sequence to obtain the patient's medical history before you perform the head-to-toe examination. In a conscious patient, the most important thing is to make sure you gather all the information you need to perform a complete patient assessment.

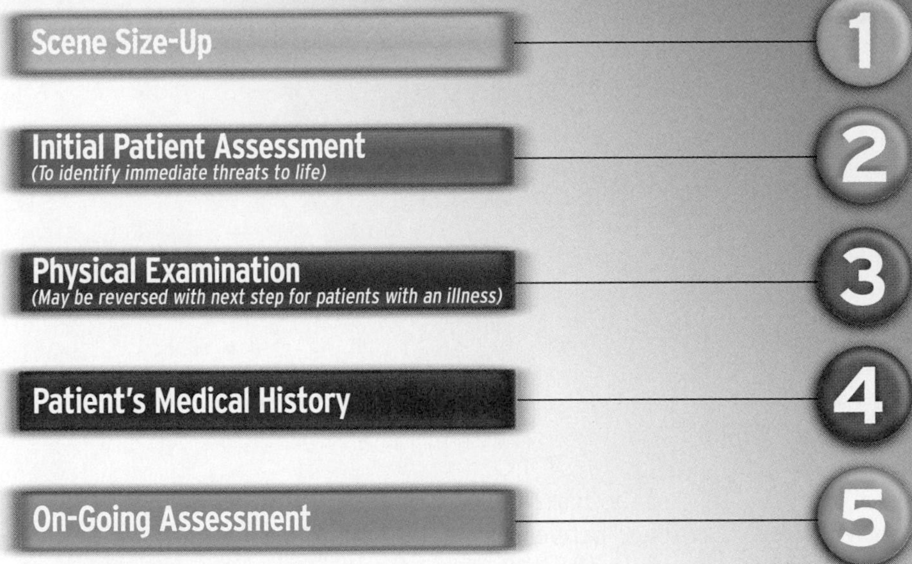

Although it is often helpful to consider whether the patient's problem is caused by trauma or sudden illness, you should avoid jumping to conclusions. Some patients will need to be treated for both trauma and sudden illness. (For example, a person who has a heart attack while driving a car needs to be treated for the heart attack and for any trauma suffered in the motor vehicle crash.) The most important factor to remember is to follow a system of patient assessment that will gather all the information you need.

7 Prep Kit

Ready for Review

Ready for Review thoroughly summarizes the chapter.

This chapter covers the five steps of the patient assessment sequence you will need to perform in the first minutes after arriving at the scene of an emergency. When you arrive, you must first determine whether the scene is safe. As a first responder, you must decide whether you will need additional equipment and personnel. You must perform an initial assessment of each patient to determine consciousness; to check airway, breathing, and circulation; and to acknowledge the chief complaints. A more thorough head-to-toe physical examination gives you additional information about any other injuries the patients may have. A medical history such as the SAMPLE history gives you needed information about patients' medical problems. Reporting the results of your assessment will give vital patient information to other emergency medical personnel.

These patient assessment steps give you a logical order for patient assessments. To perform the steps of the patient assessment, you must know the difference between signs and symptoms, as well as the importance of respiration, circulation, temperature, skin condition, pupil size and reactivity, and level of consciousness.

You will have to be somewhat flexible in assessing patients. When dealing with trauma patients, you generally perform the head-to-toe physical examination before you obtain the patient's medical history. When caring for a patient with a medical condition, you generally obtain the patient's medical history before you perform the physical examination.

The chapters that follow cover specific types of illnesses and injuries. Combining the patient assessment information from this chapter with the information on specific illnesses and injuries will enable you to assess patients who are experiencing illnesses or trauma. Good patient assessment skills will get you halfway down the road to being a good first responder.

Vital Vocabulary

The Vital Vocabulary are the key terms for this chapter.

abdomen—*page 159*
arm—*page 160*
aspiration—*page 157*
assessment-based care—*page 144*
AVPU scale—*page 149*
backboard—*page 156*
bounding pulse—*page 153*
brachial pulse—*page 153*
capillary refill—*page 153*
carotid arteries—*page 153*
carotid pulse—*page 153*
chief complaint—*page 151*
clavicle—*page 158*
cyanosis—*page 151*
exhalation—*page 158*
flail chest—*page 158*
fracture—*page 158*
illness—*page 166*
inhalation—*page 158*
initial patient assessment—*page 148*
leg—*page 161*
physical examination—*page 152*
posterior tibial pulse—*page 153*
pulse—*page 152*
pupil—*page 154*
radial pulse—*page 153*
respiratory rate—*page 152*
SAMPLE history—*page 162*
sign—*page 152*
stoma—*page 157*
symptom—*page 152*
thready pulse—*page 153*
trauma—*page 166*
vital signs—*page 152*

Ready to Respond

Ready to Respond presents a fictitious scenario to help you review what you learned in this chapter.

You are dispatched to a park for the report of an injured person. You are told that a 36-year-old woman has fallen off a bicycle.

1. The first step of the patient assessment sequence used in this situation is
- A. Obtain the patient's medical history.
- B. On-going assessment.
- C. Initial assessment.
- D Complete the first responder physical examination.
- E Scene size-up.

2. All of the following are part of this first step except
- A. Determining scene safety.
- B. Assessing mechanism of injury.
- C. Checking the patient's breathing.
- D. Considering body substance isolation.

3. Place the following parts of the second step of the patient assessment sequence in the order that you should perform them.
1. Check the patient's airway.
2. Assess responsiveness.
3. Check the patient's circulation.
4. Update responding EMS units.
5. Form a general impression of the patient.
6. Check the patient's breathing.

- A. 5, 2, 1, 6, 3, 4
- B. 6, 5, 3, 4, 1, 2
- C. 3, 2, 1, 5, 6, 4
- D. 2, 6, 3, 4, 5, 1

4. The first step in performing the first responder physical examination is
- A. Examine the patient's head
- B. Examine the patient's neck
- C. Examine the patient's extremities
- D. Determine the patient's vital signs

5. Which of the following is not usually part of the medical history gathered by a first responder?
- A. Past operations
- B. Signs and symptoms leading up to this illness or injury
- C. Current medications
- D. Allergies

6. If the patient is conscious and appears to have a broken arm, how often should you repeat the initial assessment?
- A. Every 5 minutes
- B. Every 10 minutes
- C. Every 15 minutes
- D. Every 20 minutes

7. If the patient had chest pain because of a known heart condition, how would you modify the patient assessment sequence?
- A. You never need to do a physical examination on a patient who is ill.
- B. Obtain the patient's medical history before doing the physical examination.
- C. Perform the on-going assessment before obtaining the patient's medical history.
- D. There would be no change.

Practice Points

The Practice Points are the key skills you need to know.

1. Identifying and measuring the following diagnostic signs on adult, child, and infant patients: respiration, pulse, temperature, capillary refill, skin condition (color and moisture), pupil size and reactivity, and level of consciousness.

2. Performing the following five steps of the patient assessment sequence given a real or simulated incident:
- A. Scene size-up
- B. Initial patient assessment
- C. Examining the patient from head to toe
- D. Obtaining the patient's medical history
- E. Performing on-going assessment

Chapter 8

CPR and Circulation

TECHNOLOGY

www.FirstResponderTraining.com

- Online Chapter Pretest
- Web Links
- Online Glossary
- Anatomy Review
- Online Review Manual
- CyberClass
- Interactive First Responder

Chapter FEATURES

- Skill Drills
- Vital Vocabulary
- Voices of Experience
- Signs and Symptoms
- FYI
- Special Needs
- Safety Tips
- BSI Tips
- Caution
- Check Point
- Prep Kit

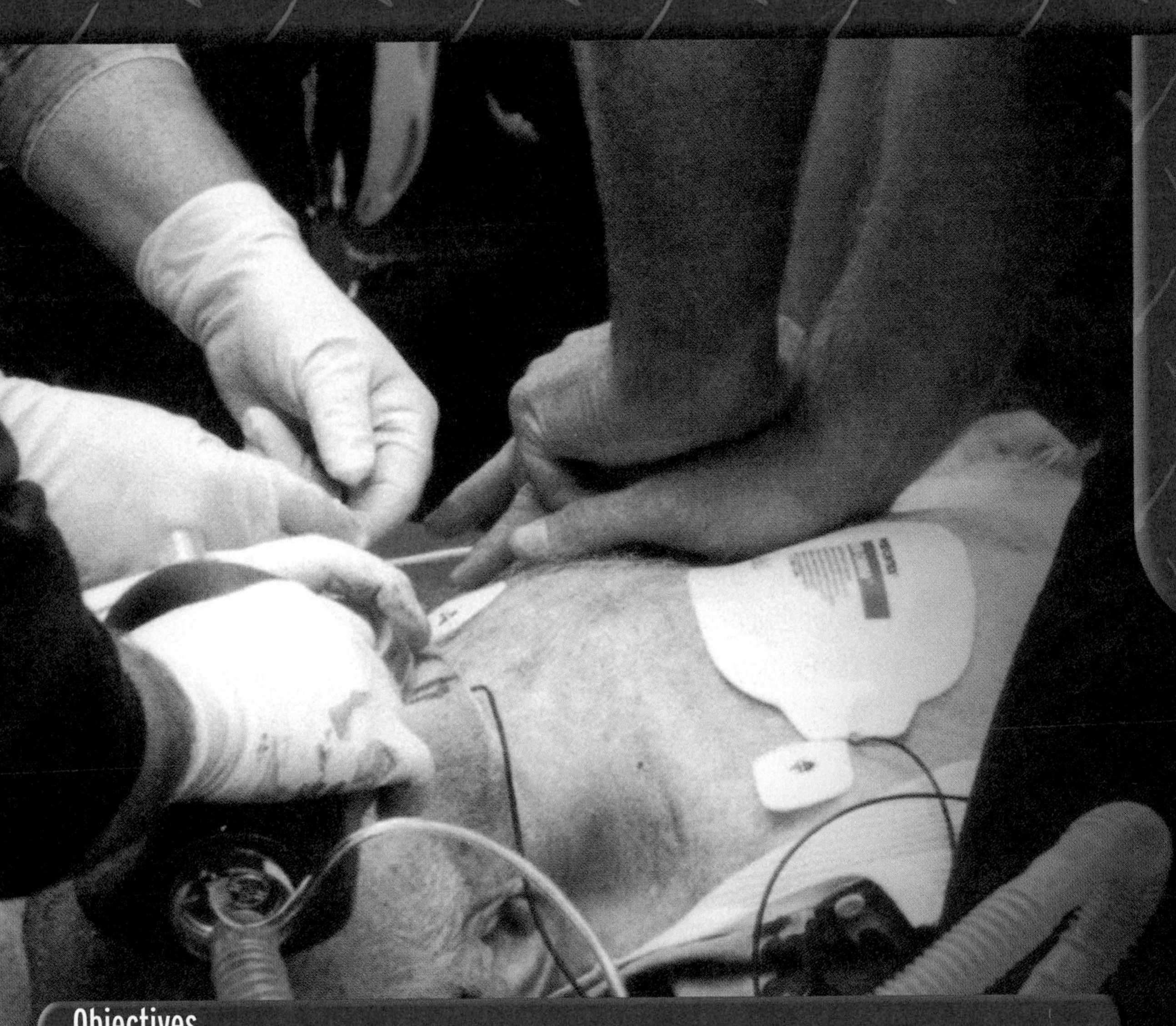

CHAPTER 8

Objectives

Knowledge and Attitude Objectives

After studying this chapter, you will be expected to:

1. Describe the anatomy and function of the circulatory system.
2. List the reasons for a heart to stop beating.
3. Describe the components of CPR.
4. Explain the links in the cardiac chain of survival.
5. Describe the conditions under which you should start and stop CPR.
6. Describe the techniques of external chest compressions on an adult, a child, and an infant.
7. Explain the steps of one-rescuer adult CPR.
8. Explain the steps of two-rescuer adult CPR.
9. Explain how to switch rescuer positions during two-rescuer adult CPR.
10. Explain the steps of infant and child CPR.
11. Describe the signs of effective CPR.
12. State the complications of performing CPR.
13. Describe the importance of creating sufficient space for CPR.
14. Describe the importance of CPR training.
15. Explain the legal implications of performing CPR.

Skill Objectives

As a first responder, you should be able to:

1. Perform one-rescuer adult CPR.
2. Perform two-rescuer adult CPR.
3. Perform infant CPR.
4. Perform child CPR.

The purpose of this chapter is to teach you the remaining skills you will need to perform cardiopulmonary resuscitation, or CPR. CPR consists of three major skills: the "A" (airway) skills, the "B" (breathing) skills, and the "C" (circulation) skills. In Chapter 6, you learned the airway and breathing skills. These airway and breathing steps may be lifesaving procedures for a patient who has just stopped breathing and whose heart is still beating. In most cases, however, by the time you arrive on the scene, the patient has not only stopped breathing, but the heart has stopped beating as well. If the patient is not breathing and has no heartbeat, rescue breathing alone will not save the patient's life. Forcing air into the lungs does no good unless the circulatory system can carry the oxygen in the lungs to all parts of the body.

In this chapter, you will learn the "C" (circulation) skills. If the patient's heart has stopped, you can maintain or restore circulation manually through the use of chest compressions (closed-chest cardiac massage). To maintain both breathing and heartbeat, rescue breathing and chest compressions must be done together. By combining the airway, breathing, and circulation skills, you will be able to perform CPR.

Anatomy and Function of the Circulatory System

circulatory system The heart and blood vessels, which together are responsible for the continuous flow of blood throughout the body.

The **circulatory system** is similar to a city water system because both consist of a pump (the heart), a network of pipes (the blood vessels), and fluid (blood). After blood picks up oxygen in the lungs, it goes to the heart, which pumps the oxygenated blood to the rest of the body.

In Chapter 4 you learned how the heart functions as a pump. The heart, which is about the size of your fist, is located in the chest between the lungs. The cells of the body absorb oxygen and nutrients from the blood and produce waste products (including carbon dioxide) that the blood carries back to the lungs. In the lungs, the blood exchanges the carbon dioxide for more oxygen. Blood then returns to the heart to be pumped out again.

Did You Know?

Without adequate blood supply, the heart muscle does not get enough oxygen and nutrients and cannot contract. The coronary arteries located on the surface of the heart supply blood to the heart muscle. These arteries are very small and can become blocked by plaque build-up. This blockage is the major cause of heart attacks.

The human heart consists of four chambers, two on the patient's right side and two on the patient's left side. Each upper chamber is called an atrium. The right atrium receives blood from the veins of the body; the left atrium receives blood from the lungs. The bottom chambers are the ventricles. The right ventricle pumps blood to the lungs; the left ventricle pumps blood throughout the body. The most muscular chamber of the heart is the left ventricle, which needs the most power because it must

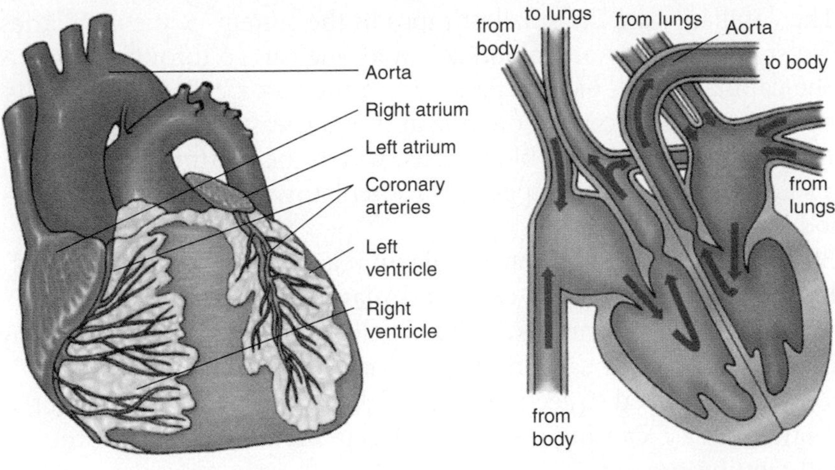

Fig. 8.1 The heart functions as the human circulatory system's pump.

force blood to all parts of the body. Together the four chambers of the heart work in a well-ordered sequence to pump blood to the lungs and to the rest of the body (**Figure 8.1**).

One-way check valves in the heart and veins allow the blood to flow in only one direction through the circulatory system. The arteries carry blood away from the heart at high pressure and are therefore thick walled. The main artery carrying blood away from the heart is quite large (about 1 inch in diameter) but arteries become smaller farther away from the heart.

The four major arteries are the neck, or carotid artery; the wrist, or radial artery; the arm, or brachial artery; and the groin, or femoral artery. The locations of these arteries are shown in **Figure 8.2**. Because these arteries lie between a bony structure and the skin, they can be used to measure the patient's **pulse**. A pulse is generated when the heart contracts and sends a wave through the artery.

pulse The wave of pressure created by the heart as it contracts and forces blood out into the major arteries.

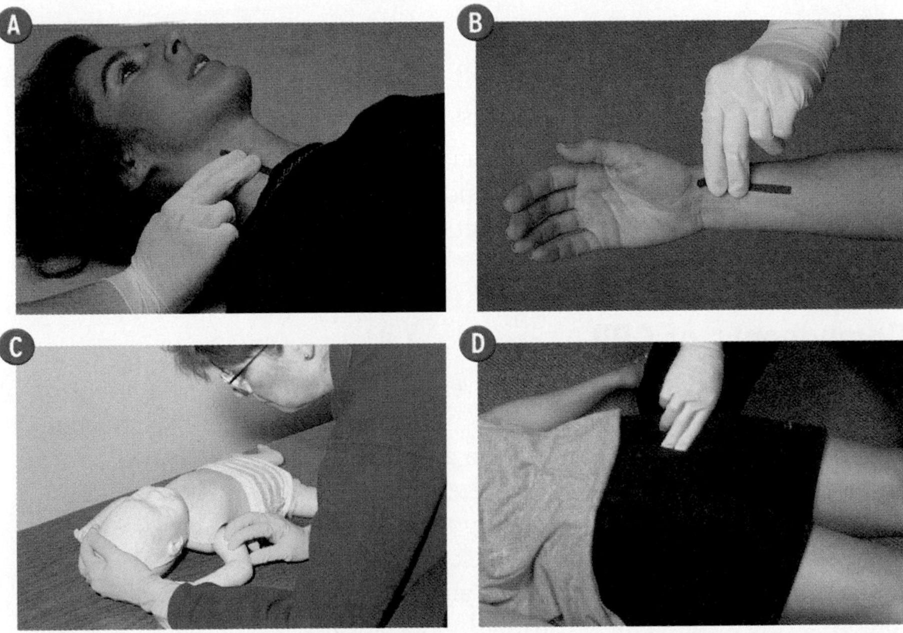

Figure 8.2 Locations for assessing the patient's pulse. **A.** Neck or carotid pulse. **B.** Wrist or radial pulse. **C.** Arm or brachial pulse. **D.** Groin or femoral pulse.

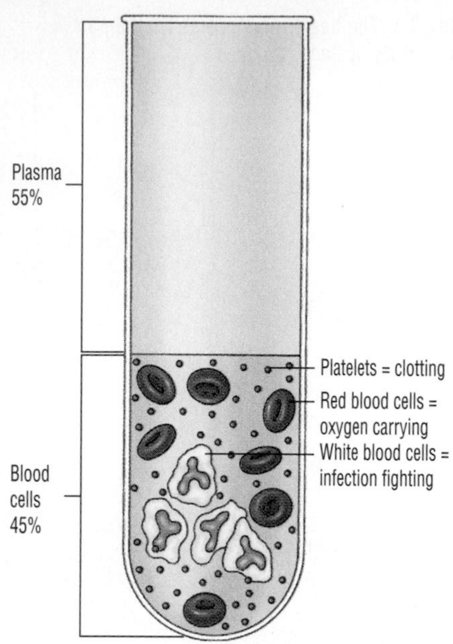

Figure 8.3 The components of blood.

The capillaries are the smallest pipes in the system. Some capillaries are so small that only one blood cell at a time can go through them. At the capillary level, oxygen passes from the blood cells into the cells of body tissues, and carbon dioxide and other waste products pass from the tissue cells to the blood cells, which then return to the lungs. Veins are the thin-walled pipes of the circulatory system that carry blood back to the heart.

Blood has several components: **plasma** (a clear, straw-colored fluid), red blood cells, white blood cells, and **platelets**. The red blood cells give blood its red coloring. Red blood cells carry oxygen from the lungs to the body and bring carbon dioxide back to the lungs. The white blood cells are called "infection fighters" because they devour bacteria and other disease-causing organisms (**Figure 8.3**). Platelets start the blood-clotting process.

plasma The fluid part of the blood that carries blood cells, transports nutrients, and removes cellular waste materials.

platelets Microscopic disc-shaped elements in the blood that are essential to the process of blood clot formation, the mechanism that stops bleeding.

Cardiac Arrest

Cardiac arrest occurs when the heart stops contracting, and no blood is pumped through the blood vessels. Without a supply of blood, the cells of the body will die because they cannot get any oxygen and nutrients and they cannot eliminate waste products. As the cells die, organ damage occurs. Some organs are more sensitive than others. Brain damage begins within four to six minutes after the patient has suffered cardiac arrest. Within eight to ten minutes, the damage to the brain may become irreversible.

Cardiac arrest may have many different causes:

1. Heart and blood vessel diseases such as heart attack and stroke
2. Respiratory arrest, if untreated
3. Medical emergencies such as epilepsy, diabetes, allergic reactions, electrical shock, and poisoning
4. Drowning
5. Suffocation
6. Trauma and shock caused by massive blood loss

A patient who has suffered cardiac arrest is unconscious and is not breathing. You cannot feel a pulse, and the patient looks dead. Regardless of the cause of cardiac arrest, the initial treatment is the same: CPR.

Components of CPR

The technique of cardiopulmonary resuscitation requires three types of skills: the A (airway) skills, the B (breathing) skills, and the C (circulation) skills. In Chapter 6, you learned the airway and breathing skills. You learned how to check patients to determine if the airway is open and to correct a blocked airway by using the head tilt–chin lift or jaw-thrust technique. You learned how to check patients to determine if they are breathing by using the look, listen, and feel technique. You learned to correct the absence of breathing by performing rescue breathing.

To perform CPR, you must combine the airway and breathing skills with circulation skills. You begin by checking the patient for a pulse. If there is no pulse, you must correct the patient's circulation by performing external chest compressions. The airway and breathing skills you know will push oxygen into the patient's lungs. External chest compressions move the oxygenated blood throughout the body. By depressing the patient's sternum (breastbone), you change the pressure in the patient's chest and force enough blood through the system to sustain life for a short period of time.

CPR by itself cannot sustain life indefinitely. However, it should be started as soon as possible to give the patient the best chance for survival. By performing all three parts of the CPR sequence, you can keep the patient alive until more advanced medical care can be administered. In many cases, the patient will need defibrillation and medication in order to recover from cardiac arrest.

The Cardiac Chain of Survival

In most cases of cardiac arrest, CPR alone is not sufficient to save lives. But it is the first treatment in the American Heart Association's "chain of survival." The links in the chain include:

1. Early access to the emergency medical services (EMS) system
2. Early CPR
3. Early defibrillation
4. Early advanced care by paramedics and hospital personnel

As a first responder, you can help the patient by providing early CPR and by making sure that the EMS system has been activated. Some first responders may also be trained in the use of automated defibrillators. By keeping these links of the chain strong, you will help keep the patient alive until early advanced care can be administered by paramedics and hospital personnel.

Just as an actual chain is only as strong as its weakest link, this CPR chain of survival is only as good as its weakest link. Your actions in performing early CPR are vital to giving cardiac arrest patients their best chance for survival (**Figure 8.4**).

Figure 8.4 The CPR chain of survival.

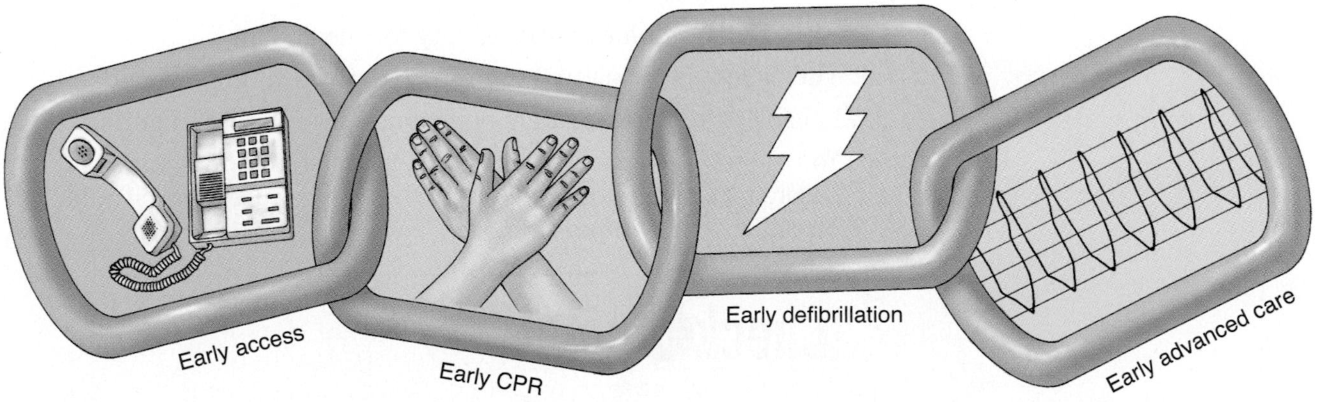

When to Start and Stop CPR

FYI

When to Start CPR

CPR should be started on all nonbreathing, pulseless patients, unless they are obviously dead or unless they have a Do Not Attempt Resuscitation (DNAR) order that is valid in your jurisdiction. (DNAR orders are discussed more fully in this chapter under Legal Implications of CPR.) Few reliable criteria exist to determine death immediately.

The following criteria are reliable signs of death and indicate that CPR should not be started.

1. *Decapitation.* Decapitation occurs when the head is separated from the rest of the body. When this occurs, there is obviously no chance of saving the patient.
2. *Rigor mortis.* This is the temporary stiffening of muscles that occurs several hours after death. The presence of this stiffening indicates the patient is dead and cannot be resuscitated.
3. *Evidence of tissue decomposition.* Tissue decomposition or actual flesh decay occurs only after a person has been dead for more than a day.
4. *Dependent lividity.* Dependent lividity is the red or purple color that appears on the parts of the patient's body that are closest to the ground. It is caused by blood seeping into the tissues on the dependent, or lower, part of the person's body. Dependent lividity occurs after a person has been dead for several hours.

If any of the preceding signs is present in a pulseless, nonbreathing person, you should not begin CPR. If none of these signs is present, you should activate the EMS system and then begin CPR. It is far better to start CPR on a person who is later declared dead by a physician than to withhold CPR from a patient whose life might have been saved.

When to Stop CPR

You should discontinue CPR only when:

1. Effective spontaneous circulation and ventilation is restored.
2. Resuscitation efforts are transferred to another trained person who continues CPR.
3. A physician assumes responsibility for the patient.
4. The patient is transferred to properly trained EMS personnel.
5. Reliable criteria for death (as previously listed) are recognized.
6. You are too exhausted to continue resuscitation, environmental hazards endanger your safety, or continued resuscitation would place the lives of others at risk.

Checkpoint

- ◯ When do you start and stop CPR?

The Technique of External Cardiac Compression in an Adult

A patient in __cardiac arrest__ is unconscious and is not breathing. You cannot feel a pulse, and the patient looks dead. If you suspect that the patient has suffered cardiac arrest, first check and correct the airway, then check and correct the breathing, and finally check for circulation. Check for circulation by feeling the carotid pulse and looking for signs of coughing or movement. To check the carotid pulse, place your index and middle fingers on the larynx (Adam's apple). Now slide your fingers into the groove between the larynx and the muscles at the side of the neck (**Figure 8.5**). Keep your fingers there for 5 to 10 seconds to be sure the pulse is absent and not just slow. As you check the pulse, look for signs of coughing or movement that may indicate circulation is present.

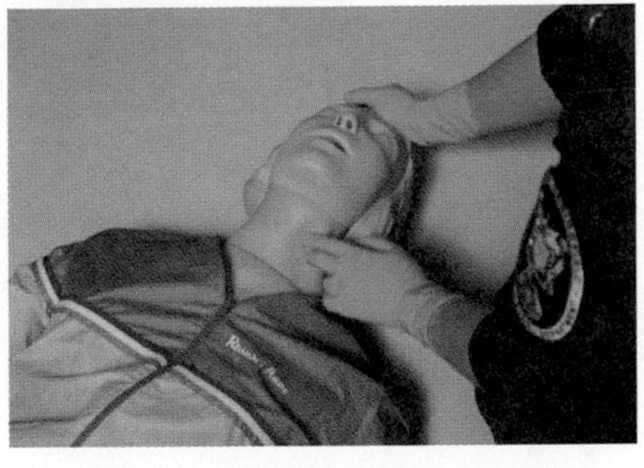

Figure 8.5 Check the patient's carotid pulse.

If there is no carotid pulse in an unresponsive patient, you must begin __chest compressions__. For chest compressions to be effective, the patient must be lying on a firm, horizontal surface. If the patient is on a soft surface, such as a bed, it is impossible to compress the chest. Immediately place all patients needing CPR on a firm, level surface.

__cardiac arrest__ A sudden ceasing of heart function.

__chest compression__ Manual chest-pressing method that mimics the squeezing and relaxation cycles a normal heart goes through; administered to a person in cardiac arrest; also called "external chest compression" and "closed-chest cardiac massage."

To perform chest compressions effectively, kneel beside the patient's chest facing the patient. Place the fingers of one hand on the notch at the upper end of the patient's sternum and run your other hand firmly down the sternum until you feel the xiphoid process. Place the heel of the first hand on the lower half of the sternum, about two finger widths above the xiphoid process (**Figure 8.6**). Place the heel of the other hand on top of the hand on the chest, and interlock your fingers.

It is important to locate and maintain the proper hand position while applying chest compressions. If your hands are too high, the force you apply will not produce adequate chest compressions. If your hands are too low, the force you apply may damage the liver. If your hands slip sideways off the sternum and onto the ribs, the compressions will not be effective, and you may damage the ribs and lungs.

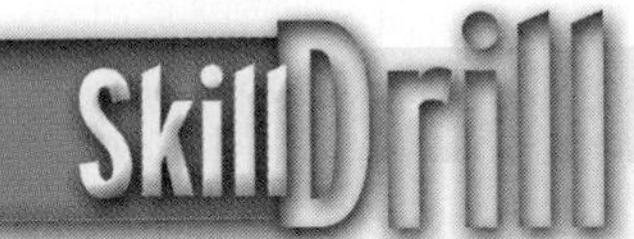

Figure 8.6 Perform Chest Compressions

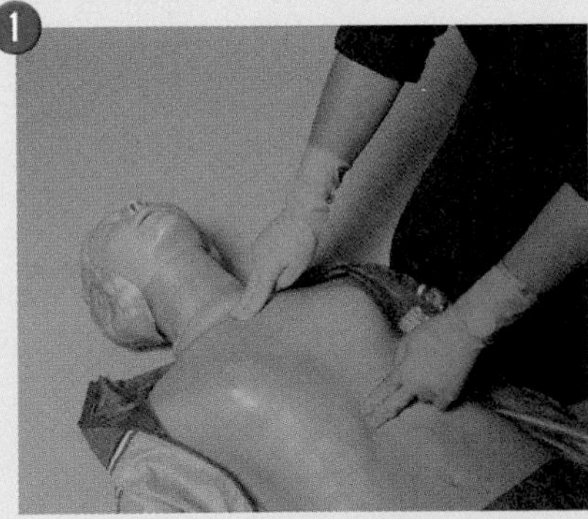

1 Locate the top and bottom of the sternum.

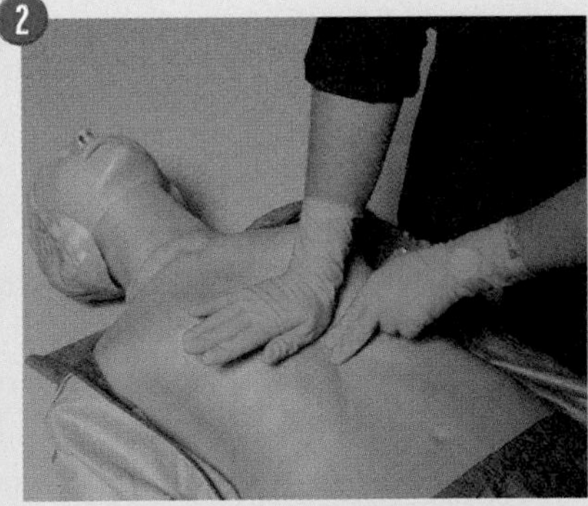

2 Place the heel of your hand on the lower half of the sternum (two finger widths above the bottom on the sternum).

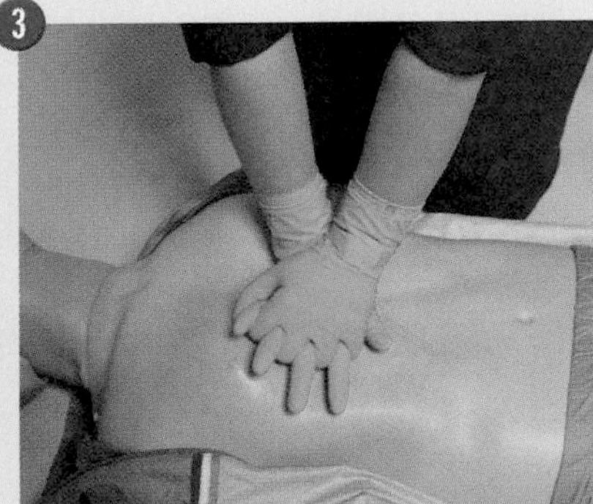

3 Place your other hand on top of your first hand.

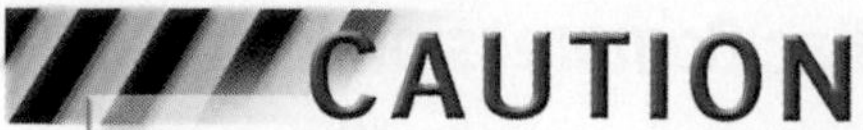

CAUTION

Do not let your fingers touch the chest wall; your fingers could dig into the patient, causing injury. Interlocking your fingers will help avoid this.

After you have both hands in the proper position, compress the chest of an adult $1\frac{1}{2}$ to 2 inches straight down. For effective compressions, kneel close to the patient's side and lean forward so that your arms are directly over the patient. Keep your back straight and your elbows stiff so you can apply the force of your whole body to each compression, not just your arm muscles. Between compressions, keep the heel of your hand on the patient's chest but completely release the pressure.

Compressions must be rhythmic and continuous. Each compression cycle consists of one downward push followed by a rest so that the heart can refill with blood. Compressions should be at the rate of 100 compressions per minute in an adult patient. After every 15 chest compressions, give two rescue breaths. Practice on a manikin until you can compress the chest smoothly and rhythmically.

External Chest Compressions on an Infant

Infants (under one year of age) who have suffered cardiac arrest will be unconscious and not breathing. They will have no pulse. To check for cardiac arrest, you first need to check and correct the airway. Remember not to tilt the head back too far because this may occlude the infant's airway. Next check for breathing by using the look, listen, and feel technique. Correct the absence of breathing by giving mouth-to-mouth-and-nose rescue breathing.

To check an infant's circulation, feel for the brachial pulse on the inside of the upper arm (**Figure 8.7**). Use two fingers of one hand to feel for the pulse, and use the other hand to maintain the head tilt. If there is no pulse, begin chest compressions. Draw an imaginary horizontal line between the two nipples, and place your index finger below the imaginary line in the middle of the chest. Place your middle and ring fingers next to your index finger. Use your middle and ring fingers to compress the sternum. Make sure you compress above the **xiphoid process**. Compress the sternum about $\frac{1}{2}$ to 1 inch (approximately one third to one half the depth of the chest). Compress the sternum at a rate of at least 100 times per minute. Give one rescue breath after every five chest compressions.

xiphoid process The flexible cartilage at the lower end of the sternum (breastbone), a key landmark in the administration of CPR and the Heimlich maneuver.

Place the infant on a solid surface such as a table, or cradle the infant in your arm, as shown in **Figure 8.8**, when doing chest compressions. You will not need to use much force to achieve adequate compressions on infants because they are so small and their chests are so pliable.

External Chest Compressions on a Child

The signs of cardiac arrest in a child (from one year to eight years of age) are the same as those for an adult and for an infant. If you suspect that a child is in cardiac arrest, first check and correct the child's airway,

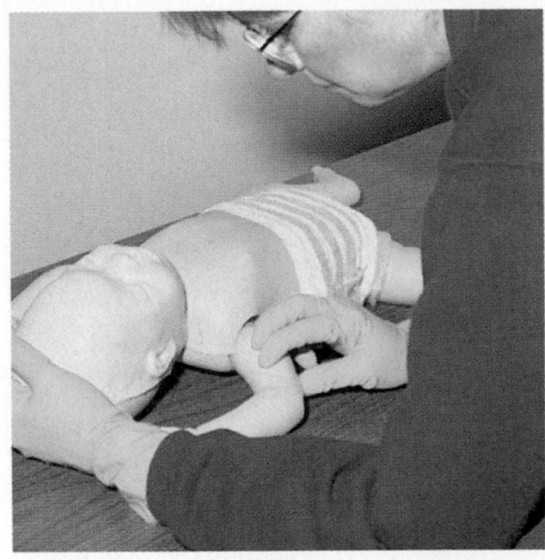

Figure 8.7 Check the brachial pulse on the inside of the infant's arm.

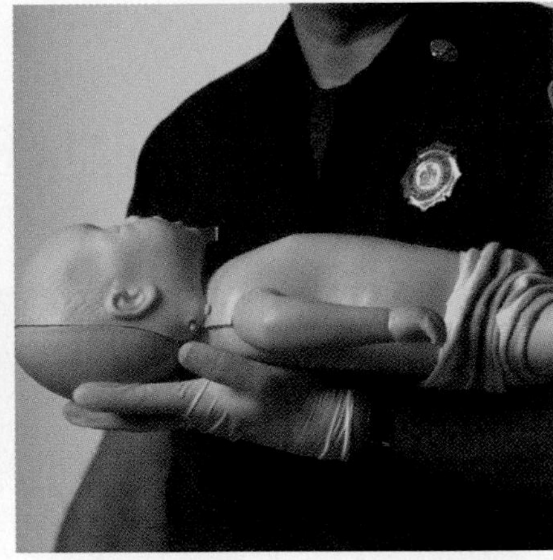

Figure 8.8 Positioning the infant patient for proper CPR.

then check and correct the child's breathing, and finally check for circulation. Check the carotid pulse by placing two or three fingers on the larynx. Slide your fingers into the groove between the Adam's apple and the muscle. Feel for the carotid pulse with one hand and maintain the head-tilt position with the other hand.

To perform chest compressions on a child, locate the proper position for your hands by placing the fingers of one hand on the upper end of the sternum and using the fingers of the other hand to locate the xiphoid process at the bottom of the sternum. Place the heel of one hand on the lower half of the sternum. Do not put the heel of your other hand on top; the force of the heel of one hand is sufficient to perform chest compressions on a child. Compress the sternum approximately one third to one half the depth of the chest, or approximately 1 to 1½ inches. Compress the chest at a rate of 100 times per minute. Give one rescue breath after every five compressions.

One-Rescuer Adult CPR

CPR consists of three skill sets: checking and correcting the airway, checking and correcting the breathing, and checking and correcting the circulation. In Chapter 6, you learned to perform the airway and breathing skill sets. Now that you have learned how to check for circulation and do chest compressions, you are ready to put all your skills together to perform CPR. If you are the only trained person at the scene, you must perform **one-rescuer CPR**. Here are the steps for one-rescuer CPR:

one-rescuer CPR Cardiopulmonary resuscitation performed by one rescuer.

1. Establish the patient's level of consciousness (**Figure 8.9, step 1**). Ask the patient, "Are you okay?" Shake the patient's shoulder. If there is no response, call for additional help by activating the EMS system. (If you are alone, phone 9-1-1 before you begin CPR. "Phone first.")
2. Turn the patient on his or her back, supporting the head and neck as you do.
3. Open the airway (**Figure 8.9, step 2**). Use the head tilt–chin lift technique or, if the patient is injured, use the jaw-thrust technique. Maintain the open airway.

Skill Drill

Figure 8.9 One-Rescuer Adult CPR

1

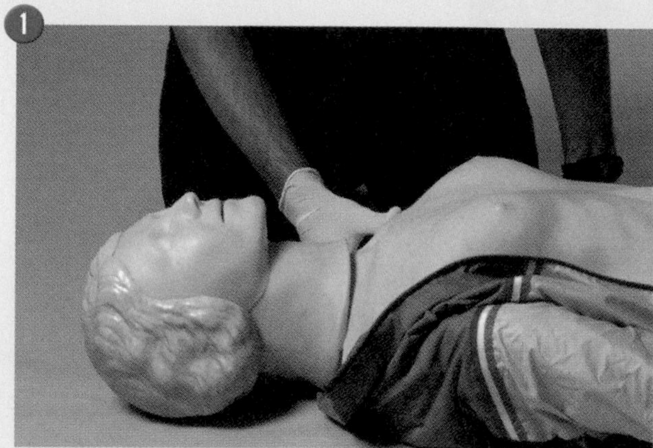

Establish responsiveness.

2

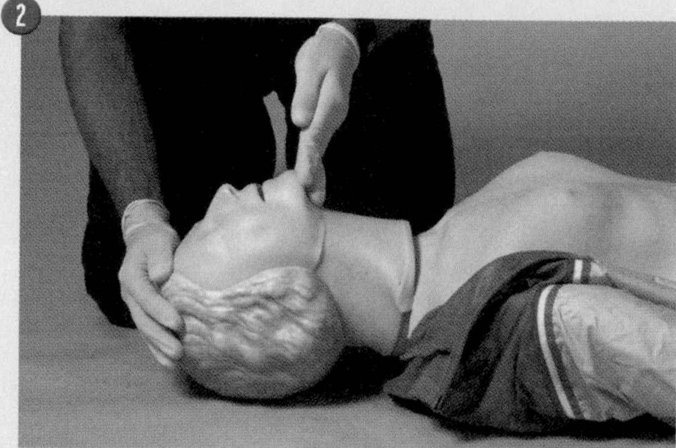

Open the airway.

3

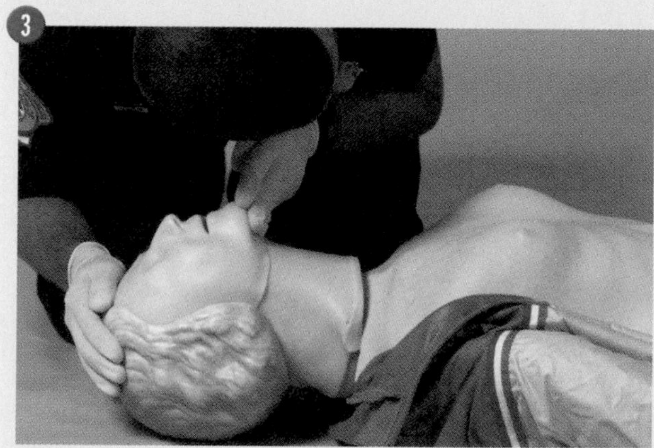

Check for breathing.

4

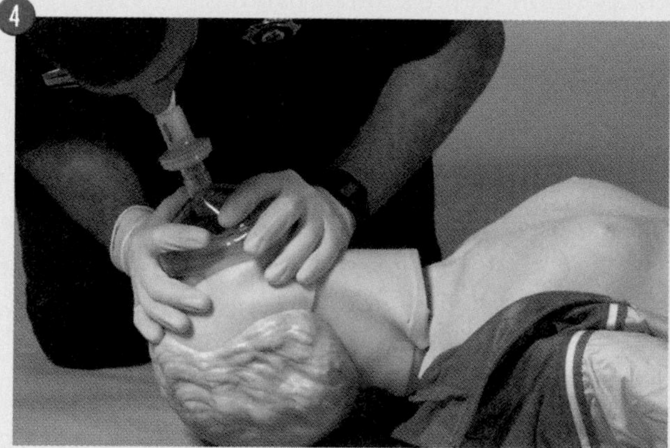

Perform rescue breathing.

5

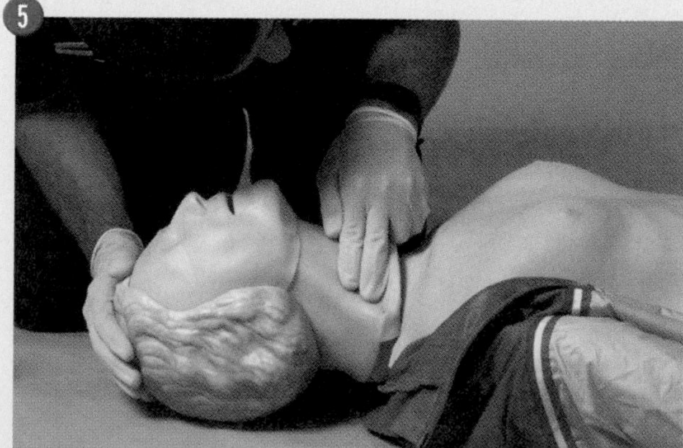

Check for circulation.

6

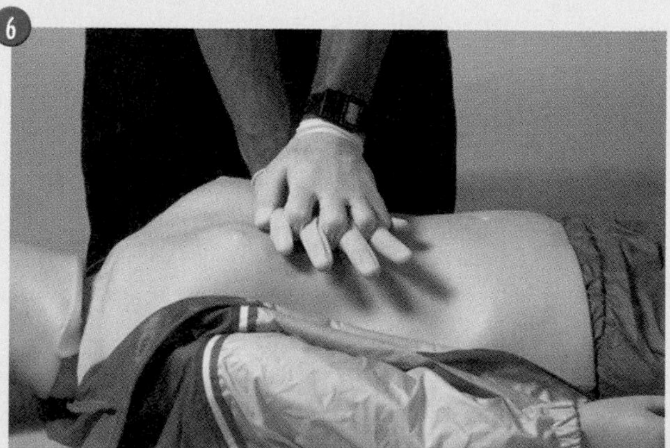

Perform chest compressions.

4. Check for breathing (**Figure 8.9, step 3**). Place the side of your face and your ear close to the nose and mouth of the patient. Look, listen, and feel for the movement of air: Look for movement of the chest, listen for sounds of air exchange, and feel for air movement on the side of your face. Your breathing check should last at least 3 to 5 seconds. If there are no signs of breathing, begin rescue breathing. Use a mouth-to-mask ventilation device, if one is available, or place your mouth over the patient's mouth, seal the patient's nose with your thumb and index finger, and begin mouth-to-mouth rescue breathing.
5. Give two breaths (**Figure 8.9, step 4**). Blow slowly for 2 seconds using just enough force to make the chest rise. Allow the lungs to deflate between breaths.
6. Check for signs of circulation by checking the carotid pulse and looking for signs of coughing or movement (**Figure 8.9, step 5**). Find the carotid pulse by locating the patient's larynx with your index and middle fingers, then sliding your fingers into the groove between the larynx and the muscles at the side of the neck. Check for 5 to 10 seconds. If the pulse is absent, proceed to the next step. (If the pulse is present, continue rescue breathing.)
7. Begin chest compressions (**Figure 8.9, step 6**). Place the heel of one hand on the lower half of the sternum, two finger widths above the xiphoid process. Place the other hand on top of the first, so the hands are parallel. Now press down to compress the chest about 1½ to 2 inches. Apply 15 compressions at the rate of 100 compressions per minute. Count the compressions out loud: "One and two and three and..."
8. After 15 chest compressions, give two full size rescue breathes.
9. Continue alternating compressions and **ventilations**. Deliver a sequence of 15 compressions followed by two ventilations.
10. Check for a pulse. After one minute and every few minutes thereafter, check for a carotid pulse.

ventilation The exchange of air between the lungs and the air of the environment; breathing.

When performing one-rescuer CPR, you must deliver chest compressions and rescue breathing at a ratio of 15 compressions to two breaths. Immediately give two lung inflations after each set of 15 chest compressions. Because you must interrupt chest compressions to ventilate, you should perform each series of 15 chest compressions in 10 seconds (a rate of 100 compressions per minute). At this rate, the patient will actually receive about 60 compressions per minute.

A skill performance sheet titled "One-Rescuer Adult CPR" is shown in **Figure 8.10**, page 184, for your review and practice.

Although one-rescuer CPR can keep the patient alive, two-rescuer CPR is preferable for an adult patient because it is less exhausting for the rescuers. Whenever possible, CPR for an adult should be performed by two rescuers.

Two-Rescuer Adult CPR

In many cases, a second trained person will be on the scene to help you perform CPR. Two-rescuer CPR is more effective than one-rescuer CPR.

Note: If you do not have help, do not wait for another rescuer to arrive. Call 9-1-1 to activate EMS and then begin one-rescuer CPR immediately!

1. As Rescuer Two tires, he or she says the following out loud (instead of counting): "We—will—switch—next—time." One word is spoken as each compression is done. These words replace the counting sequence for five compressions.
2. After 10 more chest compressions (a total of 15), Rescuer One completes two ventilations and moves to the chest to do the compressions.
3. Rescuer Two completes one last set of 15 compressions and moves to the head of the patient to maintain the airway and ventilation.
4. Rescuer Two immediately checks the carotid pulse for 5 seconds. If the carotid pulse is absent, Rescuer Two says "No pulse" and ventilates the patient twice.
5. Rescuer One then begins chest compressions.

You should practice switching until you can do it smoothly and quickly. Switching is much easier if the rescuers work on opposite sides of the patient.

One-Rescuer Infant CPR

infant Anyone under one year of age.

brachial pulse The pulse on the inside of the upper arm.

An **infant** is defined as anyone under one year of age. The principles of CPR are the same for adults and infants. In actual practice, however, you must use slightly different techniques for an infant. The steps for one-rescuer infant CPR are as follows:

1. Position the infant on a firm surface.
2. Establish the infant's level of responsiveness. An unresponsive infant is limp. Gently shake or tap the infant to determine whether he or she is unconscious. Call for additional help if the patient is unconscious. Activate the EMS system.
3. Open the airway. This is best done by the head tilt–chin lift method. Be careful as you tilt the infant's head back because tilting too far can obstruct the airway. Tilt the head back to a sniffing position, but do not tilt it back as far as it will go. Continue holding the head with one hand.
4. Check for breathing. Place the side of your face close to the mouth and nose of the infant as you would for an adult. Look, listen, and feel for at least 3 to 5 seconds.
5. Give two slow breaths, each lasting 1 to 1½ seconds. To breathe for an infant, place your mouth over the infant's mouth and nose. Because an infant has very small lungs, you should give only very small puffs of air, just enough to make the chest rise. Do not use large or forceful breaths (**Figure 8.15**).
6. Check for circulation. Check the **brachial pulse** rather than the carotid pulse. The brachial pulse is on the inside of the arm (**Figure 8.16**). You can feel it by placing your index and middle fingers on the inside of the infant's arm halfway between the shoulder and the elbow. Check for 5 to 10 seconds.
7. Begin chest compressions. An infant's heart is located relatively higher in the chest than an adult's heart. Therefore, you must deliver

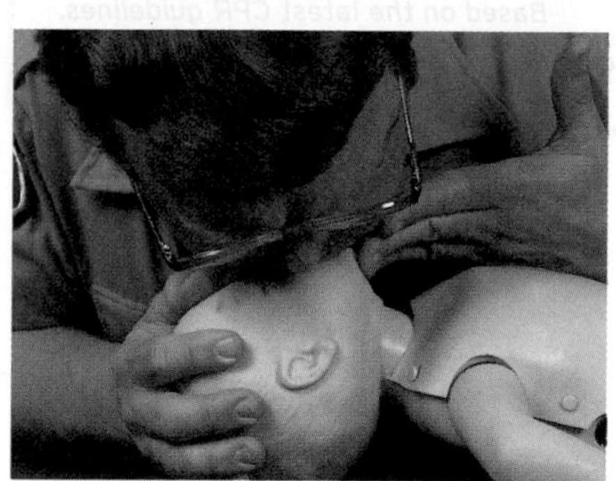

Fig. 8.15 Rescue breathing for an infant patient.

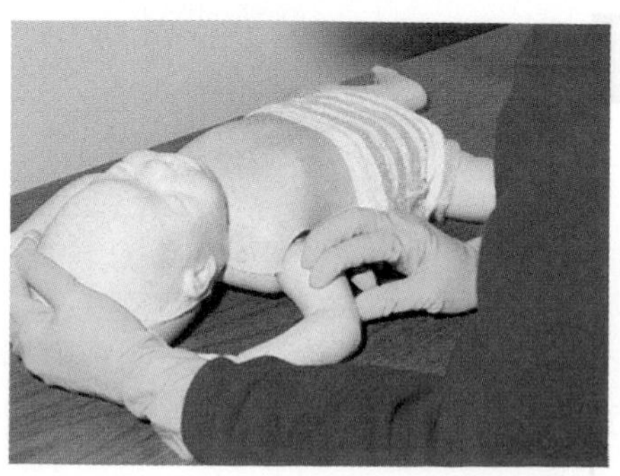

Fig. 8.16 Check the brachial pulse.

chest compressions by pressing on the middle (rather than lower) portion of the sternum. Imagine a horizontal line drawn between the infant's nipples. Place your index finger below that line in the middle of the chest. Place your middle and ring fingers next to your index finger. Use the middle and ring fingers to compress the sternum. Because the chest of an infant is smaller and more pliable than the chest of an adult, use only two fingers to compress the chest. Compress the sternum ½ to 1 inch. To achieve good results, the infant must be lying on a firm surface. Because the heart rate of an infant is faster than an adult's, you must deliver compressions at the rate of at least 100 per minute (**Figure 8.17**). The ratio of cardiac compressions to ventilations in an infant is 5 to 1 instead of the 15 to 2 ratio used for adults. The size of the infant makes it harder to perform two-rescuer CPR.

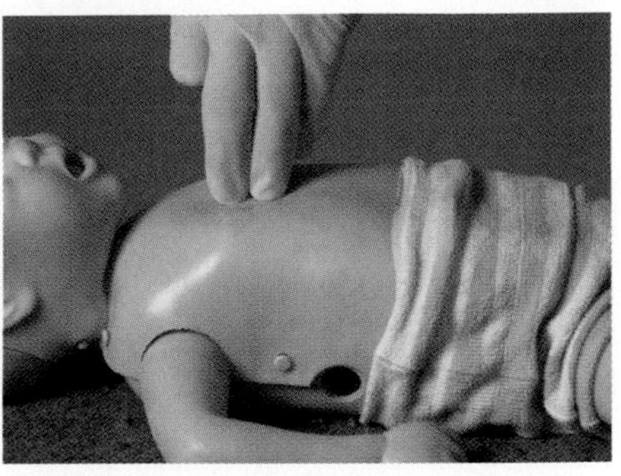

Fig. 8.17 Perform chest compressions with two or three fingers.

8. Continue compressions and ventilations. Give one slow ventilation after each set of five compressions during a 1- to 1½-second pause.
9. Reassess the patient after 20 sets of compressions and ventilations (about 1 minute) and every few minutes thereafter.

A skill performance sheet titled "One-Rescuer Infant CPR" is shown in **Figure 8.18** for your review and practice.

Figure 8.18 Skill Performance Sheet

One-Rescuer Infant CPR

Steps	Adequately Performed
1. Establish unresponsiveness. If second rescuer is available, have him or her activate the EMS system.	
2. Open airway using the head tilt-chin lift. (If trauma is present, use jaw thrust). Check breathing (look, listen, and feel).*	
3. Give two effective breaths (1 to 1½ seconds per breath); if airway is obstructed, reposition head and try to ventilate again.† Watch chest rise, allow for exhalation between breaths.	
4. Check for signs of circulation. Check brachial pulse and look for signs of coughing or movement. If breathing is absent but pulse is present, provide rescue breathing (one breath every 3 seconds, about 20 breaths per minute).	
5. If no pulse, give five chest compressions (rate at least 100 compressions per minute), followed by one slow breath.	
6. After about 1 minute of rescue support, check pulse.* If rescuer is alone, activate the EMS system. If no pulse, continue 5 to 1 cycles.	

* *If victim is unresponsive but breathing, place in recovery position.* *Based on the latest CPR guidelines.*

† *If still unsuccessful, begin the unresponsive Foreign Body Airway Obstruction (FBAO) sequence.*

Note: Your instructor may teach you another way to administer chest compressions to an infant patient. The two-thumb/encircling-hands technique is done by placing both thumbs side-by-side over the lower half of the infant's sternum and encircling the infant's chest with your hands. Compress the sternum 1/2 to 1 inch at a rate of at least 100 compressions per minute, just as you would when using your fingers for chest compressions.

child Anyone between one and eight years of age.

Checkpoint

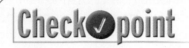

○ How is infant CPR different from one-rescuer adult CPR?

One-Rescuer Child CPR

A **child** is defined as a person between the ages of one and eight years. The steps for child CPR are almost the same as for an adult; however, some steps must be modified for a child. These variations are:

- Use less force to ventilate the child. Ventilate only until the child's chest rises.
- Use only one hand to depress the sternum 1 to 1 1/2 inches.
- Use less force to compress the child's chest.
- Give one rescue breath after every five chest compressions for a child, instead of two rescue breaths after 15 chest compressions for an adult.

Follow these steps to administer CPR to a child:

1. Establish the child's level of responsiveness. Tap and gently shake the shoulder and shout, "Are you okay?" If a second rescuer is available, have him or her activate the EMS system.
2. Turn the child on his or her back, as you support the head and neck.
3. Open the airway. Use the head tilt–chin lift technique or, if the child is injured, use the jaw-thrust technique. Maintain the open airway.
4. Check for breathing. Place the side of your face and your ear close to the nose and mouth of the child. Look, listen, and feel for the movement of air: Look for movement of the chest, listen for sounds of air exchange, and feel for air movement on the side of your face. Check for breathing for at least 3 to 5 seconds. If signs of breathing are absent, place your mouth over the child's mouth, seal the child's nose with your thumb and index finger, and begin mouth-to-mouth rescue breathing. A mouth-to-mask ventilation device may be used.
5. Give two effective breaths. Blow slowly for 1 to 1 1/2 seconds using just enough force to make the chest rise. Allow the lungs to deflate between breaths.
6. Check for circulation. Locate the larynx with your index and middle fingers. Slide your fingers into the groove between the larynx and the muscles at the side of the neck to feel for the carotid pulse. Check for at least 5 to 10 seconds. If the pulse is absent, proceed to step 7. (If the pulse is present, continue rescue breathing.)
7. Begin chest compressions. Place the heel of one hand on the lower half of the sternum, two finger widths above the xiphoid process (**Figure 8.19**). Apply five compressions, using the heel of one hand. Each compression should be about 1 to 1 1/2 inches and at the rate of 100 compressions per minute. Count the compressions out loud: "One and two and three and. . . ."

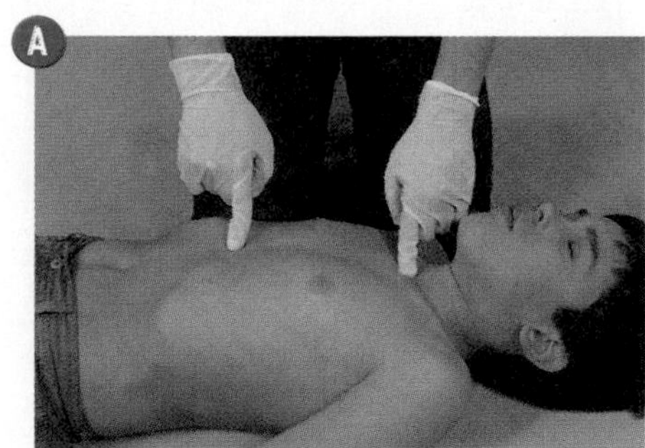

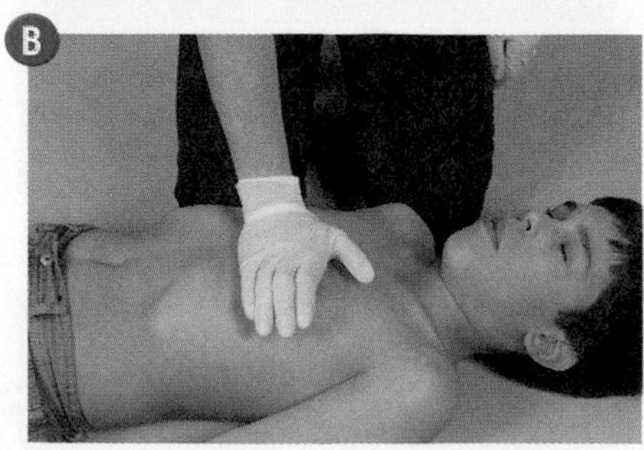

Fig. 8.19 Performing chest compressions on a child. **A.** Locate the top and bottom of the sternum. **B.** Place one hand on the lower half of the sternum, two finger widths above the xiphoid process.

Figure 8.20 Skill Performance Sheet

One-Rescuer Child CPR

Steps	Adequately Performed
1. Establish unresponsiveness. If second rescuer is available, have him or her activate the EMS system.	
2. Open airway using head tilt-chin lift. (If trauma is present, use jaw-thrust.) Check breathing (look, listen, and feel).*	
3. Give two effective breaths (1 to $1^1/_2$ seconds per breath); if airway is obstructed, reposition head and try to ventilate again.† Watch chest rise, allow for exhalation between breaths.	
4. Check for signs of circulation. Check carotid pulse and look for signs of coughing or movement. If breathing is absent but pulse is present, provide rescue breathing (1 breath every 3 seconds, about 20 breaths per minute).	
5. If no pulse, give five chest compressions (rate 100 compressions per minute), open airway with chin lift, and provide one slow breath. Repeat this cycle.	
6. After about 1 minute of rescue support, check pulse.* If rescuer is alone, activate the EMS system. If no pulse, continue 5 to 1 cycles.	

* *If victim is unresponsive but breathing, place in recovery position.* *Based on the latest CPR guidelines.*

† *If still unsuccessful, begin the unresponsive Foreign Body Airway Obstruction (FBAO) sequence.*

8. After five chest compressions, ventilate the patient's lungs. Deliver one effective breath.
9. Continue compressions and ventilations. Continue a sequence of five compressions followed by one ventilation.
10. Check for a pulse. After 1 minute and every few minutes thereafter, check for a carotid pulse.

A skill performance sheet titled "One-Rescuer Child CPR" is shown in **Figure 8.20** for your review and practice.

In large children, you may need to use two hands to achieve an adequate depth of compression.

BSI Tip

Practice good body substance isolation (BSI) when doing CPR.

Checkpoint

○ How is child CPR different from one-rescuer adult CPR?

FYI

Signs of Effective CPR

It is important to know the signs of effective CPR so you can assess your efforts to resuscitate the patient. The signs of effective CPR are:

1. A second rescuer feels a carotid pulse while you are compressing the chest.
2. The patient's pupils constrict when they are exposed to light.
3. The patient's skin color improves (from blue to pink).
4. Independent breathing begins or the patient gasps.
5. An independent heartbeat, which is the goal of CPR, begins. This does not occur often without defibrillation and other advanced life support procedures.

If some of these signs are not present, evaluate your technique to see if it can be improved.

Complications of CPR

A discussion of CPR would not be complete without mention of its complications. They can be minimized by using proper technique.

Broken Bones

If your hands slip to the side of the sternum during chest compressions, or if your fingers rest on the ribs, you may break ribs while delivering a compression. To prevent this, use proper hand position and do not let your fingers come in contact with the ribs. If you hear a cracking sound while performing CPR, check and correct your hand position but continue CPR. Sometimes you may break bones or cartilage even with proper CPR technique.

Gastric Distention

gastric distention Inflation of the stomach caused when excessive pressures are used during artificial ventilation and air is directed into the stomach rather than the lungs.

Bloating of the stomach is called **gastric distention** and is caused by too much air blown too fast and too forcefully into the stomach. A partially obstructed airway, which allows some of the air you breathe into the patient's airway to go into the stomach rather than into the lungs, can also cause gastric distention.

Gastric distention causes the abdomen to increase in size. A distended abdomen pushes up on the diaphragm, and prevents the lungs from inflating fully. Gastric distention also often causes vomiting. If vomiting occurs, quickly turn the patient to the side, wipe out the mouth with your gloved fingers, and then return the patient to a supine position.

Gastric distention is mentioned here so you will work hard to prevent it. Make sure you have completely opened the airway. Do not blow excessive amounts of air into the patient. Be especially careful if you are a large person with a large lung capacity and the patient is smaller than you are. If gastric distention is making it difficult for you to ventilate the patient, turn the patient's entire body to one side and press on the upper abdomen. This technique usually relieves the distention, but it is also likely to make the patient vomit.

Vomiting

Vomiting is common during CPR, so you must be prepared to deal with it. There is not much you can do to prevent vomiting, except to keep air out of the patient's stomach. Vomiting is likely to occur if the patient has suffered cardiac arrest. When cardiac arrest occurs, the muscle that keeps food in the stomach relaxes. If there is any food in the stomach, it backs up, causing the patient to vomit.

If the patient vomits as you are administering CPR, immediately turn the patient onto his or her side to allow the vomitus to spill out of the mouth. Then clear the patient's mouth of remaining vomitus, first with your fingers and then with a clean cloth (if one is handy). Use suction if it is available.

The patient may experience several rounds of vomiting, so you must be prepared to take these actions repeatedly. EMS units carry a suction machine that can clear the patient's mouth. As a first responder, however, you cannot wait until the suction machine arrives before beginning or resuming CPR. You must simply deal with the vomiting as it occurs.

Do your best to clear any vomitus from the patient's airway. If the airway is not cleared, three problems may arise:

1. The patient may breathe in (aspirate) the vomitus.
2. You may force vomited material into the lungs with the next artificial ventilation.
3. It takes a strong stomach and the realization that you are trying to save the patient's life to continue with resuscitation after the patient has vomited. But you must continue. Remove the vomitus with a towel, the patient's shirt, your fingers, or any other available object. As soon as you have cleared away the vomitus, take a deep breath and continue rescue breathing.

Creating Sufficient Space for CPR

As a first responder, you will frequently find yourself alone with a patient experiencing cardiac arrest. One of the first things you must do is to create or find a space where you can perform CPR. Ask yourself, "Is there enough room in this location to perform CPR?" To perform CPR effectively, you need 3 to 4 feet of space on all sides of the patient. This will give enough space so that rescuers can change places, advanced life support procedures can be implemented, and an ambulance stretcher can be brought in.

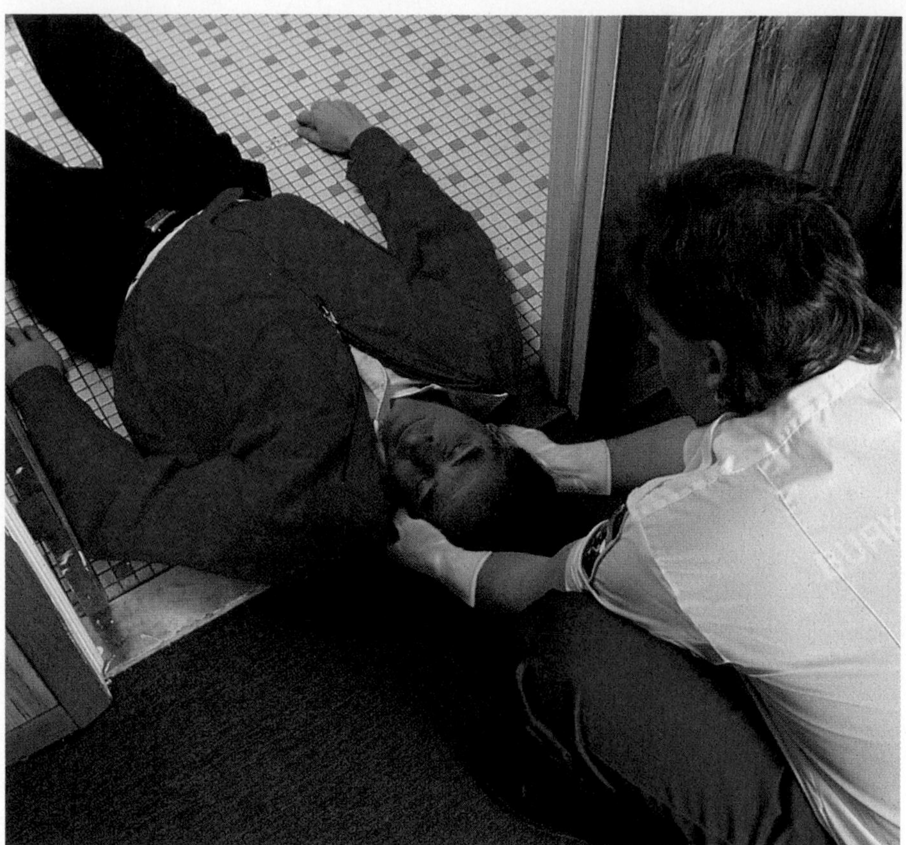

Fig. 8.21 Create sufficient space for CPR.

If there is not enough space around the patient, you have two options:

1. Quickly rearrange the furniture in the room to make space.
2. Quickly drag the patient into an area that has more room, for instance, out of the bathroom and into the living room—not the hallway (**Figure 8.21**).

Space is essential to a smooth rescue operation for a cardiac arrest patient. It only takes 15 to 30 seconds either to clear a space around the patient or to move the patient into a larger area.

CPR Training

As a first responder, you should successfully complete a CPR course through a recognized agency such the American Heart Association (AHA), the National Safety Council (NSC), or the American Red Cross (ARC). You should also regularly update your skills by successfully completing a recognized recertification course.

You cannot achieve proficiency in CPR unless you have adequate practice on adult and infant manikins. Your department should schedule periodic reviews of CPR theory and practice for all people who are trained as first responders.

Legal Implications of CPR

Living wills, advance directives, and Do Not Attempt Resuscitation (DNAR) orders are legal documents that specify the patient's wishes regarding specified medical procedures. These documents are explained in Chapter 3. First responders sometimes wonder if they should start CPR on a person who has a living will or an advance directive. Because you are not in a position to determine if the living will or advance directive is valid, CPR should be started on all patients unless they are obviously dead. If a patient has a living will or advance directive, the physician at the hospital will determine whether or not to stop CPR. You should check your department's protocols and state regulations on this matter.

Do not hesitate to begin CPR on a pulseless, nonbreathing patient. Without your help, the patient will certainly die. You may have legal problems if you begin CPR on a patient who does not need it and this action harms the patient. However, the chances of this happening are minimal if you assess the patient carefully before beginning CPR.

Another potential legal pitfall is abandonment—the discontinuing of CPR without the order of a licensed physician or without turning the patient over to someone who is at least as qualified as you are.

If you avoid these pitfalls, you need not be overly concerned about the legal implications of performing CPR. Your most important protection against a possible legal suit is to become thoroughly proficient in the theory and practice of CPR.

8 Prep Kit

Ready for Review

Ready for Review thoroughly summarizes the chapter.

CPR is one of the most important lifesaving skills that you will learn as a first responder. By combining the airway skills and the breathing skills from Chapter 6 with the circulation skills presented in this chapter, you should be able to perform effective CPR. A review of the anatomy and function of the circulatory system gives you a better understanding of the way in which the circulatory system works. This chapter also covered the problems that may cause the heart to stop beating.

It is important to understand how a first responder fits into the cardiac chain of survival. This chapter presented the techniques for performing external chest compressions in adults, infants, and children. The steps for one-rescuer and two-rescuer adult CPR, infant CPR, and child CPR are also described. It is important that you understand the signs of effective CPR so you can evaluate your performance. It is also important that you understand the complications of performing CPR so you can work to prevent these from occurring. Finally, this chapter described why you should be certified in CPR, and discussed the legal implications of CPR.

Once you have mastered CPR skills by practicing on a manikin under the watchful eye of a good instructor, you can keep those skills by practicing and refreshing your knowledge periodically. Practice as though a life depends on it, because one day it will!

Vital Vocabulary

The Vital Vocabulary are the key terms for this chapter.

brachial pulse—*page 188*
cardiac arrest—*page 179*
chest compression—*page 179*
child—*page 190*
circulatory system—*page 174*
gastric distention—*page 192*
infant—*page 188*
one-rescuer CPR—*page 181*
plasma—*page 176*
platelets—*page 176*
pulse—*page 175*
two-rescuer CPR—*page 184*
ventilation—*page 183*
xiphoid process—*page 180*

Practice Points

The Practice Points are the key skills you need to know.

1. Performing one-rescuer adult CPR.

2. Performing two-rescuer adult CPR.

3. Performing infant CPR.

4. Performing child CPR.

The Skill Drills provide a visual summary of some of the more complex skills from the skills objectives.

8.6 Perform Chest Compressions — *page 179*

8.9 One-Rescuer Adult CPR — *page 182*

8.11 Two-Rescuer Adult CPR — *page 185*

Ready to Respond

Ready to Respond presents a fictitious scenario to help you review what you learned in this chapter.

You are called to a residence for a report of an unresponsive person. Your patient is reported to be a 74-year-old male.

1. Which of the following would indicate that CPR is needed?
A. Shallow breathing
B. Dilated pupils
C. Absence of breathing and circulation
D. Shortness of breath

2. What criteria would indicate that CPR should not be started?
A. Evidence of tissue decomposition
B. Rigor mortis
C. Decapitation
D. Dilated pupils

3. Which of the following criteria would indicate that you could stop CPR?
A. A physician assumes responsibility for the patient
B. The patient vomits
C. The patient begins breathing and has a pulse
D. You are too exhausted to continue

4. When performing chest compressions on this patient, each compression should be
A. Followed by a rescue breath
B. Done quickly
C. One-half downward and one-half upward
D. Done with relaxed arms

5. The depth on compressions should be:
A. 1 to 1½ inches
B. 1½ to 2 inches
C. ½ to 1 inch
D. 2 to 2½ inches

6. If you are performing CPR on this patient by yourself, the ratio of compressions to ventilations should be
A. 5 to 1
B. 2 to 15
C. 1 to 5
D. 15 to 2

7. If you are performing CPR on this patient with a partner, the ratio of compressions to ventilations should be
A. 5 to 1
B. 2 to 15
C. 1 to 5
D. 15 to 2

8. When performing rescue breathing on this patient, each breath should be given over a period of
A. 1 second
B. 1½ seconds
C. 2 seconds
D. 2½ seconds

9. List five signs that your CPR is effective.

10. Describe three complications that could occur from administering CPR.

11. What changes would you need to make in your CPR if this patient were a 5-year-old child?

12. What changes would you need to make in your CPR if this patient were a 6-month-old infant?

MODULE 4 QuickQuiz

Circulation

1. If you are alone with a pulseless adult patient, you should
   A. Perform CPR for 1 minute before activating the EMS system
   B. Activate the EMS system before beginning CPR (phone first)
   C. Perform CPR for 3 minutes before activating the EMS system
   D. Perform CPR for 5 minutes before activating the EMS system

2. Which condition should exist before starting CPR?
   A. Dilated pupils
   B. Pale skin
   C. Shallow breathing
   D. Absence of breathing and pulse

3. When performing two-rescuer CPR on an adult patient, the ratio of chest compressions to rescue breaths is
   A. 5 to 1
   B. 15 to 1
   C. 15 to 2
   D. 1 to 15

4. To perform chest compressions on an adult patient, you should press on the
   A. lower half of the sternum
   B. middle of the sternum
   C. xiphoid process
   D. lower half of the sternum

5. The rate of chest compressions in an adult patient is
   A. at least 100 per minute
   B. 80 to 100 per minute
   C. 100 per minute
   D. 90 per minute

1. B 2. D 3. C 4. D 5. C

Illness and Injury

MODULE

5

Module CONTENTS

Chapter 9

Medical Emergencies

TECHNOLOGY

- Online Chapter Pretest
- Web Links
- Online Glossary
- Anatomy Review
- Online Review Manual
- CyberClass

www.FirstResponderTraining.com

- Interactive First Responder

Chapter FEATURES

- Skill Drills
- Vital Vocabulary
- Voices of Experience
- Signs and Symptoms
- FYI
- Special Needs
- Safety Tips
- BSI Tips
- Caution
- Check Point
- Prep Kit

Objectives

Knowledge and Attitude Objectives

After studying this chapter, you will be expected to:

1. Describe the general approach to a medical patient.
2. Explain the causes, symptoms, and treatment of a patient with altered mental status.
3. Explain the causes, symptoms, and treatment of a patient with seizures.
4. Describe the treatment of a patient who shows signs and symptoms of exposure to heat.
5. Describe the treatment of a patient who shows signs and symptoms of exposure to cold.

Note: The following objectives contain supplemental material.

6. Explain the causes of angina pectoris.
7. Describe the signs, symptoms, and initial treatment of a patient with angina pectoris.
8. Explain the major cause of a heart attack.
9. Describe the signs, symptoms, and initial treatment of a patient with a heart attack.

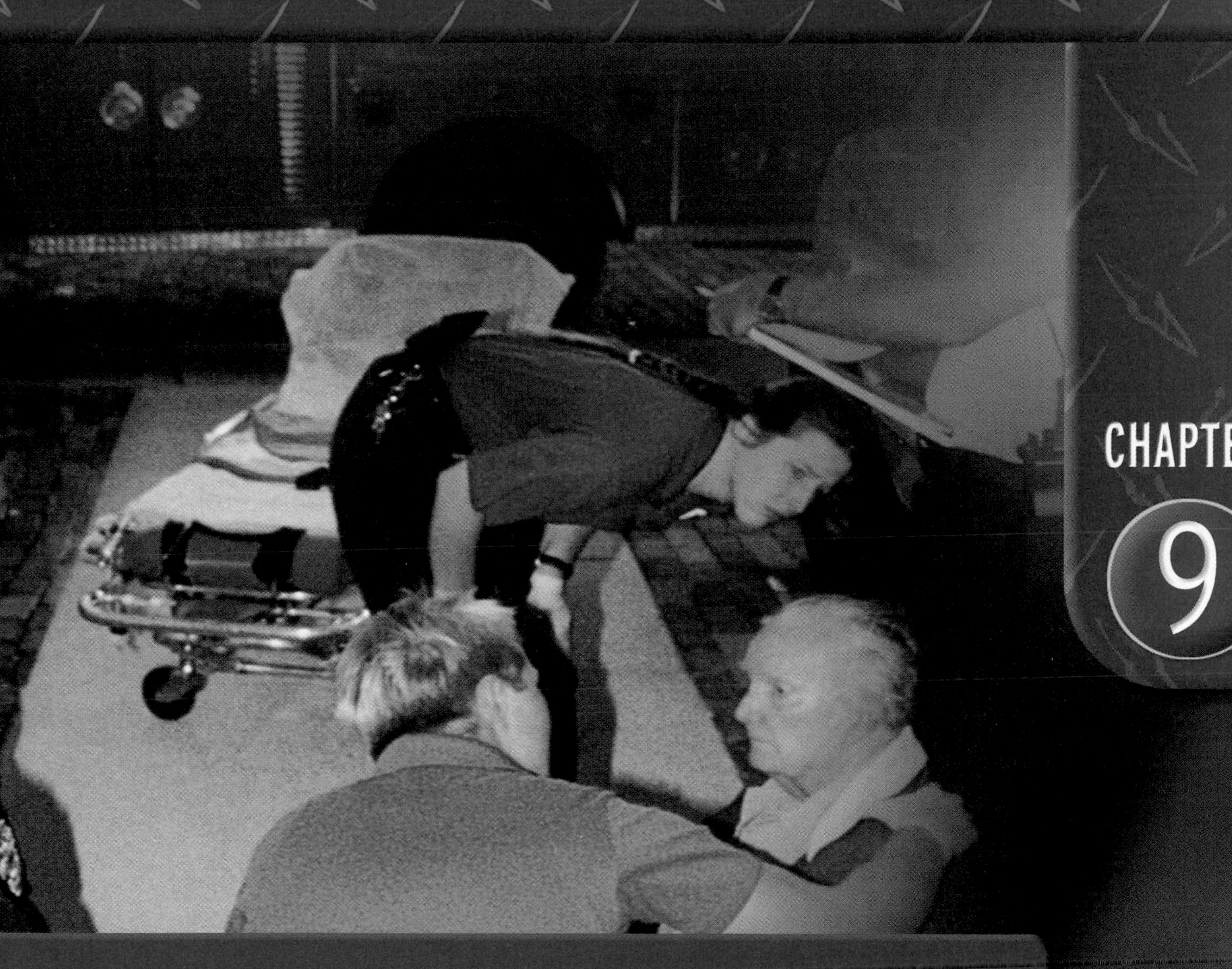

CHAPTER 9

10. Explain the cause of congestive heart failure.
11. Describe the signs, symptoms, and initial treatment of a patient with congestive heart failure.
12. Describe the causes of dyspnea.
13. Explain the signs, symptoms, and initial treatment of a patient with dyspnea.
14. Describe the major cause of a stroke.
15. Explain the signs, symptoms, and initial treatment of a patient with a stroke.
16. Describe the signs and symptoms of insulin shock.
17. Describe the initial treatment of a patient in insulin shock.
18. Describe the signs and symptoms of a patient in a diabetic coma.
19. Describe the initial treatment of a patient in a diabetic coma.
20. Describe the signs and symptoms of an abdominal problem.
21. Describe the initial treatment of a patient with abdominal pain.

Skill Objectives

As a first responder, you should be able to:

1. Perform a patient assessment on a medical patient.
2. Place an unconscious patient in the recovery position.
3. Protect a patient who is seizing from sustaining further harm.
4. Cool a patient who has suffered exposure to heat.
5. Treat a patient who has suffered exposure to cold.
6. Position a patient who has congestive heart failure.
7. Administer fluids or oral glucose to a patient who is in insulin shock.

This chapter on medical conditions has two parts. The first part covers general medical complaints, including altered mental status and seizures. General medical complaints may result from a wide variety of medical conditions. You will learn the signs, symptoms, and common treatment steps for patients with these general medical complaints.

The second part addresses some specific medical conditions you will encounter, including generalized heat emergencies, generalized cold emergencies, angina pectoris, heart attack, congestive heart failure, dyspnea, stroke, insulin shock, diabetic coma, and abdominal pain. You will learn the signs, symptoms, and treatment of patients with these specific medical conditions.

Treating patients with medical conditions can be some of the most challenging work you perform as a first responder. By carefully studying these conditions, you will be prepared to provide reassuring and sometimes lifesaving care to patients suffering from medical emergencies.

General Medical Conditions

General medical conditions may have different causes, but they result in similar signs and symptoms. By learning to recognize the signs and symptoms of these conditions as well as general treatment guidelines, you will be able to provide immediate care for patients even if you can not determine the exact cause of the problems. This initial treatment can stabilize the patient and allow other EMS and hospital personnel to diagnose and further treat the problem.

General Approaches to a Medical Patient

Your approach to a patient who has a general medical complaint should follow the systematic approach outlined in the patient assessment sequence in Chapter 7. Review your dispatch information for an idea of the possible problem. Carefully check the scene to assess your safety and that of the patient. As you perform the initial patient assessment, first try to get an impression of the patient's problem. Then determine the patient's responsiveness, introduce yourself, check the patient's ABCs, and acknowledge the patient's chief complaint.

Usually, it is best to collect a medical history on the patient experiencing a medical problem before you perform a physical examination.

The medical history should be complete and include all factors that may relate to the patient's current illness.

The SAMPLE history format will help you secure the information you need:

S = Signs/symptoms

A = Allergies

M = Medications

P = Pertinent past history

L = Last oral intake

E = Events associated with or leading to the illness or injury

Although the physical examination should focus on the areas related to the patient's current illness, you should also realize that the patient may not always be aware of all facets of his or her problem. It is better to perform a complete physical examination and find all the problems than to perform a partial examination and miss an underlying problem. Determine the patient's vital signs and do not forget to perform on-going assessment if additional EMS personnel are delayed.

As you perform the patient assessment, remember to reassure the patient. Any call for emergency medical care is a frightening experience for the patient. Many medical conditions are aggravated by stress. If you can reduce the patient's stress, you will go a long way toward making the patient more comfortable.

Altered Mental Status

Altered mental status is a sudden or gradual decrease in the patient's level of responsiveness. This change may range from a decrease in the level of understanding to unresponsiveness. Any patient who is unresponsive has suffered a severe change in mental status.

In assessing altered mental status, remember the AVPU scale:

A *Alert*. An alert patient will answer simple questions accurately and appropriately.

V *Verbal*. A patient who is responsive to verbal stimuli will react to loud voices.

P *Pain*. A patient who is responsive to a painful stimulus will react to the pain by moving or crying out.

U *Unresponsive*. An unresponsive patient will not respond to either verbal or painful stimuli.

When assessing the patient's mental status, you should consider two factors: the patient's initial level of consciousness and any change in that level of consciousness. A patient who is initially alert but later responds only to verbal stimuli has suffered a decrease in level of consciousness.

Remember

THE PATIENT ASSESSMENT SEQUENCE:

1. Scene size-up.
2. Perform an initial assessment.
   A. Form a general impression of the patient.
   B. Assess responsiveness–stabilize the spine if trauma.
   C. Assess the patient's airway.
   D. Assess the patient's breathing.
   E. Assess the patient's circulation.
   F. Update responding EMS units.
3. Examine the patient from head to toe.
4. Obtain the patient's medical history (SAMPLE).
5. Perform an on-going assessment.

Note: For medical patients reverse steps 3 and 4.

Many different conditions may cause an altered level of consciousness including:

- Head injury
- Shock
- Decreased level of oxygen to the brain
- High fever
- Infection
- Poisoning, including drugs and alcohol
- Low level of blood sugar (diabetic emergencies)
- Insulin reaction
- Psychiatric condition

Some of the specific conditions that cause altered mental status are explained in the second part of this chapter. Even if you can not determine what is causing the patient's altered level of consciousness, you can help by treating the symptoms of the problem.

You should complete the patient assessment sequence to ensure scene safety and proper assessment. Initial treatment is to maintain the patient's ABCs and normal body temperature, and to keep the patient from additional harm. If the patient is unconscious and has not suffered trauma, place the patient in the recovery position or use an airway adjunct to help maintain an open airway. Be prepared to suction if there is a chance that the patient may vomit or not be able to handle secretions.

Seizures

Seizures are characterized by random shaking movements that may involve the entire body. Most seizures last less than five minutes. Prolonged seizures may continue for more than five minutes. Patients are usually unconscious during seizures and do not remember them afterward. Although seizures are rarely life-threatening, they are a serious medical emergency and may be the sign of a life-threatening condition. When seizures occur, the patient may need help to maintain an open airway. The patient may lose bowel and/or bladder control, soiling their clothing.

There are many different types of seizures, and they can be caused by many factors including:

- Epilepsy
- Trauma
- Head injury
- Stroke
- Shock
- Decreased level of oxygen to the brain
- High fever
- Infection
- Poisoning, including drugs and alcohol
- Brain tumor
- Diabetic emergencies
- Complication of pregnancy
- Unknown causes

Many times you will not be able to determine the cause of the patient's seizure. After a seizure, the patient may be sleepy, confused, upset, hostile, or out of touch with reality for up to an hour. You must monitor the patient's ABCs and arrange for ***transport*** to an appropriate medical facility.

Usually, the seizure will be over by the time you arrive at the scene. If it has not ended, your treatment should focus on protecting the patient from injury. Do not restrain the patient's movements. If you attempt to restrain the patient, you may cause further injury. If a patient suffers a seizure while on a hard surface, control the patient's arms by grasping them at the wrists. Allow the patient's arms to move but prevent the elbows from hitting the hard surface. To prevent the patient's head from hitting a hard surface, quickly slide the toes of your shoes under the patient's head. The patient should be moved only if he or she is in a dangerous location, such as in a busy street or close to something hard, hot, or sharp.

CAUTION

Do not attempt to put anything in the mouth of a patient who is actively seizing.

During a seizure, the patient generally does not breathe and may turn blue. You cannot do anything about the patient's airway during the seizure, but once the seizure has stopped, it is essential that you ensure an open airway. This is usually best accomplished with the head tilt–chin lift technique. Observe the seizure activity and report your observations and assessment findings to other EMS providers. They may be important in determining the cause of the seizure.

After you have opened the airway, place the patient in the recovery position to help keep the airway open and to allow any secretions (saliva or blood from a bitten tongue) to drain out (**Figure 9.1**). Patients who have suffered a seizure may have excess oral secretions.

Most patients start to breathe soon after the seizure ends. If the patient does not resume breathing after a seizure or if the seizure is prolonged, begin mouth-to-mask or mouth-to-mouth breathing. (See Chapter 6.)

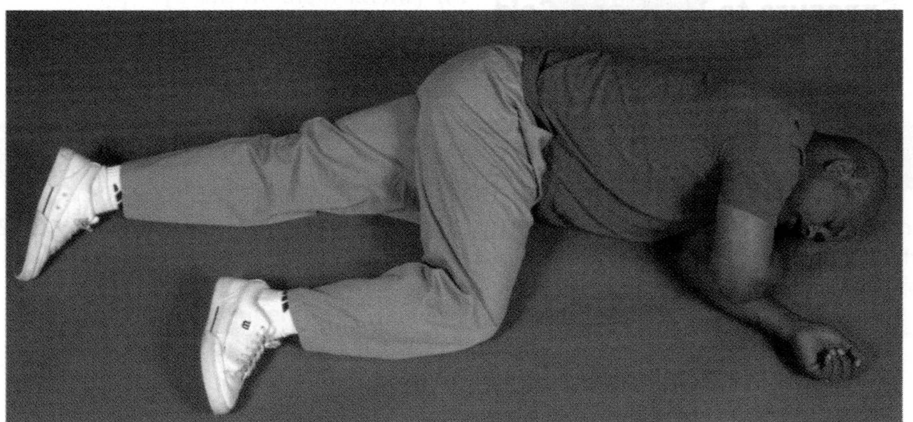

Figure 9.1 Recovery position for an unconscious patient.

TREATMENT FOR SEIZURES

- *Stay calm. You cannot stop a seizure once it has started.*
- *Do not restrain the patient.*
- *Clear the area of hard, sharp, or hot objects to protect the patient from injury.*
- *Do not force anything between the patient's teeth.*
- *Do not be concerned if the patient stops breathing temporarily during the seizure.*
- *After the seizure, turn the patient on his or her side and make sure breathing is not obstructed.*
- *If the patient does not begin breathing after a seizure, start rescue breathing.*

Remember

Although there is a st
to quickly categorize
"medical patients" or
patients," it is import
that many of the pati
encounter may have b
condition and a traum
For example, the alter
consciousness experi
diabetic in insulin sho
tribute to a motor ve
As you study this cha
imagine how you can
knowledge to treat pa
a single problem or a
problems. Remember
assess each patient a
problems that you ide

heat exhaustion A form
occurs when the body lo
water and too many elect
very heavy sweating after

heatstroke A condition
internal body temperature
the body's mechanisms fo
heat are overwhelmed. Un
can result in death.

frostbite Partial or comp
of the skin and deeper tis
by exposure to the cold.

hypothermia A conditio
internal body temperatur
95°F after prolonged exp
or freezing temperatures.

Signs & Sym

HEAT EXHAUSTIO

- Lightheadedness
- Dizziness
- Weak pulse
- Profuse sweating
- Nausea

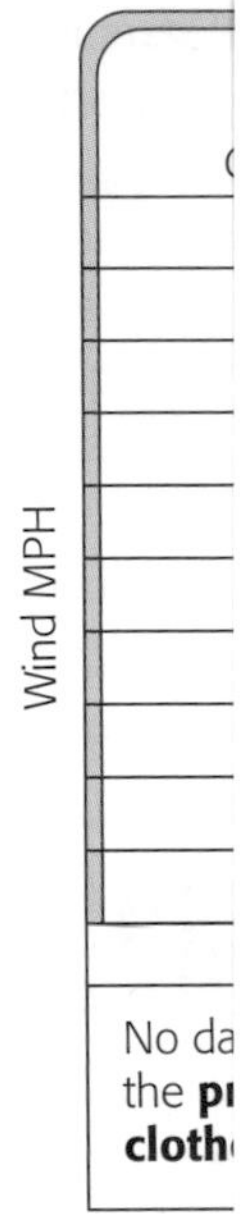

Wind MPH

No da
the **pr**
cloth

Figure 9.3 Wind chi

Note: A special example of hypothermia protecting a patient from death is an apparent drowning in water colder than 70°F (21°C). Many children who fell in cold water and apparently drowned have been resuscitated successfully. Always start CPR on apparent drowning victims pulled from cold water.

atherosclerosis A disease characterized by a thickening and destruction of the arterial walls and caused by fatty deposits within them; the arteries lose the ability to dilate and carry blood.

cardiac arrest Sudden cessation of heart function.

angina pectoris Chest pain with squeezing or tightness in the chest caused by an inadequate flow of blood to the heart muscle.

nitroglycerin A medicine used to treat angina pectoris; it increases blood flow and oxygen supply to the heart muscle and reduces or eliminates the pain of angina pectoris.

A

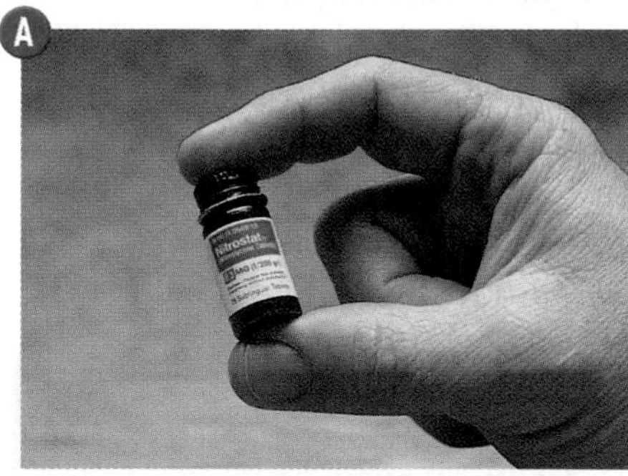

B

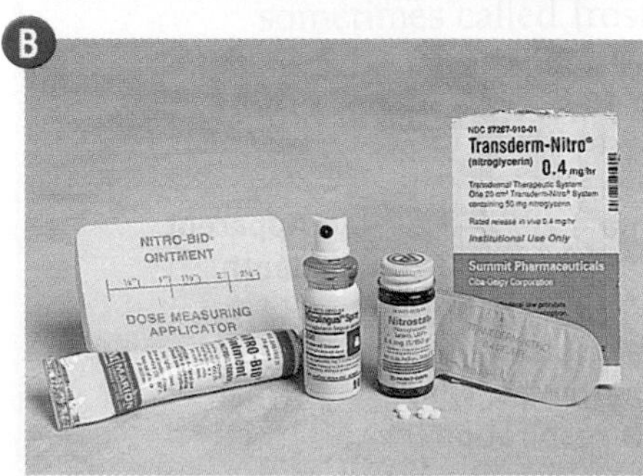

Figure 9.4 Nitroglycerin pills and spray used for relief of chest pain.

give warm fluids to drink.

If you are outdoors and cannot easily take the patient inside a building, move the patient into a heated vehicle as soon as possible. If you cannot move the patient to a warmer environment, keep the patient dry and place as many blankets and insulating materials as possible around the patient. Sometimes you can use your own body heat to warm the patient. Wrap blankets around yourself and the patient or get into a sleeping bag with the patient to use your body heat to start the warming process even during transport.

Any patient suffering from hypothermia must be examined by a physician.

Cardiac Arrest and Hypothermia

FYI

If the patient's temperature falls below 83°F (or 28°C), the heart may stop and you will need to begin CPR. Strange as it may seem, hypothermia may actually protect patients from death in some cases. Therefore, always start CPR on hypothermic patients even if you believe they have been "dead" for several hours. Hypothermic patients should never be considered dead until they have been warmed in an appropriate medical facility.

Heart Conditions

The heart must receive a constant supply of oxygen or it will die. The heart receives its oxygen through a complex system of coronary (heart) arteries. As long as these arteries continue to supply the heart with an adequate amount of oxygen, the heart can continue to function properly.

As the body ages, however, the coronary arteries may narrow as a result of a disease process called **atherosclerosis**. Atherosclerosis causes layers of fat to coat the inner walls of the arteries. Progressive atherosclerosis can cause angina pectoris, heart attack, and even **cardiac arrest**.

Angina Pectoris

As atherosclerosis progresses, it can reduce the blood (oxygen) supply to the heart enough to cause pain or pressure in the chest. This pain is known as **angina pectoris**, or simply "angina." The heart simply needs more oxygen than the narrowed coronary arteries can deliver.

When a patient has chest pain, you should first ask the person to describe the pain. Angina is often described as pressure or heavy discomfort. The patient may say something like, "It feels like an elephant is sitting on my chest." Angina attacks are usually brought on by exertion, emotion, or eating. Crushing pain may be felt in the chest and may radiate to either or both arms, the neck, jaw, or any combination of these sites. The patient is often short of breath and sweating, is extremely frightened, and has a sense of doom.

Ask whether the patient is already being treated for a diagnosed heart condition. If the answer is "yes," ask if the patient has a pill or spray to take for angina pain. A patient who has suffered previous bouts of angina usually has medication that can be taken (placed or sprayed under the tongue) to relieve the pain. The most common medication of this type is **nitroglycerin**, and the patient may have already taken a dose by the time you arrive on the scene (**Figure 9.4**).

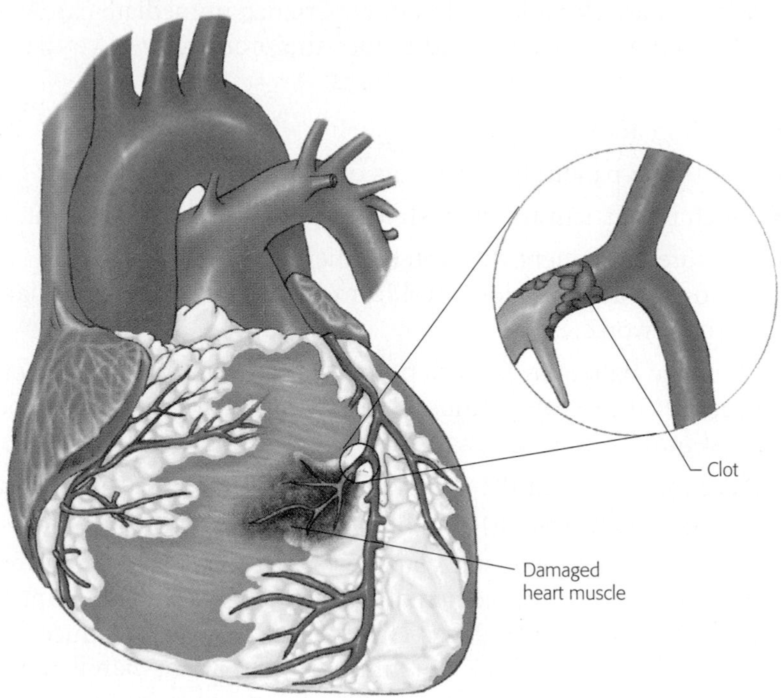

Figure 9.5 Blocked cardiac artery results in heart attack.

If the patient has nitroglycerin but has not taken it during the past five minutes, help place one of the tiny pills under the patient's tongue or help the patient administer the aerosol spray. You should follow your local protocols regarding the administration of nitroglycerin.

Nitroglycerin usually relieves angina pain within five minutes. If the pain has not diminished after five minutes, help the patient take a second dose. If the pain still has not lessened five minutes after the second dose, assume the patient is having a heart attack.

Heart Attack

A heart attack (myocardial infarction) results when one or more of the coronary arteries is completely blocked. The two primary causes of coronary artery blockage are severe atherosclerosis and a blood clot from somewhere else in the circulatory system that has broken free and become lodged in the artery. If one of the coronary arteries becomes blocked, the part of the heart muscle served by that artery is deprived of oxygen and dies (**Figure 9.5**).

Blockage of a coronary artery causes the patient to suffer immediate and severe pain. The pain of angina pectoris and heart attack may be similar at first. Most heart attack patients describe the pain as crushing. The pain may radiate from the chest to the left arm or to the jaw (**Figure 9.6**). The patient is usually short of breath, weak, sweating, nauseated, and may vomit. The pain of heart attack is not relieved by nitroglycerin pills, and it will persist, unlike the pain of angina that rarely lasts more than five minutes.

If the area of heart muscle supplied by the blocked artery is either critical or large, the heart may stop completely. Complete cessation of heartbeat is called cardiac arrest. CPR is your first emergency treatment for cardiac arrest. (See Chapters 6 and 8.)

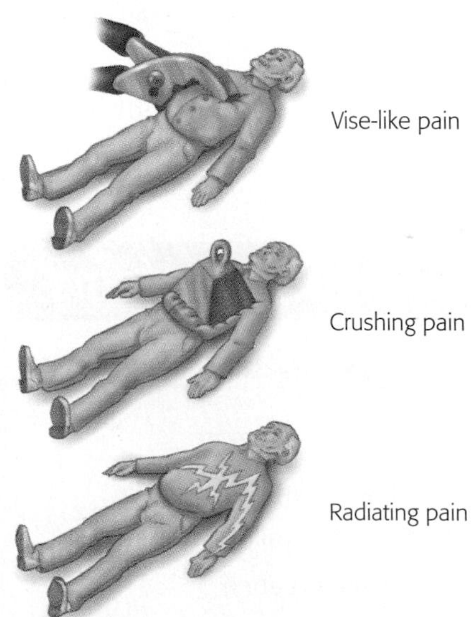

Figure 9.6 Descriptions of pain caused by heart attack.

Signs & Symptoms

CARDIAC ARREST

- Unconscious
- Absence of respirations
- Absence of carotid pulse

Did You Know?

Within the last ten years, the use of "clot busting" drugs has been an important advance in treating heart attack patients. Clot buster drugs can often open the blocked coronary vessels and prevent the need for costly and painful operations. Because clot busters must be administered by a specially trained physician within a few hours of the start of a heart attack to be effective, your prompt response and thoughtful care of a heart attack patient may be the first step in returning that patient to a comfortable, healthy, and productive life.

Signs & Symptoms

CONGESTIVE HEART FAILURE

- Shortness of breath
- Rapid, shallow breathing
- Moist or gurgling respirations
- Profuse sweating
- Enlarged neck veins
- Swollen ankles
- Anxiety

Most heart attack patients do not experience immediate cardiac arrest. To support the patient and reduce the probability of cardiac arrest, you can take the following actions:

- Summon additional help.
- Talk to the patient to relieve his or her anxiety.
- Touch the patient to establish a bond. Hold the person's hand.
- Reassure the patient that you are there to help. The person is afraid that death is close, and fear can create tension and make the pain worse.
- Move the patient as little as possible and do not allow the person to move! If the patient must be moved, you and other bystanders must move the patient.
- Place the patient in the position he or she finds most comfortable. This is usually a semi-reclining or sitting position.
- If oxygen is available and you are trained to use it, administer it to the patient. Supplemental oxygen increases the amount of oxygen the blood can carry. The increase in oxygen reduces pain and anxiety. It also eases the minds of the patient's family and friends to see that something is being done to relieve the patient's physical distress.

Because you do not have extensive equipment available to help the heart attack patient, your primary role is to provide psychological support and arrange for T ***prompt transportation*** to an appropriate medical facility. Because the patient's emotional state can affect his or her physical condition, psychological support is valuable. It can prevent cardiac arrest.

Congestive Heart Failure

Congestive heart failure (CHF) is not directly caused by narrow or blocked coronary arteries, but by failure of the heart to pump adequately.

As explained in Chapters 4 and 8, the heart has two sides. The right side receives "used" blood from the body and sends it to the lungs; the left side receives "fresh" oxygenated blood from the lungs and pumps it to the body. If one side of the heart becomes weak and cannot pump as well as the other side, the circulatory system becomes unbalanced, resulting in circulatory congestion. In CHF, the failure is in the heart muscle, but the congestion is in the blood vessels.

Figure 9.7 shows what happens if CHF occurs on the left side of the heart, which sends blood to the body. Because the left side cannot send blood to the body as efficiently as the right side can send blood to the lungs, more blood goes to the lungs than to the body. This results in congestion (overload) in the blood vessels of the lungs.

The major symptom of CHF is breathing difficulty, not chest pain. If you are called to assist a patient who has respiratory problems but no signs of injury or airway obstruction are present, look for the signs and symptoms of CHF.

As blood pressure builds in the vessels of the lungs, fluid is forced into lung tissue, causing it to swell. The patient may make a gurgling sound when breathing and start spitting up a white or pink froth or foamy fluid. At this point, the patient is actually "drowning" in his or

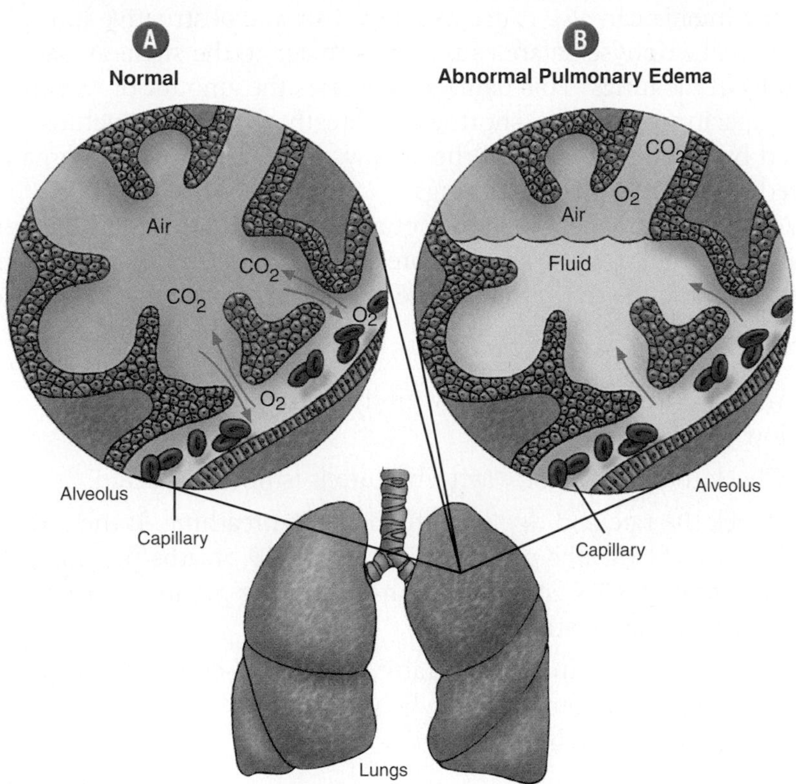

Figure 9.7 A. Normal exchange of oxygen and carbon dioxide between a capillary and an alveolus. **B.** Pulmonary edema: congestive heart failure causes fluid to leak from the capillary and build in the alveolus, impeding oxygen and carbon dioxide exchange.

CAUTION

Patients who are short of breath or receiving oxygen should have their breathing and pulse monitored at least every five minutes. Underlying illness or trauma may cause certain patients to stop breathing and require you to begin rescue breathing.

her own body fluids. The patient is very anxious but is usually in little or no pain (unless he or she is suffering a heart attack coupled with CHF).

As soon as you determine that the patient is suffering from CHF, take these simple, lifesaving actions:

1. Place the patient in a sitting position, preferably on a bed or chair. Having the legs hang down over the edge of the bed or chair helps drain some of the fluid back into the lower parts of the body and may improve breathing.
2. Administer oxygen, if it is available and you are trained to give it, in large quantities and at a high flow rate.
3. Summon additional help.
4. Arrange for Ⓣ ***prompt transportation*** to an appropriate medical facility.

The most important action is to place the patient in a sitting position with the legs down. This position helps relieve CHF symptoms until more highly trained EMS personnel arrive.

Remember

The major symptom of heart attack is chest pain; the major symptom of CHF is difficulty breathing.

Dyspnea (Shortness of Breath)

Dyspnea means shortness of breath or difficulty breathing. Although healthy people may experience shortness of breath during intense physical exertion or at high altitudes, this condition is usually associated with serious heart or lung disease. Heart-related causes of dyspnea include angina pectoris, heart attack, and CHF. These conditions have already been discussed. Pulmonary (lung) diseases such as **chronic obstructive lung disease (COLD)**, emphysema, chronic **bronchitis**,

dyspnea Difficulty or pain with breathing.

chronic obstructive lung disease (COLD) A slow process of destruction of the airways, alveoli, and pulmonary blood vessels caused by chronic bronchial obstruction (emphysema). This condition is also known as chronic obstructive pulmonary disease (COPD).

bronchitis Inflammation of the airways in the lungs.

and pneumonia can also cause dyspnea. Chronic obstructive lung disease and emphysema are caused by damage to the small air sacs (alveoli) in the lungs. This damage decreases the amount of working lung capacity, resulting in shortness of breath. Chronic bronchitis is caused by an inflammation of the airways in the lungs. Pneumonia is caused by an infection in the lungs.

As a first responder, you will not always be able to determine what is causing a patient to be short of breath. Do not spend too much time trying to determine the specific cause, but focus on treating the symptoms of dyspnea.

General treatment for patients with dyspnea consists of the following steps:

1. Check the patient's airway to be sure it is not obstructed.
2. Check the rate and depth of the patient's breathing. If the rate is below eight breaths per minute or above 40 breaths per minute, be prepared to assist with mouth-to-mask or mouth-to-barrier-device rescue breathing.
3. Place the patient in a comfortable position. A conscious patient is usually most comfortable when sitting.
4. Provide reassurance.
5. Loosen any tight clothing.
6. Administer oxygen, if it is available and you are trained to do so.

Stroke

Strokes are a leading cause of brain injury in adults. Each year millions of adults suffer strokes. Nearly a quarter of them die. Most strokes are caused by a blood clot that lodges in an artery of the brain. The clot blocks the blood supply to part of the brain. Without treatment, that part of the brain will be damaged or die. You can think of a stroke as a "brain attack" similar to a heart attack.

The signs and symptoms of stroke vary depending on which portion of the brain is affected. A stroke patient may be alert, confused or unresponsive. Responsive patients may not be aware that they have signs of a stroke. Some stroke patients are unable to speak. The patient may have a headache, and may describe it as "the worst headache of my life." Some stroke patients suffer seizures.

Your first priority is to maintain an open airway. Administer oxygen (if available and you are trained to use it) using a nonrebreathing facemask. If the patient is having convulsions, try to prevent further injury from occurring. Be prepared to administer rescue breathing if the patient stops breathing. Place unresponsive patients in the recovery position to help them maintain an open airway (see **Figure 9.1**, page 205). This is especially important since some stroke patients are unable to swallow. Give psychological support by talking to and touching the patient. Be especially careful if you must move a patient because some patients may not be able to feel one side of their body.

Some stroke patients can be treated with special drugs to dissolve the blood clot in their brain. These "clot buster" drugs must be given in the hospital within the first few hours after the stroke. For this reason, it important for you to determine the time the stroke began from the

Signs & Symptoms

STROKE

- Headache
- Numbness or paralysis on one side of the body
- Dizziness
- Confusion
- Drooling
- Inability to speak
- Difficulty seeing
- Unequal pupil size
- Unconscious
- Convulsions
- Respiratory arrest
- Incontinence

Table 9.3

The Cincinnati Prehospital Stroke Scale

The Cincinnati Prehospital Stroke Scale is a tool you can use to tell if there is a high probability that a patient has suffered a stroke. This scale requires you to quickly assess three things: Facial Droop, Arm Drift, and Abnormal Speech.

FACIAL DROOP	*have patient show teeth or smile.*
Normal	Both sides of the face move equally.
Abnormal	One side of the face does not move as well as the other side.
ARM DRIFT	*patient closes eyes and holds both arms straight out for 10 seconds.*
Normal	Both arms move the same or both arms do not move the same.
Abnormal	One arm does not move or one arm drifts down compared to the other.
ABNORMAL SPEECH	*have patient say, "you can't teach an old dog new tricks."*
Normal	Patient uses correct words with no slurring.
Abnormal	Patient slurs words, uses the wrong words, or is unable to speak.

NOTE: If any of these three signs is abnormal, the probability of a stroke is 72 percent.

Note: A stroke patient may be able to hear what you are saying even if he or she cannot speak or appears to be unconscious. Do not say anything that would increase the patient's anxiety.

patient, family or bystanders. If the patient has signs or symptoms of a stroke, it is important for you to arrange for ***prompt transportation*** of the patient to a medical facility that is equipped to treat stroke patients. Some EMS services use the Cincinnati Prehospital Stroke Scale to determine if a patient is showing signs or symptoms of a stroke (See **Table 9.3**).

Diabetes

Diabetes is caused by the body's inability to process and use the type of sugar that is carried by the bloodstream to the body's cells.

Sugar is an essential nutrient. The body's cells need both oxygen and sugar to survive. The body produces a hormone (chemical) called insulin, which enables sugar carried by the blood to move into individual cells, where it is used as fuel.

If the body does not produce enough insulin, the cells become "starved" for sugar. This condition is called diabetes. Many diabetics (people with diabetes) must take supplemental insulin injections to bring their insulin levels up to normal. Mild diabetes can sometimes be treated by oral medicine rather than insulin.

Diabetes is a serious medical condition. Therefore, all diabetic patients who are sick must be evaluated and treated in an appropriate medical facility. Two specific things can go wrong in the management of diabetes: **insulin shock** and **diabetic coma**. Both are medical emergencies that you must deal with as a first responder.

diabetes A disease in which the body is unable to use sugar normally because of a deficiency or total lack of insulin; often called "sugar diabetes."

insulin shock Condition that occurs in a diabetic who has taken too much insulin or has not eaten enough food. (Also referred to as a low blood sugar reaction or just "a reaction.")

diabetic coma A state of unconsciousness that occurs when the body has too much sugar and not enough insulin.

Remember

During your initial examination of every patient, look for an emergency medical alerting device to find out whether the patient has a pre-existing medical condition, such as diabetes.

Insulin Shock

Insulin shock occurs if the body has enough insulin but not enough blood sugar. A diabetic may take insulin in the morning and then alter his or her usual routine by not eating or by exercising vigorously. In either case, the level of blood sugar drops and the patient suffers insulin shock.

The signs and symptoms of insulin shock are similar to those of other types of shock. Suspect insulin shock if a patient has a history of diabetes or is wearing medical emergency information, such as a MedicAlert® tag (**Figure 9.8**).

Insulin shock is a serious medical emergency that can occur quickly, often within a few minutes. If insulin shock is not diagnosed and corrected by the administration of sugar in some form, the patient may die.

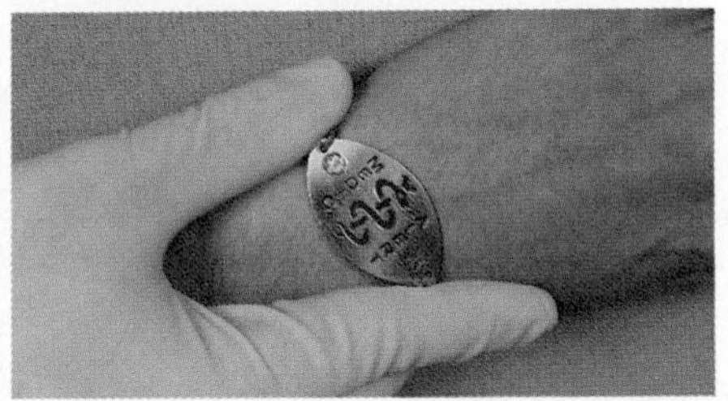

Figure 9.8 MedicAlert® tag.

Signs & Symptoms

INSULIN SHOCK

- Pale, moist, cool skin
- Rapid pulse
- Dizziness or headache
- Confusion or unconsciousness
- Rapid onset of symptoms (within minutes)

A person experiencing insulin shock may appear to be drunk. You must keep this fact in mind. Mistakes have been and will continue to be made by first responders and others who misinterpret insulin shock as intoxication. If you suspect that a patient is suffering from insulin shock, try to get answers to the following questions:

- Are you a diabetic?
- Did you take your insulin today?
- Have you eaten today?

If the patient is diabetic and has taken insulin that day, but has not yet eaten, you should suspect that the patient is going into insulin shock.

If the patient is partly conscious, attempt to get the patient to eat or drink something sweet. For example, you could use a drink such as a cola, orange juice, or honey that has a high sugar concentration.

Note: Be sure that the drink you give to a person suffering from insulin shock is not "sugar free" or "diet."

If the patient is unconscious, do not try to administer fluids by mouth because the patient may choke and aspirate the fluid into the lungs. Summon help immediately. Open the patient's airway and assist breathing and circulation, if necessary. The patient must have sugar administered intravenously as soon as possible. This can be done by a paramedic or a physician. Some first responders carry a tube of oral glucose that can be placed inside the cheek. This can be administered to unconscious patients and may be effective in providing the patient with the needed sugar (**Figure 9.9**).

Even though the patient's body may absorb only a small amount of sugar as a result of your efforts, it may be enough to prolong consciousness until the patient receives further medical treatment.

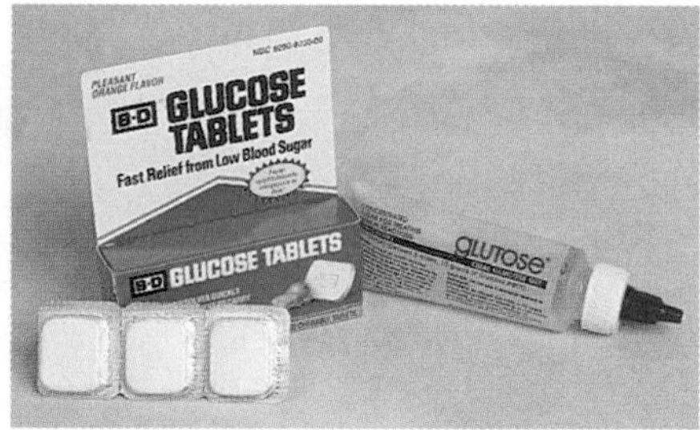

Figure 9.9 Instant glucose provides high concentrations of sugar.

Diabetic Coma

Diabetic coma occurs when the body has too much blood sugar and not enough insulin. A person with diabetes may fail to take insulin for several days. Blood sugar builds to higher and higher levels, but there is no insulin to process it for use by body cells.

The patient may be unresponsive or unconscious. A patient suffering from diabetic coma may appear to have the flu (influenza) or a severe cold. As with insulin shock, misdiagnosis is common. It is not always easy to tell the difference between insulin shock and diabetic coma (**Table 9.4**).

If the patient is conscious or partly conscious, if you cannot get definite answers to your questions, or if you are not sure whether the patient is suffering from insulin shock or diabetic coma, you can do

Table 9.4

Comparing Insulin Shock and Diabetic Coma

Insulin Shock	Diabetic Coma
Pale, moist, cool skin	Warm, dry skin
Rapid, weak pulse	Rapid pulse
Normal breathing	Deep, rapid breathing
Dizziness or headache	–
Confusion or unconsciousness	Unresponsiveness or unconsciousness
Rapid onset of symptoms (minutes)	Slow onset of symptoms (days)

no harm by administering a liquid sugar substance. Sugar may improve the condition of a patient suffering from insulin shock, and will not raise blood sugar levels enough to do further harm to the patient entering a diabetic coma.

In general, give conscious diabetic patients sugar by mouth and arrange for Ⓣ ***prompt transport*** to an appropriate medical facility. If the diabetic patient is unconscious, arrange for Ⓣ ***prompt transport*** to an appropriate medical facility and administer oral glucose only if approved by your medical director. Every sick diabetic patient must be transported by ambulance to an appropriate medical facility for further treatment and examination.

Check✓point

- ◯ Compare the treatment for insulin shock and diabetic coma.

Signs & Symptoms

DIABETIC COMA

- History of diabetes
- Warm, dry skin
- Rapid, weak pulse
- Deep, rapid breathing
- Fruity odor on the patient's breath
- Slow onset of symptoms (days)

Note: Progression into insulin shock is rapid and may be fatal; progression into diabetic coma usually takes several days.

Abdominal Pain

Separated from the chest by the diaphragm, the abdomen is a crossroads for several body systems, including the circulatory, skeletal, nervous, digestive, and genitourinary systems. For example, the aorta carries blood from the heart through the abdomen to the lower parts of the body while a large vein, the vena cava, carries blood back to the heart. The spine, with its large trunks of nerves, runs through this area, and parts of the rib cage surround the abdominal cavity. Most of the digestive system including the stomach, small intestine, large intestine, liver, gall bladder, and pancreas are in the abdomen. The kidneys and ureters are located in the abdominal area as well as parts of the male and female reproductive systems.

The contents of the abdomen are divided into hollow and solid structures. Hollow structures, such as the small intestine, are really tubes through which contents pass. Solid structures, such as the pancreas and the liver, produce substances. The structures in the abdomen are sometimes identified by quadrant, according to their location. As a first responder, you do not have to learn the names, types, and locations of all the abdominal structures.

The abdomen occupies a large part of the body, and abdominal pain is a common complaint. Because of the number of body systems and organs located in the abdomen, even physicians may have a difficult time identifying the cause of abdominal pain. As a first responder, you need to be able to recognize that a patient has an abdominal problem. You are not expected to determine the cause of the abdominal pain.

One condition you may encounter is called an **acute abdomen**, which is caused by irritation of the abdominal wall. The irritation may be due to infection or to the presence of blood in the abdominal cavity as the result of disease or trauma. A patient with an acute abdomen may have referred pain in other parts of the body such as the shoulder. The abdomen may feel as hard as a board.

If a patient has abdominal pain, monitor their vital signs, treat symptoms of shock, keep the patient comfortable, and arrange for Ⓣ ***transportation*** to an appropriate medical facility. It is important for these patients to be examined by a physician.

Signs & Symptoms

ACUTE ABDOMEN

- Nausea and vomiting
- Loss of appetite
- Pain in the abdomen
- Distention
- Shock

acute abdomen The sudden onset of abdominal pain caused by disease or trauma which irritates the lining of the abdominal cavity, and requires immediate medical or surgical treatment.

9 Prep Kit

Ready for Review

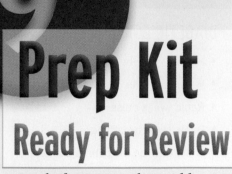

Ready for Review thoroughly summarizes the chapter.

This chapter discusses some of the more common medical problems encountered by first responders. The first part of this chapter covers general medical conditions. These conditions—altered mental status and seizures—can be caused by a variety of problems. When you encounter general medical conditions, it is not necessary to determine their cause. Base your treatment on the symptoms the patient displays.

The second part of this chapter covers some specific medical conditions. By learning about the causes and knowing the signs and symptoms of these conditions, you may be able to provide more specific care for the patient. Although these conditions must be diagnosed and treated by a physician, you can greatly improve the patient's chances of survival by taking the simple actions described here until more highly trained EMS personnel arrive on the scene to assist you.

Vital Vocabulary

The Vital Vocabulary are the key terms for this chapter.

acute abdomen—*page 217*
angina pectoris—*page 210*
atherosclerosis—*page 210*
bronchitis—*page 213*
cardiac arrest—*page 210*
chronic obstructive lung disease (COLD)—*page 213*
diabetes—*page 215*
diabetic coma—*page 215*
dyspnea—*page 213*
frostbite—*page 206*
heat exhaustion—*page 206*
heatstroke—*page 206*
hypothermia—*page 206*
insulin shock—*page 215*
nitroglycerin—*page 210*

Practice Points

The Practice Points are the key skills you need to know.

1. How to perform a patient assessment sequence on a medical patient.
2. How to place an unconscious patient in the recovery position.
3. How to prevent a patient who is seizing from further harm.
4. How to treat a patient who has suffered exposure to heat.
5. How to treat a patient who has suffered exposure to cold.
6. How to position a patient who has congestive heart failure.
7. How to administer fluids or oral glucose to a patient who is in insulin shock.

Ready to Respond

Ready to Respond presents a fictitious scenario to help you review what you learned in this chapter.

You are dispatched to a bus station for the report of a sick person. As you arrive on the scene, the station manager reports that the woman had been confused and became unresponsive just before you arrived.

1. Your first concern is
   A. The patient's airway
   B. The patient's level of consciousness
   C. Scene safety
   D. The cause of the problem
2. As you begin to examine the patient you should first check for
   A. The status of the patient's airway
   B. The patient's radial pulse
   C. The patient's brachial pulse
   D. The patient's level of responsiveness
3. The best position for this patient would be
   A. Sitting up
   B. Lying on the back
   C. The position in which you find her
   D. The recovery position
4. Your patient becomes restless and starts to seize. You should
   A. Open the patient's airway
   B. Insert something between the patient's teeth
   C. Insert an oral airway
   D. Protect the patient from further harm
5. After the patient stops seizing, you should
   A. Place her in the recovery position
   B. Insert an oral airway
   C. Assure that her airway is open
   D. Preserve her body temperature
6. In order to try to obtain some medical history, you should
   A. See if there are any friends or family with the patient
   B. Ask the station manager
   C. Check for a medic alert symbol
   D. All of the above
7. This patient's seizure could be caused by
   A. A stroke
   B. A diabetic emergency
   C. Epilepsy
   D. All of the above

Chapter 10

Medical Emergencies–Poisoning

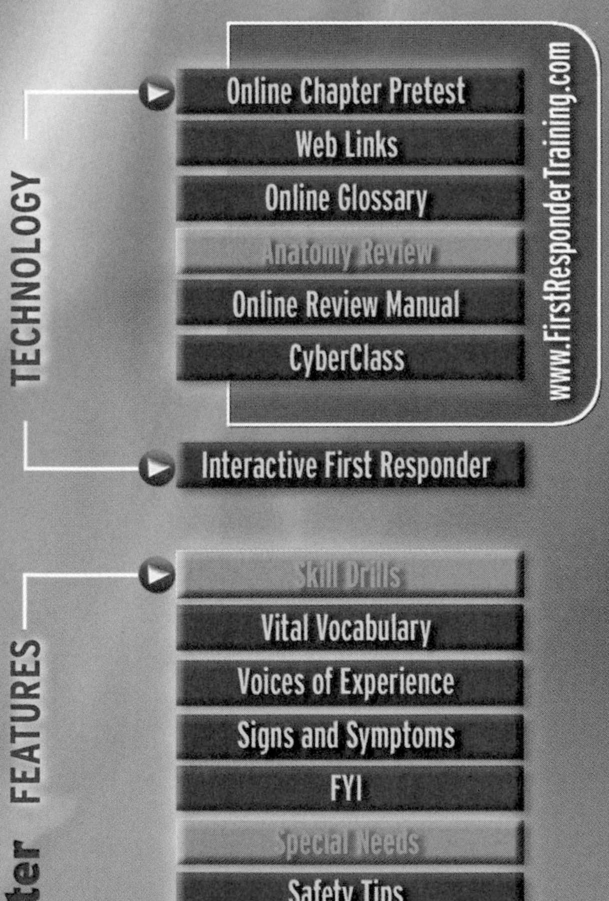

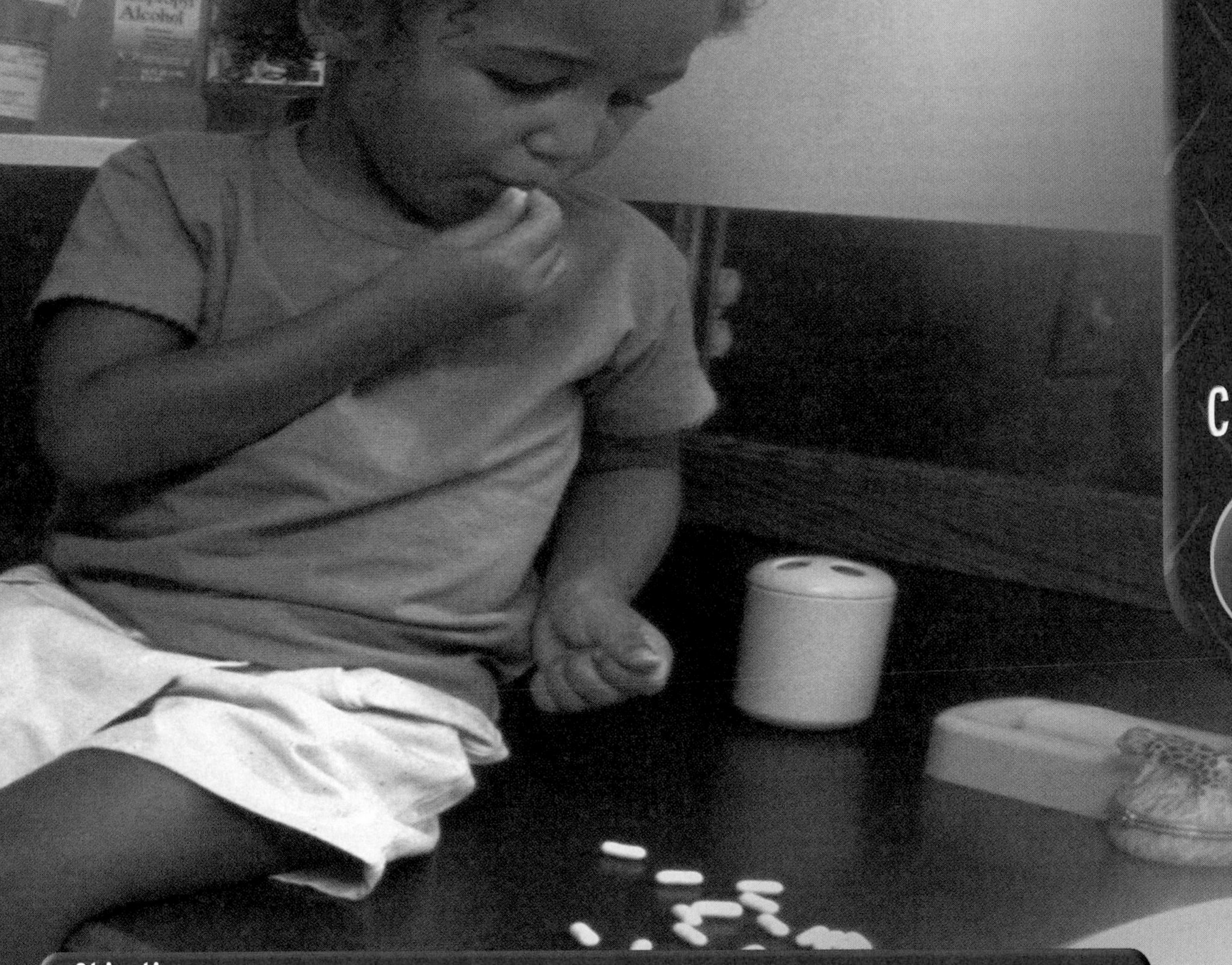

CHAPTER 10

Objectives

Knowledge and Attitude Objectives

After studying this chapter, you will be expected to:

1. Understand what a poison is.
2. Describe the signs and symptoms of ingested poisons.
3. Describe how to treat a patient who has ingested a poison.
4. Describe the signs and symptoms of inhaled poisons.
5. Describe how to treat a patient who has inhaled a poison.
6. Describe the signs and symptoms of injected poisons.
7. Describe how to treat a patient who has injected a poison.
8. Describe the signs and symptoms of absorbed poisons.
9. Describe how to treat a patient who has absorbed a poison.
10. Describe the signs and symptoms of a drug overdose caused by uppers, downers, hallucinogens, and abused inhalants.
11. Describe the general treatment for a patient who has suffered a drug overdose.

Skill Objectives

As a first responder, you should be able to:

1. Use water to flush a patient who has come in contact with liquid poison.
2. Brush a dry chemical off the patient and then flush with water.

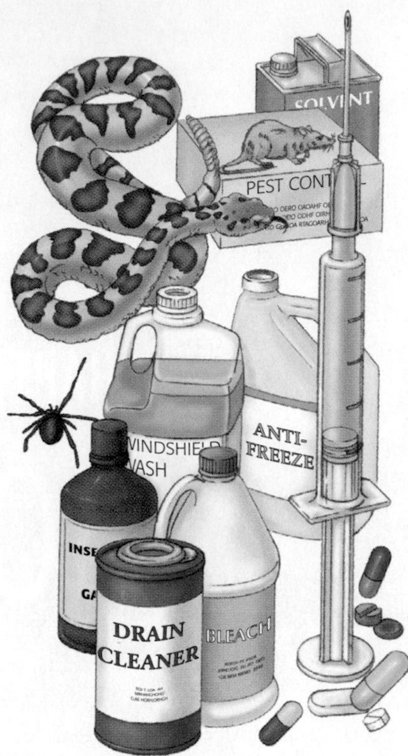

Figure 10.1 Sources of poisons.

poison Any substance that may cause injury or death if relatively small amounts are ingested, inhaled, or absorbed, or applied to, injected into, or developed within the body.

A poison is a substance that causes illness or death when eaten, drunk, inhaled, injected, or absorbed in relatively small quantities. This chapter covers signs, symptoms, emergency care, and treatment of patients suffering from accidental or intentional poisoning, bites, stings, or alcohol or substance abuse. Typical sources of poison are shown in **Figure 10.1**. *You can save a patient's life by quickly recognizing and promptly treating a serious poisoning.*

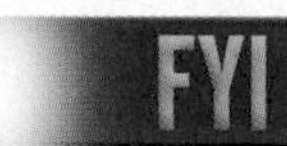

All material in this chapter is supplemental to the First Responder DOT curriculum.

General Considerations

As a first responder, you need to be a good detective when dealing with patients who have come in contact with **poisons**. Poisoning can be classified according to the way the poison enters the body.

Poisons can enter the body by four primary routes:

- ***Ingestion*** occurs when a poison enters the body through the mouth and is absorbed by the digestive system.
- ***Inhalation*** occurs when a poison enters the body through the mouth or nose and is absorbed by the mucous membranes lining the respiratory system.
- ***Injection*** occurs when a poison enters the body through a small opening in the skin and spreads through the circulatory system. Injection can occur as a result of an insect sting, a snake bite, or the intentional use of a hypodermic needle to inject a poisonous substance into the body.
- ***Absorption*** occurs when a poison enters the body through intact skin and spreads through the circulatory system.

Even though poisons can be introduced into the body by different routes, some of the effects of the poison on the body may be very similar.

In general, to assess and treat patients who have been poisoned, begin with a thorough assessment that follows the patient assessment sequence. If you suspect poisoning, obtain a thorough history from the patient or from bystanders. A good history of the incident will help guide you in your patient assessment.

Be alert for any visual clues that may indicate the patient has been in contact with a poison. These include traces of the substance on the patient's face and mouth (ingested poisons), traces of the substance on the skin (absorbed poisons), needle pricks or sting marks (injected poisons), and respiratory distress (inhaled poisons).

Much of the emergency care you give will be based on the patient's symptoms. A patient with a poisonous substance on the skin needs to have the substance removed. A patient who is showing signs of respiratory distress needs to receive respiratory support. A patient who is exhibiting signs of digestive distress needs to receive support for that problem. Sometimes the patient's signs and symptoms may be less specific, and you will have to base your treatment on general signs and symptoms. The general signs and symptoms of poisoning are shown in the box on the right.

Ingested Poisons

An ingested poison is taken by mouth. More than 80 percent of all poisoning cases are caused by ingestion. Often, there are chemical burns, odors, or stains around the mouth. The person may also be suffering from nausea, vomiting, abdominal pain, or diarrhea. Later symptoms may include abnormal or decreased respirations, unconsciousness, or seizures.

Treatment for Ingested Poisons

To treat a person who has ingested a poison:

- Identify the poison.
- Call the poison control center for instructions and follow instructions. If you are unable to contact the poison control center, dilute the poison by giving water.
- Arrange for T ***prompt transport*** to a hospital.

Before treating a person who has ingested a poison, attempt to identify the substance that has been ingested. Question the patient's family or bystanders and look for empty containers such as empty pill bottles that may indicate what the patient ate or drank.

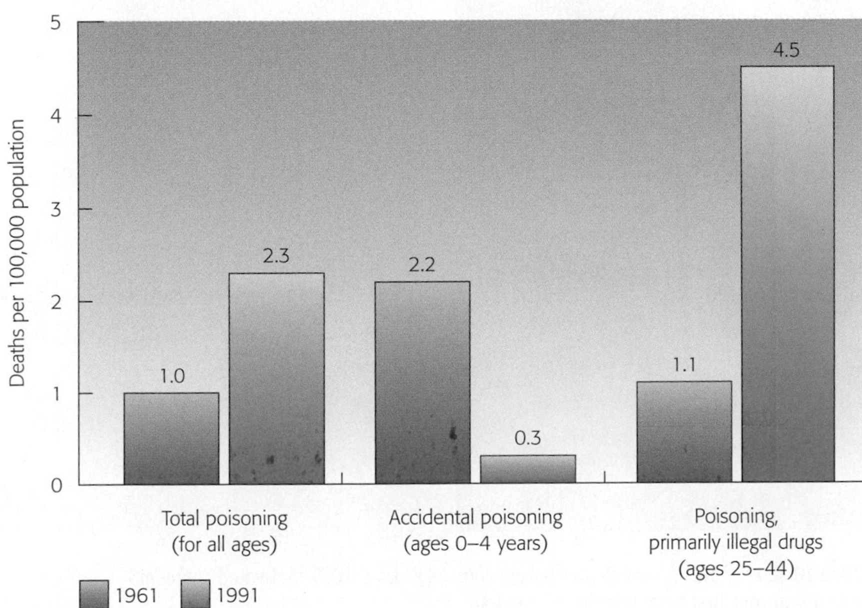

Figure 10.2 Deaths from poisoning are highest in people 25 to 44 years of age.

Safety Tips

Be especially careful when performing an overview of the scene to determine if it is safe to enter. Be alert for odors. Look for containers close to the patient. If you believe the scene is unsafe, stay a safe distance away and call for specialized assistance.

Signs & Symptoms

POISONING–GENERAL

History	History of ingesting, inhaling, injecting, or absorbing a poison
Respiratory	Difficulty breathing or decreased respirations
Digestive	Nausea and vomiting Abdominal pain Diarrhea
Central Nervous System	Unconsciousness or altered mental status Dilation or constriction of the pupils Convulsions
Other	Excess salivation Sweating Cyanosis Empty containers

Note: Accidental poisonings can occur in people of all ages. In the past, the rate of deaths from accidental poisonings was highest in children between birth and four years of age. The advent of child-proof caps and other safety containers have significantly decreased poisoning deaths among children. Today, deaths from accidental poisonings are highest in adults between 25 and 44 years of age, primarily because of the increase in the use of illegal drugs. According to the National Safety Council, a person between 25 and 44 years of age is now fifteen times more likely to die from poisoning than a child between birth and four years of age. (See **Figure 10.2**.)

Signs & Symptoms

INGESTED POISONS

- Unusual breath odors
- Discoloration or burning around the mouth
- Nausea and vomiting
- Abdominal pain
- Diarrhea
- Any of the other general signs and symptoms of poisoning shown on page 223.

If there will be a delay in transporting the patient, contact the poison control center in your community. You should have the number of your local poison control center accessible in your first responder life support kit (**Figure 10.4**). The poison control center can tell you if you should start any treatment before the patient is transported to the hospital.

Dilution

Most poisons can be diluted by giving the patient large quantities of water.

Activated Charcoal

Administering activated charcoal is another method of treating ingested poisons (**Figure 10.5**). Activated charcoal is a finely ground powder that is mixed with water to make it easier to swallow. It works by binding to the poison, thereby preventing the poison from being absorbed in the patient's digestive tract.

Activated charcoal may be used by some first responder systems to treat poisonings if the nearest medical facility is a long distance away. However, you should give activated charcoal only if you are trained in its use and have approval from your medical director or your poison control center. Do not give it if the patient has ingested an **acid** or an alkali such as liquid drain cleaner, or if the patient is unconscious. The usual dose for an adult patient is 25 to 50 grams. The usual dose for a pediatric patient is 12.5 to 25 grams. Because the mixture looks like mud, you can serve the mixture in a covered cup and give the patient a straw. This may make it easier for the patient to drink.

acid A chemical substance with a pH of less than 7.0 that can cause severe burns.

Vomiting

The third method of treating ingested poisonings is to induce vomiting. Vomiting may be induced if the person is far from a medical facility, if the poisoning occurred less than one hour before your arrival, and if the person is totally alert. You should induce vomiting in a patient only if you have been instructed to do so by your medical director or local poison control center.

THREE GENERAL TREATMENTS FOR POISONING BY INGESTION

- *Dilution using water*
- *Activated charcoal*
- *Vomiting*

Remember

Place an unconscious patient in the recovery position to help keep the airway open and to facilitate the drainage of mucus and vomitus from the mouth and nose (**Figure 10.3**).

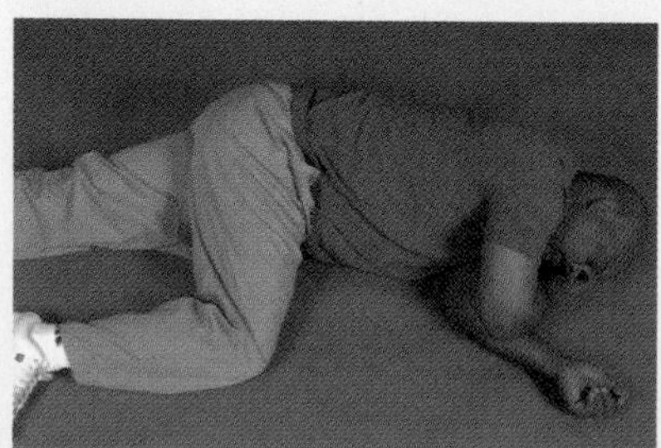

Figure 10.3 Position for an unconscious patient.

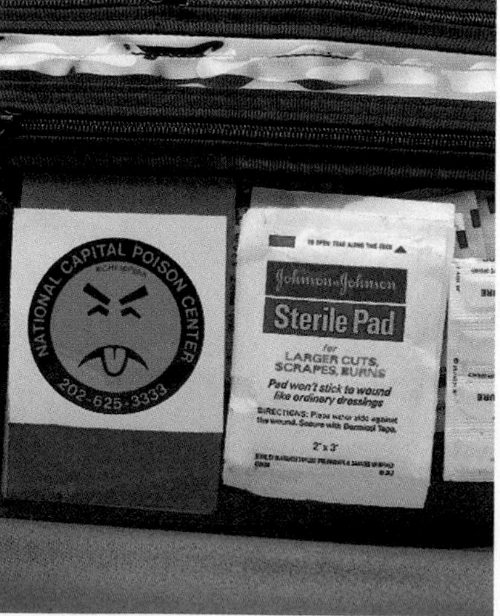

Figure 10.4 Post the number of your poison control center in your first responder life support kit.

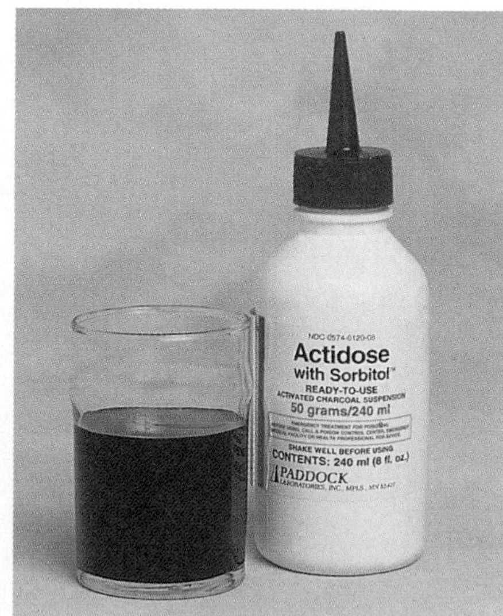

Figure 10.5 Activated charcoal.

Vomiting should not be induced if the person has ingested a strong acid, a strong alkaline substance, or an oil-based product such as gasoline or kerosene. Vomiting in these cases may cause additional chemical burns as the poison is vomited, or it may result in inhalation of vapors, which can damage the lungs.

CAUTION

Do not induce vomiting if the patient has a history of heart disease.

To induce vomiting, administer syrup of ipecac. This drug can be obtained from a pharmacy without a prescription. Give two tablespoons of syrup of ipecac to an adult, and one tablespoon to a child. Then have the patient drink as many glasses of warm water as possible.

CAUTION

You should not induce vomiting unless you have been instructed in how to use syrup of ipecac and you have received permission from your medical director or local poison control center.

Ipecac will produce vomiting in approximately 95 percent of patients within 30 minutes. Watch the patient carefully to be sure that he or she remains conscious and that the induced vomiting does not cause any respiratory problems.

Inhaled Poisons

Poisoning by inhalation occurs if a **toxic** substance is breathed in and absorbed through the lungs. Some toxic substances such as **carbon monoxide (CO)** are very poisonous but are not irritating. Carbon monoxide is an odorless, colorless, tasteless gas that cannot be detected by your normal senses. Other toxic gases such as chlorine gas and ammonia are very irritating and will cause coughing and severe respiratory distress. These gases can be classified as irritants. General signs and symptoms of inhaled poisons are shown.

Carbon Monoxide

One of the most common causes of carbon monoxide poisoning is an improperly vented heating appliance. Carbon monoxide is present in smoke. People caught in building fires often suffer carbon monoxide poisoning.

Inhaling relatively small quantities of carbon monoxide gas can result in severe poisoning because carbon monoxide combines with red blood cells about 200 times more readily than oxygen. Therefore, a small quantity of carbon monoxide can "monopolize" the red blood cells and prevent them from transporting oxygen to all parts of the body.

The signs and symptoms of carbon monoxide poisoning are shown in the box at right. Low levels of carbon monoxide poisoning have signs and symptoms that are just like the flu. If you find several

Signs & Symptoms

INHALED POISONS

- Respiratory distress
- Dizziness
- Cough
- Headache
- Hoarseness
- Confusion
- Chest pain
- Any other general signs and symptoms of poisoning listed on page 223.

toxic Poisonous.

carbon monoxide (CO) A colorless, odorless, poisonous gas formed by incomplete combustion, such as in a fire.

Signs & Symptoms

CARBON MONOXIDE POISONING

- Headache
- Nausea
- Disorientation
- Unconscious

Note: Residential carbon monoxide detectors are being installed in many homes. These detectors are designed to sound an alarm before the residents of the house show signs and symptoms of carbon monoxide poisoning. Once the residential carbon monoxide detector is activated, specially trained and equipped personnel must be summoned to investigate the source of the carbon monoxide.

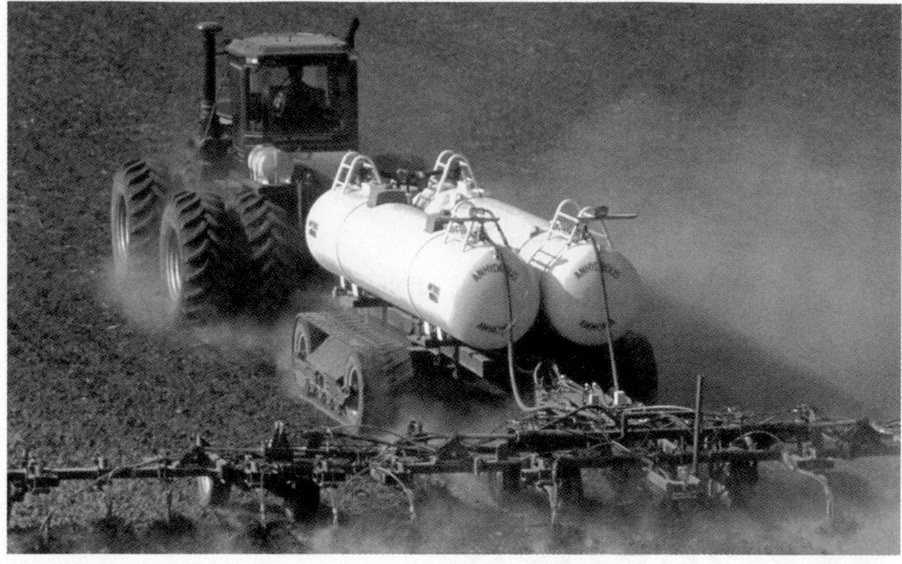

Figure 10.6 Fertilizer trucks on farms often contain ammonia.

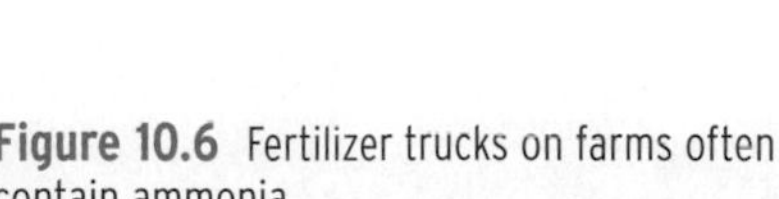

Safety Tips

Do not venture into areas where poisonous gases are present. Call an agency (such as the fire department) that is equipped with a self-contained breathing apparatus (SCBA). You should be especially aware of the hidden dangers found in farm silos, sewers, and other below-ground structures. Every year, rescuers lose their lives by venturing into a silo, sewer, or pit to save a person who may already be dead.

self-contained breathing apparatus (SCBA) A complete unit for delivery of air to a rescuer who enters a contaminated area; contains a mask, regulator, and air supply.

patients together who all have these symptoms (especially in winter), suspect carbon monoxide poisoning and remove everyone from the structure or vehicle.

Irritants

Many gases irritate the respiratory tract. Two of the more frequently encountered gases are:

1. *Ammonia*. Inhalation of ammonia usually occurs in agricultural settings where it is used as a fertilizer (**Figure 10.6**). It has a strong, irritating odor that is highly toxic. Inhaling large amounts of ammonia gas deadens the sense of smell and severely irritates the lungs and upper respiratory tract, causing violent coughing. Ammonia can also severely burn the skin. Anyone who enters an environment containing ammonia must wear a proper encapsulating suit with a **self-contained breathing apparatus (SCBA)** (**Figure 10.7**).

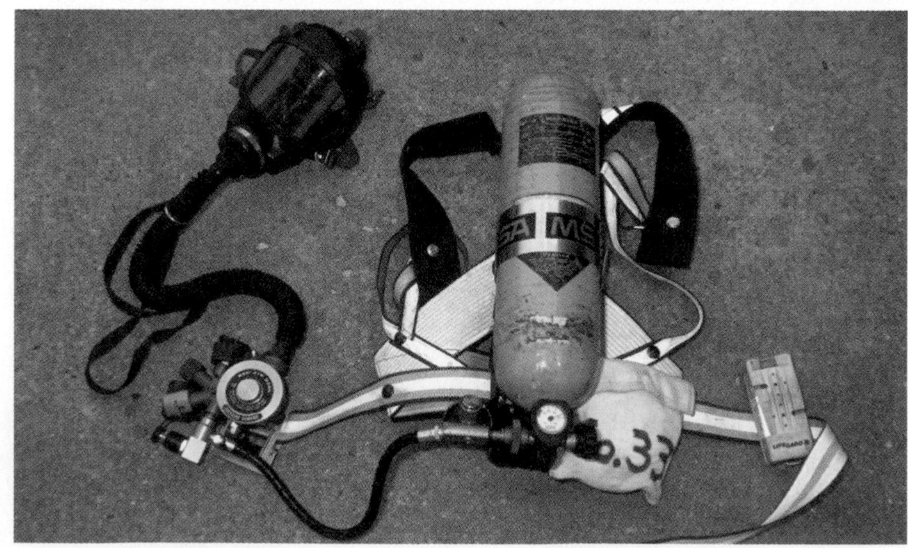

Figure 10.7 Self-contained breathing apparatus (SCBA).

2. *Chlorine*. Chlorine gas is commonly found in large quantities around swimming pools and water treatment plants. The odor of chlorine is familiar to anyone who has used chlorine bleach or been in a swimming pool or hot tub. Chlorine can severely irritate the lungs and the upper respiratory tract, causing violent coughing (**Figure 10.8**). Chlorine gas can also cause skin burns. Anyone who enters an environment containing chlorine must wear a proper encapsulating suit with an SCBA.

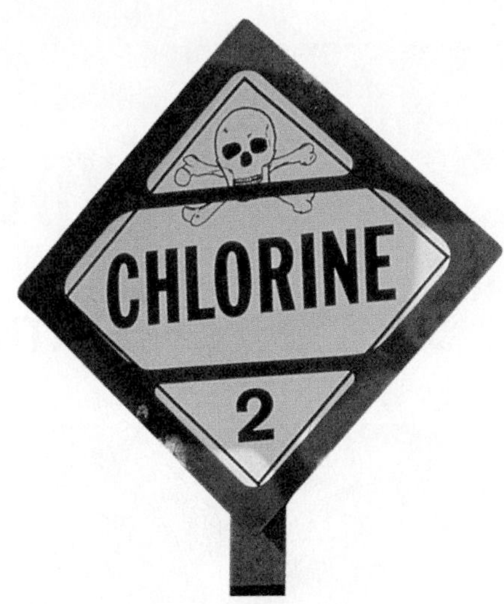

Figure 10.8 Placard used to identify the presence of chlorine.

Treatment for Inhaled Poisons

The first step in treating a patient who has inhaled any poison gas is to remove him or her from the source of the gas. If the patient is not breathing, begin mouth-to-mask breathing. If the patient is breathing, administer large quantities of oxygen (if available). Any patient who has inhaled a poisonous gas should be T ***transported promptly*** to a medical facility for further examination because there may be a delayed reaction to the poison.

In some situations, your first response is to evacuate people. If you are called to the scene of a large poison gas leak (or other hazardous material leak), you may have to evacuate large numbers of people to prevent further injuries. Once this has been done, begin to treat the evacuees as necessary.

○ How would you treat a patient who has inhaled carbon monoxide?

Injected Poisons

The two major causes of poisoning by injection are animal bites and stings and toxic injection. This section covers animal bites and stings; toxic injection will be discussed later, as part of substance abuse. The signs and symptoms of poisonous stings and bites are shown in the right column.

If a person has received a large amount of poison (for example, multiple bee stings) or if a person is especially sensitive to this poison (has an anaphylactic reaction), he or she may collapse and become unconscious.

Treatment for Insect Stings and Bites

A person who has been bitten or stung by an insect should be kept quiet and still. This will help slow the spread of the poison throughout the body. A light constricting band (NOT a tourniquet) may be used if there is severe swelling. Apply the band between the sting or bite and the patient's heart. It should be snug, but not so snug that it cuts off circulation. (Check for a distal pulse after application.) Ice packs may help reduce local swelling and pain.

Signs & Symptoms

INJECTED POISONS (BITES OR STINGS)

- Obvious injury site (bite or sting marks)
- Tenderness
- Swelling
- Red streaks radiating from injection site
- Weakness
- Dizziness
- Localized pain
- Itching
- Any other general signs and symptoms of poisoning listed on page 223.

Voices of Experience

Scene Assessment Critical in Geriatric Poisonings

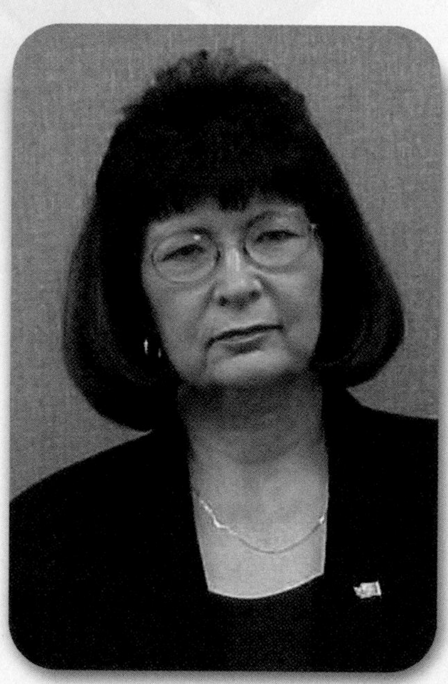

I have a background in Emergency Department nursing and now am the Director of the Department of EMS for a rural county that is a wonderful area for persons to retire. There is a large geriatric population for which we provide care.

As the age of the population increases, we respond to increased number of accidental "poisonings" of elderly patients. This sometimes results from an individual failing to inform the physician that they are seeing another physician and are already taking medication. They may also "doctor shop;" since they may not feel that one physician is helping them, they go to another, which can increase the likelihood of medication being misprescribed or overprescribed. Many of these events are indeed accidental, as the patient may not or cannot remember if they have taken their prescribed medications. They may not take them at all, or may take another dose, thereby creating a medical event that often requires intervention.

"...the patient's environment...will produce the most clues to the possible reasons for the symptoms presented."

First responders are the most important link in the care of this kind of patient. The first responder will find the patient's environment at a time when it will produce the most clues to possible reasons for the symptoms presented. Take a look around—often the major clues will be right in front of you. Are there medication containers on the counter, in the bathroom, at the bedside? These include prescribed and over-the-counter medications. Are there pills on the floor that may have been dropped? Look at the date of refill and the number of tablets left in the container. Gather all medications found and take them with the patient.

As first responders, it is important to assess the patient—the primary concern. However, it takes just a minute to assess the scene and that assessment may be as important as the patient care. ❖

Nina Conn, RN, BS Health Care Administration
EMS Director
Walla Walla County
Walla Walla, WA

Some people suffer an extreme allergic reaction to stings and bites and may go into **anaphylactic shock** (See Chapter 12). The signs and symptoms of anaphylactic shock are shown on the right. The patient's blood pressure drops, and the patient may even suffer cardiac arrest.

Elevating the patient's legs (shock treatment) may help in some cases. If the patient's condition progresses to the point of respiratory or cardiac arrest, begin mouth-to-mask breathing or CPR.

If a patient appears to be going into anaphylactic shock, immediately arrange for T ***rapid transport*** to a medical facility where the patient can receive treatment with specific medications. Medication may also be started by a paramedic who is working under the direction of a physician.

Signs & Symptoms

ANAPHYLACTIC SHOCK

- Itching all over the body
- Hives, swelling
- Generalized weakness
- Unconsciousness
- Rapid, weak pulse
- Rapid, shallow breathing

anaphylactic shock Severe shock caused by an allergic reaction to food, medicine, or insect stings.

hives An allergic skin disorder marked by patches of swelling, redness, and intense itching.

Snakebite

There are four kinds of poisonous snakes in the United States: rattlesnake, cottonmouth, copperhead, and coral snake. The snake injects its poison into the skin and muscles with its fangs. This poison can cause local injury to the skin and muscle and may even involve the entire extremity. Signs and symptoms may affect the entire body. A bite from a poisonous snake is rarely fatal; although nearly 7,000 people are bitten by snakes each year in the United States, fewer than 20 will die from the bite. However, permanent injury can sometimes result.

The bite of the coral snake delivers a slightly different poison that may cause these additional problems:

- Respiratory difficulties
- Slurred speech
- Paralysis
- Coma
- Seizures

Treatment for Snakebite

The field treatment for snakebite is basically the same as the treatment for shock. (See Chapter 12.) Keep the patient quiet; have the patient lie down and try to relax. Wash any venom off the patient's skin with soap and water.

Depending on your local protocols or medical control directions, you could apply a light constricting band to the extremity above the bite site if less than thirty minutes have passed since the bite occurred. Use a band from your first responder life support kit, or improvise one with a shoelace or rubber glove. Do not use a rubber band! It will probably be too tight. The band should be snug but not tight enough to stop the flow of blood. You should be able to slip your finger under the band. Treat the patient carefully and arrange for T ***prompt transport*** to the hospital or medical facility. The only effective treatment for poisonous snakebites is the administration of antivenin in the hospital.

Signs & Symptoms

SNAKEBITES

- Immediate pain at the bite site
- Swelling and tenderness around the bite site
- Fainting (from the emotional shock of the bite)
- Sweating
- Nausea and vomiting
- Shock

Signs & Symptoms

ABSORBED POISONS

- Traces of powder or liquid on the skin
- Inflammation or redness of the skin
- Chemical burns
- Skin rash
- Burning
- Itching
- Nausea and vomiting
- Dizziness
- Shock
- Any other general signs and symptoms of poisoning listed on page 223.

Note: When in doubt in absorbed-poison situations, have the patient remove all clothing so that he or she is no longer in contact with the toxic substance.

Note: A person who appears intoxicated may be suffering instead from any one of a number of serious illnesses or injuries. Insulin shock, diabetic **coma**, head injury, traumatic shock, and drug reactions may all display the same symptoms as alcohol intoxication.

coma A state of unconsciousness from which the patient cannot be aroused.

alcohol A liquid obtained by fermentation of carbohydrates with yeast.

Absorbed Poisons

Poisoning by absorption occurs when a poisonous substance enters the body through the skin. Insecticides and toxic industrial chemicals are two common poisons absorbed through the skin. A person suffering from absorption poisoning may have both localized and systemic signs and symptoms, as shown in the box on the left.

Treatment for Absorbed Poisons

The first step in treating a patient who has absorbed a poisonous substance is to ensure that the patient is no longer in contact with the toxic substance. You may have to ask the patient to remove all clothing. Then brush—do not wash—any dry chemical off the patient. Contact with water may activate the dry chemical and result in a burning or caustic reaction.

After removing all the dry chemical, wash the patient completely for at least 20 minutes. Use any water source that is available: an industrial shower, a home shower, a garden hose, or even a fire engine's booster hose. Do not forget to wash out the patient's eyes if they have been in contact with the poison. If additional EMS personnel are delayed, contact the poison control center or your medical director for additional treatment information.

If the patient is suffering from shock, have the patient lie down and elevate the legs. If the patient is having difficulty breathing, administer oxygen if it is available and you are trained to use it.

Substance Abuse

Alcohol

Alcohol is the most commonly abused drug in our society. Alcohol intoxication may be seen in people of any age, including children and teenagers. Alcohol usage is involved in more than one half of all traffic fatalities, more than one half of all murders, and more than one third of all suicides. Deaths as a result of alcohol abuse are two and one half times as numerous as deaths from motor vehicle crashes. But because the symptoms of alcohol intoxication are similar to those of other medical illnesses or severe injuries, you should never assume that an apparently intoxicated person is "just another drunk."

In addition, people who have been drinking can be injured or suddenly develop a serious illness. You cannot assume that the symptoms (including the smell of alcohol on someone's breath) are caused by drunkenness. If you are unsure about whether a patient who appears to be intoxicated has a serious injury or illness, be extra careful with your examination. You should arrange for T ***prompt transport*** to an appropriate medical facility, where a physician can make a complete assessment.

Alcohol is an addictive, depressant drug. A person who is physically dependent on alcohol and then is suddenly deprived of it may develop withdrawal symptoms, such as convulsions or seizures. The most severe withdrawal symptoms are called **delirium tremens (DTs)**. The signs and symptoms of DTs include shaking, restlessness, confusion, hallucinations, gastrointestinal distress, chest pain, and fever. These signs and symptoms usually appear three to four days after the person stops drinking. **T** ***Transport*** a person suffering from DTs to an appropriate medical facility. DTs are a serious medical emergency and can be fatal.

Drugs

In today's society, people of all ages abuse many different prescription and street drugs. Drugs may be ingested, inhaled, or injected into the body. As a first responder, you may not be able to identify the type of drug used, although this information will be helpful to medical providers. When you do your scene assessment, look for clues that can indicate what type of drug was used and how it was administered. Today, the most popular drugs fall into four categories: **uppers**, downers, hallucinogens, and inhalants (**Figure 10.9**).

Uppers

Uppers are drugs that stimulate the **central nervous system (CNS)**. They include **amphetamines** (speed, ice, or crystal) and **cocaine** (coke). People using these substances show signs of restlessness, irritability, and talkativeness. They may need to be kept from harming themselves and should be taken to a facility where they can be monitored until the effects of the drug wear off.

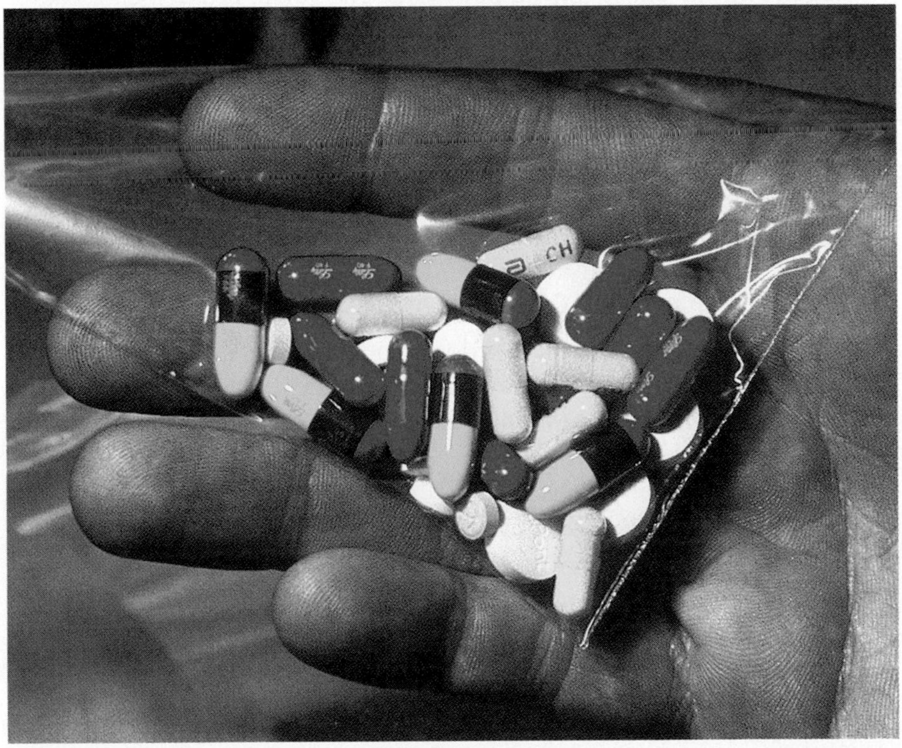

Figure 10.9 Types of drugs that are commonly abused.

delirium tremens (DTs) A severe, often fatal, complication of alcohol withdrawal that can occur from one to seven days after withdrawal. It is characterized by restlessness, fever, sweating, confusion, disorientation, agitation, hallucinations, and convulsions.

uppers Drugs that stimulate the central nervous system. These include amphetamines and cocaine.

central nervous system (CNS) The brain and spinal cord.

amphetamines Stimulants that produce a general mood elevation, improve task performance, suppress appetite, or prevent sleepiness.

cocaine A powerful stimulant that induces an extreme state of euphoria. Legitimately, it is a potent local anesthetic. On the street, it is commonly known as "coke." Synthetic cocaine is known as "crack."

downners Depressants; barbiturates.

barbiturates Drugs that depress the nervous system; they can alter the state of consciousness so that the individual may appear drowsy or peaceful.

hallucinogens Chemicals that cause a person to see visions or hear sounds that are not real.

Downers

Like alcohol, **downers** are depressants. Downers include **barbiturates**, tranquilizers, opiates, and marijuana. An overdose of one of these drugs can result in respiratory depression or arrest. A person who has overdosed on downers may be breathing shallowly or not at all. If the person is not breathing, begin mouth-to-mask resuscitation. If cardiac arrest occurs, begin CPR immediately.

Hallucinogens

Hallucinogens include PCP, LSD, peyote, mescaline, and some types of mushrooms. Hallucinogens cause people to see things that are not there. A patient who is hallucinating may become frightened and unable to distinguish between reality and fantasy.

One hallucinogen, PCP, also blocks the body's pain receptors. People on PCP may feel no pain and may seriously injure themselves or others. Large doses of PCP can produce convulsions, coma, heart and lung failure, or stroke.

Abused Inhalants

Recently the intentional inhaling of volatile chemicals has increased, especially among teenagers who are seeking an alcohol-like high. Many of these substances can be bought in hardware stores and include gasoline, paint thinners, cleaning compounds, lacquers, and a wide variety of substances used as aerosol propellants. Users put the chemical in a plastic bag, and inhale from the bag. The combination of a lack of oxygen and the effects of the poisonous substance inhaled can lead to unconsciousness. Some abused inhalants cause drowsiness or unresponsiveness. Some cause seizures. Others overstimulate the heart and produce sudden cardiac death from ventricular fibrillation.

Treat these patients carefully. Try to keep them from struggling. Support their airway, breathing, and circulation. Give high-flow oxygen as soon as it is available. Carefully monitor their vital signs and arrange for T ***prompt transport*** to an appropriate medical facility.

Treatment for a Drug Overdose

As a first responder to a drug overdose, you can provide basic life support (clear the airway and perform mouth-to-mask breathing or CPR) and arrange for T ***prompt transport*** to an appropriate medical facility.

Once you have determined that a patient is suffering from a drug overdose, your job is to:

- Provide basic life support (clear the airway and perform mouth-to-mask breathing or CPR, as necessary).
- Keep the patient from hurting himself or herself and others.
- Provide reassurance and psychological support.
- Arrange for T ***prompt transport*** to a medical facility for treatment.

The effects of some drugs can only be counteracted by other drugs administered by a paramedic or a physician. If a patient is acting out, speak to him or her in a calm, reassuring tone of voice and try to keep the patient from harming anyone.

If a person reports seeing things that are not there, say, "I believe you are seeing those things; however, I do not see them myself." This statement lets the patient know that you understand his or her experience, but that in reality, the perceived object is not present.

Patients who are suffering adverse reactions from drug overdose require specialized treatment. You and other EMS personnel should be aware of local facilities equipped to deal with such cases. Keep in mind that a person suffering from a drug overdose may also have other injuries or medical conditions that require medical treatment. Try to avoid classifying the patient as "just another overdose."

Toxic Injection from Drugs

Drugs that are injected into the bloodstream can result in toxic injection. The patient's reaction depends on the quantity and type of drug injected. Because street drugs may be diluted, or "cut," with sugar or other substances that should not be injected into the bloodstream, the patient may be unaware of exactly what has been injected. After a toxic injection, the patient may complain of weakness, dizziness, fever, or chills. This type of emergency requires you to support the patient, treat the symptoms, and provide T ***transport*** to an appropriate medical facility.

You should also check the injection site for redness, swelling, and increased skin temperature. The presence of any of these signs may indicate an infection that will require medical care.

Intentional Poisoning

Intentional self-poisoning is attempted suicide, and may involve ingested poisons (or drugs) or inhaled poisons (such as carbon monoxide). Regardless of whether the poisoning was accidental or intentional, medical treatment is the same.

A patient who has attempted suicide needs both medical and psychological support. The patient may not want your help and may be difficult to treat. Nevertheless you and all other EMS personnel must make every effort to preserve life and offer reassurance.

BSI Tip

People who use intravenous drugs have a high incidence of blood-borne diseases such as hepatitis B and AIDS. Use body substance isolation (BSI) techniques to reduce your chances of coming in contact with blood-borne pathogens.

10 Prep Kit

Ready for Review

Ready for Review thoroughly summarizes the chapter.

This chapter discusses common poisoning problems that you will encounter as a first responder. Poisons may be ingested, inhaled, injected, or absorbed. Alcohol abuse, drug overdose, and attempted suicide are also discussed. Although you will not always be able to identify the poisonous substance, you can treat the patient's symptoms. As you approach the scene of a poisoning, follow the patient assessment steps you learned in Chapter 7. Pay special attention to scene safety and do not enter a hazardous environment without the proper training and equipment.

Vital Vocabulary

The Vital Vocabulary are the key terms for this chapter.

acid—*page 224*
alcohol—*page 230*
amphetamines—*page 231*
anaphylactic shock—*page 229*
barbiturates—*page 232*
carbon monoxide (CO)—*page 225*
central nervous system (CNS)—*page 231*
cocaine—*page 231*
coma—*page 230*
delirium tremens (DTs)—*page 231*
downers—*page 232*
hallucinogens—*page 232*
hives—*page 229*
poison—*page 222*
self-contained breathing apparatus (SCBA)—*page 226*
toxic—*page 225*
uppers—*page 231*

Practice Points

The Practice Points are the key skills you need to know.

1. How to use water to flush a patient who has come in contact with liquid poison.
2. How to brush a dry chemical off a patient and then flush with water.

Ready to Respond

Ready to Respond presents a fictitious scenario to help you review what you learned in this chapter.

As part of your training, you are an observer at your local poison control center. You are listening to the calls over a speaker phone. The first call comes from a mother who is home with three children ages 7, 5, and 4. She says that her children all seem to have the flu. They are complaining of headaches and feeling sick, and two of the children have vomited. She pressed the wrong button on her speed dial; she meant to call the children's doctor.

1. You should

A. Tell her to hang up and call her doctor.

B. Tell her to call the emergency department

C. Tell her she has the wrong number

D. Tell her to get her children out of the house and call EMS

2. The second call comes from a man who says he has been stung by a yellow jacket. In dealing with this patient you would be most concerned about

A. Infection

B. Swelling

C. Heart attack

D. Anaphylactic shock

3. The third call is from a mother who says her 2-year-old child has swallowed several of her birth control pills. You think that the poison control center might recommend all but which of the following?

A. Drinking lots of water

B. Taking activated charcoal

C. Doing nothing

D. Taking syrup of ipecac

4. The last call is from a teenager who says her boyfriend has intentionally inhaled fumes from a plastic bag that contained gasoline. Which of the following symptoms would you not expect from this?

A. Unconsciousness

B. Cardiac arrest

C. Respiratory arrest

D. Unequal pupils

5. In looking over the records of the cases of poisoning for the last two years, which age group would you expect to have the highest incidence of poisoning?

A. 0 to 4 years old

B. 4 to 8 years old

C. 12 to 18 years old

D. 25 to 44 years old

Chapter 11

Behavioral Emergencies–Crisis Intervention

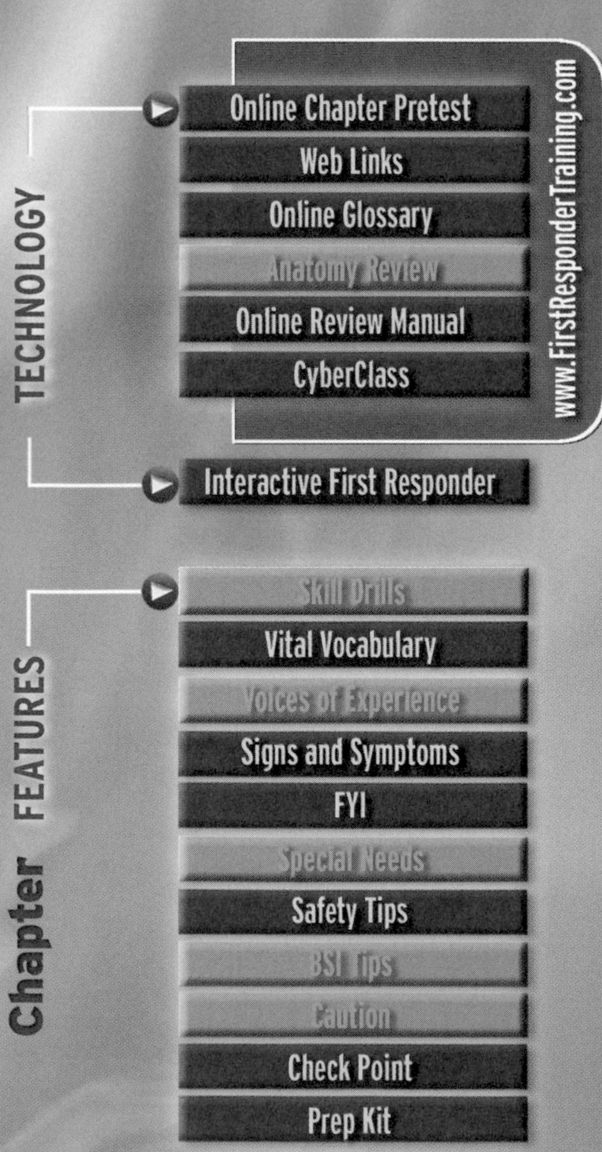

CHAPTER 11

Objectives

Knowledge and Attitude Objectives

After studying this chapter, you will be expected to:

1. Identify patients experiencing signs of a behavioral crisis.
2. List the five factors that may cause behavioral emergencies.
3. Describe the phases of a situational crisis.
4. Explain the role of a first responder in dealing with a patient experiencing a behavioral emergency.
5. Describe the principles for assessing behavioral emergency patients.
6. Explain the following communication skills:
   A. Restatement
   B. Redirection
   C. Empathy
7. Describe the method for assessing potentially violent patients.
8. Describe the method for dealing with domestic violence situations.
9. Describe the safety precautions that should be taken when dealing with a potentially violent patient.
10. Describe the first responder's role in dealing with an armed patient.
11. Explain the medical/legal considerations related to dealing with behavioral emergencies.
12. Describe the approaches to be used when dealing with:
    A. Suicide crisis
    B. Sexual assault
    C. Death and dying
13. Explain the purpose of critical incident stress debriefing.

Skill Objectives

As a first responder, you should be able to:

1. Master the following communication techniques:
   A. Restatement
   B. Redirection
   C. Empathy
2. Calm a patient experiencing a behavioral crisis.

Every emergency situation, whether it is an illness or an injury, has emotional and psychological effects on everyone involved—you, the patient, the patient's family and friends, and even bystanders. As a first responder to a behavioral emergency, you will need to give psychological support as well as necessary emergency medical care. This chapter explains the five major factors that cause behavioral crises.

The simple intervention techniques addressed in this chapter will help prepare you to deal with patients and their families during the stressful experience of a medical emergency. You will also be better able to identify and understand the reactions to the grief that you observe.

Many patients experience high anxiety, denial, anger, remorse, and grief during a situational crisis. Three skills that are useful when communicating with patients in crisis are restatement, redirection, and empathy. This chapter also provides information on how to deal with crowd control, domestic violence, violent patients, armed patients, suicide crisis, sexual assault, and death and dying. Medical/legal considerations and the role of critical incident stress debriefings are also covered.

Behavioral Crises

As a first responder, you will encounter situations where patients exhibit abnormal behavior. Sometimes this abnormal behavior is the primary reason that you were called, and sometimes it is a secondary reaction to another situation such as an accident or illness. **Behavioral emergencies** are defined as situations in which a person exhibits abnormal, unacceptable behavior that cannot be tolerated by the patients themselves or by family, friends, or the community. Some behavioral emergencies involve your patient and others involve the patient's family or friends.

behavioral emergencies Situations where a person exhibits abnormal behavior that is unacceptable or cannot be tolerated by the patients themselves or by family, friends, or the community.

psychotic behavior Mental disturbance characterized by defective or lost contact with reality.

Five main factors contribute to behavioral changes:

1. ***Medical conditions*** such as uncontrolled diabetes that causes low blood sugar, respiratory conditions that prevent the patient's brain from receiving enough oxygen, high fevers, and excess cold.
2. ***Physical trauma*** conditions such as head injuries and injuries that result in shock and an inadequate blood supply to the brain.
3. ***Psychiatric illnesses*** such as depression, panic, or **psychotic behavior**.
4. ***Mind-altering*** substances such as alcohol and a wide variety of chemical substances.
5. ***Situational stresses*** from a wide variety of emotional trauma such as death or serious injury to a loved one.

To better understand a behavioral crisis, you need to look at the stages a person passes through when experiencing a situational crisis.

What Is a Situational Crisis?

Simply put, a **situational crisis** is a state of emotional upset or turmoil. It is caused by a sudden and disruptive event such as a physical illness, a traumatic injury, or the death of a loved one. Every emergency creates some form of situational crisis for the patient and those persons close to the patient. You will often encounter this type of crisis as a first responder. Some of the concepts covered here are similar to the concepts covered in Chapter 2.

Most situational crises are sudden and unexpected (such as an automobile crash), cannot be handled by the person's usual coping mechanisms, last only a short time, and can cause socially unacceptable, self-destructive, or dangerous behavior.

situational crisis A state of emotional upset or turmoil caused by a sudden and disruptive event.

emotional shock A state of shock caused by sudden illness, accident, or death of a loved one.

Phases of a Situational Crisis

There are four emotional phases to each situational crisis. Although a person may not experience every phase during a crisis, he or she will certainly experience one or more. If you understand what these phases are and why they occur, you can better understand how to help people who are experiencing an emotional crisis.

EMOTIONAL PHASES OF A SITUATIONAL CRISIS

- *High anxiety or emotional shock*
- *Denial*
- *Anger*
- *Remorse and grief*

High Anxiety or Emotional Shock

In the first phase of a situational crisis, a person exhibits high anxiety or **emotional shock**. High anxiety is characterized by rather obvious signs and symptoms: flushed (red) face, rapid breathing, rapid speech, increased activity, loud or screaming voice, and general agitation. Emotional shock is often the result of sudden illness, accident, or sudden death of a loved one. Like most other types of shock, emotional shock is characterized by cool, clammy skin; a rapid, weak pulse; vomiting and nausea; and general inactivity and weakness.

Denial

The next phase of a situational crisis may be denial—refusal to accept the fact that an event has occurred. For example, a child who has just lost a parent may refuse to accept the death by telling everyone that the parent is sleeping or has gone away.

Allow the patient to express denial. Do not argue with the patient, but try to understand the emotional and psychological trauma that he or she is experiencing.

Anger

Anger is a normal human response to emotional overload or frustration. Anger may follow denial or, in some cases, may occur instead of denial. For example, the spouse of a patient may, for no apparent reason, begin screaming at you, calling you incompetent, or using foul language or racial slurs. Although it may be difficult, you should remain calm and not respond angrily as well.

Remember

Virtually every emergency call requires some degree of psychological intervention.

In crisis situations, it is often easier to vent angry feelings on an unknown person (the first responder) or an authority figure (a law enforcement officer) than on a friend or family member. Anger is perhaps the most difficult emotion to deal with objectively because the angry person seems to be directing their anger at you. Do not take the person's anger personally, but acknowledge that it is a reaction to stress.

Frustration and a sense of helplessness can often build to anger. If these emotions are not released, the anger may be expressed by aggressive physical behavior. For example, in a serious crash involving a school bus, you may have to demonstrate to bystanders that you and other rescue personnel are indeed removing children. If little activity is apparent to the bystanders, they may become angry, hostile, and even violent. In such situations, show confidence. Demonstrate that you are making progress. Be professional and do not react to anger by becoming angry yourself. If necessary, a member of the EMS team may have to explain the situation—what is being done and why it appears to be taking so long. Acknowledge anger by saying something like, "What's the matter? Can you tell me what I can do to help?" Then allow the person to express his or her anger.

Remorse or Grief

An acceptance of the situation may lead to remorse or grief. People may feel guilty or apologetic about their behavior or actions during an incident. They may also express grief about the incident itself.

Checkpoint

- ◯ List and explain the types of behavior you would expect to encounter from a patient experiencing each phase of a situational crisis.

Crisis Management

As a first responder, you should consider how you can deal with the patient's emotional concerns or crises. You need to approach patients who are experiencing behavioral or situational crises using the same general framework for patient assessment that applies to other types of patients. In this section, you will learn about some additional skills that you can use for patients who are exhibiting behavioral crises or emotional stress.

CRISIS INTERVENTION TIPS

- *Remain calm.*
- *Reassure the patient.*
- *Take your time.*
- *Use eye contact.*
- *Touch the patient.*
- *Talk in a calm, steady voice.*
- *Demonstrate confidence.*
- *Do not take the patient's comments personally.*
- *Keep your sense of humor*

Role of the First Responder

As a first responder, your approach to a patient who may be exhibiting abnormal behavior is to follow the steps of your patient assessment sequence:

1. Perform a scene size-up.
2. Perform an initial patient assessment.
3. Examine the patient from head to toe—first responder physical examination.
4. Obtain the patient's medical history (SAMPLE).
5. Perform on-going assessment.

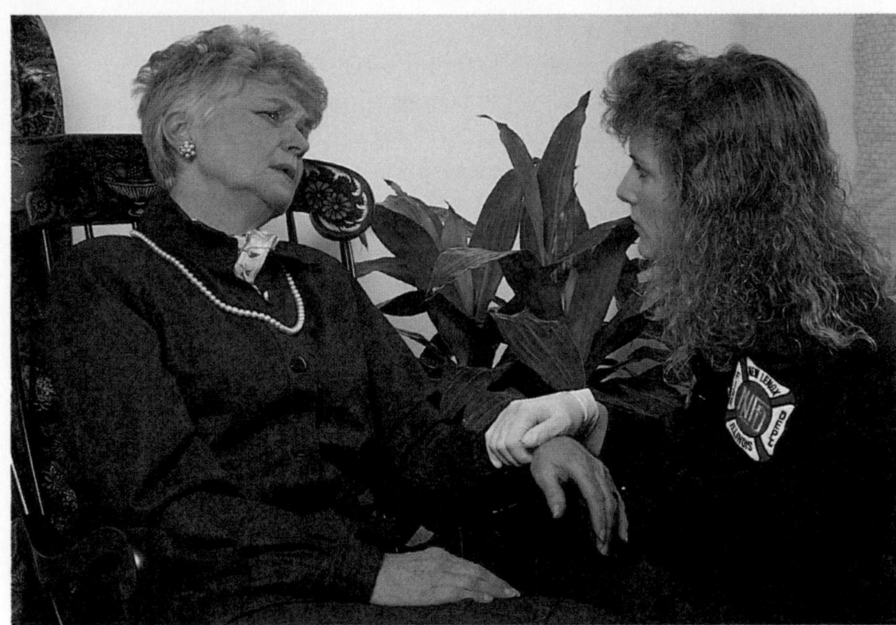

Figure 11.1 Crouch or seat yourself at the same level as the patient.

After you have completed the initial patient assessment, you may need to perform a physical examination or obtain the patient's medical history, depending on the needs of that individual patient. As you perform these steps, it is important that you remain calm and reassuring to the patient.

Your most important assessment skill may be your ability to communicate with the patient. Your communication skills will help you obtain needed information from the patient as you calm and reassure the patient.

Note: Body language is very important.

Communicating with the Patient

The first and most important step in crisis management is to talk with the person. Talking lets the person know that someone cares. When communicating with the patient, be honest, warm, caring, and empathetic.

When you begin talking with the patient, your body language is as important as your words. Try to position yourself so you are at the patient's eye level (**Figure 11.1**). If the person is lying down, kneel beside him or her. If the person is sitting, move down to his or her level. Do not stand above the person with your hands on your hips. This is a threatening position and communicates an uncaring attitude and indifference to the patient's problem (**Figure 11.2**).

Establish eye contact. This assures the person that you are, indeed, interested in helping. Use a calm, steady voice when you talk to the person and provide honest reassurance. Avoid making false statements or giving false assurances. The patient does not want to be told that everything is all right when it obviously is not.

Try not to let negative personal feelings about the person or about the person's behavior interfere with your attempt to assist. Your function is to help the person deal with the events that caused the crisis. You should remain neutral and avoid taking sides in any situation or argument.

Sometimes a simple act, such as offering a tissue or a warm blanket, defuses the person's immediate crisis reaction. Simple acts of kindness can comfort and reassure the person that you are there to help.

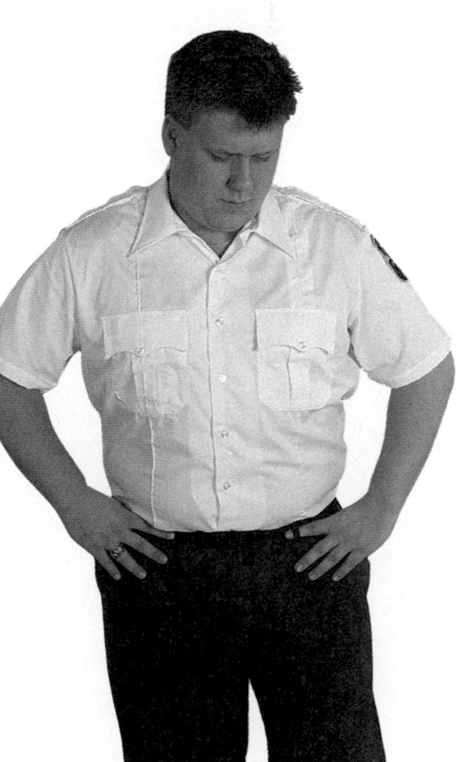

Figure 11.2 This body language communicates an uncaring attitude.

restatement Rephrasing a patient's own statement to show that he or she is being heard and understood by the rescuer.

redirection A means of focusing the patient's attention on the immediate situation or crisis.

empathy The ability to participate in another person's feelings or ideas.

Restatement

To show the person that you understand what he or she is saying, you can use a technique known as **restatement**. This means rephrasing a person's own words and thoughts and repeating them back to the person. Here is one example of restatement:

Patient with broken arm: "I can't take any more of this pain!"

First responder: "The pain seems unbearable to you now, but it will ease up when we finish applying this splint."

It is not usually helpful simply to say, "I know what you mean," or "I know how you feel." You do not know exactly how the patient is feeling, even though you may have been through a similar experience. Be honest and give the patient hope, but do not give false hope.

Redirection

Sometimes, a patient may be embarrassed about being the center of attention, or may be concerned about others involved in the situation. **Redirection** helps focus a patient's attention on the immediate situation or crisis. This is an attempt to alleviate the patient's expressed concerns and draw his or her attention back to the immediate situation. An example of redirection follows:

Patient involved in a motor vehicle crash: "Oh my God! Where are my children? What's wrong with my children?"

First responder: "Your children are being taken care of by my partner; they are in good hands. Now, we must take care of you."

If the patient is in a public place such as on a sidewalk or in the lobby of a building, move the patient to a location that is quieter and more private, if the injury or illness permits.

Empathy

The ability to empathize involves imagining yourself in another person's situation, sharing their feelings or ideas. **Empathy** helps you understand the emotional or psychological trauma the patient is experiencing. Ask yourself, "How would I feel if I were lying on the sidewalk with my clothes all torn and bloody, and strangers looking down at me?" Empathy is one of the most helpful concepts you can use in dealing with patients in crisis situations.

By using these communication skills, you will be able to deal more effectively with the patient's problems. Practice these skills with another person until you are able to use them comfortably. Some principles you can use when assessing patients with a behavioral problem are listed below.

1. Identify yourself and let the patient know you are there to help.
2. Inform the patient of what you are doing.
3. Ask questions in a calm, reassuring voice.
4. Allow the patient to tell what happened. Do not be judgmental.
5. Show you are listening by using restatement and redirection.
6. Acknowledge the patient's feelings.
7. Assess the patient's mental status:
   a. Appearance
   b. Activity
   c. Speech
   d. Orientation to person, place, and time

Checkpoint

- Explain how the use of restatement, redirection, and empathy can improve your communication with a patient.

Crowd Control

FYI

Simple crowd control may help reduce a patient's anxiety when there are too many people around. Encourage bystanders to leave. Sometimes too many emergency personnel have been dispatched to the scene. The presence of many uniformed personnel in a small apartment, for instance, is overwhelming or threatening to some people. Any emergency personnel who are not needed right away should leave the room or immediate vicinity until the patient calms down.

During your initial overview of the emergency scene, look to see if there is a crowd that may become hostile. It is better to ask for help early to deal with an unhappy crowd than it is to wait until the situation is unsafe for you and your patient.

Domestic Violence

FYI

Domestic violence is a common occurrence in our society. Its different forms include elder abuse, child abuse, spouse abuse, and abuse against gay or lesbian lovers. As a first responder, you need to be able to recognize the signs and symptoms of abuse and to understand the three phases in the cycle of abuse. When you respond to a situation involving domestic violence, you will have to maintain safety for yourself and for the patient and be able to perform effective assessment and treatment. Finally, you need to understand the requirements for reporting abuse in your state.

The signs and symptoms of abuse include physical injuries, the emotional state of the victim and the personality indicators of the abuser. Physical injuries from domestic violence include broken bones, cuts, head injuries, bruises, burns, and scars from old injuries. Internal injuries may also be caused by abuse. In some cases, injuries will be in varying stages of healing. The abused person's emotional scars may include depression, suicide attempts, and abuse of alcohol or drugs. The patient may have feelings of anxiety, distress, and hopelessness. Persons who are abusers may be paranoid, overly sensitive, obsessive or threatening. They often abuse alcohol or drugs, and have access to weapons.

Abuse has been described as a three-part cycle. In the tension phase, the abuser becomes angry and often blames the victim. If the victim has been in the relationship for some time, he or she may recognize the tension build up and react by trying to placate the abuser. The victim may also try to minimize or deny the abuse. The tension phase is usually the longest part of the abuse cycle.

The second stage is the explosive phase, when the batterer becomes enraged and loses control as well as the ability to think clearly. Most injuries to the victim occur during this stage. The third phase is the make-up phase. During this stage, the abuser may make all sorts of promises, which are seldom kept. This phase helps keep the abused

Note: Most violent patients calm down as time passes. The longer you can keep the patient talking, the better your chances are of resolving the situation without violence. Time is on your side.

person in the relationship with the abuser. As a first responder, you may enter a domestic scene anywhere in this cycle. Understanding this cycle will help you to anticipate the actions of both abuser and victim.

If you suspect abuse, your responsibility is to maintain safety for yourself and for the patient. Dealing with a violent person is covered below. To diffuse a tense situation, try to separate the patient from the person who may have been the abuser. This will create a safe place for the patient, give you a chance to gather needed information, and allow you to treat the patient's injuries. As you question the patient, express your concern. Ask the patient if she or he is all right. Try to keep from judging the patient. If the patient refuses to be transported, some agencies provide information about domestic abuse shelters. In some cases, the presence of law enforcement personnel will be helpful. Finally, learn the requirements for reporting cases of suspected abuse in your state.

Violent Patient

If you must treat an unarmed patient who is or may become violent, immediately attempt to establish verbal and eye contact with the patient. This begins the process of establishing rapport with the patient, and is important for communicating with a potentially violent person.

If family members or friends are present, check with them about the patient's past history of violence. A patient with a past history of violence is more likely to become violent again. Listen to the patient for yelling or verbal threatening. Loud, obscene, or bizarre speech indicates emotional instability. Assess the patient's posture to determine if he or she shows threatening behavior (**Figure 11.3**). A person who is pacing, cannot sit still, or tries to protect personal space is more likely to become violent. Patients who have been abusing alcohol or drugs are also at high risk for developing violent behavior. Do not force the patient into a corner, and do not allow yourself to be cut off from a route of retreat.

In situations like this, it is usually best to have only one person talk with the patient. Having more than one rescuer attempt conversation is often very threatening. The communicator should be the rescuer with whom the patient seems to have the best initial rapport.

If all other means of approach and intervention fail, it may be necessary to summon law enforcement personnel to control a violent patient.

Remember

If you have any doubts about your safety at a scene, wait at a safe distance and request help from law enforcement officials.

Violence Against First Responders

According to the National Institute for Occupational Safety and Health, the following factors increase the risk of violence in the workplace:

- working alone or in small numbers
- working late at night or early in the morning hours
- working in high crime areas
- working in community settings

All of those factors describe your job as a first responder. You come in contact with all kinds of people at all hours of the day and night. You work in the community, and may be called to high crime areas. You should be alert when you respond to a call that has an increased chance for violence. These include: crime scenes, incidents involving

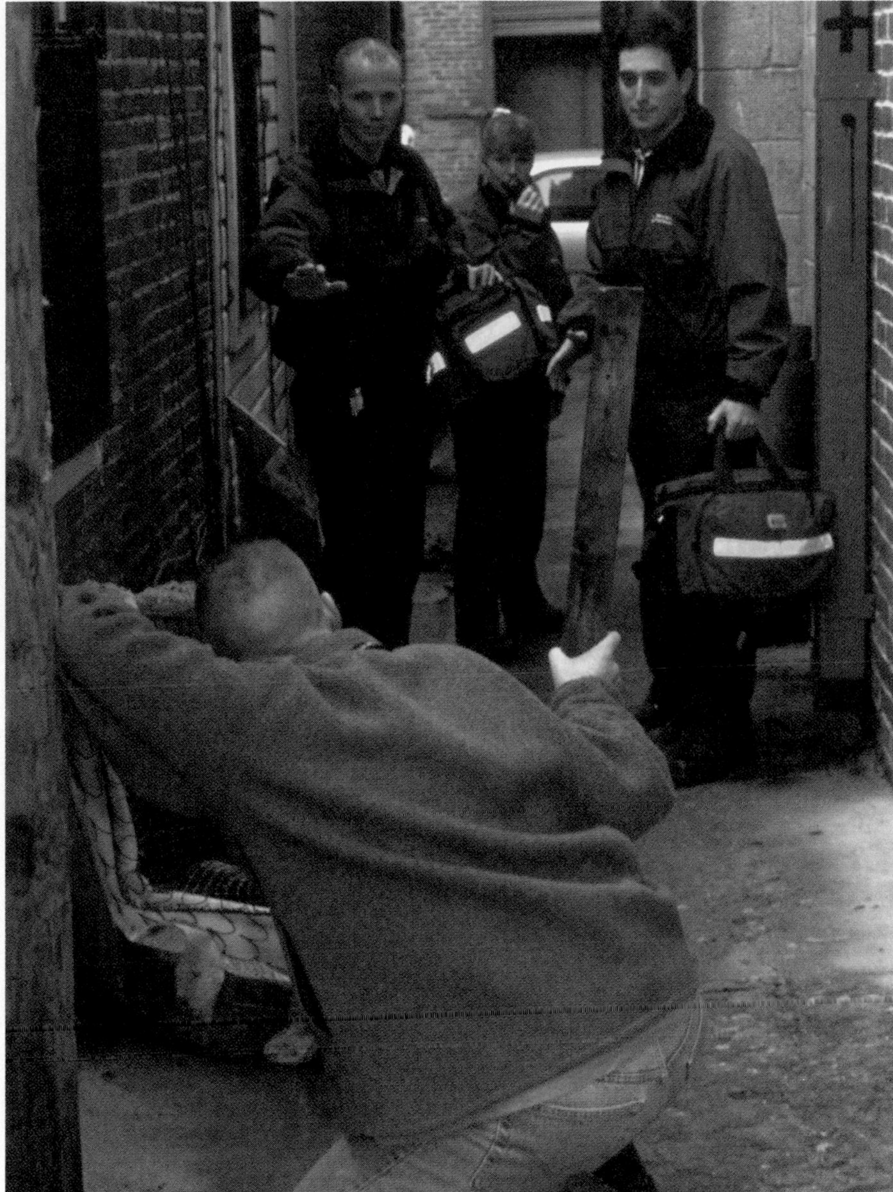

Figure 11.3 A patient's posture will indicate the potential for violent behavior.

gangs, large gatherings of hostile or potentially hostile people, and domestic disputes (previously discussed).

But even though you are more likely to be involved in potentially violent situations than the average citizen, there are steps you can take to minimize the chance of injury to you and to patients.

Prevention is the best way to avoid violence. It is far better to avoid or prevent an incident of violence than to have to deal with actual violence. You may have several different opportunities for preventing violence. Can you learn anything from the dispatch information? As you arrive at the scene use your personal "antenna" to pick up any signs that you may be approaching a violent situation. (Review the section on scene safety in Chapter 2). Be sure you have an escape route in mind as you approach any suspicious scene.

Your ability to use good interpersonal communications skills will help prevent many situations from becoming violent. Empathy can defuse tense situations. Practice the communications skills reviewed in this chapter. If you think you need backup or law enforcement personnel, request it early. If you are unable to handle a situation by yourself, remember your escape route. Learn your local protocols for violent situations and avail yourself of additional training for handling this type of situation.

The Armed Patient

You may encounter a person who is armed with a gun, knife, or other weapon. It is not your role to handle this situation unless you are a law enforcement officer.

Be alert for potentially threatening situations, and summon assistance if you think the person is armed. Do not proceed into an area where there may be an armed person without assistance from law enforcement personnel. If you must wait for the arrival of law enforcement personnel, stay with your vehicle in a safe location.

If, despite caution, you are confronted by an armed person, immediately attempt to withdraw. Your best defense is to avoid confronting a person who is armed!

Safety Tips

If you cannot withdraw from the scene:

- Stay calm.
- Do not turn your back on the patient.
- Do not make threatening moves.
- Try to talk with the person and explain that you are there to give emergency medical assistance.

Medical/Legal Considerations

To protect the rights of the patient and to protect yourself from any possible legal action, you must understand the laws of your state and community that relate to dealing with emotionally disturbed patients. If an emotionally disturbed patient agrees to be treated, there should be few legal issues. However, if a patient who appears to be disturbed refuses to accept treatment, it may be necessary to provide care against the patient's will. To do this, you must have a reasonable belief that the patient would harm himself, herself, or others.

Usually, if patients are a threat to themselves or to others, it is possible to treat and transport them without their consent. As a first responder, you will usually not be responsible for transporting the patient, but you should know what the laws permit you to do. This direction should come from your medical director and from legal counsel.

There may be times when it is necessary for you to apply reasonable force to keep patients from injuring themselves or others. If you are required to restrain a patient, you should consider the following factors: the patient's size and strength, the sex of the patient, the type of abnormal behavior, the mental state of the patient, and the method of restraint. Whenever possible, you should avoid acts of physical force that may injure the patient. You may, however, use reasonable force to defend yourself against an attack by an emotionally disturbed patient.

To prevent problems if you must restrain a patient, seek assistance from law enforcement officials or from your medical director. It is also important to document the conditions present in cases where you must restrain or subdue a patient. To prevent accusations of sexual misconduct by emotionally disturbed patients, a caregiver of the same sex should take primary responsibility for the care of the patient, whenever possible.

Three other types of emotional crises—attempted suicide, sexual assault, and death and dying—also require good communications skills from the first responder. Each of these is difficult for the patient and for the first responder.

Attempted Suicide

FYI

Each year, thousands of people, from teenagers to the elderly, attempt **suicide**. People attempt suicide by ingesting poisons, jumping from heights or in front of cars or trains, cutting their wrists or neck, and shooting or hanging themselves. Not all suicide attempts result in death, and many patients who fail at first will attempt suicide again. Most people who attempt suicide have a serious psychiatric illness, such as depression or alcohol or substance abuse. Many people attempt suicide while under the influence of alcohol or drugs. The underlying psychiatric disease is usually treatable, however, and with proper treatment the patient will no longer be suicidal. However, until that treatment is carried out, the patient must at all times be considered suicidal. All suicide attempts should be taken seriously.

suicide Self-inflicted death.

Management of an attempted suicide consists of the following steps:

1. Get a complete history of the incident.
2. Support the patient's ABCs, as needed.
3. Dress open wounds.
4. Treat the patient for spinal injuries, if indicated.
5. Do not judge the patient. Treat him or her for the injuries or conditions you discover.
6. Provide emotional support for the patient and family.

Talk with the patient during treatment. Remember that many suicide attempts are cries for help. In addition to treating the patient, you should provide emotional support for the patient's family. Help the family understand that a suicide attempt usually indicates an underlying psychiatric illness, and that it is not the fault of the family or friends. It is not your role as a first responder to pass judgment on a patient; it is your role to provide a caring attitude and good medical care.

Sexual Assault

Special consideration should be given to any victim of sexual assault. Such victims may be male or female, old or young. Because sexual assault creates an emotional crisis, the psychological aspects of treatment are important.

The patient may have a hard time dealing with a rescuer who is the same sex as the person who has committed the assault. You may have to delay all but the most essential treatment until a rescuer of the same sex as the victim arrives. Your first priority is the medical well-being of the patient, so you will need to treat any injuries the person may have (knife wounds, gunshot wounds, and so forth). However, because sexual assault is a crime, you should not remove clothing except to give medical care. Try to convince the victim not to bathe. Keep the scene and any evidence as undisturbed and intact as possible, and avoid aggressively questioning the patient as to what happened.

In addition to giving medical care, treat the patient with empathy. Maintain the patient's privacy by covering her or him with a sheet or blanket and do not leave the patient alone. Contact your local law enforcement agency and rape crisis center, if one is available in your community.

Remember

Your primary role as a first responder is to give emergency medical care.

Death and Dying

As a first responder, you will encounter death and dying from natural, accidental, and intentional causes. How well you can help the dying patient and the person's family or relatives largely depends on your own feelings about death. The material presented here expands on the material introduced in Chapter 2.

In some situations, there is nothing you can do, and the patient dies. In other situations, the patient dies despite everyone's best efforts. In yet other situations, the patient's death is completely unexpected. In every case, you must do whatever you can to meet the patient's medical needs. Your attempts to save or give comfort to the patient help everyone (the patient, the family, and you) to deal emotionally with the patient's death.

Most human beings are afraid of dying. Witnessing the death of another human being brings that fear to the forefront, if only for a brief time. You must work through your personal feelings about death so you can confront it in the field. Although you may be somewhat uncomfortable about bringing up the subject, it helps to discuss it with others in the emergency care field. If you are uncomfortable talking with your peers, talk to a member of your hospital's emergency department staff.

Once you have done everything you can to treat a patient medically, consider the psychological needs of the patient and his or her family. Just being there as an empathetic caregiver is helpful. Do not be afraid to touch. Putting an arm around a shoulder or holding the hand of the patient or a member of the family helps everyone, including you.

Do not make false statements about the situation, but it is just as important not to destroy hope. Even if, in your judgment, the situation is hopeless, try to give comfort by making such positive statements as, "We're here to help you, and we are doing everything we can. The ambulance is on its way, and you will be at the hospital as soon as possible."

Dealing with the deaths of others is a routine aspect of your job as a first responder. You must, therefore, constantly be on guard to prevent any callousness from entering into your interactions with patients and their families.

One specific type of death, **sudden infant death syndrome (SIDS)**, is discussed in Chapter 15.

sudden infant death syndrome (SIDS) Death from unknown cause that occurs during sleep in an otherwise healthy infant; also called crib death.

Signs & Symptoms

EXTREME STRESS

- Depression
- Inability to sleep
- Weight changes
- Increased alcohol consumption
- Inability to get along with family and co-workers
- Lack of interest in food or sex

Critical Incident Stress Debriefing

Providing emergency care is stressful for you as well as for the patient. As a first responder, you will deal with patients experiencing high levels of stress and anxiety. In emergency situations, you may not always be able to help patients. Some types of situations, such as rescue missions involving children or mass-casualty incidents, tend to produce more stress than others. You may need counseling to deal with these stresses.

If you let stress build up without releasing it in healthy ways, it can begin to have negative effects on you and your performance. Signs and symptoms of extreme stress include depression, inability to sleep, weight change, increased alcohol consumption, inability to get along with family and co-workers, and lack of interest in food or sex.

To help prevent excess stress and to relieve stress caused by critical incidents, psychologists have developed a process called **critical incident stress debriefing (CISD)**. CISD brings rescuers and a trained person together to talk about the rescuers' feelings. CISD helps rescuers understand the signs and symptoms of stress and to receive reassurance from the group leader. It also allows people to obtain more help from trained professionals, if needed. Many public safety agencies have set up CISD teams to handle stressful events. These teams have been helpful to rescuers who have been through an overwhelming or stressful event. Additional information about critical incident stress debriefing was presented in Chapter 2. Check with your agency to see what resources are available (**Figure 11.4**).

critical incident stress debriefing (CISD) A system of psychological support designed to reduce stress on emergency personnel.

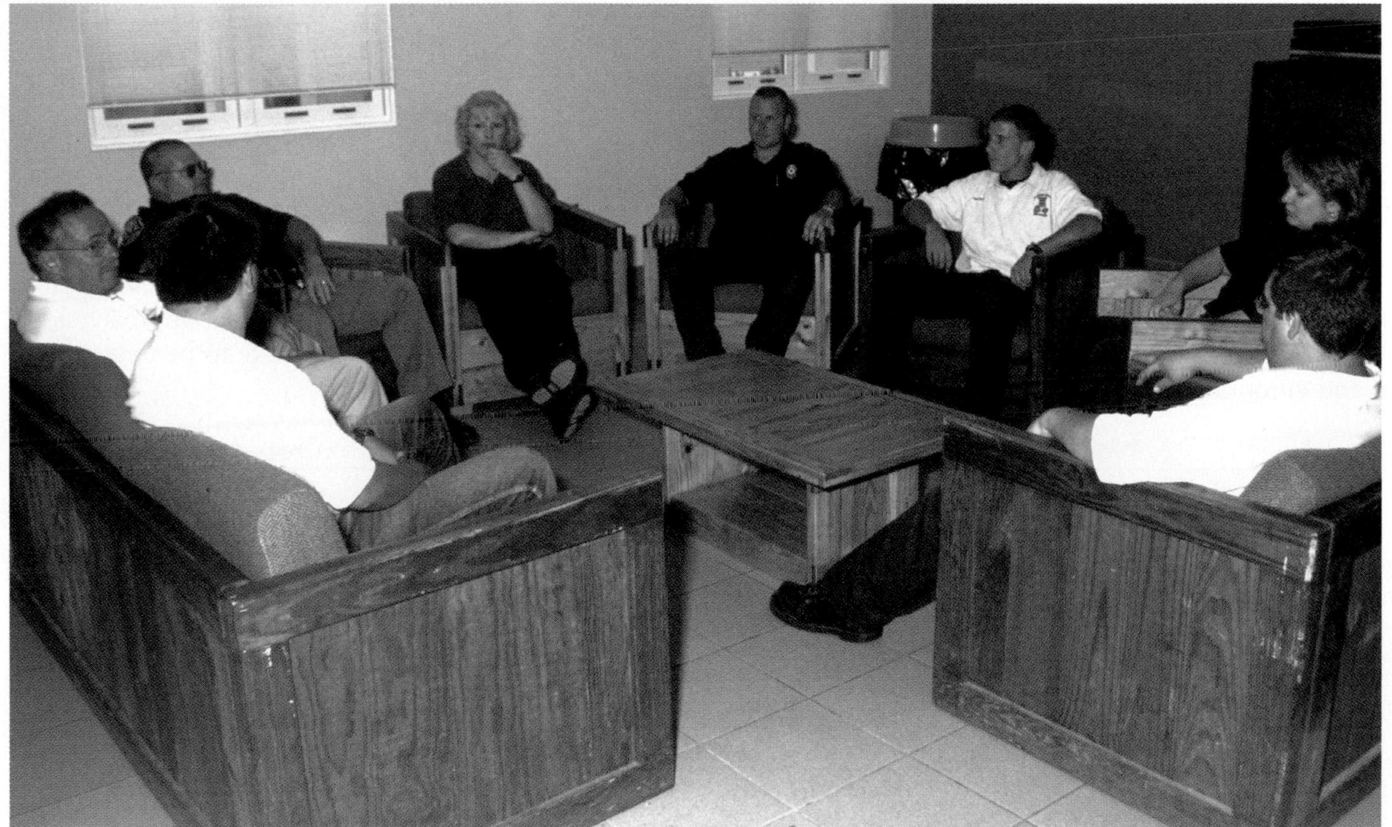

Fig. 11.4 A critical incident stress debriefing session.

11

Prep Kit

Ready for Review

Ready for Review thoroughly summarizes the chapter.

Only a small percentage of the patients you treat are severely mentally disturbed, but almost every patient you deal with is experiencing some degree of mental and emotional crisis. Even "normal" people react to stress in unexpected ways. No matter what the incident or crisis, your response must be to help the patient. This chapter presents you with some tools to help you deal with patients who are experiencing a stressful medical emergency or a behavioral emergency.

This chapter covers five major factors that cause behavioral crises: medical conditions, physical trauma, psychiatric illnesses, mind-altering substances, and emotional trauma. Your role as a first responder consists of assessing the patient and providing physical and emotional care. Because many patients experience anxiety, denial, anger, remorse, or grief during an emotional crisis, it is important to understand how to use restatement, redirection, and empathy. These concepts will help you be a more effective and caring first responder.

Understanding how to deal with crowds, violent patients, domestic violence, violence against first responders, armed patients, attempted suicides, sexual assaults, and death and dying is an important part of being an effective first responder. This chapter presents medical/legal considerations and the role of critical incident stress debriefing. Even with these tools for managing behavioral crises, it is important to remember that sometimes the best approach is to ask yourself, "How would I like to be treated if I were in this situation?"

Vital Vocabulary

The Vital Vocabulary are the key terms for this chapter.

behavioral emergencies—*page 238*
critical incident stress debriefing (CISD)—*page 249*
emotional shock—*page 239*
empathy—*page 242*
psychotic behavior—*page 238*
redirection—*page 242*
restatement—*page 242*
situational crisis—*page 239*
sudden infant death syndrome (SIDS)—*page 248*
suicide—*page 247*

Practice Points

The Practice Points are the key skills you need to know.

1. The following communication techniques:
   A. Restatement
   B. Redirection
   C. Empathy

2. How to calm a patient experiencing a behavioral crisis.

Ready to Respond

Ready to Respond presents a fictitious scenario to help you review what you learned in this chapter.

You are called to a fast-food restaurant for the report of a disturbed patient. As you arrive, you note a man who is about 45 years old, pacing back and forth between some of the tables. He is muttering to himself. As you approach him, you introduce yourself by name and by title.

1. Which of the following conditions is least likely to be causing the man's behavior?
   A. Situational crisis
   B. Physical trauma
   C. Medical conditions
   D. Myocardial infarction

2. His behavior is best described as
   A. Unusual
   B. Psychotic
   C. Depressed
   D. Violent

3. As you attempt to approach this man you should be most concerned about
   1. The potential of him becoming violent
   2. A way to get out of harms way
   3. His current medications
   4. The safety of other people in the restaurant

   A. 2,3,4
   B. 1,3,4
   C. 1,2,4
   D. 1,2,3,4

4. If this patient continues to get more agitated in spite of your efforts to calm him, you should
   A. Ask about his recent medical history
   B. Begin to examine him
   C. Consider calling for backup
   D. Ask him to leave

5. Describe the condition under which you could take a disturbed patient to a medical facility against his or her will.

6. Which part of the domestic violence cycle is most likely to filled with promises?
   A. Honeymoon
   B. Make-up phase
   C. Tension phase
   D. Explosive phase

7. The signs and symptoms of domestic abuse include all but which of the following?
   A. Physical injuries
   B. Emotional state of the victim
   C. Location of the incident
   D. Personality indicators of the abuser

Chapter 12

Bleeding, Shock, and Soft-Tissue Injuries

TECHNOLOGY

- Online Chapter Pretest
- Web Links
- Online Glossary
- Anatomy Review
- Online Review Manual
- CyberClass

www.FirstResponderTraining.com

- Interactive First Responder

Chapter FEATURES

- Skill Drills
- Vital Vocabulary
- Voices of Experience
- Signs and Symptoms
- FYI
- Special Needs
- Safety Tips
- BSI Tips
- Caution
- Check Point
- Prep Kit

CHAPTER 12

Objectives

Knowledge and Attitude Objectives

After studying this chapter, you will be expected to:

1. Establish the relationship between body substance isolation and bleeding.
2. Describe the function and relationship between the following parts of the circulatory system:
   A. Pump (heart)
   B. Pipes (blood vessels)
   C. Fluid (blood)
3. Explain how shock is caused by pump failure, pipe failure, and fluid loss.
4. List three types of shock caused by pipe failure.
5. List signs and symptoms of internal bleeding.
6. List signs and symptoms of shock.
7. List the general treatment for internal bleeding and shock.
8. Differentiate among arterial, venous, and capillary bleeding.
9. Explain the emergency care for external bleeding.
10. Describe the use of the femoral and brachial pressure points.
11. Explain the relationship between body substance isolation and soft-tissue injuries.
12. List and explain four types of soft-tissue injuries.
13. Describe the principles of treatment for soft-tissue injuries.
14. Explain the functions of dressings and bandages.
15. Discuss the emergency medical care for patients with the following injuries:
   A. Face wounds
   B. Nosebleeds
   C. Eye injuries
   D. Neck wounds
   E. Chest and back wounds
   F. Impaled objects
   G. Closed abdominal wounds
   H. Open abdominal wounds
   I. Genital wounds
   J. Extremity wounds
   K. Gunshot wounds
   L. Bites
16. Describe why the use of a tourniquet is to be discouraged.
17. Describe how the seriousness of a burn is related to the depth of the burn.
18. Describe how the seriousness of a burn is related to the extent of the burn.
19. Describe the signs, symptoms, and possible complications associated with each of the following types of burns:
   A. Thermal
   B. Respiratory
   C. Chemical
   D. Electrical
20. Explain the emergency treatment for each of the following types of burns:
   A. Thermal
   B. Respiratory
   C. Chemical
   D. Electrical

Skill Objectives

As a first responder, you should be able to:

1. Perform body substance isolation procedures for patients with wounds.
2. Treat patients with signs and symptoms of internal bleeding or shock.
3. Control bleeding using the following techniques:
   A. Direct pressure
   B. Elevation
   C. Femoral pressure point
   D. Brachial pressure point
4. Dress and bandage the following types of wounds:
   A. Face wounds
   B. Nosebleeds
   C. Eye injuries
   D. Neck wounds
   E. Chest and back wounds
   F. Impaled objects
   G. Closed abdominal wounds
   H. Open abdominal wounds
   I. Genital wounds
   J. Extremity wounds
   K. Gunshot wounds
   L. Bites
5. Perform emergency medical care for patients suffering the following types of burns:
   A. Thermal
   B. Respiratory
   C. Chemical
   D. Electrical

This chapter presents the skills you need to recognize and care for patients who are suffering from shock, bleeding, or soft-tissue injuries. Because most soft-tissue injuries result in bleeding, maintaining good body substance isolation (BSI) is important when you are caring for these injuries. The chapter describes four types of wounds: abrasions, lacerations, punctures, and avulsions. Techniques for controlling external bleeding are stressed. It is important that you learn the techniques for dressing and bandaging wounds presented here.

Damage to internal soft tissues and organs can cause life-threatening problems. Internal bleeding causes the patient to lose blood in the circulatory system and results in shock. More trauma patients die from shock than any other reason. Your ability to recognize the signs and symptoms of shock and to take simple measures to aid shock patients will give them the best chance for survival. This chapter explains the causes and types of shock using an analogy of a pump, pipes, and fluid. You will learn how a failure of any part of the system can cause shock.

Burns are another type of soft-tissue injury. Burns may be caused by heat, chemicals, or electricity. They may damage any part of the body and are especially harmful if they occur inside the respiratory tract. This chapter examines the extent, depth, and cause of burns. As you study this chapter, keep in mind the importance of maintaining good BSI techniques to prevent the spread of disease-carrying organisms.

BSI Tip

Most soft-tissue injuries involve some degree of bleeding. Any time you approach a patient with a potential soft-tissue injury, you need to consider your BSI strategy.

Body Substance Isolation and Soft-Tissue Injuries

The BSI concept assumes that all body fluids are potentially dangerous. Therefore, you must take appropriate measures to prevent contact with the patient's body fluids. When dealing with patients who have soft-tissue injuries, wear gloves to prevent contact with the patient's blood. At times, you may also need to wear a surgical mask and eye protection if there is danger of blood splatter from a massive wound or if the patient is coughing or vomiting bloody material.

THREE PARTS OF THE CIRCULATORY SYSTEM

1. *Pump (heart)*
2. *Pipes (arteries, capillaries, and veins)*
3. *Fluid (blood cells and other blood components)*

Review of the Parts and Function of the Circulatory System

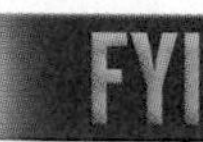

Figure 12.1 presents a schematic illustration of the circulatory system.

The Pump

The heart functions as the human circulatory system's pump. The heart consists of four separate chambers, two on top and two on the bottom.

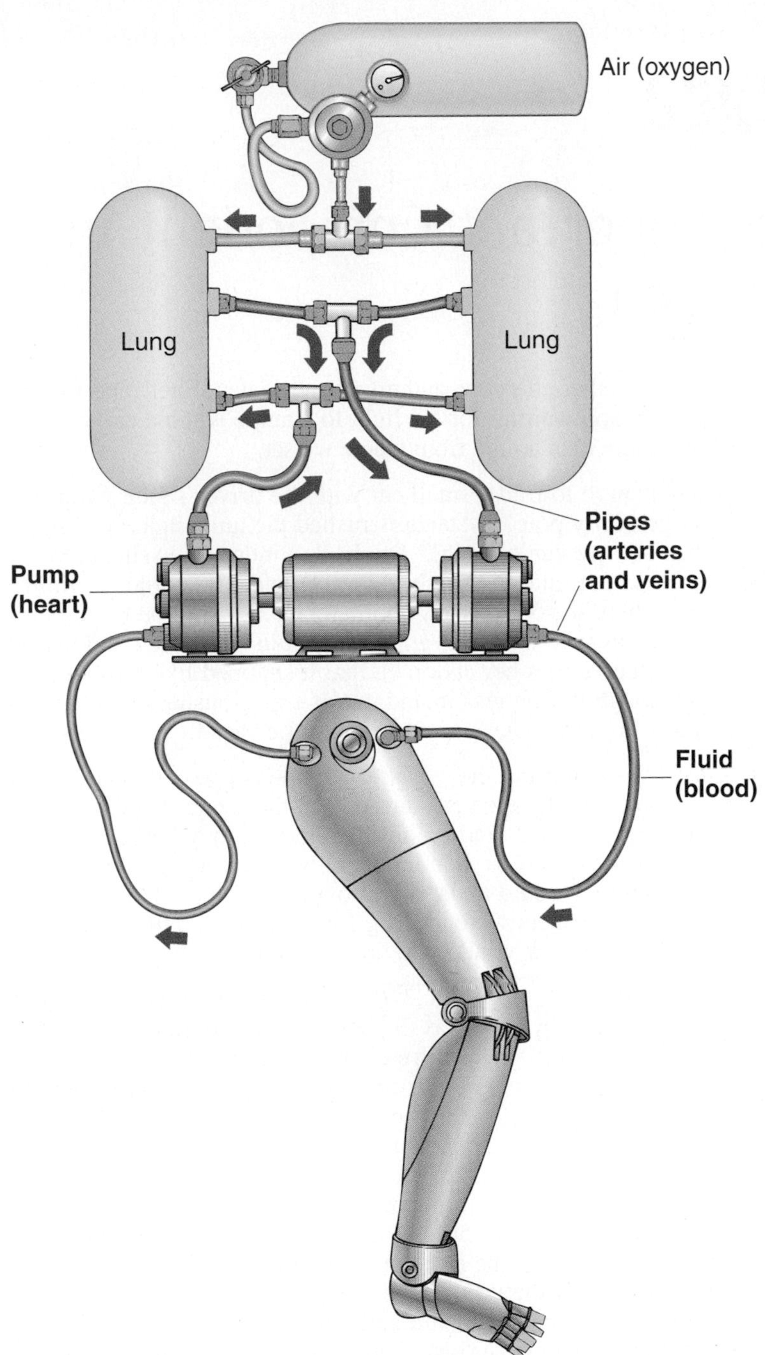

Figure 12.1 A schematic representation of the parts of the circulatory system.

The lower chambers are the left and right **ventricles**, and the upper chambers are the left and right atria (a single chamber is called an **atrium**). The ventricles are the larger chambers and do most of the actual pumping. The atria are somewhat less muscular and serve more as reservoirs for blood flowing into the heart from the body and the lungs (**Figure 12.2**, page 257).

ventricle Either of the two lower chambers of the heart.

atrium Either of the two upper chambers of the heart.

Voices of Experience

Teamwork the Most Important Component in Complicated Extrication

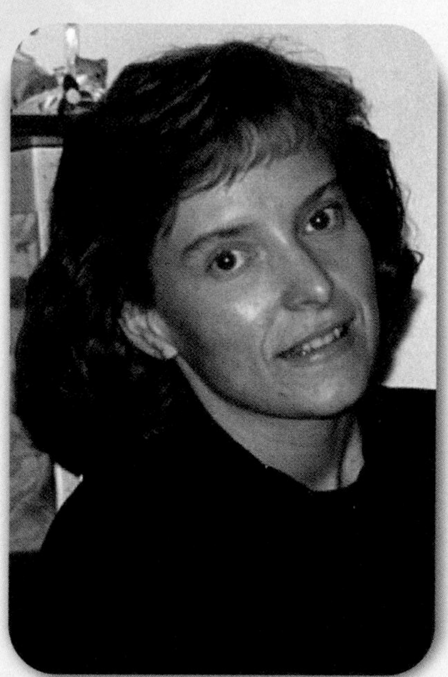

It was a hot summer afternoon and my partner, Lucas Shell, and I were sitting at an intersection waiting for the light to change when a call came for a wreck not more than a mile from where we sat.

We rounded a curve to find a small car with the driver's side wrapped around a large utility pole. Bystanders rushed the ambulance yelling, "She's bleeding bad and we can't get in!" The back window was shattered, so two of the men lifted me onto the trunk of the car and I was able to climb into the backseat where the 58-year-old woman lay, still strapped into her seatbelt. The pole was where the driver's seat should have been and the seatbelt was pulled so taut across her abdomen that it snapped like a rubber band when I cut through it. She was in and out of consciousness and the bleeding was coming from a large gash on the back of her head.

While Lucas was gathering the necessary supplies I would need, the fire department and several police cars arrived on the scene. All of the firemen are trained first responders and before I could ask, they had brought me a nonrebreather mask and oxygen tank and were taking the driver's side back door off so they could assist me, providing a much needed pair of hands. The police officers were helping Lucas set up IV lines and one even crawled through the back window to hold C-spine so I could start the IVs.

"The pole was where the driver's seat should have been and the seatbelt was pulled so taut across her abdomen that it snapped like a rubber band when I cut through it."

The extrication, though long and tedious, was the best job of communication and skill I have ever seen. I was inside the vehicle for thirty-nine minutes. The doors were removed, the top lifted off and the dash rolled, but the patient remained trapped. When the wrecker arrived, one of the men immediately rushed to the patient and asked how he could assist while the other two set up according to instructions from myself and the fire department. The car had to be removed from the pole and the door pried off the patient. As soon as she was free, there must have been twelve sets of hands lifting her onto the backboard and wrapping MAST around her broken body. The patient would never have had a chance had it not been for the skill of the first responders, the police officers, the bystanders, and the men on the wrecker who all knew their jobs and proved what teamwork can do.

I am happy to say that despite femur fractures, pelvic fractures, rib fractures, arm fractures, a head injury and massive bleeding, the patient spent a week in the hospital and two weeks at rehab before going home with the prognosis of a complete recovery. ❖

Rhonda J. Beck, NREMT-P
Houston County EMS
Warner Robins, GA

EMT/Paramedic Instructor
Central Georgia Technical College
Macon, GA

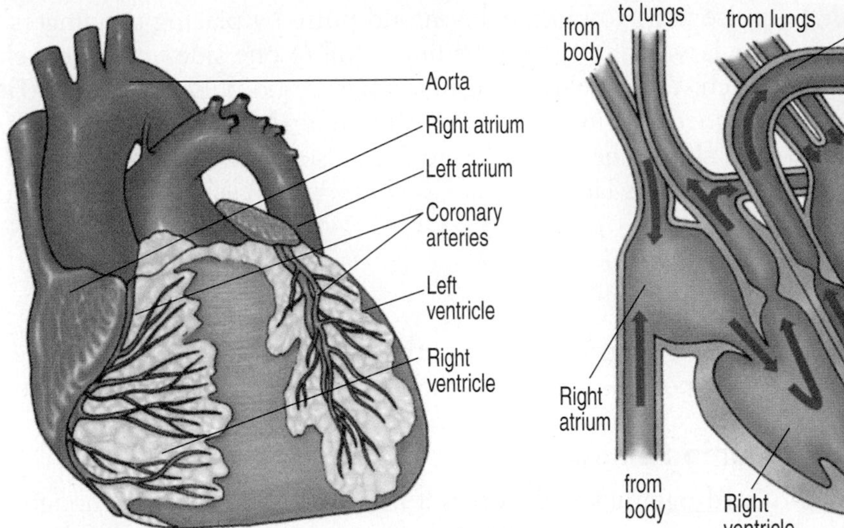

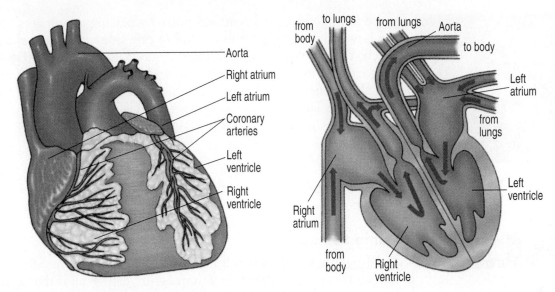

Figure 12.2 The heart functions as the pump of the human circulatory system.

Pipes

The human body has three main types of blood vessels: arteries, capillaries, and veins. The arteries (big-flow, heavy-duty, high-pressure pipes) carry blood away from the heart. The capillaries (distribution pipes), the smallest of the blood vessels, form a network that distributes blood to all parts of the body. The smallest capillaries are so narrow that blood cells have to flow through them "single file." The veins return the blood from the capillaries to the heart, where it is pumped to the lungs. There, the blood gives off carbon dioxide and takes on oxygen.

The Fluid

Fluid consists of blood cells and other blood components, each with a specific function. The liquid part of the blood is known as plasma. Plasma serves as the transporting medium for the "solid" parts of the blood, which are the red blood cells, white blood cells, and platelets. Red blood cells carry oxygen and carbon dioxide (**Figure 12.3**). White blood cells have a "search and destroy" function. They consume bacteria and viruses to combat infections in the body. Platelets interact with each other and with other substances in the blood to form clots that help stop bleeding.

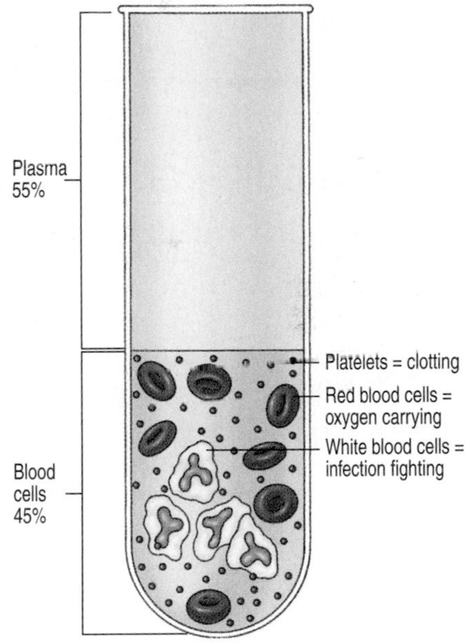

Figure 12.3 The components of blood.

Pulse

A pulse is the pressure wave generated by the pumping action of the heart. The beat you feel is caused the surge of blood from the left ventricle as it contracts, and pushes blood out into the main arteries of the body. In counting the number of pulsations per minute, you also count heartbeats per minute. In other words, the pulse rate reflects the heart rate.

Usually you can feel a patient's radial and carotid pulses. In a conscious patient, you can easily find the radial (wrist) pulse at the base of the thumb. If the patient is unconscious, suffering from <u>**shock**</u>, or both, it may be impossible for you to feel a radial pulse. Therefore, it is vital that you know how to locate the carotid (neck) pulse. If the patient appears to be in shock or is unconscious, attempt to locate the carotid

<u>**shock**</u> A state of collapse of the cardiovascular system; the state of inadequate delivery of blood to the organs of the body.

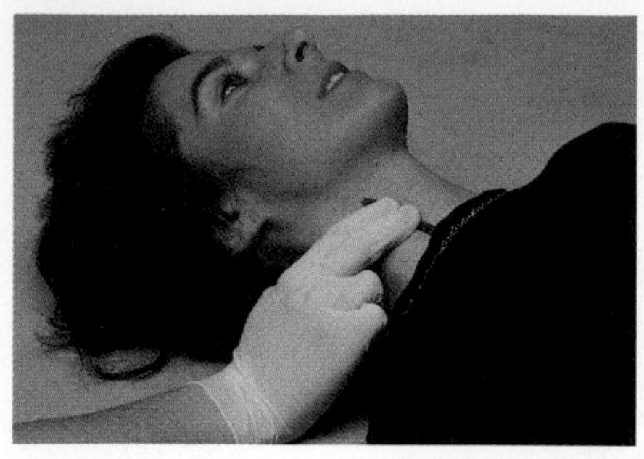

Figure 12.4 Taking the carotid pulse.

pulse first. You locate the carotid pulse by placing two fingers lightly on the larynx and sliding the fingers off to one side until you feel a slight notch. You should be able to feel the carotid pulse at this spot (**Figure 12.4**). Practice locating the carotid pulse of another person in a dark room. You should be able to locate the pulse within three seconds of touching the person's larynx.

Special Needs

CHILDREN

In an infant, you should check the brachial (upper arm) pulse instead of the carotid pulse.

Shock

Shock is defined as failure of the circulatory system. Circulatory failure has many possible causes, but the three primary causes are discussed here.

PRIMARY CAUSES OF CIRCULATORY FAILURE

1. *Pump failure*
2. *Pipe failure*
3. *Fluid loss*

Pump Failure

Cardiogenic shock occurs if the heart cannot pump enough blood to supply the needs of the body. Pump failure can result if the heart has been weakened by a heart attack. Inadequate pumping of the heart can cause blood to back up in the vessels of the lungs, resulting in a condition known as **congestive heart failure (CHF)**.

Pipe Failure

Pipe failure is caused by the expansion (dilation) of the capillaries to as much as three or four times their normal size. This causes blood to pool in the capillaries, instead of circulating throughout the system. When blood pools in the capillaries, the rest of the body, including the heart and other vital organs, is deprived of blood. **Blood pressure** falls, and shock results.

In shock caused by sudden expansion of the capillaries, blood pressure may drop so rapidly that you are unable to feel either a radial or a carotid pulse.

Three types of shock caused by capillary expansion are:

1. Shock induced by fainting
2. Anaphylactic shock
3. Spinal shock

The least serious type of "shock" caused by pipe failure is fainting. Fainting (**psychogenic shock**) is the body's response to a major psychological or emotional stress. The capillaries suddenly expand to three or four times their normal size. Fainting is a short-term condition that corrects itself once the patient is placed in a horizontal position.

Anaphylactic shock is caused by an extreme allergic reaction to a foreign substance, such as venom from bee stings (see Chapter 10), penicillin, or certain foods. Shock develops very quickly following exposure. The patient may suddenly start to itch, a rash or hives may appear, the face and tongue may swell very quickly, and a blue color may appear around the mouth. The patient appears flushed (reddish), and breathing may quickly become difficult, with wheezing sounds coming from the chest.

Blood pressure drops rapidly as the blood pools in the expanded capillaries. The pulse may be so weak that you cannot feel it.

cardiogenic shock Shock resulting from inadequate functioning of the heart.

congestive heart failure (CHF) Heart disease characterized by breathlessness, fluid retention in the lungs, and generalized swelling of the body.

blood pressure The pressure of the circulating blood against the walls of the arteries.

psychogenic shock Commonly known as fainting; caused by a temporary reduction in blood supply to the brain.

anaphylactic shock Severe shock caused by an allergic reaction to food, medicine, or insect stings.

Pipe failure has occurred, and death will result if prompt action to counteract the toxin is not taken.

Spinal shock may occur in patients who have suffered a spinal cord injury. The injury to the spinal cord allows the capillaries to expand, and blood pools in the lower extremities. The brain, heart, lungs and other vital organs are deprived of blood, resulting in shock.

hemorrhage Bleeding.

Fluid Loss

The third general type of shock is caused by fluid loss. Fluid loss caused by excessive bleeding (**hemorrhage**) is the most common cause of shock. Blood escapes from the normally closed circulatory system through an internal or external wound, and the system's total fluid level (blood volume) drops until the pump cannot operate efficiently. To compensate for fluid loss, the heart begins to pump faster to maintain pressure in the pipes. But as the fluid continues to drain out, the pump eventually "loses its prime" and stops pumping altogether.

External bleeding is not difficult to detect because you can see blood escaping from the circulatory system to the outside. With internal bleeding, blood escapes from the system, but you cannot see it. Even though the escaped blood remains inside the body, it cannot reenter the circulatory system and is not available to be pumped by the heart. Whether external or internal, unchecked bleeding causes shock, eventual pump failure, and death.

An average adult has about 12 pints of blood circulating in the system. Losing a single pint of blood will not produce shock in a healthy adult. In fact, one pint per donor is the amount that blood banks collect. However, the loss of two or more pints of blood can produce shock. This amount of blood can be lost as a result of injuries such as a fractured femur. **Figure 12.5** shows the amount of blood that can be lost as a result of various injuries.

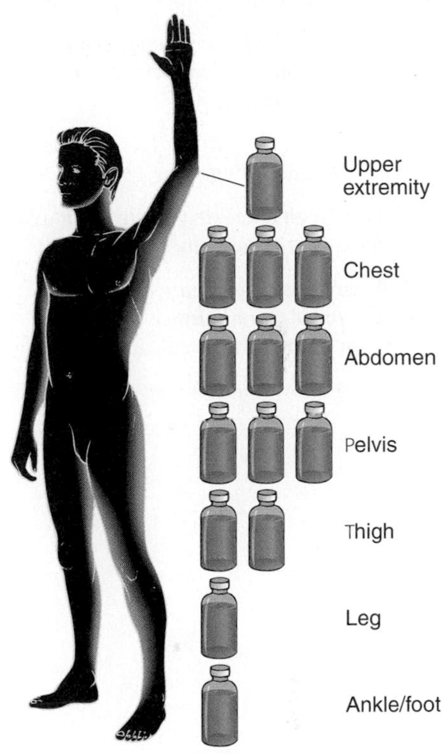

Figure 12.5 Potential blood loss from injuries in various parts of the body. Each bottle equals one pint.

Signs and Symptoms of Shock

Shock deprives the body of sufficient blood to function normally. As shock progresses, the body alters some of its functions in an attempt to maintain sufficient blood supply to its vital parts. A patient who is suffering from shock may exhibit some or all of the signs and symptoms shown in the box on the next page. Initially, the patient's breathing may be rapid and deep, but as shock progresses in severity, breathing becomes rapid and shallow.

Changes in mental status may be the first signs of shock, so monitoring the overall mental status of a patient can help you detect shock. Any change in mental status may be significant. In severe cases, the patient loses consciousness. If a trauma patient who has been quiet suddenly becomes agitated, restless, and vocal, you should suspect shock. If a trauma patient who has been loud, vocal, and belligerent becomes quiet, you should also suspect shock and begin treatment. If the patient has dark skin, you will not be able to use skin color changes to help you detect shock. Therefore you must be especially alert for other signs of shock. The capillary refill test and the condition of the skin (cool and clammy) will help you recognize shock in patients who have dark skin.

Signs & Symptoms

SHOCK

- Confusion, restlessness, or anxiety
- Cold, clammy, sweaty, pale skin
- Rapid breathing
- Rapid, weak pulse
- Increased capillary refill time
- Nausea and vomiting
- Weakness or fainting
- Thirst

GENERAL TREATMENT FOR SHOCK

1. *Position the patient correctly.*
2. *Maintain the patient's ABCs.*
3. *Treat the cause of shock, if possible.*
4. *Maintain the patient's body temperature by placing blankets under and over the patient.*
5. *Make sure the patient does not eat or drink anything.*
6. *Assist with other treatments (such as administering oxygen, if available).*
7. *Arrange for immediate and* T *prompt ambulance transport to an appropriate medical facility.*

CAUTION

A quiet patient is often a patient in shock. Watch carefully!

General Treatment for Shock

As a first responder, you can combat shock from any cause and keep it from getting worse by taking several simple but important steps.

Position the Patient Correctly

If there is no head injury, extreme discomfort, or difficulty breathing, lay the patient flat on the back on a horizontal surface. Place the patient on a blanket, if available. Elevate the patient's legs 12 to 18 inches off the floor or ground (**Figure 12.6**). This enables some blood to drain from the legs back into the circulatory system. If the patient has a head injury, do not elevate the legs.

If the patient is having chest pain or difficulty breathing (which is likely to occur in cases of heart attack and emphysema), place the patient in a sitting or semi-reclining position.

CAUTION

Do not allow the patient to stand!

Maintain the Patient's ABCs

Check the patient's airway, breathing, and circulation at least every five minutes. If necessary, open the airway, perform rescue breathing, or begin CPR.

Treat the Cause of Shock If Possible

Most causes of shock must be treated in the hospital. Often this treatment consists of surgery by specially trained physicians. However, you will be able to treat one common cause of shock—external bleeding. By controlling external bleeding with direct pressure, elevation, or pressure

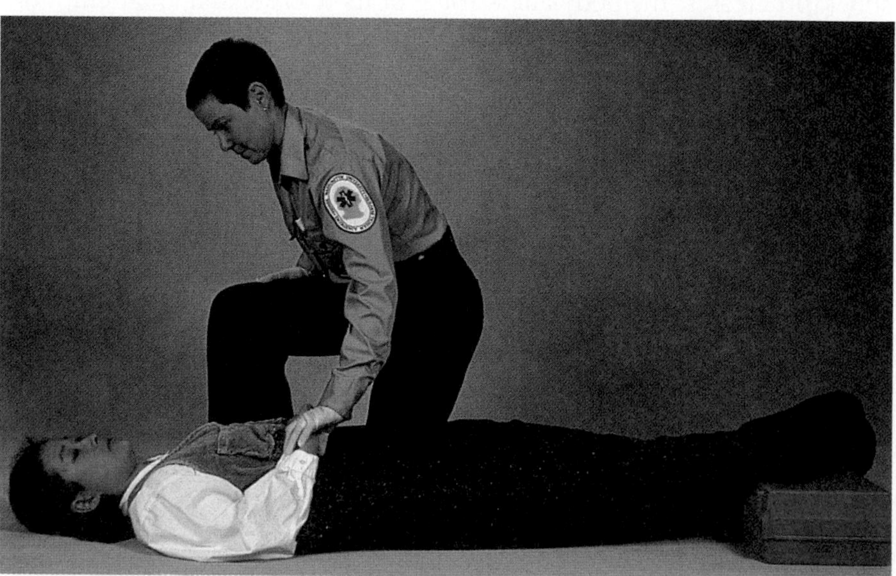

Figure 12.6 Position for treatment of shock if there is no head injury. Note the elevated legs. If the patient is experiencing difficulty breathing, place the patient in a sitting or semi-reclining position.

points, you will be able to temporarily treat this cause of shock until the patient can be transported to an appropriate medical facility for more advanced treatment.

Note: In the summer or in hot rooms, it is not necessary to cover every shock patient with blankets. You are trying to maintain body heat, not produce more.

Maintain the Patient's Body Temperature

Attempt to keep the patient comfortably warm. A patient with cold, clammy skin should be covered. It is as important to place blankets under the patient to keep body heat from escaping into the ground as it is to cover the patient with blankets.

Make Sure the Patient Does Not Eat or Drink Anything

Even though a patient in shock is very thirsty, do not give liquids by mouth. There are two reasons for this:

1. A patient in shock may be nauseated, and eating or drinking may cause vomiting.
2. A patient in shock may need emergency surgery. Patients should not have anything in their stomachs before surgery.

If you are working in an area where ambulance response time is more than 20 minutes, you may give patients a clean cloth or gauze pad that has been soaked in water to suck. This relieves dryness of the mouth but does not quench thirst. No matter how thirsty patients are, do not permit them to drink anything.

FYI

Assist with Other Treatments

When a basic life support (BLS) or advanced life support (ALS) unit arrives on the scene, be ready to assist unit personnel with further treatment. Patients may be given oxygen or **intravenous (IV) fluids; pneumatic antishock garments (PASGs)** may be used.

If you are trained in the administration of oxygen and have it available, give it to shock patients. Oxygen benefits such patients by ensuring that the reduced number of red blood cells are as oxygen-saturated as they can be.

EMTs or paramedics can administer IV solutions. Adding fluid to the body combats the loss of blood volume.

Some EMS personnel use PASGs in the field to treat pelvic fractures and to treat shock. PASGs are placed around the patient's legs and abdomen and inflated with air. As the PASG inflates, it exerts pressure around the legs and abdomen. Although you, as a first responder, will not use these devices yourself, you should know their purpose and function. It is also important to understand that PSAGs must not be removed in the field. Removing PSAGs must be done in a hospital and under the direct supervision of a physician.

Arrange for Prompt Ambulance Transport to an Appropriate Medical Facility

As soon as you realize that you have a patient who is suffering from shock, you should make sure that an ambulance has been dispatched. When the ambulance arrives, give the EMS personnel a concise hand-off report emphasizing the signs and symptoms of shock that you noted. The EMTs or paramedics should make sure that the patient is quickly prepared for immediate and Ⓣ *prompt transport* to a medical facility

intravenous (IV) fluid Fluid other than blood or blood products infused into the vascular system to maintain an adequate circulatory blood volume.

pneumatic antishock garment (PASG) A trousers-like device placed around a shock victim's legs and abdomen and inflated with air. Also called military antishock trousers (MAST).

pressure points Points where a blood vessel lies near a bone; pressure can be applied to these points to help control bleeding.

that can handle a patient with these severe problems. The cure for shock is usually surgical repair, and the sooner the patient gets to the hospital, the better the chance of survival will be.

Treatment for Shock Caused by Pump Failure

Patients suffering from pump failure may be confused, restless, anxious, or unconscious. Their pulse is usually rapid and weak. Their skin is cold and clammy, sweaty, and pale. Their respirations are often rapid and shallow.

Pump failure is a serious condition. Your proper treatment and prompt transport by ambulance to a medical center will give these patients their best chance for survival. See the box at right for treatment.

Treatment for Shock Caused by Pipe Failure

Patients who have fainted, who are suffering from anaphylactic shock, or who have suffered a severe spinal cord injury will have pipe failure. The size of their capillaries may increase three or four times, causing signs and symptoms of shock. See the box at right for treatment.

Treatment for Anaphylactic Shock

The initial treatment for anaphylactic shock (shock caused by an allergic reaction) is similar to the treatment for any other type of shock. Anaphylactic shock is an extreme emergency and the patient must be transported as soon as possible. Paramedics, nurses, and doctors can give medications that may reverse the allergic reaction. See the box at right for treatment.

Signs & Symptoms

INTERNAL BLEEDING

- Coughing or vomiting of blood
- Abdominal tenderness, rigidity, or distention
- Rectal bleeding
- Vaginal bleeding in women
- Classic signs of shock

Treatment for Shock Caused by Fluid Loss

Shock may be caused by internal blood loss (blood that escapes from damaged blood vessels and stays inside the body) or by external blood loss (blood that escapes from the body). Excessive bleeding is the most common cause of shock. See the box at right for treatment.

Shock Caused by Internal Blood Loss

Patients die quickly and quietly from internal bleeding following abdominal injuries that rupture the spleen, liver, or large blood vessels. You must be alert to catch the earliest signs and symptoms of internal bleeding and to begin treatment for shock. If you are treating several injured patients, those with internal bleeding should be T ***transported promptly*** to the medical facility first, as immediate surgery may be needed. (Chapter 16 discusses how to decide which patients should receive care first.)

Bleeding from stomach ulcers, ruptured blood vessels, or tumors can all cause internal bleeding and shock. This bleeding can be spontaneous, massive, and rapid, often leading to the loss of large quantities of blood by vomiting or bloody diarrhea.

It is important that you recognize the signs and symptoms of internal bleeding and take prompt corrective action. In addition to the classic signs of shock (confusion, rapid pulse, cold and clammy skin, and rapid breathing), patients with internal bleeding may show some of the signs and symptoms depicted in the box.

Remember

You cannot stop internal bleeding. You can only treat its symptoms and arrange for prompt ambulance transport to an appropriate medical facility.

TREATMENT FOR SHOCK CAUSED BY PUMP FAILURE

1. *Keep the patient lying down unless breathing is better in a sitting position.*
2. *Maintain the patient's ABCs. Be prepared to do CPR, if necessary.*
3. *Conserve the patient's normal body temperature.*
4. *Make sure the patient does not eat or drink anything.*
5. *Keep the patient quiet and do any necessary moving for him or her.*
6. *Provide reassurance.*
7. *Arrange for (T) prompt ambulance transport to an appropriate medical facility.*
8. *Provide high-flow oxygen as soon as it is available*

TREATMENT FOR SHOCK CAUSED BY PIPE FAILURE

Fainting

1. *Examine the patient to make sure there is no injury.*
2. *Keep the patient lying down with legs elevated 12 to 18 inches off the floor or ground. This enables the blood to drain from the legs back into the central circulatory system.*
3. *Maintain the ABCs.*
4. *Maintain the patient's normal body temperature.*
5. *Provide reassurance.*

Anaphylactic Shock

1. *Keep the patient lying down. Elevate the legs 12 to 18 inches off the floor or ground.*
2. *Maintain the patient's ABCs. Anaphylactic shock may cause airway swelling. In severe reactions, the patient may require mouth-to-mask breathing or full CPR.*
3. *Maintain the patient's normal body temperature.*
4. *Provide reassurance.*
5. *Arrange for (T) rapid transport by ambulance to an appropriate medical facility.*

Spinal Shock

1. *Place the patient on his or her back. Because the spine may be injured, keep the patient's head and neck stabilized to protect the spinal cord (Chapter 13). Do not elevate the patient's feet because this will make breathing more difficult.*
2. *Maintain the patient's ABCs and stabilize the neck.*
3. *Maintain the patient's body temperature.*
4. *Make sure the patient does not eat or drink anything.*
5. *Assist with other treatments. Help other medical providers to place the patient on a backboard.*

TREATMENT FOR SHOCK CAUSED BY FLUID LOSS

Internal Blood Loss

1. *Keep the patient lying down. Elevate the legs 12 to 18 inches off the floor or ground.*
2. *Maintain the patient's ABCs.*
3. *Maintain the patient's normal body temperature.*
4. *Make sure the patient does not eat or drink anything.*
5. *Provide reassurance.*
6. *Keep the patient quiet and do any necessary moving for him or her.*
7. *Provide high-flow oxygen as soon as it is available.*
8. *Monitor the patient's vital signs at least every five minutes.*
9. *Arrange for (T) prompt transportation by ambulance to an appropriate medical facility.*

External Blood Loss

1. *Control bleeding by applying direct pressure on the wound, elevating the injured part, and using* ***pressure points*** *(compressing a major artery against the bone). This is the most important step.*
2. *Make sure the patient is lying down. Elevate the legs 12 to 18 inches off the floor or ground.*
3. *Maintain the patient's ABCs.*
4. *Maintain the patient's body temperature.*
5. *Make sure the patient does not eat or drink anything.*
6. *Provide reassurance.*
7. *Provide high-flow oxygen as soon as it is available.*
9. *Arrange for (T) prompt transportation by ambulance to an appropriate medical facility.*

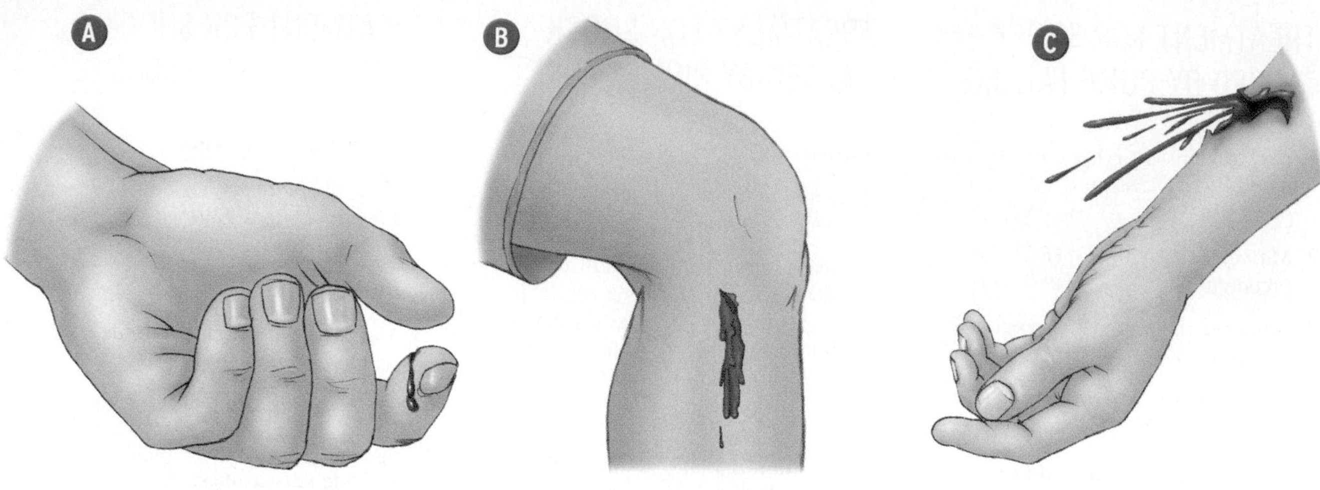

Figure 12.7 Recognizing the three types of external bleeding. **A.** Capillary **B.** Venous **C.** Arterial

Check✓point

- Describe the three major causes of shock and outline the treatment for each.

Bleeding

Controlling External Blood Loss

There are three types of external blood loss: capillary, venous, and arterial (**Figure 12.7**).

The most common type of external blood loss is **capillary bleeding**. In capillary bleeding, the blood oozes out (such as from a cut finger). You can control capillary bleeding simply by applying direct pressure to the site.

The next most common type of bleeding is venous bleeding. This bleeding has a steady flow. Bleeding from a large vein may be profuse and life threatening. To control **venous bleeding**, apply direct pressure.

The most serious type of bleeding is **arterial bleeding**. Arterial blood spurts or surges from the laceration or wound with each heartbeat. Blood pressure in arteries is higher than in capillaries or veins, and unchecked arterial bleeding can result in death from loss of blood in a short time. To control arterial bleeding, exert direct pressure and, if necessary, apply pressure to a pressure point. This is done by compressing a major artery against the underlying bone, as explained below.

Because many injured patients actually die from shock caused by blood loss, it is vitally important that you control external bleeding quickly.

Direct Pressure

Most external bleeding can be controlled by applying direct pressure to the wound. Place a dry, sterile **dressing** directly on the wound and press on it with your gloved hand (**Figure 12.8**). Wear the gloves from your first responder life support kit. If you do not have a sterile dressing or gauze bandage, use the cleanest cloth available.

capillary bleeding Bleeding from the capillaries in which blood oozes from the open wound.

venous bleeding External bleeding from a vein, characterized by steady flow; the bleeding may be profuse and life threatening.

arterial bleeding Serious bleeding from an artery in which blood frequently pulses or spurts from an open wound.

dressing A bandage.

Remember

Veins carry blood to the heart, and arteries carry blood away from the heart. Capillaries are tiny, thin-walled vessels that connect arteries and veins.

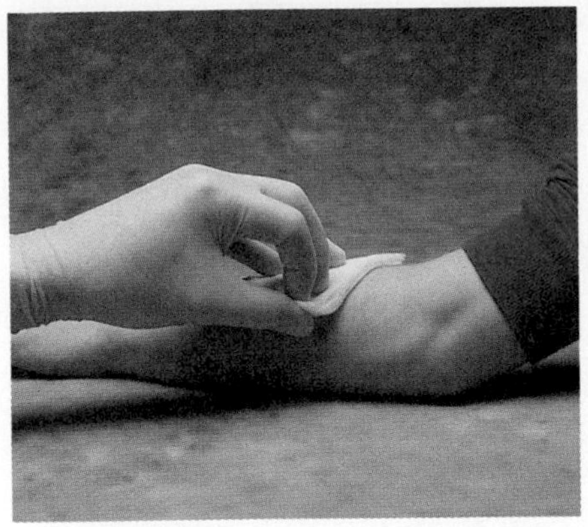

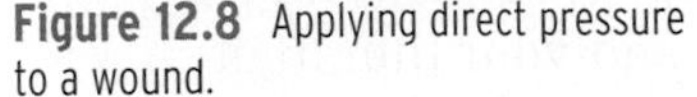

Figure 12.8 Applying direct pressure to a wound.

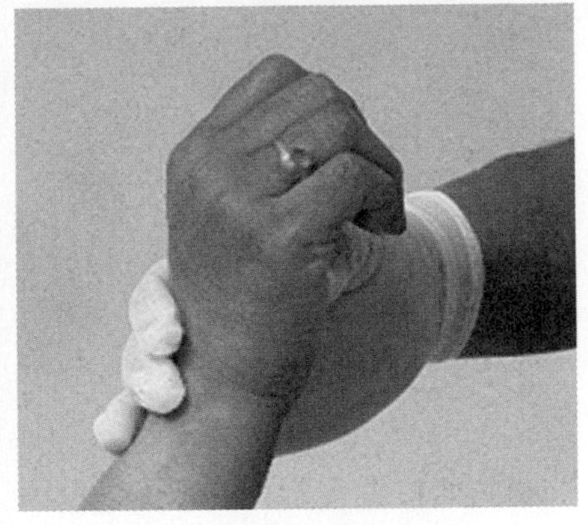

Figure 12.9 Elevate an arm while maintaining direct pressure to control external bleeding.

To maintain direct pressure on the wound, wrap the dressing and wound snugly with a roller gauze bandage. Do not remove a dressing after you have applied it, even if it becomes blood-soaked. Place another dressing on top of the first and keep them both in place.

According to the American Medical Association, it is extremely unlikely that you—as a first responder providing emergency care—will contract AIDS from a patient who is bleeding. For more information, call the Centers for Disease Control National AIDS Hotline at 1-800-342-AIDS. Direct exposure to blood must be reported to the emergency physician.

Elevation

If direct pressure does not stop external bleeding from an extremity, elevate the injured arm or leg as you maintain direct pressure. Elevation, in conjunction with direct pressure, will usually stop severe bleeding (**Figure 12.9**).

Pressure Points

If the combination of direct pressure and elevation does not control bleeding from an arm or leg wound, you must try to control it indirectly by preventing blood from flowing into the limb. This is accomplished by compressing a major artery against the bone at a pressure point.

> Compressing the artery at a pressure point stops blood flow in much the same way that stepping on a garden hose stops the flow of water. Although there are several pressure points in the body, the **brachial artery pressure point** (in the upper arm) and the **femoral artery pressure point** (in the groin) are the most important (**Figure 12.10**).

In applying pressure to the brachial artery, you should remember the words "slap, slide, and squeeze." Proceed as follows:

1. Position the patient's arm so the elbow is bent at a right angle (90°) and hold the upper arm away from the patient's body.
2. Gently "slap" the inside of the biceps with your fingers halfway between the shoulder and the elbow to push the biceps out of the way.
3. "Slide" your fingers up to push the biceps away.
4. "Squeeze" (press) your hand down on the humerus (upper arm bone). You should be able to feel the pulse as you press down.

THREE METHODS OF CONTROLLING EXTERNAL BLEEDING

1. *Applying direct pressure*
2. *Elevating the body part*
3. *Applying pressure at a pressure point*

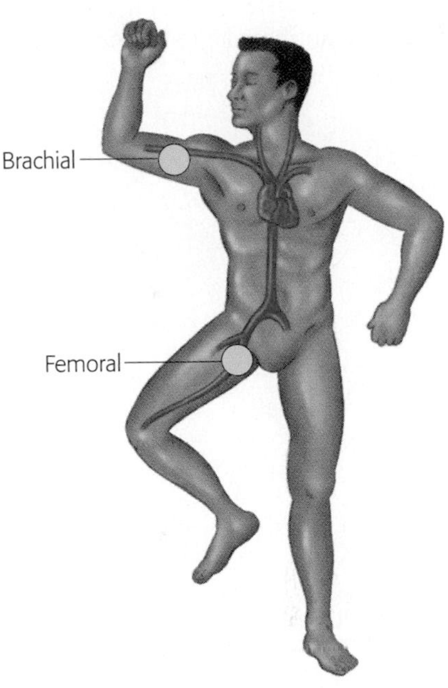

Figure 12.10 The location of the brachial and femoral pressure points.

BSI Tip

Before you touch blood, put on gloves and other precautionary devices as necessary.

brachial artery pressure point Pressure point located in the arm between the elbow and the shoulder; also used in taking blood pressure and for checking the pulse in infants.

femoral artery pressure point Pressure point located in the groin, where the femoral artery is close to the skin.

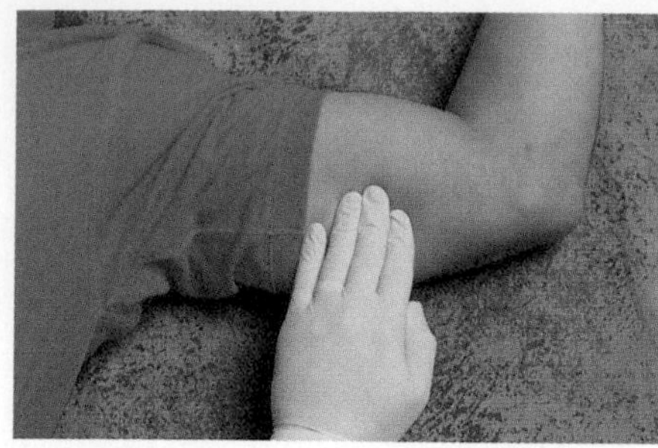

Figure 12.11 Applying pressure to the brachial artery.

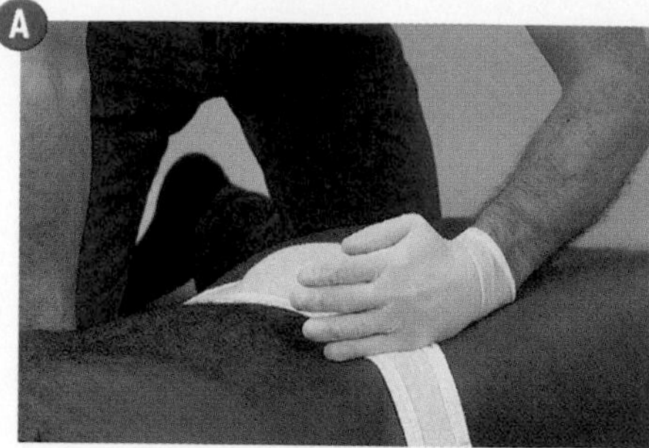

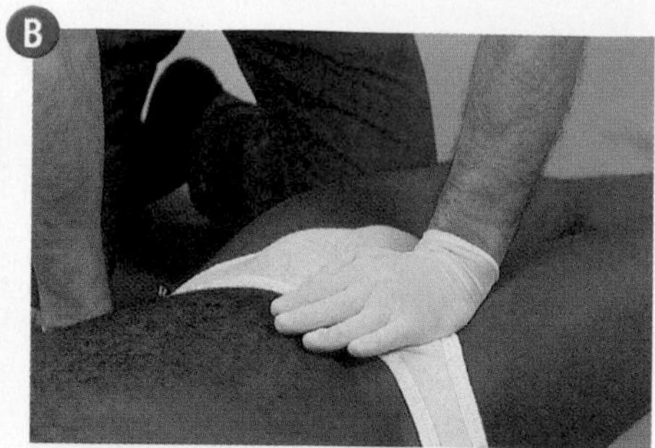

Figure 12.12 Locating and applying pressure to the femoral artery. A. Locate the femoral pressure point. B. Apply pressure to the femoral artery.

Note: Do not hesitate to lean into the pressure point.

If the patient is sitting down, "squeeze" by placing your fingers halfway between the shoulder and the elbow and your thumb on the opposite side of the patient's arm. If done properly, this technique (in combination with direct wound pressure and elevation) will quickly stop any bleeding below the point of application (**Figure 12.11**).

The femoral artery pressure point is more difficult to locate and squeeze. Proceed as follows:

1. Position the patient on his or her back and kneel next to the patient's hips, facing the patient's head. You should be on the side of the patient opposite the extremity that is bleeding.
2. Find the pelvis and place the little finger of your hand closest to the injured leg along the anterior crest on the injured side (**Figure 12.12A**).
3. Rotate your hand down firmly into the groin area between the genitals and the pelvic bone. This compresses the femoral artery and usually stops the bleeding, when combined with elevation and direct pressure over the bleeding site (**Figure 12.12B**).
4. If the bleeding does not slow immediately, reposition your hand and try again.

Body Substance Isolation and Bleeding Control

Certain communicable diseases such as hepatitis or AIDS can be spread by contact with blood from an infected person. This risk is greatly increased when the infected blood contacts a cut or an open sore on your skin. Although the risk of contracting hepatitis or AIDS through intact skin is small, you should minimize this risk as much as possible by wearing vinyl or latex gloves whenever you might come in contact with a patient's blood or bodily fluids (**Figure 12.13**). Carry your gloves on top of your first responder life support kit or in a pouch on your

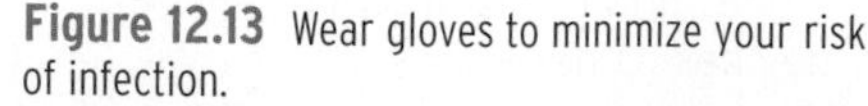

Figure 12.13 Wear gloves to minimize your risk of infection.

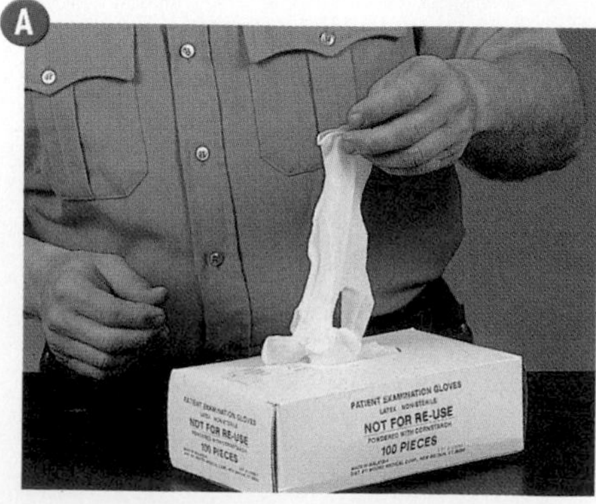

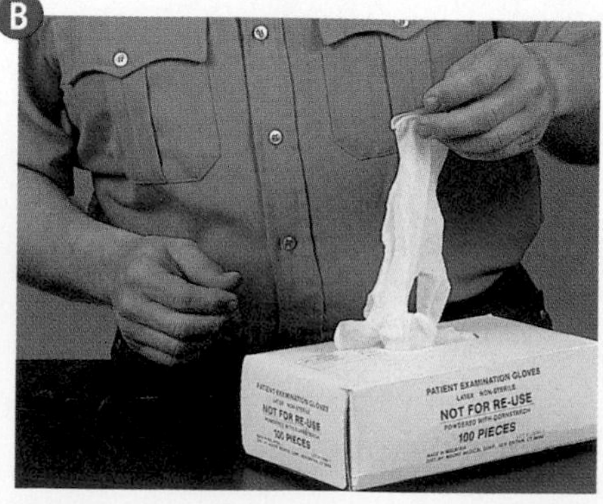

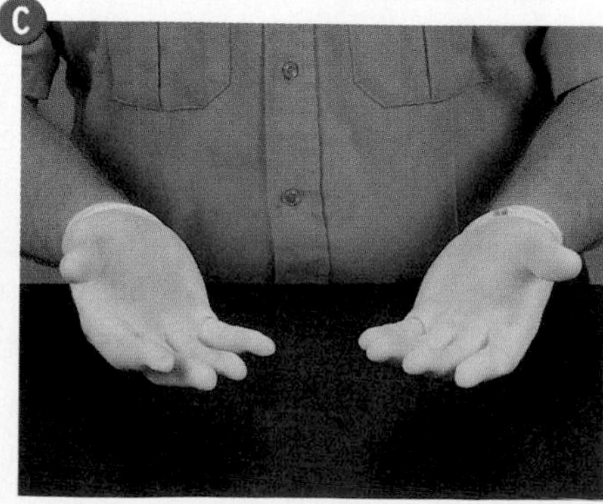

belt for quick access (**Figure 12.14**). If you do get blood on your hands, wash it off as soon as possible with soap and water. If you are in the field and cannot wash your hands, you can use a waterless hand-cleaning solution that contains an effective germ-killing agent.

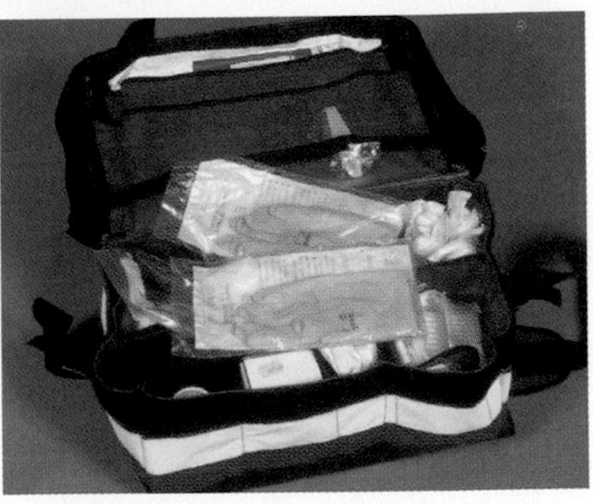

Figure 12.14 Keep your gloves on top in your first responder life support kit.

CAUTION

A word about tourniquets: No!
Tourniquets are mentioned only to discourage their use. A tourniquet is made of a band of material that is placed around an arm or leg above a wound and tightened to stop severe bleeding. Tourniquets are difficult to make from improvised materials. They are also difficult to apply properly. If a tourniquet is applied improperly, it can actually increase bleeding. Tourniquets are almost never needed to control external bleeding. You should concentrate on using a combination of direct pressure, elevation of arms or legs, and pressure points to control bleeding. Be careful not to move the neck or head!

Wounds

A wound is an injury caused by any physical means that leads to damage of a body part. Wounds are classified as closed or open. In a **closed wound**, the skin remains intact; in an **open wound**, the skin is disrupted.

closed wound Injury in which soft-tissue damage occurs beneath the skin but there is no break in the surface of the skin.

open wound Injury that breaks the skin or mucous membrane.

Closed Wounds

The only closed wound is the **bruise** (contusion). A bruise is an injury of the soft-tissue beneath the skin. Because small blood vessels are broken, the injured area becomes discolored and swells. The severity of these closed soft-tissue injuries varies greatly. A simple bruise heals quickly. In contrast, bruising and swelling following an injury may also be a sign of an underlying fracture that could take months to heal. Whenever you encounter a significant amount of swelling or bruising, suspect the possibility of an underlying fracture.

bruise Injury caused by a blunt object striking the body and crushing the tissue beneath the skin. Also called a contusion.

abrasion Loss of skin as a result of a body part being rubbed or scraped across a rough or hard surface.

road rash An abrasion caused by sliding along a highway. Usually seen after motorcycle or bicycle accidents.

Open Wounds

Abrasion

Abrasions are commonly called scrapes, **road rashes**, or rug burns. They occur when the skin is rubbed across a rough surface (**Figure 12.15**).

A

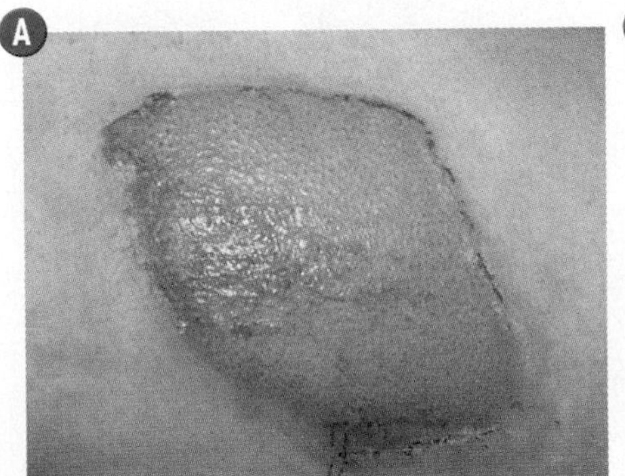

B

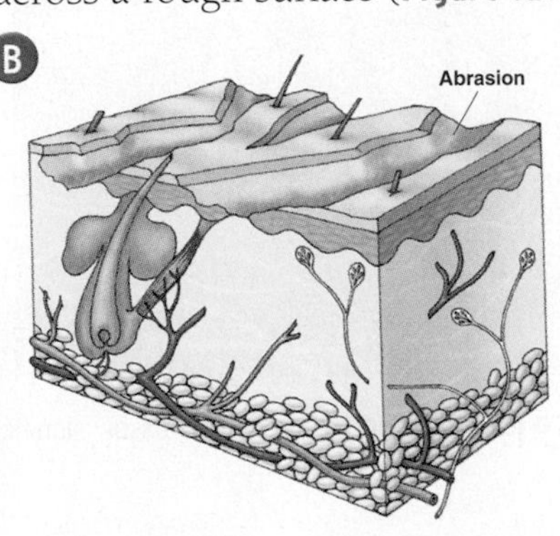

Figure 12.15 Abrasions involve variable depth of the skin; they are often called scrapes or road rashes.

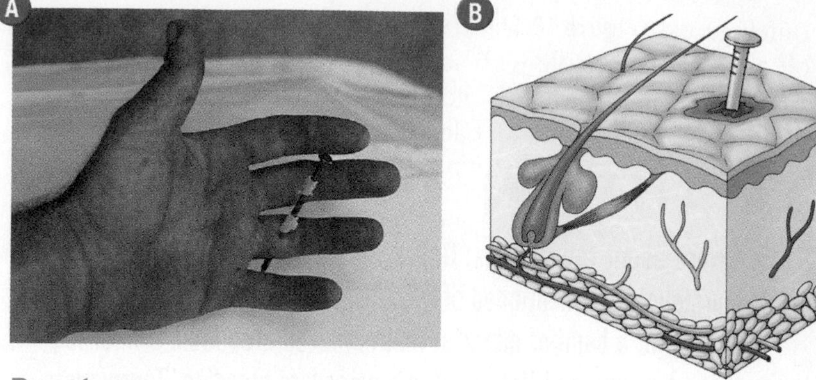

Figure 12.16 Puncture wounds may penetrate the skin to any depth.

puncture A wound resulting from a bullet, knife, ice pick, splinter, or any other pointed object.

impaled object An object such as a knife, splinter of wood, or glass that penetrates the skin and remains in the body.

gunshot wound A puncture wound caused by a bullet or shotgun pellet.

entrance wound Point where an injurious object such as a bullet enters the body.

exit wound Point where an injurious object such as a bullet passes out of the body.

laceration An irregular cut or tear through the skin.

avulsion An injury in which a piece of skin is either torn completely loose from all of its attachments or is left hanging as a flap.

Puncture

Puncture wounds are caused by a sharp object that penetrates the skin (**Figure 12.16**). These wounds may cause significant deep injury that is not immediately recognized. Puncture wounds do not bleed freely. If the object that caused the puncture wound remains sticking out of the skin, it is called an **impaled object**.

A **gunshot wound** is a special type of puncture wound. The amount of damage done by a gunshot depends on the type of gun used and the distance between the gun and the victim. A gunshot wound may appear as an insignificant hole but can do massive damage to internal organs. Some gunshot wounds are smaller than a dime, and some are large enough to destroy significant amounts of tissue. Gunshot wounds usually have both an **entrance wound** and an **exit wound**. The entrance wound is usually smaller than the exit wound. Most deaths from gunshot wounds result from internal blood loss caused by damage to internal organs and major blood vessels as the bullet passes through the body. There is often more than one gunshot wound. A thorough patient examination is important to be sure that you have discovered all of the entrance and exit wounds.

Laceration

The most common type of open wound is a **laceration** (**Figure 12.17**). Lacerations are commonly called cuts. Minor lacerations may require little care, but large lacerations can cause extensive bleeding and even be life-threatening.

Avulsion

An **avulsion** is a tearing away of body tissue (**Figure 12.18**). The avulsed part may be totally severed from the body or it may be attached by a flap

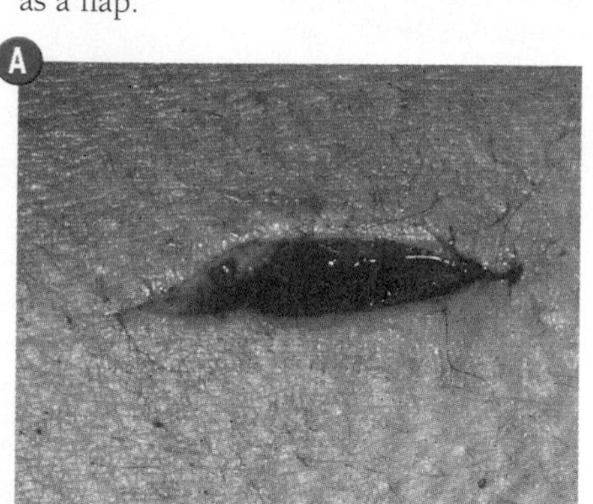

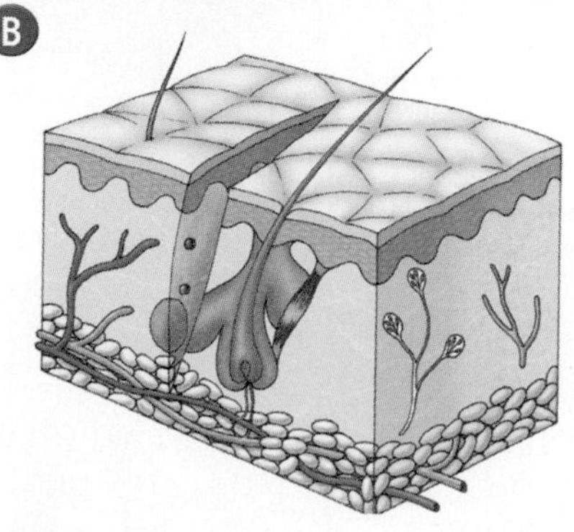

Figure 12.17 Lacerations are cuts produced by sharp objects.

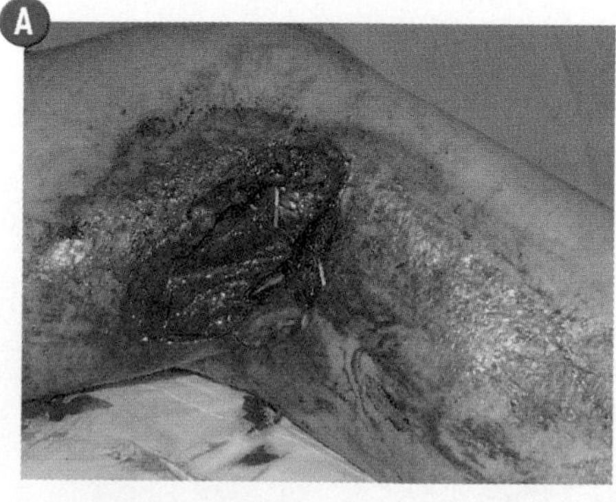

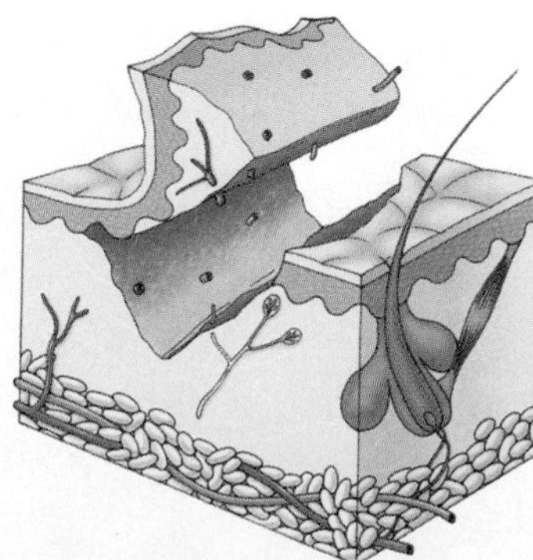

Figure 12.18 Avulsions raise flaps of tissue; significant bleeding is common.

of skin. Avulsions may involve small or large amounts of tissue. If an entire body part is torn away, the wound is called a traumatic amputation (**Figure 12.19**). Any amputated body part should be located, placed in a clean plastic bag, kept cool, and taken with the patient to the hospital for possible reattachment (reimplantation). If a clean plastic bag is not available, you can use a surgical glove turned inside out. Cold pacs or iced water can be used to keep the detached body parts cold.

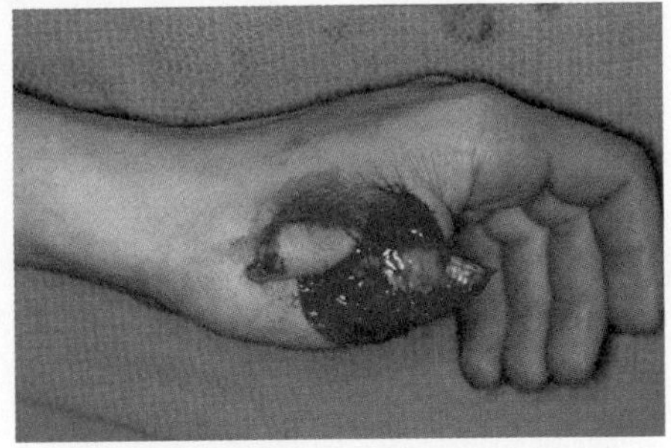

Figure 12.19 An amputated thumb. Amputated parts can often be reattached. You should attempt to locate the part and transport it to the hospital with the patient.

Principles of Wound Treatment

Very minor bruises need no treatment. Other closed wounds should be treated by applying ice and gentle compression, and by elevating the injured part. Because extensive bruising may indicate an underlying fracture, all contusions should be **splinted**. (See Chapter 13.)

splinting Immobilizing an injured part by using a rigid or soft support splint.

immobilize To reduce or prevent movement of a limb, usually by splinting.

The major principles of open-wound treatment are to:

- Control bleeding
- Prevent further contamination of the wound
- **Immobilize** the injured part
- Stabilize any impaled object

It is important to stop bleeding as quickly as possible using the cleanest dressing available. You can usually control bleeding by covering an open wound with a dry, clean, or sterile dressing and applying pressure to the dressing with your hand. If the first dressing does not control the bleeding, reinforce it with a second layer. Additional ways to control bleeding include elevating an extremity and using pressure points.

A dressing should cover the entire wound to prevent further contamination. Do not attempt to clean the contaminated wound in the field, because cleaning will only cause more bleeding. A thorough cleaning will be done at the hospital. All dressings should be secured in place by a compression bandage.

Learning to dress and bandage wounds requires practice. As a trained first responder, you should be able to bandage all parts of the body quickly and competently (**Figure 12.20**).

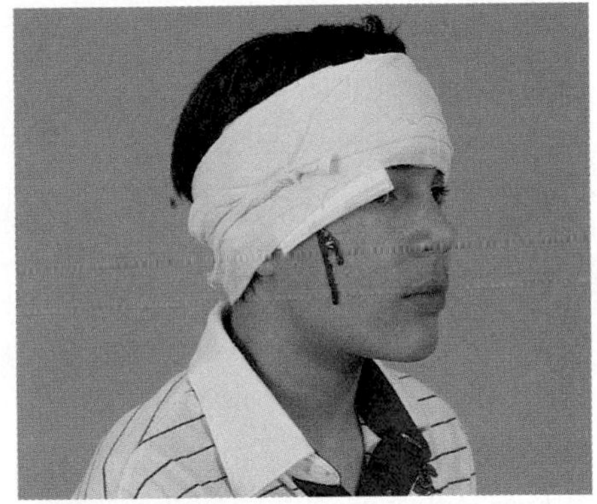

Figure 12.20 Head bandage.

Dressing and Bandaging Wounds

Dressing and bandaging are done to:

- Control bleeding
- Prevent further contamination
- Immobilize the injured area
- Prevent movement of impaled objects

Dressings

A dressing is an object placed directly on a wound to control bleeding and prevent further contamination. Once a dressing is in place, apply firm direct manual pressure on it to stop the bleeding. It is important to stop severe bleeding as quickly as possible using the cleanest dressing

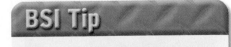

BSI Tip

Direct exposure to blood must be reported to the emergency physician.

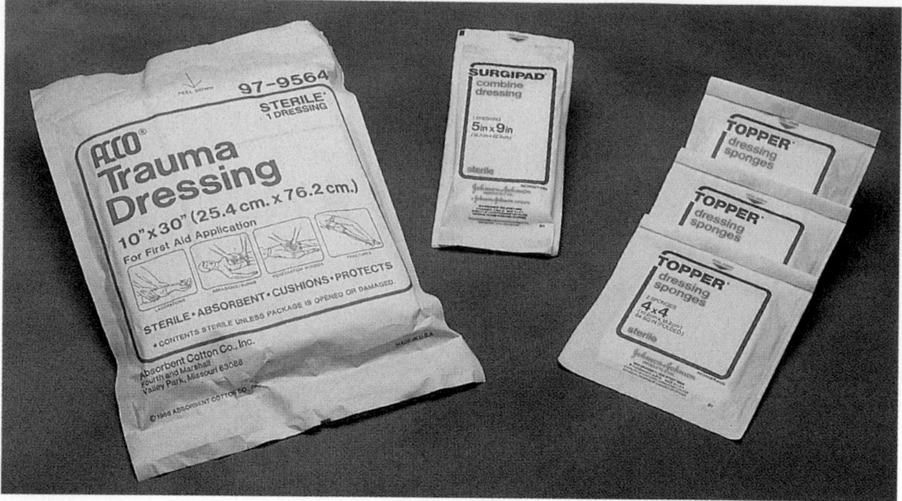

Figure 12.21 Common sizes of wound dressings are 10 inches x 30 inches, 5 inches x 9 inches and 4 inches x 4 inches.

available. If no equipment is available, you may have to apply direct pressure with your hand to a wound that is bleeding extensively, even though you should normally wear gloves.

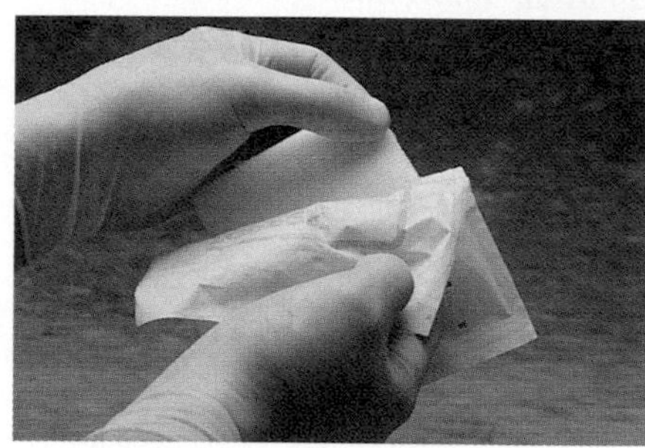

Figure 12.22 Open the package containing a sterile dressing carefully.

Sterile dressings come packaged in many different sizes. Three of the most common sizes are 4 inches by 4 inches gauze squares (commonly known as 4x4s). Heavier pads measure 5 inches by 9 inches (5x9s). A trauma dressing is a thick sterile dressing that measures 10 inches by 30 inches. Use a trauma dressing to cover a large wound on the abdomen, neck, thigh, or scalp—or as padding for splints (**Figure 12.21**).

When you open a package containing a sterile dressing, touch only one corner of the dressing (**Figure 12.22**). Place it on the wound without touching the side of the dressing that will be next to the wound. If bleeding continues after you have applied a compression dressing to the wound, put additional gauze pads over the original dressing. Do not remove the original dressing because the blood-clotting process will have already started and should not be disrupted.

When you are satisfied that the wound is sufficiently dressed, proceed to bandage.

Improvise

If commercially prepared dressings are not available, use the cleanest cloth object available, such as a clean handkerchief, wash cloth, disposable diaper, or article of clothing (**Figure 12.23**).

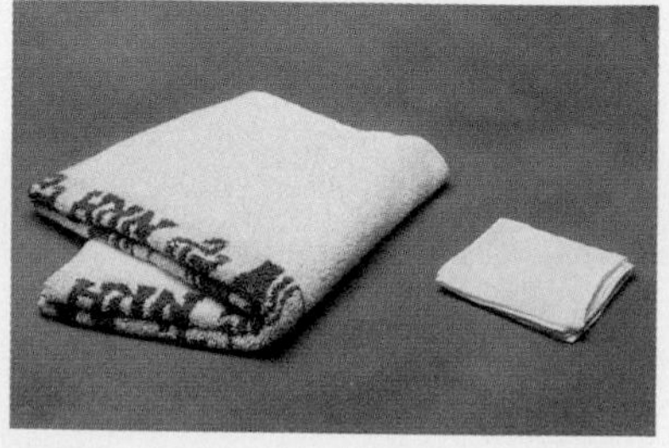

Figure 12.23 Improvised dressings may include a towel or clean handerchief.

Bandaging

A bandage is used to hold the dressing in place. Two types of bandages commonly used in the field are roller gauze and triangular bandages. The first type, conforming roller gauze, stretches slightly and is easy to wrap around the body part (**Figure 12.24**). Triangular bandages are usually 36 inches across (**Figure 12.25**). A triangular bandage can be folded and

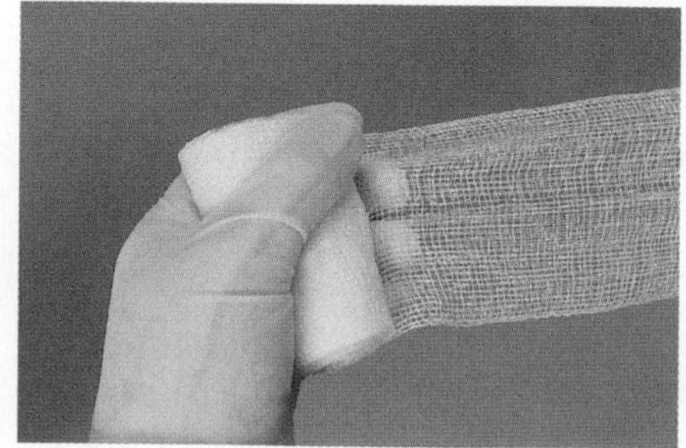

Figure 12.24 Roller gauze bandage.

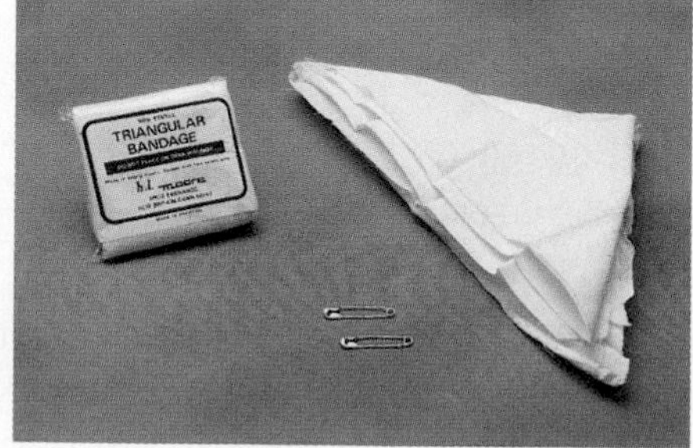

Figure 12.25 Triangular bandage.

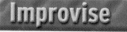

used as a wide **cravat**, or it can be used without folding (**Figure 12.26**). Roller gauze is easier to apply and stays in place better than a triangular bandage, but a triangular bandage is very useful for bandaging scalp lacerations and lacerations of the chest, back, or thigh.

cravat A triangular swathe of cloth that is used to hold a body part splinted against the body.

You must follow certain principles if the bandage is to hold the dressing in place, control bleeding, and prevent further contamination. Before you apply a bandage, check to ensure that the dressing completely covers the wound and extends beyond all sides of the wound (**Figure 12.27**). Wrap the bandage just tightly enough to control bleeding. Do not apply it too tightly because it may cut off all circulation. It is important to regularly check circulation at a point further away from the heart than the injury itself because swelling may make the bandage too tight. If this happens while the patient is under your care, remove the roller gauze or triangular bandage and reapply it, making sure that you do not disturb the dressing beneath.

Once bandaging is complete, secure the bandage so it cannot slip. Tape, tie or tuck in any loose ends. Figures 12.29 through 12.36 show how to dress and bandage wounds of various parts of the body. Practice these bandaging techniques for several types of wounds using both roller gauze and triangular bandages. Although the principles of bandaging are simple, some parts of the body are difficult to bandage. It is important to practice bandaging different parts of the body, to assure competency in emergency situations.

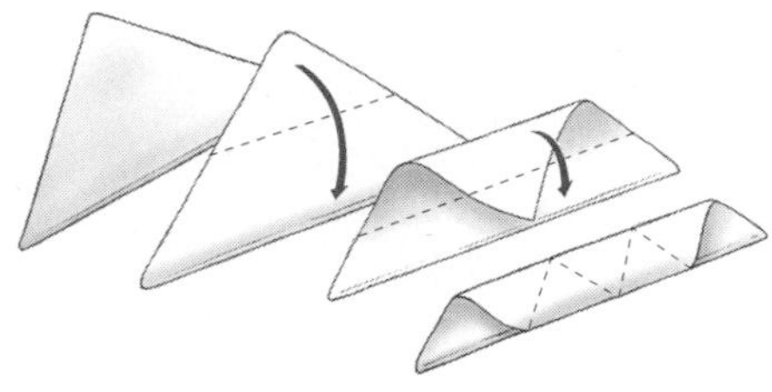

Figure 12.26 Folding a triangular bandage to make a cravat.

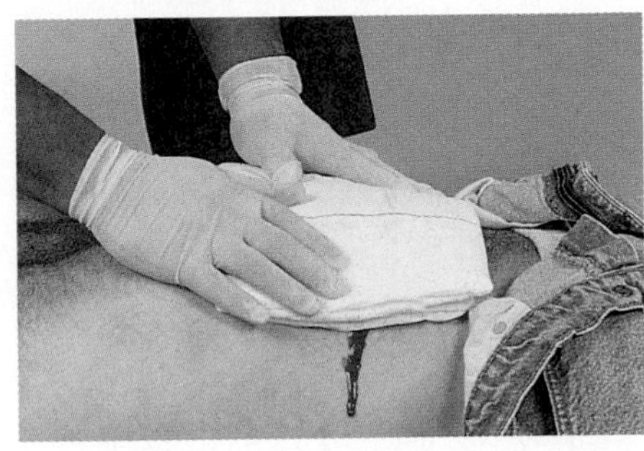

Figure 12.27 Check to make sure the dressing completely covers the wound.

Body Substance Isolation Techniques for the First Responder

Some infectious disease organisms, including the hepatitis and AIDS viruses, can be transmitted if blood from an infected person enters the bloodstream of a healthy person through a small cut or opening in the skin. Because you may have such a cut, it is important that you wear gloves to avoid contact with patients' blood (**Figure 12.28**). Using gloves also protects wounds from being contaminated by dirt or infectious organisms you may have on your hands. Vinyl or latex medical gloves can be stored on the top of your first responder life support kit or in a pouch on your belt, where they will be readily available. (See Chapter 2 for more information on infectious diseases.)

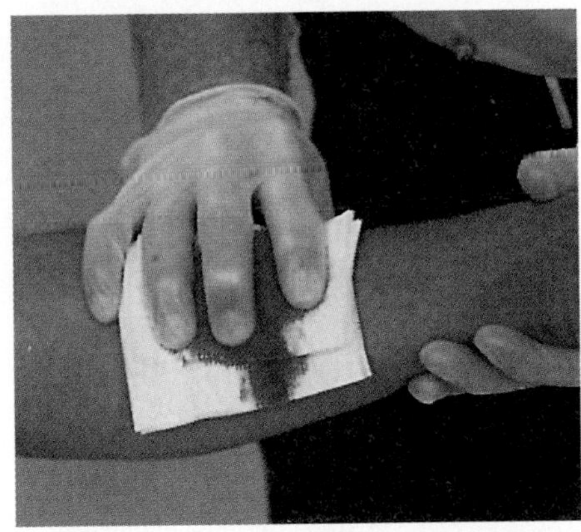

Figure 12.28 Always wear gloves when in contact with body fluids.

Specific Wound Treatment

FYI

Face and Scalp Wounds

The face and scalp have many blood vessels. Because of this generous blood supply, a relatively small laceration can result in a large amount of bleeding. Although face and scalp lacerations may not be life threatening, they are always bloody and cause much anxiety for the patient and the first responder.

You can control almost all facial or scalp bleeding by applying direct manual pressure. Direct pressure is effective because the bones of the skull are so close to the skin. Direct pressure compresses the blood vessels against the skull and stops the bleeding. If bleeding continues, do not remove the dressing. Instead, reinforce it with a second layer

BSI Tip

Providing for your own safety and that of patients is always a high priority when you are examining and treating open wounds.

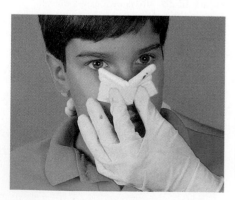

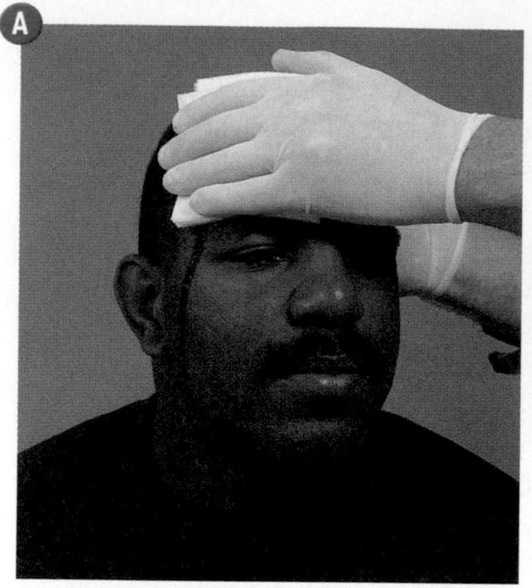

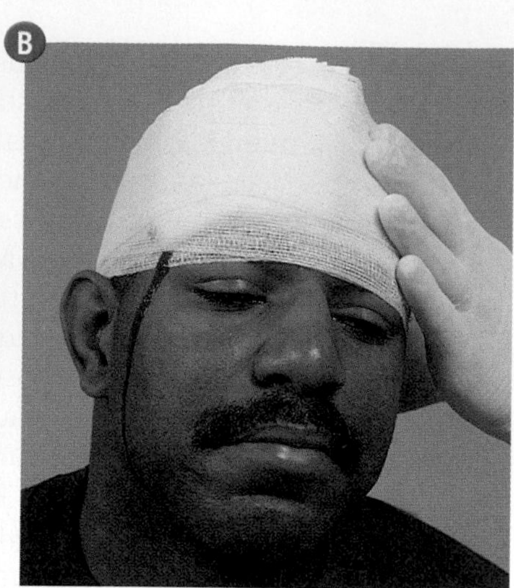

Figure 12.29 Bandaging a head wound. **A.** Apply direct pressure until bleeding stops. **B.** Wrap the head with a bandage.

and continue to apply manual pressure. After the bleeding stops, wrap the head with a bandage (**Figure 12.29**).

For wounds inside the cheek, hold a gauze pad inside the cheek (in the mouth). If necessary, you can also apply a pad outside the cheek. Always keep the airway open.

Severe scalp lacerations may be associated with skull fractures or even brain injury. If any brain tissue or bone fragments are visible, do not apply pressure to the wound. Instead, cover the wound loosely, being careful not to exert direct pressure on the brain or the bone fragments.

If the patient has a head injury, the neck and spine may also be injured. Move the head as little as possible and stabilize the neck. (Treatment of spinal injuries is discussed in Chapter 13.) In cases of head injury, always evaluate the patient's level of consciousness. Carefully monitor the patient's airway and breathing and protect the spine.

Note: Any patient you think may have high blood pressure must be evaluated in the hospital.

Nosebleeds

Nosebleeds can result from injury or high blood pressure. In some cases, there is no apparent cause. A nosebleed with no apparent cause is called a **spontaneous nosebleed**. In a patient with high blood pressure, increased pressure in the small blood vessels of the nose may cause one to rupture, resulting in bleeding. A patient with high blood pressure should be seen and treated by a physician.

spontaneous nosebleed A nosebleed with no apparent cause.

Most nosebleeds can be controlled easily. Unless the patient is suffering from shock, seat the person and tilt the head slightly forward. This position keeps the blood from dripping down the throat. Swallowing blood may cause coughing or vomiting, and make the nosebleed worse.

After the patient is seated correctly, pinch both nostrils together for at least five minutes. The patient may wish to do this without assistance. This treatment usually controls nosebleeds (**Figure 12.30**). If a nosebleed persists or is very severe, arrange to have the patient transported to an appropriate medical facility. Instruct the patient to avoid blowing his or her nose because this will often cause additional bleeding.

Figure 12.30 Pinch nostrils together to control a nosebleed.

Eye Injuries

All eye injuries are potentially serious and require medical evaluation. When an eye laceration is suspected, cover the entire eye with a dry gauze pad. Have the patient lie on his or her back and arrange for ***transport*** to an appropriate medical facility.

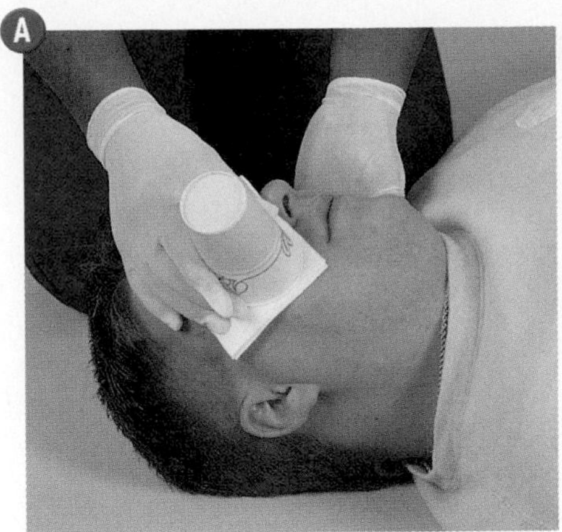

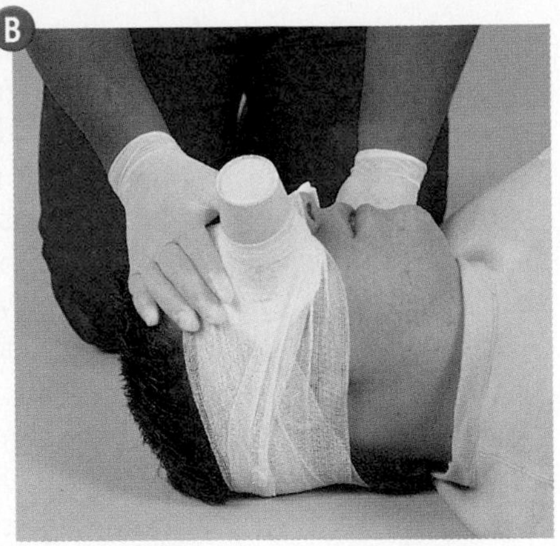

Figure 12.31 Bandaging an eye impaled by an object. **A.** Use a cup to cover an impaled object. **B.** Bandage both eyes to minimize eye movement.

Occasionally an object will be impaled in the eye. Immediately place the patient on his or her back and cover the injured eye with a dressing and a paper cup so the impaled object cannot move. Bandage both eyes. This is important because both eyes move together, and if the patient attempts to look at something with the uninjured eye, the injured eye will move also, aggravating the injury (**Figure 12.31**). Arrange for *transport* of the patient to the hospital.

Note: Whenever you must bandage both eyes, explain to the patient why you are doing so. Having both eyes covered can be very distressing. Stay with the patient to help reassure him or her.

Neck Wounds

The neck contains many important structures: the trachea, the esophagus, large arteries, veins, muscles, vertebrae, and the spinal cord. Because an injury to any of these structures may be life threatening, all neck injuries are serious.

Use direct pressure to control bleeding neck wounds. Once bleeding is controlled, bandage the neck (**Figure 12.32**). In rare cases, you may have to exert finger pressure above and below the injury site to prevent further neck bleeding.

Always keep in mind that major trauma to the neck may be associated with airway problems and with neck fracture or spinal cord injury. Therefore, maintain the patient's airway and stabilize the head and neck.

Chest Wounds and Back Wounds

The major organs affected by chest wounds and back wounds are the lungs, large blood vessels, and heart. Any wound involving these organs is a life-threatening injury. Place the patient with a chest injury in a comfortable position (usually sitting). (See Chapter 13.)

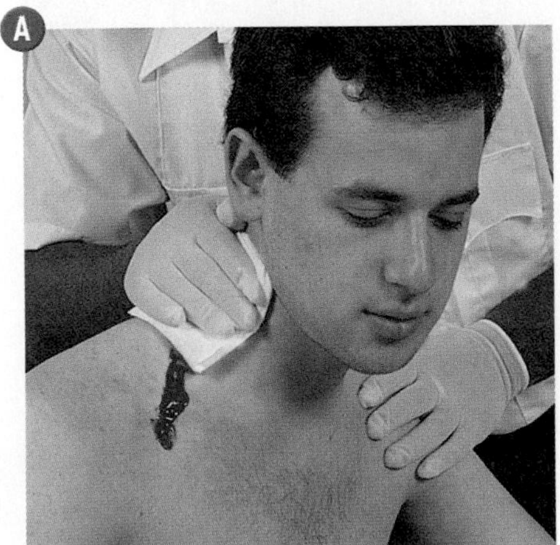

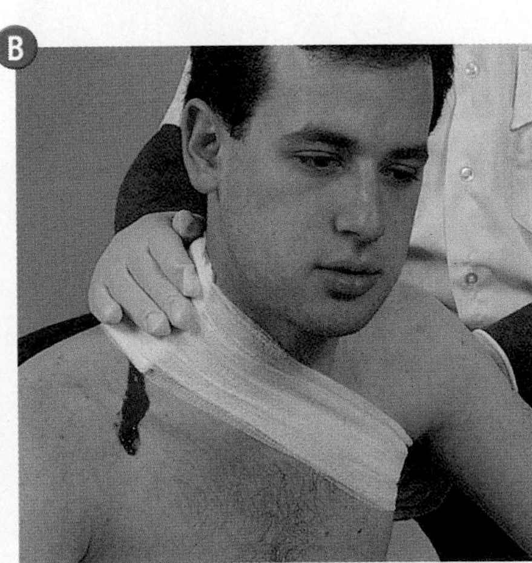

Figure 12.32 Bandaging a neck wound. **A.** Place dressing over wound. **B.** Place bandage over wound and under the arm on the opposite side.

Improvise

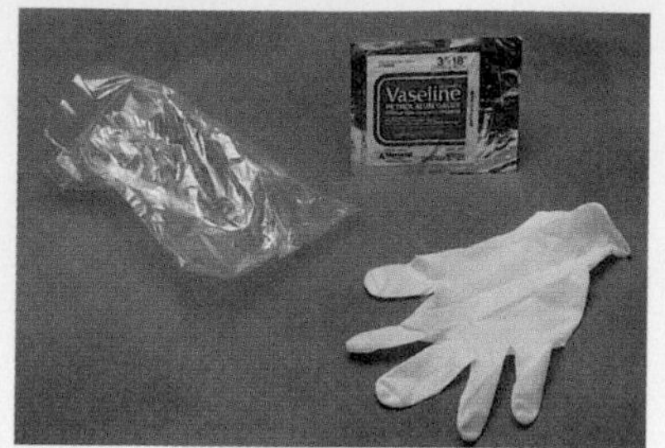

Figure 12.33 For occlusive dressings, use plastic, petroleum jelly, or gloves.

If a lung is punctured, air can escape, and the lung will collapse. The patient may cough up bright red blood. To help maintain air pressure in the lung, your first act should be to cover any open chest wound with airtight material, sealing it. This covering is called an **occlusive dressing**. Use a clear plastic cover from your medical supplies, aluminum foil, plastic wrap, or a special dressing that has been impregnated with petroleum jelly (Vaseline™). Any material that will occlude (seal off) the wound is sufficient (**Figure 12.33**).

Administering oxygen is important early treatment for an injured lung. It should be given by EMS personnel when they arrive or by first responders who are trained and have the equipment available.

Chest wounds may also damage the heart. Seal the wound in the manner described. Monitor the patient's airway, breathing, and circulation. Treat the patient for shock and perform CPR, if necessary.

occlusive dressing An airtight dressing or bandage for a wound.

Impaled Objects

If an object is impaled in the patient, apply a stabilizing dressing and arrange for the patient's immediate and Ⓣ ***prompt transport*** to an appropriate medical facility. Sometimes an impaled object is too long to permit the patient to be removed from the accident scene and transported to an appropriate medical facility. In these cases, it may be necessary to stabilize the impaled object and carefully cut it close to the patient's body. If you encounter a situation like this, stabilize the impaled object as well as you can and immediately request a specialized rescue team that has the tools and training to handle such a situation.

If you find the patient with a knife or other object protruding from the abdomen, do not attempt to remove it. Instead, support the impaled object so it cannot move. Place a large roll of gauze on either side of the object and secure the rolls with additional gauze wrapped around the body. It is important to stabilize the object so it will not move while the patient is being transported to the hospital (**Figure 12.34**). Any movement of the object may cause further internal damage.

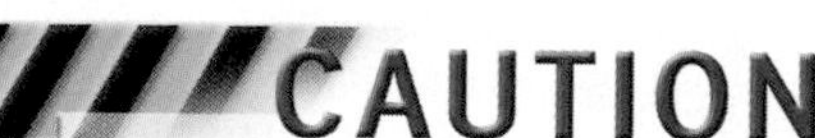

Never remove an impaled object.

Figure 12.34 Bandaging an impaled object. **A.** Do not attempt to remove or move an impaled object. **B.** Stabilize the object in place with dressings. **C.** Place a bandage over the dressings.

A

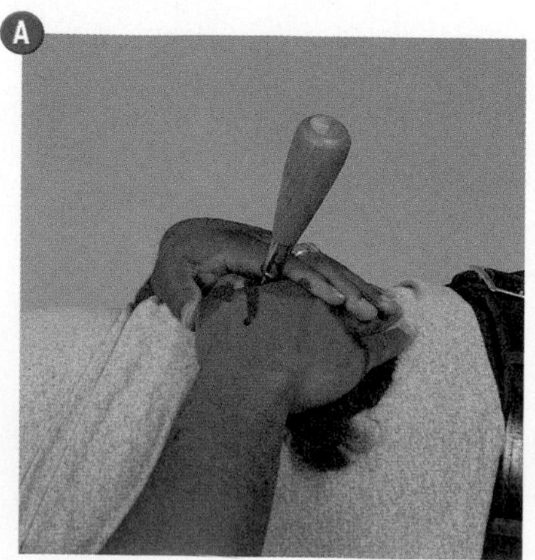

B

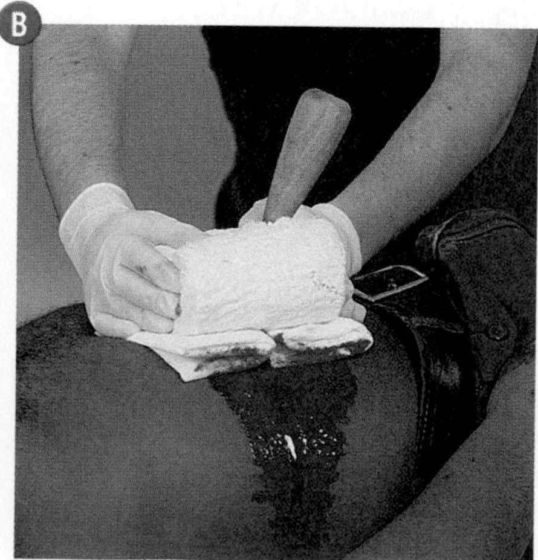

C

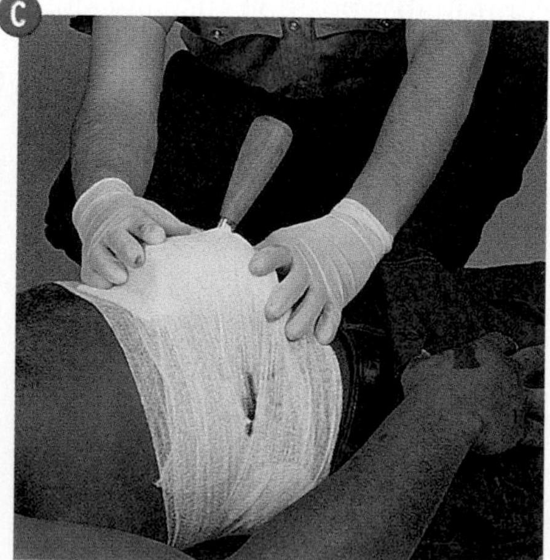

FYI

Closed Abdominal Wounds

Closed abdominal wounds commonly occur as the result of a direct blow from a blunt object. You should check for a closed abdominal wound whenever force has been applied to the abdomen. Look for bruises or other marks on the abdomen that indicate blunt injury.

Any time an injured patient is suffering from shock, you should remember that there may be internal abdominal injuries accompanied by bleeding. When there is internal bleeding, the abdomen may become swollen, rigid, or hard like a board.

Treat patients with closed abdominal injuries and signs of shock by placing them on their backs and elevating their legs at least six inches (unless they are having difficulty breathing). Conserve their body heat.

If the patient is vomiting blood (ranging in color from bright red to dark brown), it may be an indication of bleeding from the esophagus or stomach. Monitor the patient's vital functions carefully because shock may result. Give the patient nothing by mouth. Arrange for T ***prompt transport*** to an appropriate medical facility.

Open Abdominal Wounds

Open abdominal wounds usually result from slashing with a knife or other sharp object and are always serious injuries.

To treat an open abdominal wound follow these steps:

1. Apply a dry, sterile dressing to the wound.
2. Maintain the patient's body temperature.
3. Place the patient on his or her back with the legs elevated.
4. Place the patient who is having difficulty breathing in a semireclining position.
5. Administer oxygen, if it is available, and you are trained to administer it.

If the intestines are protruding from the abdomen, place the patient on his or her back with the knees bent, to relax the abdominal muscles. Cover the injured area with a sterile dressing (**Figure 12.35**). Do not attempt to replace the intestines inside the abdomen.

You can make a bandage to cover intestines protruding from the abdomen from a large trauma pad (10 inches x 30 inches) and several cravats. Position the trauma pad to cover the whole area of the wound. Tie two or three wide cravats loosely over the trauma pad, just tightly

Figure 12.35 Bandaging an open abdominal wound. **A.** Open abdominal wounds are serious injuries. **B.** Cover with a moist, sterile dressing or occlusive dressing, depending on local protocol. **C.** Secure the dressing.

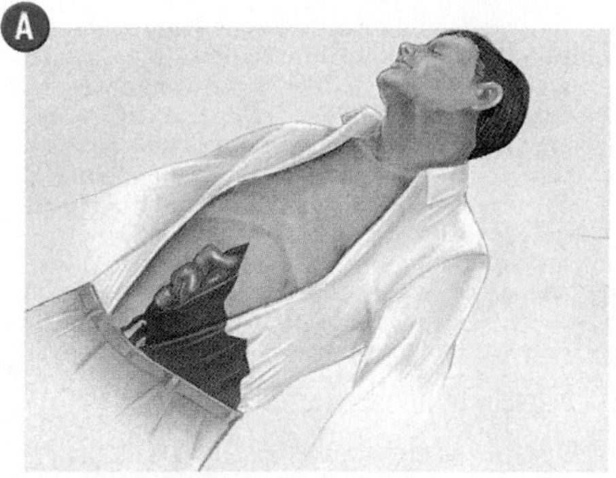

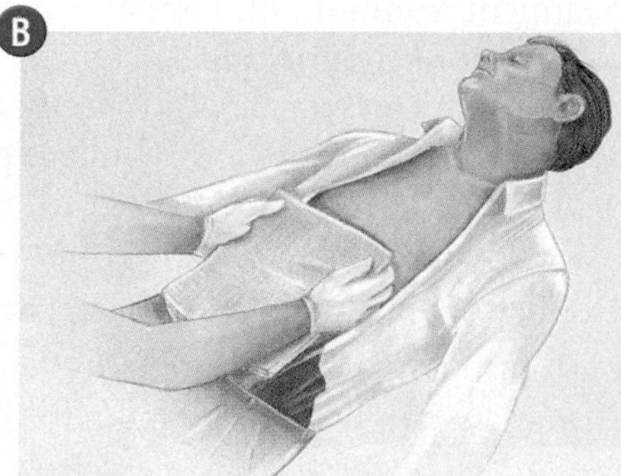

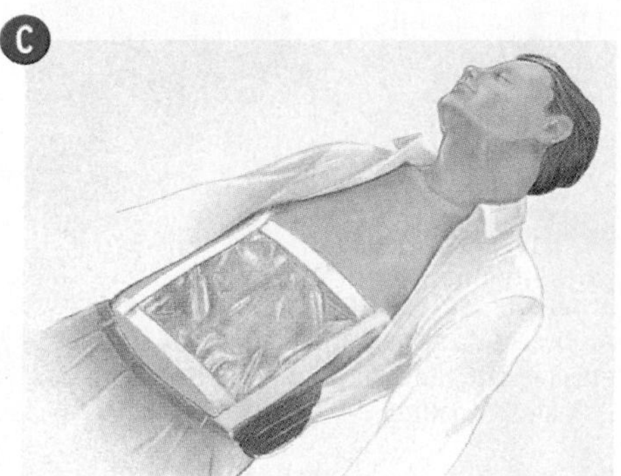

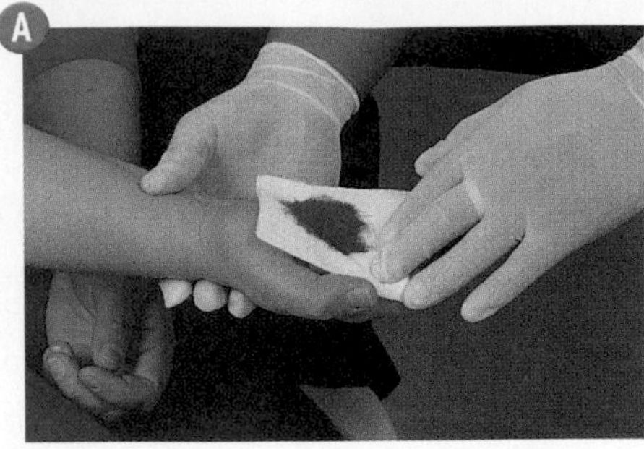
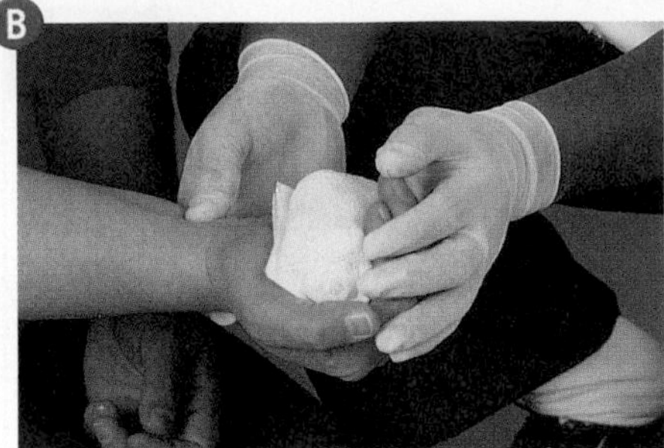
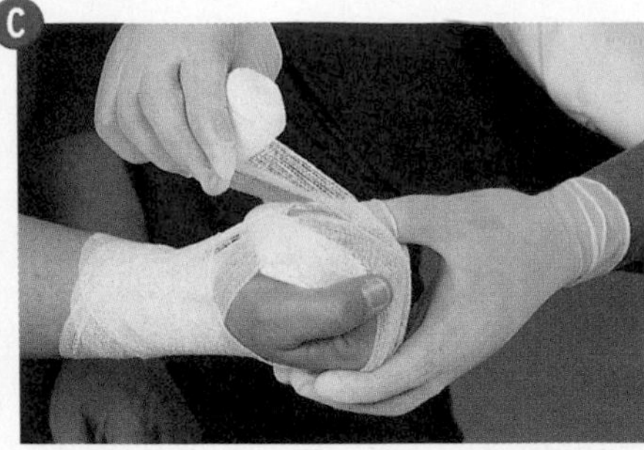

Figure 12.36 Bandaging a hand wound. A. Place a dressing over the wound. B. Place a gauze roll in the palm of the hand to apply pressure. C. Secure the dressing with a gauze roller bandage.

enough to keep it firmly in place, but not tightly enough to push the intestines back into the abdomen.

EMTs and paramedics carry sterile **saline** (salt water), which can be poured on the dressing to keep the protruding organs moist so they do not dry out. Only sterile saline should be used.

saline Salt water.

FYI

Genital Wounds

Both male and female genitals have a rich blood supply. Injury to the genitals can often result in severe bleeding. Apply direct pressure to any genital wound with a dry, sterile dressing. Direct pressure usually stops the bleeding. Although it may be embarrassing to examine the patient's genital area to determine the severity of the injury, you must do so if you suspect such injuries. The patient can suffer a critical loss of blood if you do not find the injury and control the bleeding.

Extremity Wounds

To treat all open extremity wounds, apply a dry, sterile compression dressing and bandage it securely in place (**Figures 12.36** and **12.37**). Elevating the injured part decreases bleeding and swelling. You should splint all injured extremities prior to transport because there may be an underlying fracture.

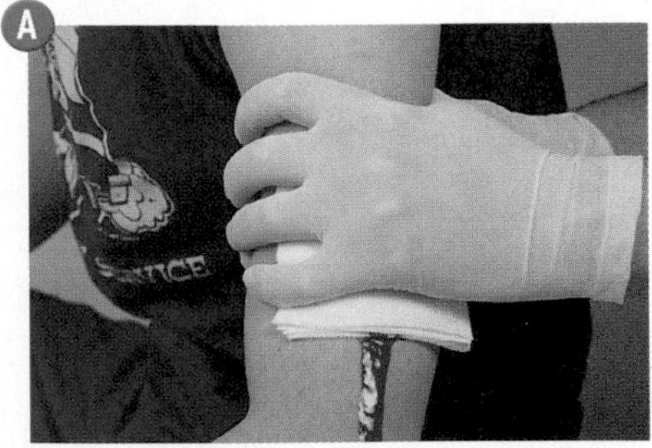
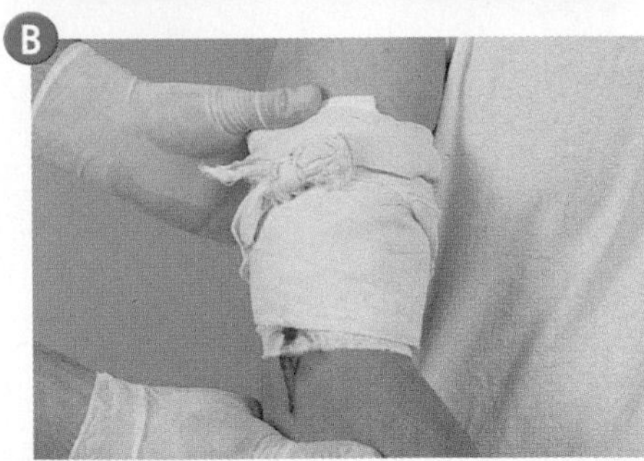
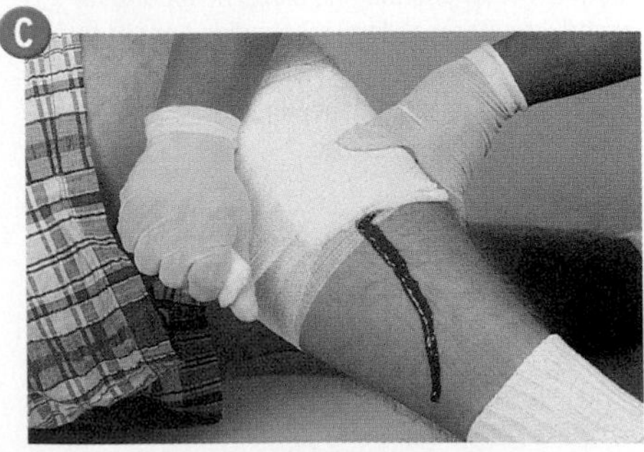

Figure 12.37 Bandaging an extremity wound. A. Place a dressing over the wound B. Secure the dressing with a cravat C. Secure the dressing with a roller gauze.

Gunshot Wounds

Some gunshot wounds are easy to miss unless you perform a thorough patient examination (**Figure 12.38**). Most deaths from gunshot wounds result from internal blood loss caused by damage to internal organs and major blood vessels. Because gunshot wounds are so serious, prompt and effective treatment is important. Gunshot wounds of the trunk and neck are a major cause of spinal cord injuries. Because you cannot see the bullet's path through the body, you should treat these patients for spinal cord injuries.

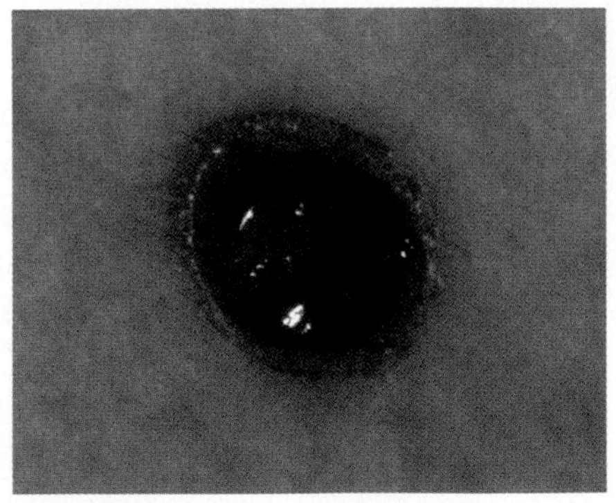

Figure 12.38 Bullet entry wound.

To treat a gunshot wound, follow these steps:

1. Open the airway and establish adequate ventilation and circulation.
2. Control any external bleeding by covering wounds with sterile dressings and applying pressure with your hand or a bandage.

3. Examine the patient thoroughly to be sure you have discovered all entrance and exit wounds.
4. Treat for symptoms of shock by:
   a. Maintaining the patient's body temperature.
   b. Placing the patient on his or her back with the legs elevated 6 inches.
   c. Placing a patient who is having difficulty breathing in a semireclining position.
   d. Administering oxygen, if available.
5. Arrange for **T** ***prompt transportation*** of the patient to an appropriate medical facility.
6. Perform CPR if the patient's heart stops as a result of loss of blood.

Bites

Bites from animals or humans may range from minor to severe. All bites have a high chance of causing infection. Bites from an unvaccinated animal may cause **rabies**. Minor bites can be washed with soap and water, if it is available. Major bite wounds should be treated by controlling the bleeding and applying a suitable dressing and bandage.

All patients who have been bitten by an animal or another person must be treated by a physician. In most states, EMS personnel are required to report animal bites to the local health department or a law enforcement agency. You should check the laws in your local area to determine requirements.

rabies An acute viral infection of the central nervous system transmitted by the bite of an infected animal.

superficial burns Burns in which only the superficial part of the skin has been injured; an example is a sunburn.

- List and describe the four principles of wound treatment.

Burns

The skin serves as a barrier that prevents foreign substances, such as bacteria, from entering the body. It also prevents the loss of body fluids. When the skin is damaged, such as by a burn, it can no longer perform these essential functions.

Burn Depth

There are three classifications of burns by depth: superficial (first-degree) burns, partial-thickness (second-degree) burns, and full-thickness (third-degree) burns. Although it is not always possible to determine the exact degree of a burn injury, it is important for you to understand this concept.

Superficial burns (first-degree burns) are characterized by reddened and painful skin. The injury is confined to the outermost layers of skin, and the patient experiences minor to moderate pain. An example of a superficial burn is a sunburn, which usually heals in about a week, with or without treatment (**Figure 12.39**).

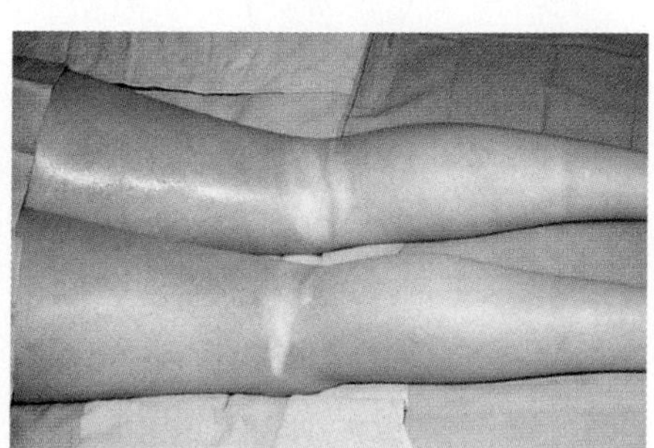

Figure 12.39 Superficial, or first-degree burn

CHARACTERISTICS FOR BURN CLASSIFICATION

- *Depth*
- *Extent (amount of the body injured by the burn)*
- *Cause or type*

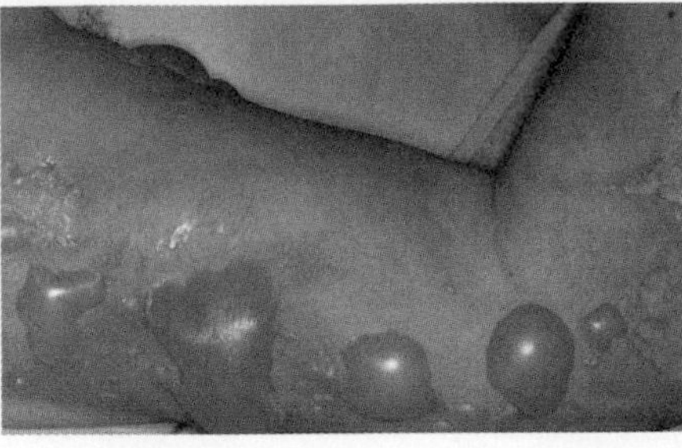

Figure 12.40 Partial-thickness, or second-degree burn.

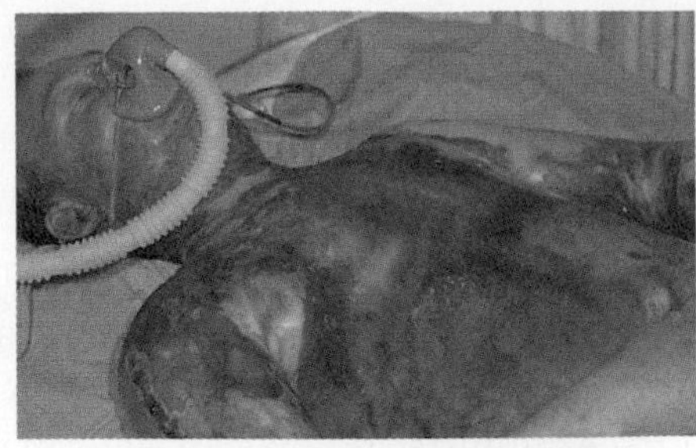

Figure 12.41 Full-thickness, or third-degree burn.

partial-thickness burns Burns in which the outer layers of skin are burned; these burns are characterized by blister formation.

full-thickness burns Burns that extend through the skin and into or beyond the underlying tissues; the most serious class of burn.

Rule of Nines A way to calculate the amount of body surface burned; the body is divided into sections, each of which constitutes approximately 9 percent or 18 percent of the total body surface area.

Partial-thickness burns (second-degree burns) are somewhat deeper but do not damage the deepest layers of the skin (**Figure 12.40**). Blistering is present, although blisters may not form for several hours in some cases. There may be some fluid loss and moderate to severe pain because the nerve endings are damaged. Partial-thickness burns require medical treatment. They usually heal within two to three weeks.

Full-thickness burns (third-degree burns) damage all layers of the skin. In some cases the damage is deep enough to injure and destroy underlying muscles and other tissues (**Figure 12.41**). Pain is often absent because the nerve endings have been destroyed. Without the protection provided by the skin, patients with extensive full-thickness burns lose large quantities of body fluids and are susceptible to shock and infection.

Extent of Burns

FYI

The **Rule of Nines** is a method for determining what percentage of the body has been burned. Although this rule is most useful for EMTs and paramedics who report information to the hospital from the field, first responders should be able to roughly estimate the extent of a burn.

Figure 12.42 shows how the Rule of Nines divides the body. In an adult, the head and arms each equal 9 percent of the total body surface. The front and back of the trunk and each leg are equal to 18 percent of the total body surface.

For example, if one-half of the back and all of the right arm of a patient are burned, the burn involves about 18 percent of the total body area. The Rule of Nines is slightly modified for young children, but the adult figures serve as an adequate guide.

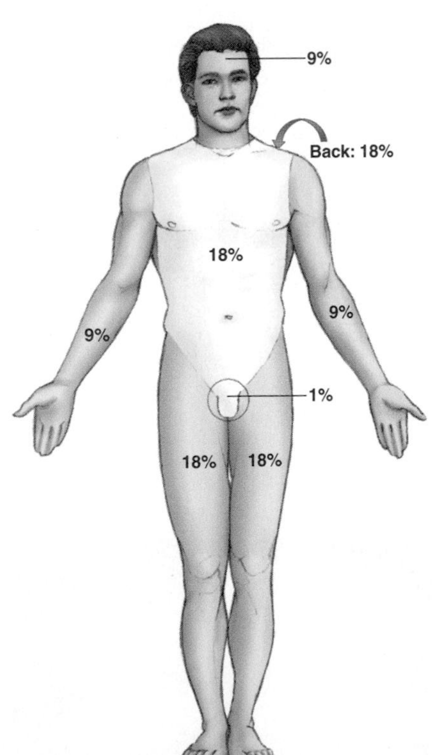

Figure 12.42 Use the Rule of Nines to determine the extent of burns.

Cause or Type of Burns

Burns are caused by exposure to the following elements:

- Heat (thermal burns)
- Chemicals
- Electricity

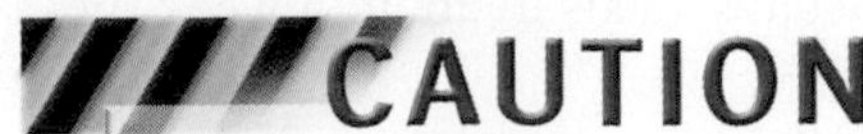

Do not apply burn ointments, butter, grease, or cream to any burn!

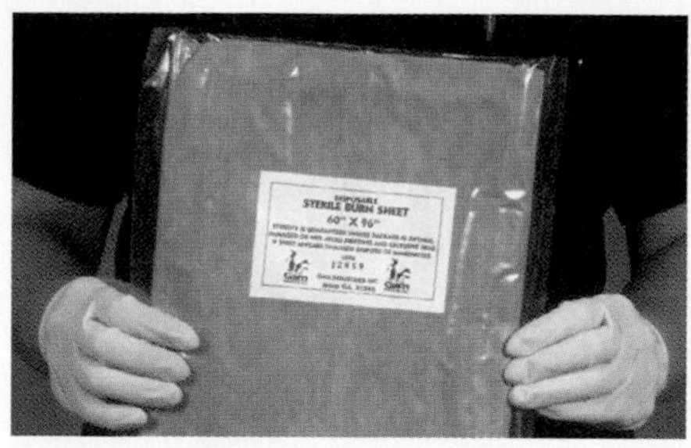

Figure 12.43 Sterile burn sheet.

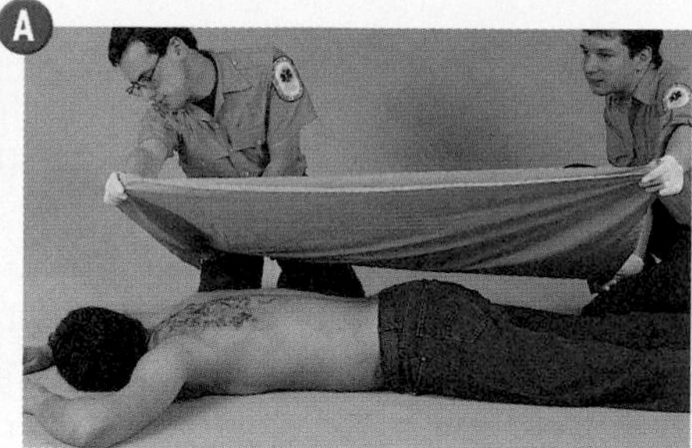

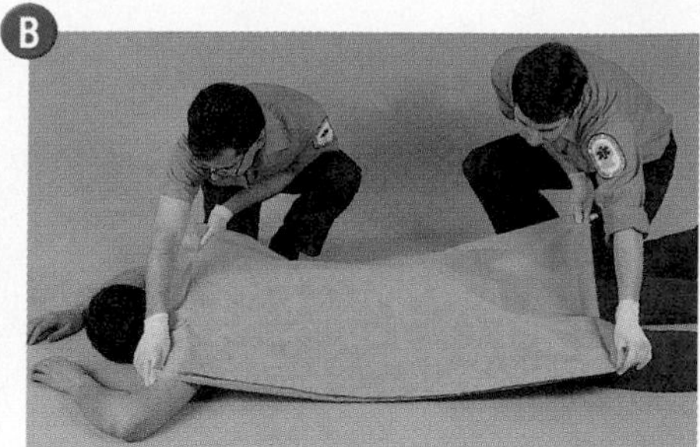

Figure 12.44 Applying a sterile burn sheet.

Thermal Burns

thermal burns Burns caused by heat; the most common type of burn.

respiratory burns Burns to the respiratory system resulting from inhaling superheated air.

chemical burns Burns that occur when any toxic substance comes in contact with the skin. Most chemical burns are caused by strong acids or alkalis.

Thermal burns are caused by heat. The first step in treating thermal burns is to cool the skin by "putting out the fire." Superficial burns can be quite painful, but if there is clean, cold water available, you can place the burning area in cold water to help reduce the pain. You can also wet a clean towel with cold water and put it on superficial burns. After the burned area is cooled, cover it with a dry, sterile dressing or the large sterile cloth (found in your first responder life support kit) called a burn sheet (**Figure 12.43**).

Partial-thickness burns should be cooled if the burn area is still warm. Cooling helps reduce pain, stops the heat from cooking the skin, and helps stop the swelling caused by partial-thickness burns.

If blisters are present, be very careful not to break the blisters. Intact skin, even if blistered, provides an excellent barrier against infection. If the blisters break, the danger of infection increases. Cover partial-thickness burns with a dry, sterile dressing or burn sheet.

Full-thickness burns, if still warm, should also be cooled with water to keep the heat from damaging more skin and tissue. Cut any clothing away from the burned area, but leave any clothing that is stuck to the burn. Cover full-thickness burns with a dry, sterile dressing or burn sheet (**Figure 12.44**).

Patients with large superficial burns or any partial-thickness or full-thickness burns must be treated for shock and transported to a hospital.

Respiratory Burns

FYI

A burn to any part of the airway is a **respiratory burn**. If a patient has been burned around the head and face or while in a confined space (such as in a burning house), you should look for the signs and symptoms of respiratory burns, listed in the box on the next page.

Watch the patient carefully. Breathing problems that result from this type of burn can develop rapidly or slowly over several hours. Administer oxygen as soon as it is available and be prepared to perform CPR. If you suspect that a patient has suffered respiratory burns, arrange for *prompt transport* to a medical facility.

If the patient has injuries in addition to the burn, treat the injuries before transporting the patient. For example, if a patient who has a partial-thickness burn of the arm and has also fallen off a ladder and fractured both legs, splint the fractures and place the patient on a backboard, in addition to treating the burn injury.

Signs & Symptoms

RESPIRATORY BURN

- Burns around the face
- Singed nose hairs
- Soot in mouth and nose
- Difficulty breathing
- Pain while breathing
- Unconscious as a result of fire

Chemical Burns

Many strong substances can cause **chemical burns** to the skin. These substances include strong acids such as battery acid or strong alkalis such as drain cleaners. Some chemicals cause damage even if they are on the

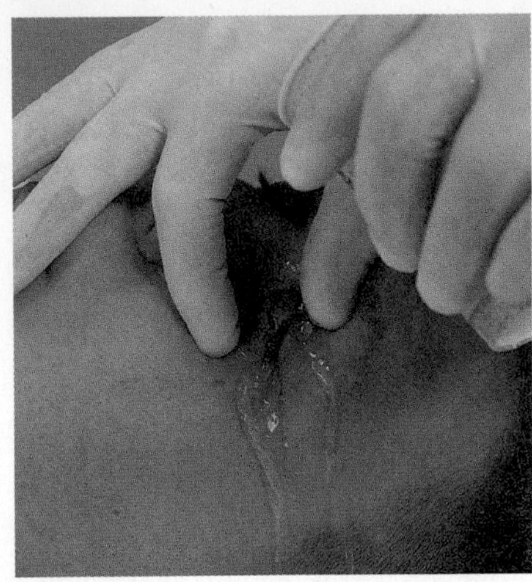

Figure 12.45 Flushing the eyes with water.

skin or in the eyes for only a short period of time. The longer the chemical remains in contact with the skin, the more it damages the skin and underlying tissues. Chemicals are extremely dangerous to the eyes and can cause superficial, partial-thickness, or full-thickness burns to the skin.

The initial treatment for chemical burns is to remove as much of the chemical as possible from the patient's skin. Brush away any dry chemical on the patient's clothes or skin, being careful not to get any on yourself. You may have to ask the patient to remove all clothing.

After you have removed as much of the dry chemical as possible, flush the contaminated skin with abundant quantities of water. You can use water from a garden hose, a shower in the home or factory, or even the booster hose of a fire engine. It is essential that the chemical be washed off the skin quickly to avoid further injury. Flush the affected area of the body for at least 10 minutes, then cover the burned area with a dry, sterile dressing or a burn sheet and arrange for T ***prompt transport*** to an appropriate medical facility.

Chemical burns to the eyes cause extreme pain and severe injury. Gently flush the affected eye or eyes with water for at least 20 minutes (**Figure 12.45**). You must hold the eye open to allow water to flow over its entire surface. Direct the water from the inner corner of the eye to the outward edge of the eye. You may have to put the patient's face under a shower, garden hose, or faucet so that the water flows across the patient's entire face. Flushing the eyes can continue while the patient is being transported.

After flushing the eyes for 20 minutes, loosely cover the injured eye or eyes with gauze bandages and arrange for T ***prompt transport*** to an appropriate medical facility. All chemical burns should be examined by a physician.

Electrical Burns

electrical burns Burns caused by electric current.

Electrical burns can cause severe injuries or even death, but they leave little evidence of injury on the outside of the body. These burns are caused by an electrical current that enters the body at one point (for example, the hand that touches the live electrical wire), travels through the body tissues and organs, and exits from the body at the point of ground contact (**Figure 12.46**).

Electricity causes major internal damage, rather than external damage. A strong electrical current can actually "cook" muscles, nerves, blood vessels, and internal organs, resulting in major damage. Patients who have been subjected to a strong electrical current can also suffer irregularities of cardiac rhythm or even full cardiac arrest and death.

Children often suffer electrical burns by chewing on an electrical cord or by pushing something into an outlet. Although the burn may

Figure 12.46 Electrical burns. **A.** An entrance wound is often small. **B.** An exit wound can be extensive and deep.

A

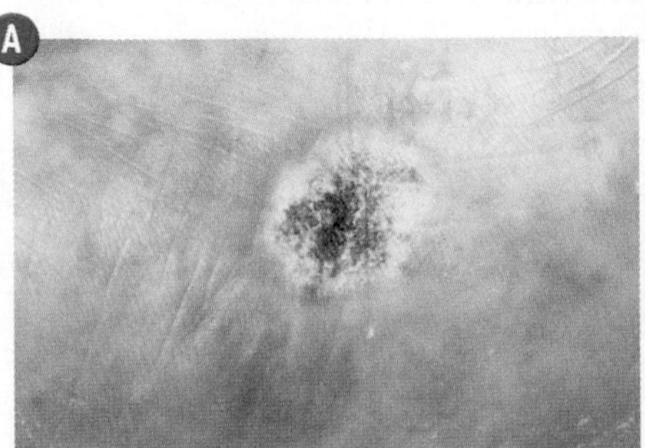

B

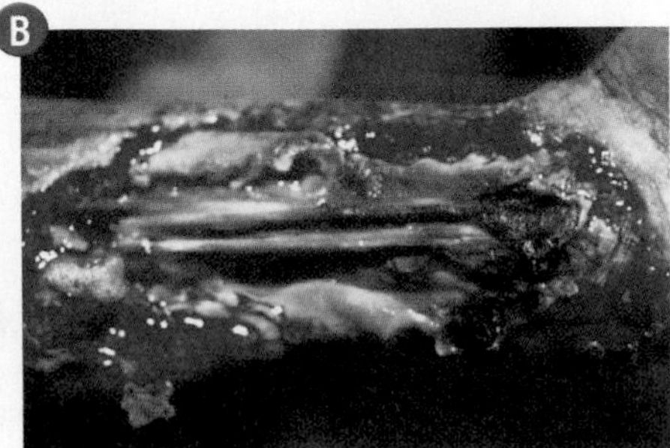

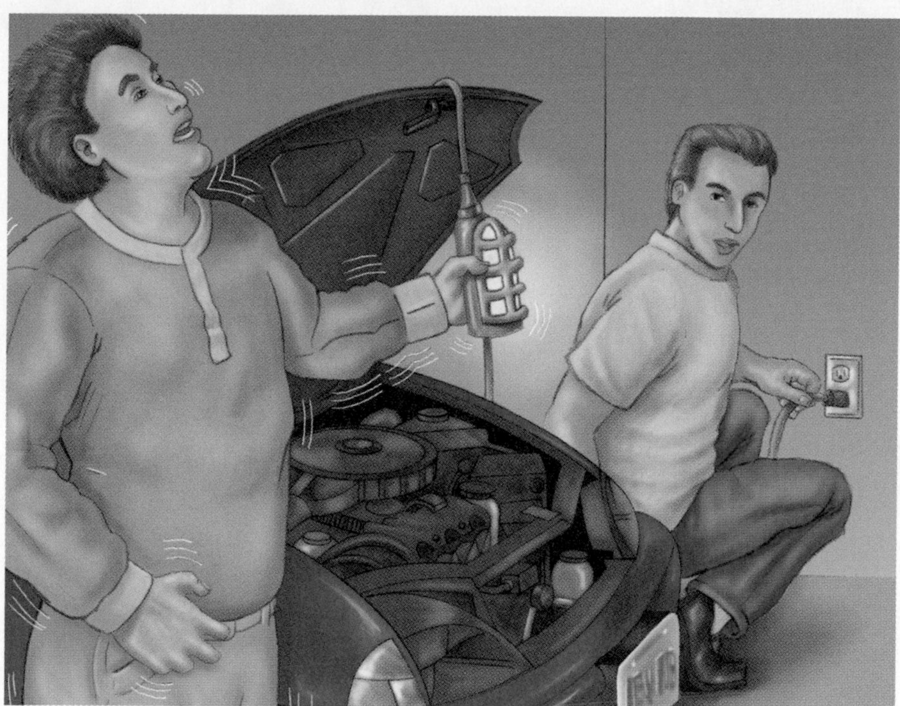

Figure 12.47 Do not touch the patient without unplugging, disconnecting, or turning off the power first.

not look serious at first, it is often quite severe because of underlying tissue injury.

Persons who have been hit or nearly hit by lightning frequently suffer electrical burns. Treat these patients as you would electrical burn patients. Evaluate them carefully because they may also suffer cardiac arrest. Arrange for Ⓣ ***prompt transport*** to an appropriate medical facility.

Before you touch or treat a person who has suffered an electrical burn, be certain that the patient is not still in contact with the electrical power source that caused the burn. If the patient is still in contact with the power source, anyone who touches him or her may be electrocuted.

If the patient is touching a live power source, your first act must be to unplug, disconnect, or turn off the power (**Figure 12.47**). If you cannot do this alone, call for assistance from the power company or from a qualified rescue squad or fire department.

If a power line falls on top of a motor vehicle, the people inside the vehicle must be told to stay there until qualified personnel can remove the power line or turn the power off.

After ensuring that the power has been disconnected, examine each electrical burn patient carefully, assess the ABCs, and treat the patient for visible, external burns. Cover these external burns with a dry, sterile dressing and arrange for Ⓣ ***prompt transport*** to an appropriate medical facility.

Monitor the airway, breathing, and circulation of electrical burn patients closely and arrange to have such patients transported promptly to an emergency department for further treatment.

Safety Tips

Avoid direct or indirect contact with live electrical wires. Direct contact occurs when you touch a live electrical wire. Indirect contact occurs when you touch a vehicle, a patient, a fence, a tree, or any other object that is in contact with a live electrical wire.

Check✓point

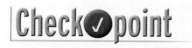

- ◯ Describe the importance of body substance isolation as it relates to the treatment of soft-tissue injuries.

12 Prep Kit

Ready for Review

Ready for Review thoroughly summarizes the chapter.

This chapter covered the knowledge and skills you need to treat patients suffering shock, bleeding, and soft-tissue injuries. It reviewed the functions of the pump (heart), the pipes (blood vessels), and the fluid (the blood). If you understand the role of each component of the circulatory system, you can understand how shock is caused by pump failure, pipe failure, or fluid loss. Because shock is the silent killer of trauma patients, it is important to learn its signs and symptoms. You also need to understand the general treatment for shock.

The chapter defined and explained the four types of open wounds. You need to understand how to control external bleeding, the principles of wound treatment, and how to dress and bandage the types of wounds you may encounter as a first responder. Body substance isolation techniques need to be used any time you are at risk for contact with a patient's bodily fluids.

Burns are a special type of soft-tissue injury. You should understand how burns can be caused by heat, chemicals, or electricity and the complications that may go along with specific types of burns. As a first responder, you need to be able to recognize respiratory burns and provide initial care for them. The severity of burns is related to the depth and extent of the burn. It is important that you be able to estimate the severity of burns.

By learning to recognize and provide initial emergency treatment for patients suffering shock, soft-tissue injuries, and bleeding, you will be able to provide physical and emotional assistance to these patients in their time of need. And, at times, your prompt recognition and treatment will make a real difference.

Vital Vocabulary

The Vital Vocabulary are the key terms for this chapter.

abrasion—*page 267*
anaphylactic shock—*page 258*
arterial bleeding—*page 264*
atrium—*page 255*
avulsion—*page 268*
blood pressure—*page 258*
brachial artery pressure point—*page 265*
bruise—*page 267*
capillary bleeding—*page 264*
cardiogenic shock—*page 258*
chemical burns—*page 279*
closed wound—*page 267*
congestive heart failure (CHF)—*page 258*
cravat—*page 271*
dressing—*page 264*
electrical burns—*page 280*
entrance wound—*page 268*
exit wound—*page 268*
femoral artery pressure point—*page 265*
full-thickness burns—*page 278*
gunshot wound—*page 268*
hemorrhage—*page 259*
immobilize—*page 269*
impaled object—*page 268*
intravenous (IV) fluid—*page 261*
laceration—*page 268*
occlusive dressing—*page 274*
open wound—*page 267*
partial-thickness burns—*page 278*
pneumatic antishock garment (PASG)—*page 261*
pressure points—*page 262*
psychogenic shock—*page 258*
puncture—*page 268*
rabies—*page 277*
respiratory burns—*page 279*
road rash—*page 267*
Rule of Nines—*page 278*
saline—*page 276*
shock—*page 257*
splinting—*page 269*
spontaneous nosebleed—*page 272*
superficial burns—*page 277*
thermal burns—*page 279*
venous bleeding—*page 264*
ventricle—*page 255*

Practice Points

The Practice Points are the key skills you need to know.

1. Performing body substance isolation procedures for patients with wounds.

2. Treating patients with signs and symptoms of internal bleeding or shock.

3. Controlling bleeding using the following techniques

A. Direct pressure
B. Elevation
C. Femoral pressure point
D. Brachial pressure point

4. Dressing and bandaging the following types of wounds

A. Face wounds
B. Nosebleeds
C. Eye injuries
D. Neck wounds
E. Chest and back wounds
F. Impaled objects
G. Closed abdominal wounds
H. Open abdominal wounds
I. Genital wounds
J. Extremity wounds
K. Gunshot wounds
L. Bites

5. Performing emergency medical care for patients suffering the following types of burns

A. Thermal burns
B. Respiratory burns
C. Chemical burns
D. Electrical burns

Ready to Respond

Ready to Respond presents a fictitious scenario to help you review what you learned in this chapter.

On a Friday afternoon you are called to a factory for an injured worker. On the way, your radio dispatcher informs you that your patient is inside building one, that the factory is a sheet metal fabricating facility, and that the worker is 32 years old.

1. Which of the following factors is least important when making an initial overview of this scene?

A. Electrical hazards
B. Sharp metal
C. The time of day
D. Visible blood

As you examine the patient, you notice an actively bleeding wound on the patient's thigh and skin scraped off the patient's lower arm.

2. Which wound should be treated first?

A. Thigh wound
B. Arm wound

3. What is the proper order of use for the following bleeding control measures?

1. Elevation	A. 3, 1, 2
2. Pressure points	B. 2, 3, 1
3. Direct pressure	C. 3, 2, 1

4. Which treatments for shock would you consider for this patient? (Circle all that apply.)

A. Water by mouth
B. Lay the patient down
C. Preserve the patient's body temperature
D. Intravenous fluids
E. Control of external bleeding

5. Which body substance isolation measures should you use?

A. Hand washing
B. Medical gloves
C. Face shield
D. Surgical gown

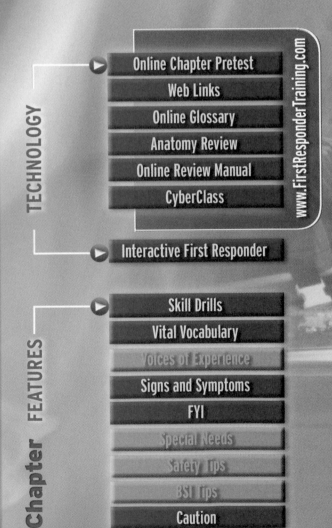

Chapter 13

Injuries to Muscles and Bones

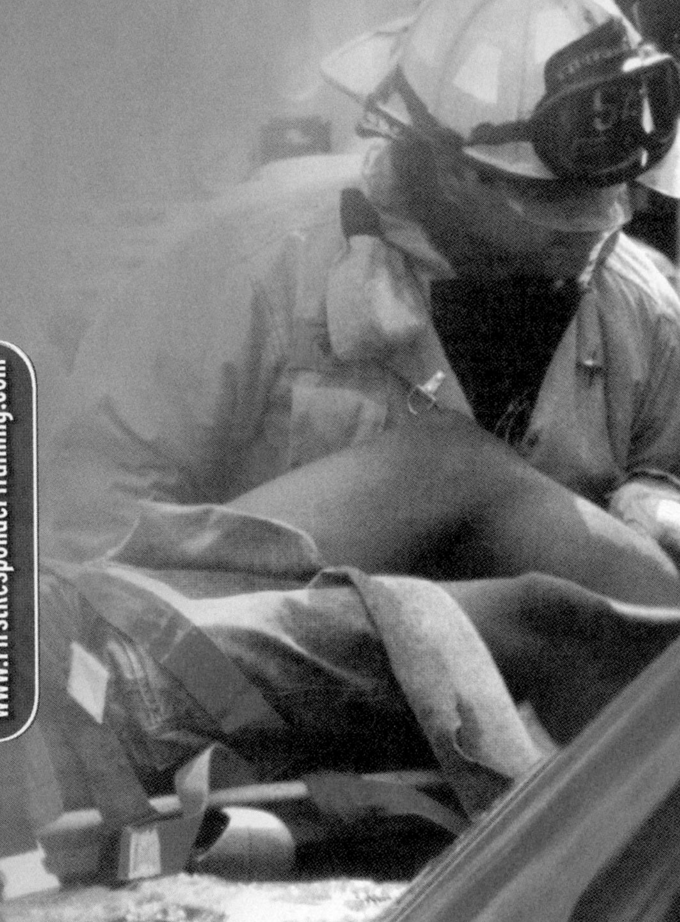

TECHNOLOGY

www.FirstResponderTraining.com

- Online Chapter Pretest
- Web Links
- Online Glossary
- Anatomy Review
- Online Review Manual
- CyberClass

- Interactive First Responder

Chapter FEATURES

- Skill Drills
- Vital Vocabulary
- Voices of Experience
- Signs and Symptoms
- FYI
- Special Needs
- Safety Tips
- BSI Tips
- Caution
- Check Point
- Prep Kit

CHAPTER 13

Objectives

Knowledge and Attitude Objectives

After studying this chapter, you will be expected to:

1. Describe the anatomy and functions of the parts of the musculoskeletal system.
2. Describe the mechanisms of injury for musculoskeletal injuries.
3. Define fracture, dislocation, and sprain.
4. Describe the need for body substance isolation techniques when examining or treating patients with musculoskeletal injuries.
5. Describe the importance of the following three steps when examining patients with musculoskeletal injuries:
   A. General assessment of the patient
   B. Examination of the injured part
   C. Evaluation of circulation and sensation
6. Describe the general principles of splinting.
7. Explain how to splint the following sites and injuries:
   A. Shoulder girdle
   B. Dislocation of the shoulder
   C. Elbow injury
   D. Injury to the forearm
   E. Injury to the hand, wrist, or fingers
   F. Pelvic fracture
   G. Hip injury
   H. Injury to the thigh
   I. Knee injury
   J. Leg injury
   K. Injury to the ankle or foot
8. Describe the mechanism for head and spine injuries.
9. Explain the two types of head injuries.
10. Describe the signs and symptoms of head injuries.
11. Describe the treatment of patients with head injuries.
12. Describe the treatment of facial injuries.
13. Explain the mechanism of spine injuries.
14. Describe the signs and symptoms of spinal cord injuries.
15. Describe the treatment of spine injuries.
16. Describe the signs, symptoms, and treatment of the following injuries:
    A. Fractured ribs
    B. Flail chest
    c. Penetrating chest wound

Skill Objectives

As a first responder, you should be able to:

1. Perform body substance isolation techniques when treating a patient with musculoskeletal injuries.
2. Examine a patient with musculoskeletal injuries.
3. Evaluate the circulation and sensation of a patient with an extremity injury.
4. Splint the following musculoskeletal injuries:
   A. Shoulder girdle injury
   B. Dislocation of the shoulder
   C. Elbow injury
   D. Injury to the forearm
   E. Injury to the hand, wrist, or fingers
   F. Pelvic fracture
   G. Hip injury
   H. Injury to the thigh
   I. Knee injury
   J. Leg injury
   K. Injury to the ankle or foot
5. Treat injuries of the face.
6. Stabilize spine injuries.
7. Treat the following injuries of the chest:
   A. Fractured ribs
   B. Flail chest
   C. Penetrating chest injuries

As a first responder, you will encounter many types of musculoskeletal injuries, including fractures, dislocations, sprains, head injuries, spinal cord injuries, and chest injuries. You need to understand the anatomy and functioning of the musculoskeletal system, and to study the causes, or mechanisms of injury. This will give you a better understanding of the results of various injuries.

Before you can treat musculoskeletal injuries, you must be able to recognize their signs and symptoms and to differentiate between open and closed injuries. Giving proper care at the scene can prevent additional injury or disability. This chapter describes how to manage injuries to the upper and lower extremities, the head, the spinal cord, and the chest. It also provides information on body substance isolation techniques and their relation to musculoskeletal injuries.

The Anatomy and Function of the Musculoskeletal System

The musculoskeletal system has two parts: the skeletal system, which provides support and form for the body, and the muscular system, which provides both support and movement.

The Skeletal System

The skeletal system consists of 206 bones and is the supporting framework for the body.

The four functions of the skeletal system are:

- To support the body
- To protect vital structures
- To assist in body movement
- To manufacture red blood cells

The skeletal system (**Figure 13.1**) is divided into seven areas:

1. Head, skull, and face
2. Spinal column
3. Shoulder girdle
4. Upper extremities
5. Rib cage (thorax)
6. Pelvis
7. Lower extremities

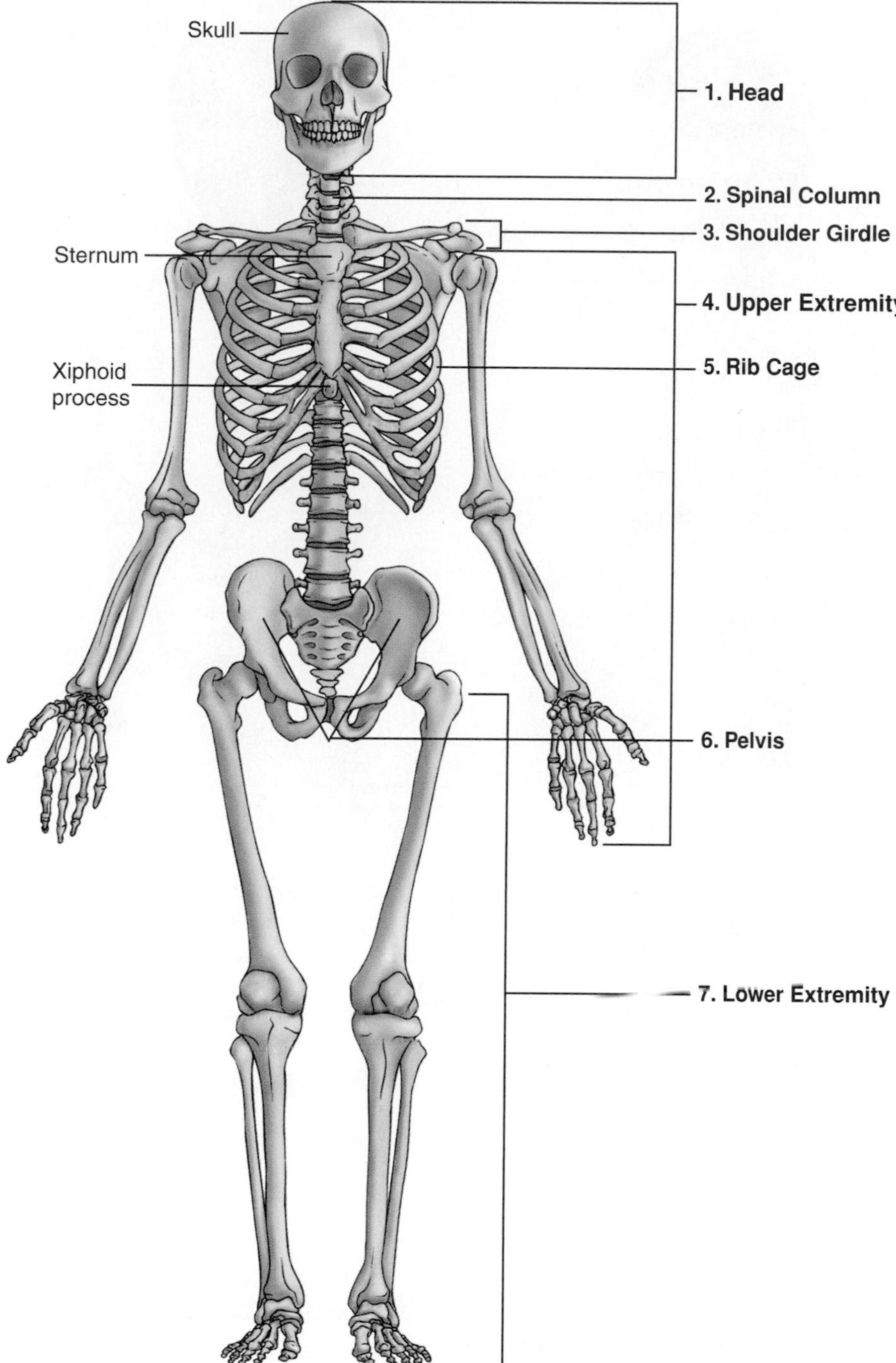

Figure 13.1 The seven major areas of the human skeleton.

The bones of the head include the skull and the lower jawbone. The skull is actually many bones fused together to form a hollow sphere that contains and protects the brain. The jawbone is a movable bone attached to the skull that completes the structure of the face.

The spine consists of a series of separate bones called vertebrae. The spinal vertebrae are stacked on top of each other and are held together by muscles, tendons, disks, and ligaments. The spinal cord, a group of nerves that carry messages to and from the brain, passes through a hole in the center of each vertebra.

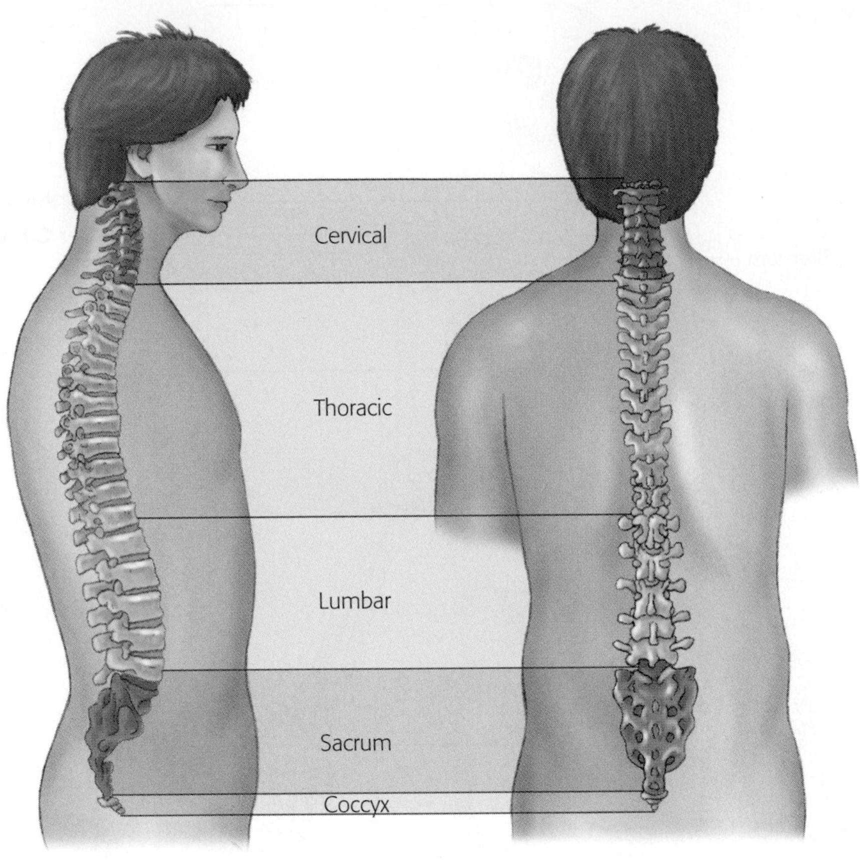

Figure 13.2 The five sections of the spine.

In addition to protecting the spinal cord, the spine is the primary support structure for the entire body.

The spine has five sections (**Figure 13.2**):

- Cervical spine (neck)
- Thoracic spine (upper back)
- Lumbar spine (lower back)
- Sacrum
- Coccyx (tailbone)

The shoulder girdles form the third area of the skeletal system. Each shoulder girdle supports an arm and consists of the collarbone (clavicle) and the shoulder blade (scapula).

The fourth area of the skeletal system, the upper extremities, consists of three major bones as well as the wrist and hand. The arm has one bone (the humerus), and the forearm has two bones (the radius and the ulna). The radius is located on the thumb side of the arm; the ulna is located on the little-finger side. There are several bones in the wrist and hand. However, you do not need to learn their names and you can consider them as one unit for the purposes of emergency treatment.

The fifth area of the skeletal system is the rib cage, or chest (thorax). The 12 sets of ribs protect the heart, lungs, liver, and spleen. All the ribs are attached to the spine (**Figure 13.3**). The upper five rib sets connect directly to the sternum (breastbone). A bridge of cartilage connects the

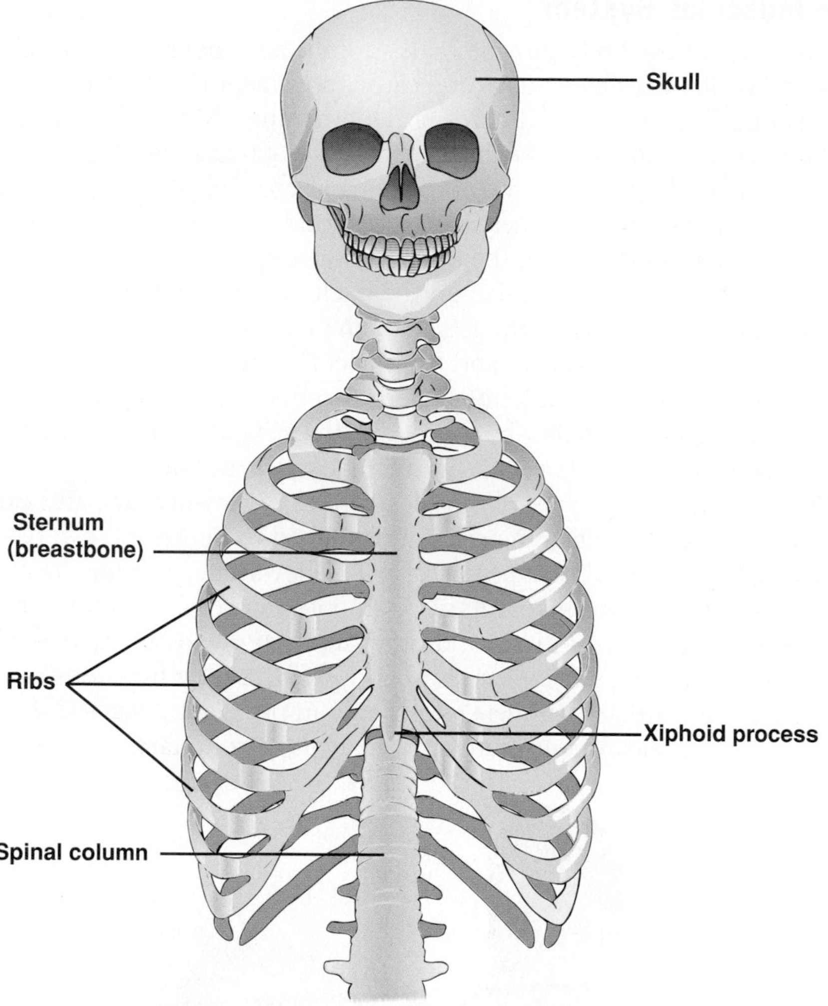

Figure 13.3 The rib cage.

ends of the sixth through tenth rib sets to each other and to the sternum. The eleventh and twelfth rib sets are called floating ribs because they are not attached to the sternum. The sternum is located in the front of the chest. The pointed structure at the bottom of the sternum is called the xiphoid process. The xiphoid process is an important location to remember because it is a body landmark used for proper hand placement during cardiopulmonary resuscitation (CPR).

The sixth area of the skeletal system is the pelvis, which links the body and the lower extremities. The pelvis also protects the reproductive organs and the other organs located in the lower abdominal cavity.

The lower extremities (the thigh and the leg) form the seventh area of the skeletal system. The thigh bone (femur) is the longest and strongest bone in the entire body. The leg consists of two major bones, the tibia and fibula, as well as the ankle and foot. The kneecap (patella) is a small, relatively flat bone that protects the front of the knee **joint**. Like the wrist and hand, the ankle and foot contain a large number of smaller bones that can be considered as one unit.

A vital but often overlooked function of the skeletal system is to produce red blood cells. Red blood cells are manufactured primarily within the spaces inside the bone called the marrow.

Note: A protective bony structure surrounds each of the body's essential organs. The skull protects the brain. The vertebrae protect the spinal cord. The ribs protect the heart and lungs. The pelvis protects the lower abdominal and reproductive organs.

joint The place where two bones come in contact with each other.

The Muscular System

The muscles of the body provide both support and movement. Muscles are attached to bones by tendons and cause movement by alternately contracting (shortening) and relaxing (lengthening). Muscles are usually paired in opposition: as one member of the pair contracts, the other relaxes. This mechanical opposition moves bones and enables you to open and close your hand, turn your head, and bend and straighten your knee or other joints. To straighten the elbow, for example, the biceps muscle relaxes, and an opposing muscle on the back of the arm contracts.

The musculoskeletal system gets its name from the coordination between the muscular system and the skeletal system to produce movement. Movement occurs at joints, where two bones come together. The bones are held together by ligaments, thick bands that arise from one bone, span the joint, and insert into the adjacent bone.

The body has three types of muscles: voluntary, involuntary, and cardiac. Voluntary, or skeletal, muscles are attached to bones and can be contracted and relaxed by a person at will. They are responsible for the movement of the body. Involuntary, or smooth, muscles are found on the inside of the digestive tract and other internal organs of the body. They are not under conscious control and perform their functions automatically. Cardiac muscle is found only in the heart (**Figure 13.4**). Most musculoskeletal injuries involve skeletal, or voluntary, muscles.

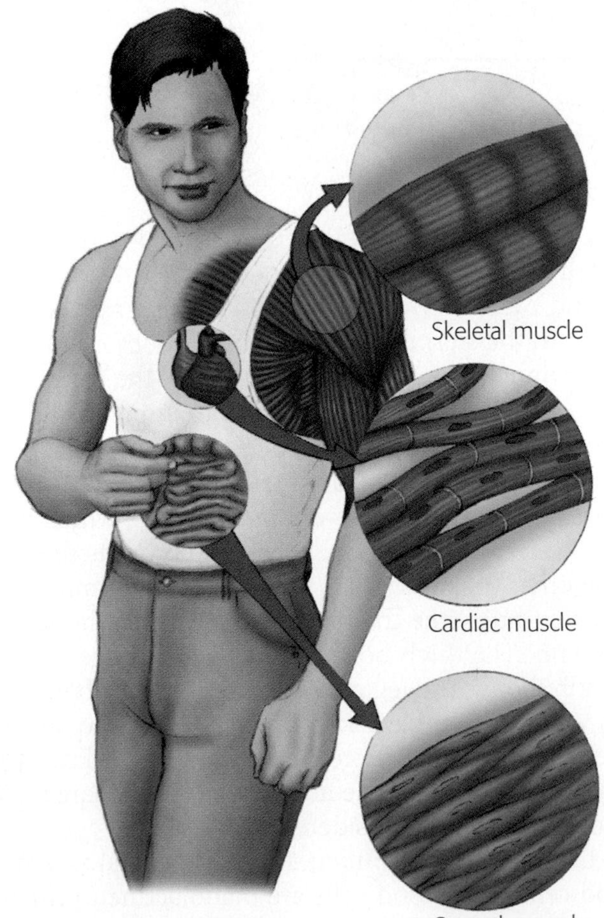

Figure 13.4 Three types of muscle in the human body.

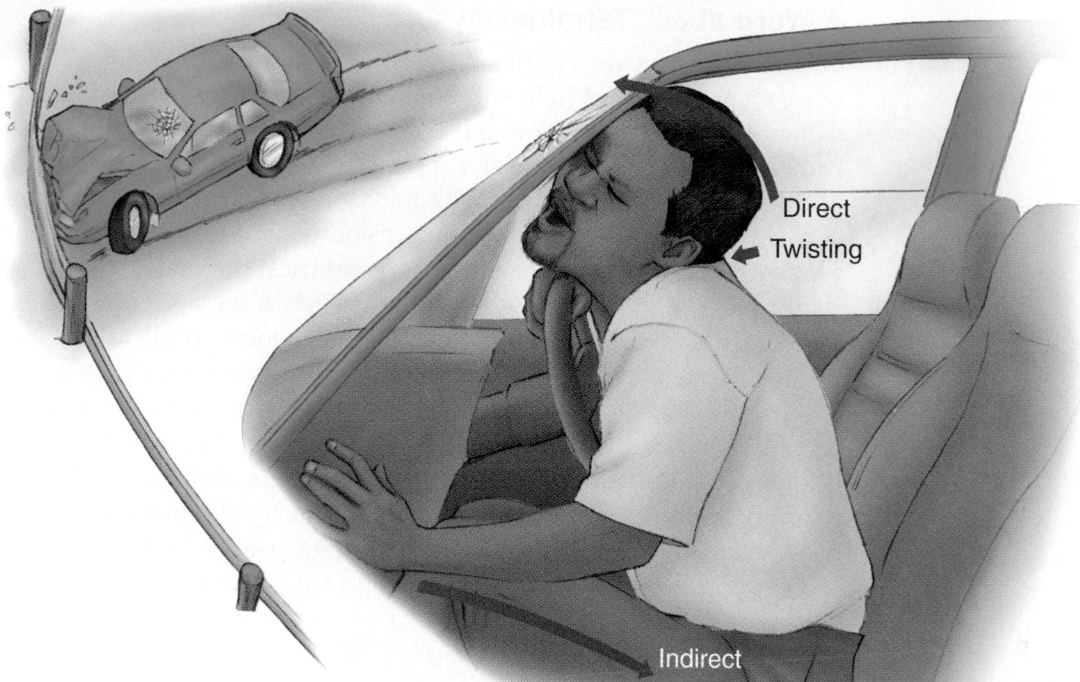

Figure 13.5 Three types of mechanisms of injury cause musculoskeletal injuries: direct force, indirect force, and twisting force.

Mechanism of Injury

As a first responder, you must understand the **mechanism of injury**, or how injuries occur. Musculoskeletal injuries are caused by three types of mechanisms of injury: direct force, indirect force, and twisting force (**Figure 13.5**).

mechanism of injury The means by which a traumatic injury occurs.

Examples of each mechanism and the type of injury it causes are:

- *Direct force:* A car strikes a pedestrian on the leg. The pedestrian sustains a broken leg.
- *Indirect force:* A woman falls on her shoulder. The force of the fall transmits energy to the middle of the collarbone (clavicle), and the excess force breaks the bone.
- *Twisting force:* A football player is tackled as he is turning. He twists his leg, causing a severe injury to his knee.

Injuries can be caused by direct force at the site of impact or can be caused by indirect force at an impact site removed from the site of the injury.

As a first responder, you will see many different types of traumatic injuries. Some of these will be the result of motor vehicle crashes or auto/pedestrian accidents; others will be the result of athletic activities, work-related accidents, or violence. You will see injuries in people of all ages, from very young children to elderly people. Use the information provided by your dispatcher and gathered from your overview of the scene to identify the possible mechanisms of injury. You will gain additional information from examining and questioning the patient. By understanding the mechanism of injury (how the injury occurred), you will be better able to assess the patient and provide the needed treatment.

A Word about Terminology

FYI

There are different ways to describe a patient's injuries. You must rely on your senses of sight and touch to determine the type of injury the patient has experienced. You must also listen to the information that the patient can give you. However, keep in mind that, as a first responder, you do not have the training or tools to diagnose an injury as a physician can.

The next section defines fractures, dislocations, and sprains. Although you are not expected to diagnose these injuries, the patient's signs and symptoms will lead you to suspect that a certain injury is most probable. Some instructors and medical directors may choose to identify musculoskeletal injuries strictly in terms of the signs and symptoms present, such as a painful, swollen, deformed extremity. Others may choose to use terms such as suspected fracture, dislocation, or sprain. To meet the needs of both groups of instructors and medical directors, this text uses "PSDE" (painful, swollen, deformed extremity) after each relevant term. Regardless of the terminology used, the most important part of the first responder's job is to provide the best assessment and treatment for the patient.

THREE MAJOR TYPES OF MUSCULOSKELETAL INJURIES:

- *Fractures*
- *Dislocations*
- *Sprains*

Types of Injuries

It is often difficult to distinguish one type of musculoskeletal extremity injury from another. All three types are serious, and all extremity injuries must be identified so they can receive appropriate medical treatment.

Fractures

A fracture is a broken bone. Fractures can be caused by a variety of mechanisms, but almost always require a significant force. Fractures are generally classified as either closed or open (**Figure 13.6**). In the more common **closed fracture**, the bone is broken but there is no break in the skin.

In an **open fracture**, the bone is broken and the overlying skin is lacerated. The open wound can be caused by a penetrating object, such as a bullet, or by the fractured bone end itself protruding through the skin. Open fractures are contaminated by dirt and bacteria that may lead to infection. Both open and closed fractures injure adjacent soft tissues, resulting in bleeding at the fracture site. Fractures can also injure nearby nerves and blood vessels, causing severe nerve injury and excessive bleeding. Open fractures result in more bleeding than do closed fractures.

closed fracture A fracture in which the overlying skin has not been damaged.

open fracture Any fracture in which the overlying skin has been damaged.

dislocation Disruption of a joint so that the bone ends are no longer in alignment.

sprain A joint injury in which the joint is partially or temporarily dislocated, and some of the supporting ligaments are either stretched or torn.

Dislocations

A **dislocation** is a disruption that tears the supporting ligaments of the joint. The bone ends that make up the joint separate completely from each other and can lock in one position. Any attempt to move a dislocated joint is very painful. Because many nerves and blood vessels lie near joints, a dislocation can damage these structures, also.

Sprains

A **sprain** is a joint injury caused by excessive stretching of the supporting ligaments. It can be thought of as a partial dislocation.

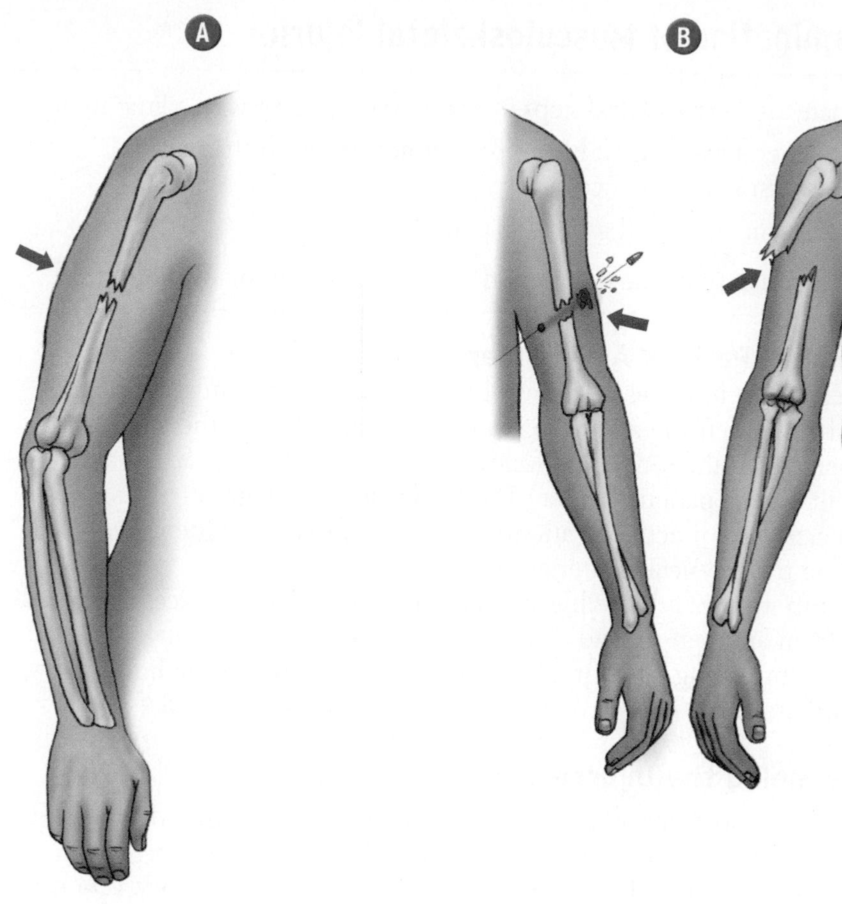
A
B

Figure 13.6 Closed and open fractures. **A.** Closed fracture. **B.** Two types of open fractures: gunshot and exposed bone.

Body Substance Isolation and Musculoskeletal Injuries

As you examine and treat patients with musculoskeletal injuries, you need to practice body substance isolation (BSI). These patients may have open wounds related to the musculoskeletal injury or to a separate, open soft-tissue injury. You should assume that trauma patients have open wounds that pose a threat of infection. Wear approved gloves. When responding to motor vehicle crashes or other situations that may present a hazard from broken glass or other sharp objects, it is wise to wear heavy rescue gloves that provide protection from sharp objects. Some first responders wear latex or vinyl gloves under the heavy rescue gloves for added BSI protection. If the patient has active bleeding that may splatter, you should have protection for your eyes, nose, and mouth as well.

Signs and Symptoms of Extremity Injuries

- Pain at the injury site
- An open wound
- Swelling and discoloration (bruising)
- The patient's inability or unwillingness to move the extremity
- Deformity or angulation
- Tenderness at the injury site

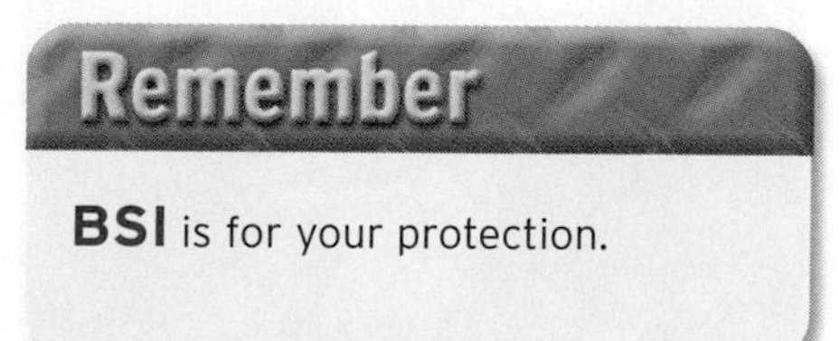
Remember
BSI is for your protection.

Note: Listen to the patient. He or she is usually right about the location and type of injury.

Examination of Musculoskeletal Injuries

There are three essential steps in examining a patient with a limb injury:

1. General assessment of the patient according to the patient assessment sequence
2. Examination of the injured part
3. Evaluation of the circulation and sensation in the injured limb

General Patient Assessment

A general, primary assessment of the injured patient must be carried out before focusing attention on any injured limb. All the steps in the patient assessment must be followed. Once you have checked and stabilized the patient's airway, breathing, and circulation (ABCs), you can then direct your attention to the injured limb identified during the physical examination.

Limb injuries are not life-threatening unless there is excessive bleeding from an open wound. Therefore, it is essential that you stabilize the airway, breathing, and circulation before you focus on the limb injury, regardless of the pain or deformity that may be present at that injury site.

Examining the Injured Limb

As a first responder, you should initially inspect the injured limb and compare it to the opposite, uninjured limb. To do this, gently and carefully cut away any clothing covering the wound, if necessary. (Do not ever hesitate to cut clothing in order to uncover a suspected injury.)

When you examine the limb, you may find any one of the following:

- An open wound
- Deformity
- Swelling
- Bruising

After you have uncovered and looked at the injured limb, you should gently feel it for any points of tenderness. Tenderness is the best indicator of an underlying fracture, dislocation, or sprain (PSDE).

To detect limb injury, start at the top of each limb (where it connects to the body) and, using both hands, squeeze the entire limb in a systematic, firm (yet gentle) manner, moving down the limb and away from the body. Make sure you examine the entire extremity.

As you carry out your hands-on examination, it is important to ask the patient where it hurts most; the location of greatest pain is probably the injury site. Also ask if the patient feels tingling or numbness in the extremity because this may indicate nerve damage or lack of circulation.

Careful inspection and a gentle hands-on examination will identify most musculoskeletal injuries (**Figure 13.7**). After you have made a careful visual and hands-on examination, and if the patient shows no sign of injury, ask the patient to move the limb carefully. If there is an injury, the patient will complain of pain and refuse to move the limb.

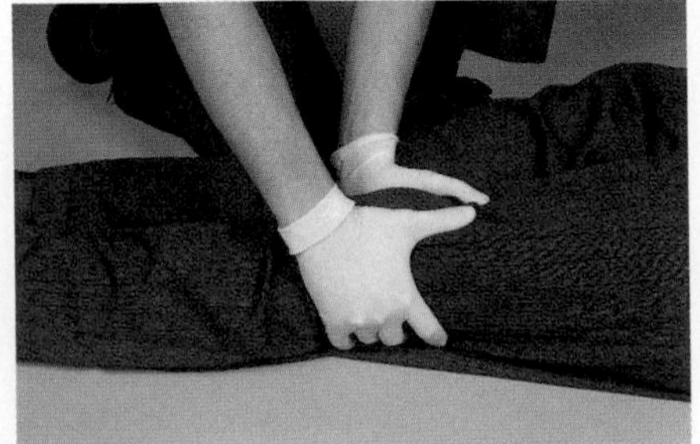

Figure 13.7 Examine the extremities.

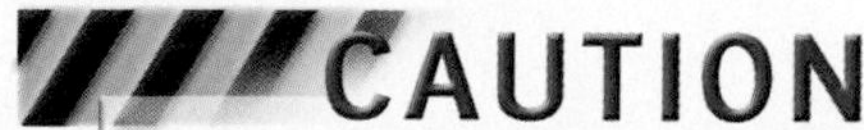

If even the slightest motion causes pain, NO further motion should be attempted.

Any of the signs or symptoms described earlier (deformity, swelling, bruising, tenderness, or pain with motion) indicate the presence of a limb injury (PSDE). Only one sign is necessary to indicate an "injury to the limb." All limb injuries, regardless of type or severity, are managed in the same way.

Evaluation of Circulation, Sensation, and Movement

Once you suspect limb injury, you must evaluate the circulation and sensation in that limb (**Figure 13.8**, page 296). Many important blood vessels and nerves lie close to the bones, especially around major joints. Therefore, any injury may have associated blood vessel or nerve damage.

It is also essential to check circulation and sensation after any movement of the limb (such as for splinting). Moving the limb during splinting might have caused a bone fragment to press against or even cut a blood vessel or nerve.

FACTORS TO EXAMINE FOR EACH INJURED LIMB

- *Pulse*
- *Capillary refill*
- *Sensation*
- *Movement*

Pulse

Feel the pulse distal to the point of injury. If the patient has an upper extremity injury, check the radial (wrist) pulse (see **Figure 13.8, step 1**). If the patient has a lower extremity injury, check the tibial (posterior ankle) pulse (see **Figure 13.8, step 2**).

Capillary Refill

Test the capillary refill in a finger or toe of any injured limb. Firm pressure on the tip of the nail causes the nail bed to turn white (see **Figure 13.8, steps 3 and 4**). Release the pressure and the normal pink color should return by the time it takes to say "capillary refill". If the pink color does not return in this two-second interval, it is considered to be delayed or absent and indicates a circulation problem in the limb. A cold environment will naturally delay capillary refill, so in that situation, do not use capillary refill to assess an injured limb.

The absence of a pulse or capillary refill indicates that a limb is in immediate danger. Impaired circulation demands prompt transportation and prompt medical treatment at an appropriate medical facility.

Sensation

The patient's ability to feel your light touch on the fingers or toes is a good indication that the nerve supply is intact. In the hand, check sensation by touching lightly the tips of the index and little fingers. In the foot, the tip of the big toe and the top of the foot should be checked for sensation (see **Figure 13.8, steps 5 and 6**).

Movement

If the hand or foot is injured, do not have the patient do this part of the test. When the injury is between the hand or foot and the body, have the patient open and close the fist or wiggle the toes of the injured limb (see **Figure 13.8, steps 7, 8, 9, and 10**). These simple movements indicate that the nerves to these muscles are working. Sometimes any attempt

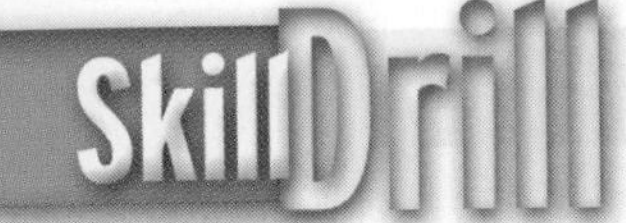

Figure 13.8 Checking Circulation, Sensation, and Movement in an Injured Extremity

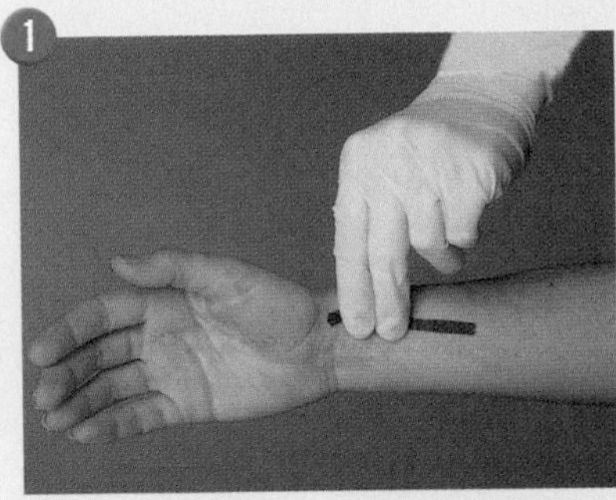

1 Check for circulation. If upper extremity injury, check radial pulse.

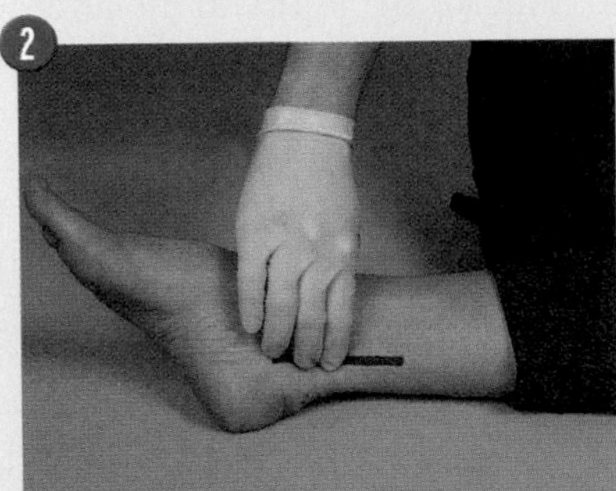

2 If lower extremity injury, check posterior ankle pulse.

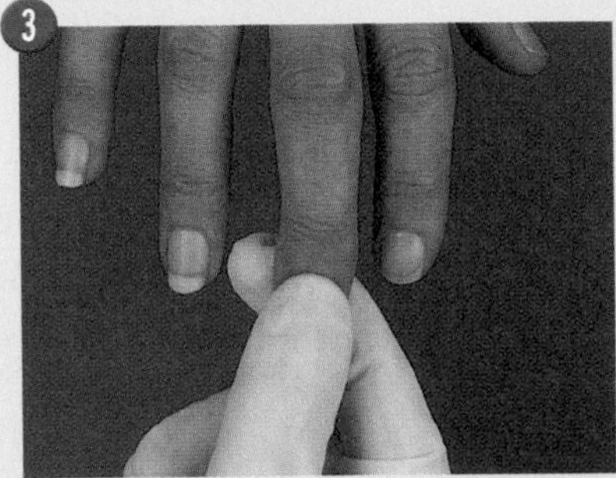

3 Test capillary refill on finger/toe of injured limb.

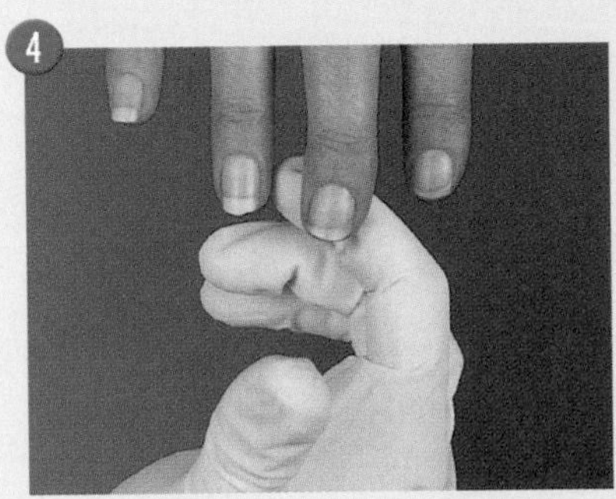

4 Release pressure. Pink color should return.

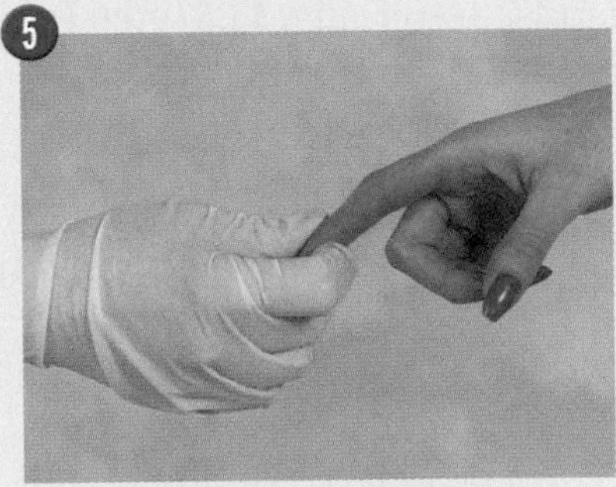

5 Check for sensation at fingertips.

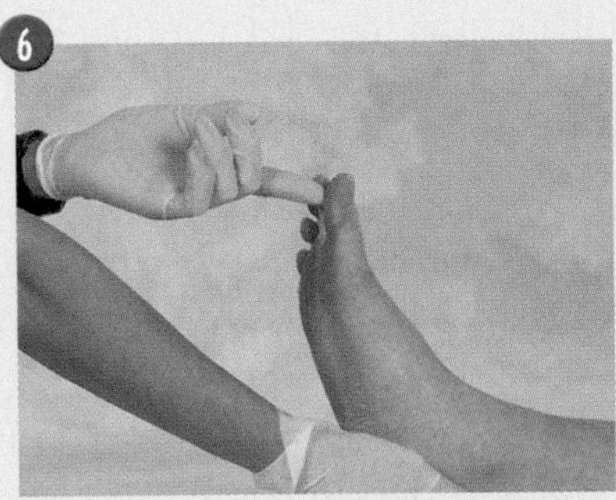

6 Check for sensation at toes.

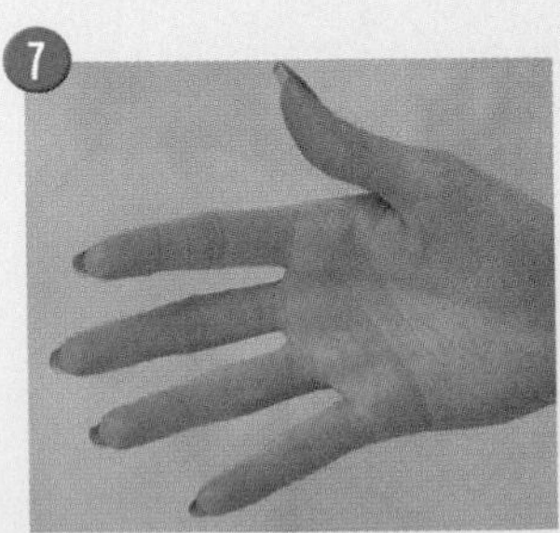

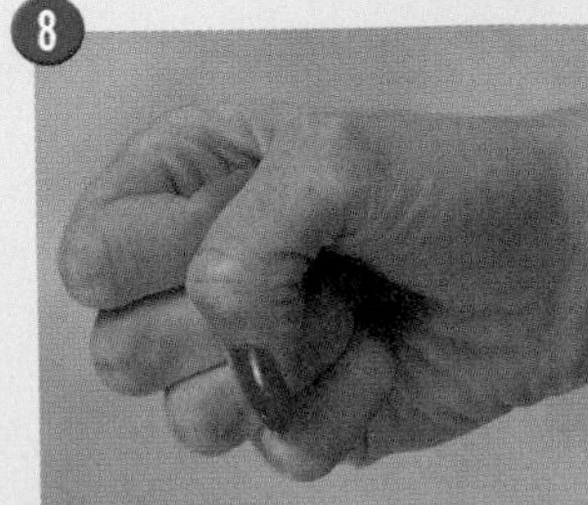

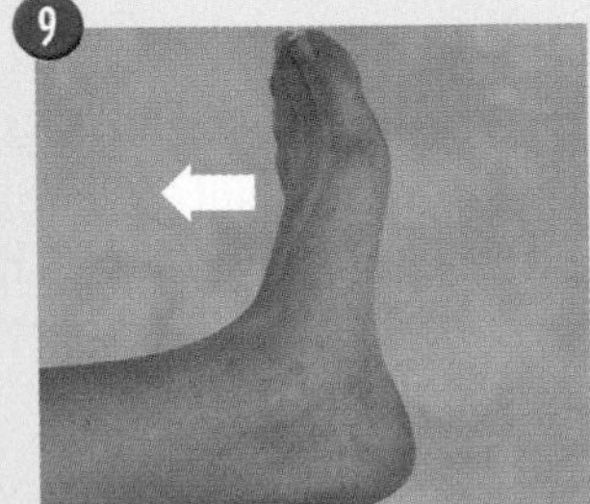

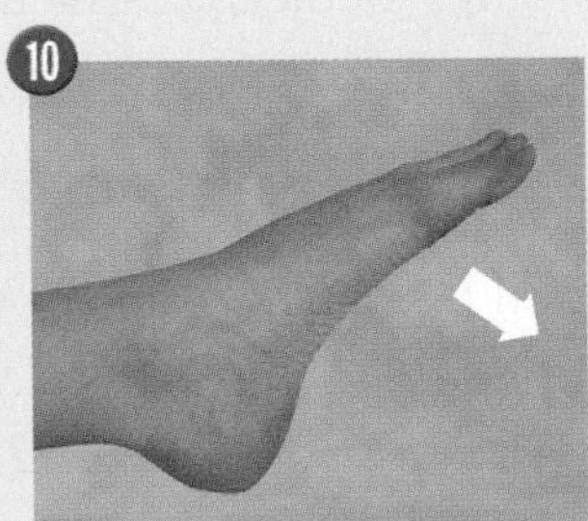

7–10 Check for movement of extremities.

at motion will produce pain. In this case, do not ask the patient to move the limb any further.

Any open wound, deformity, swelling, or bruising of a limb should be considered evidence of a possible limb injury and treated as such.

Checkpoint

- ◯ Describe the three major steps of examining a patient for musculoskeletal injuries.
- ◯ Describe the components in each part of the examination.

Treatment of Musculoskeletal Injuries

Regardless of their extent or severity, all limb injuries are treated in the same way in the field. For all open extremity wounds, first cover the entire wound with a dry, sterile dressing and then apply firm but gentle pressure to control bleeding, if necessary. The sterile compression dressing protects the wound and underlying tissues from further contamination. The injured limb should then be splinted.

General Principles of Splinting

All limb injuries (PSDE) should be splinted before a patient is moved, unless the environment prevents effective splinting or threatens the patient's life (or that of the rescuer). Splinting prevents the movement of broken bone ends, a dislocated joint, or damaged soft tissues and thereby reduces pain. With less pain, the patient relaxes and the trip to the medical facility is easier.

Splinting also helps to control bleeding and decreases the risk of damage to the nearby nerves and vessels by sharp bone fragments. Splinting prevents closed fractures (PSDE) from becoming open fractures (PSDE) during movement or transportation.

All first responders should know the following general principles of splinting:

1. In most situations, remove clothing from the injured limb (PSDE) to inspect the limb for open wounds, deformity, swelling, bruising, and capillary refill.
2. Note and record the pulse, capillary refill, sensation, and movement distal to the point of injury.
3. Cover all open wounds with a dry, sterile dressing before applying the splint.
4. Do not move the patient before splinting, unless there is an immediate danger to the patient or the first responder.
5. Immobilize the joint above and the joint below the injury site.
6. Pad all rigid splints.
7. When applying the splint, use your hands to support the injury site and minimize movement of the limb until splinting is completed.
8. Splint the limb in the position in which it is found.
9. When in doubt, splint.

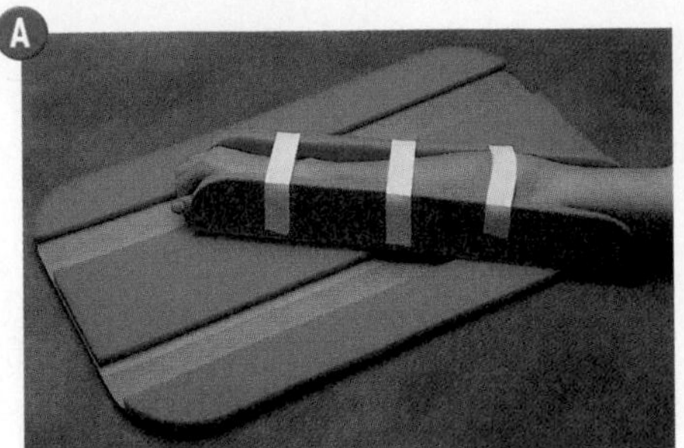

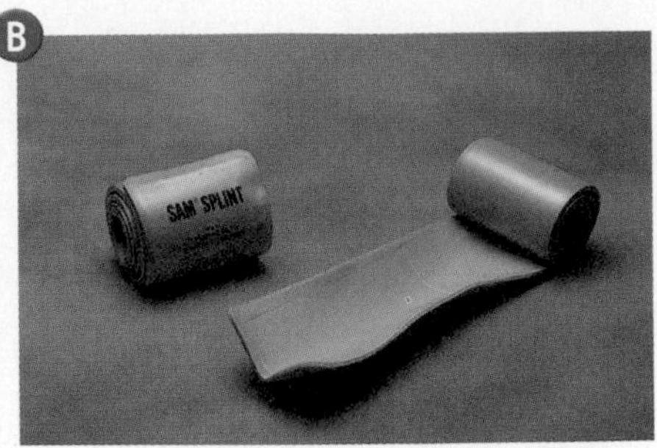

Figure 13.9 Different kinds of splints. A. Rigid cardboard splints. B. SAM® splint.

THREE BASIC TYPES OF SPLINTS

- *Rigid*
- *Soft*
- *Traction*

Materials Used for Splinting

Many different materials can be used as splints, if necessary. Even when standard splints are not available, the arm can be bound to the chest and an injured leg can be secured to the other, uninjured lower extremity for temporary stability.

Rigid Splints

Rigid splints are made from firm material and are applied to the sides, front, or back of an injured extremity. Common types of rigid splints include padded board splints, molded plastic or aluminum splints, padded wire ladder splints, SAM® splints, and folded cardboard splints (**Figure 13.9**). Padded wire ladder or SAM® splints can be molded to the shape of the limb to splint it in the position found.

rigid splints Splints made from firm materials such as wood, aluminum, or plastic.

soft splint A splint made from soft material that provides gentle support.

Soft Splints

The most commonly used **soft splint** is the inflatable, clear plastic air splint. This splint is available in a variety of sizes and shapes and with or without a zipper that runs the length of the splint (**Figure 13.10**). After it is applied, the splint is inflated by mouth—never by using a pump or air cylinder. The air splint is comfortable for the patient and provides uniform pressure to a bleeding wound.

The air splint has some disadvantages, particularly if it must be used in cold, dirty areas. The zipper can stick, clog with dirt, or freeze. After it is inflated, the splint can be punctured by sharp fragments of glass or other objects. Temperature and altitude changes can increase or decrease the pressure in the air splint, so careful monitoring by emergency care personnel is required.

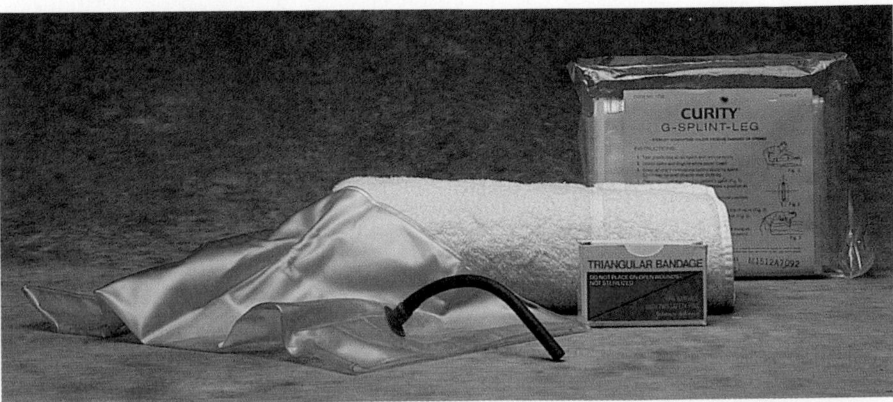

Figure 13.10 Soft splints.

Traction Splints

A **traction splint** holds a lower extremity fracture (PSDE) in alignment by applying a constant, steady pull on the extremity. Properly applying a traction splint requires two well-trained EMTs working together; one person cannot do it alone. First responders do not learn the skills necessary to apply this type of splint. However, you may be asked to assist trained medical personnel in the placement of a traction splint, and you should be familiar with the general techniques, as shown later in **Figure 13.26**, on page 306.

traction splint A splint used to immobilize a fractured thigh bone that produces a longitudinal pull on the extremity.

sling A triangular bandage or material tied around the neck to support the weight of an injured upper extremity.

FYI

Splinting Specific Injury Sites

The treatment techniques described here can be carried out by a person with your level of training and with materials readily available to you. Most splinting techniques are two-person operations. One person stabilizes and supports the injured limb, while the other person applies the splint.

Shoulder Girdle Injuries

The easiest way to splint most shoulder injuries is to apply a **sling** made of a triangular bandage and to secure the sling (and arm) to the body with swathes around the arm and chest. Apply the sling by tying a knot in the point of the triangular bandage, placing the elbow into the cup formed by the knot, and passing the two ends of the bandage up and around the patient's neck. Tie the sling so the wrist is slightly higher than the elbow (**Figure 13.12**).

To keep the arm immobilized, fold another triangular bandage until you have a long swathe that is 3 to 4 inches wide (**Figure 13.13**). Tie one or two swathes around the upper arm and chest of the patient. This easily applied splint adequately immobilizes fractures of the collar bone (clavicle), most shoulder injuries, and fractures of the arm (upper humerus).

Dislocation of the Shoulder

The dislocated shoulder is the only shoulder girdle injury that is difficult to immobilize with a sling and swathe. In a shoulder dislocation, there is often a space between the upper arm and the chest wall. Fill this space with a pillow or a rolled blanket and before applying a sling and swathe as for other shoulder injuries (see **Figure 13.13**).

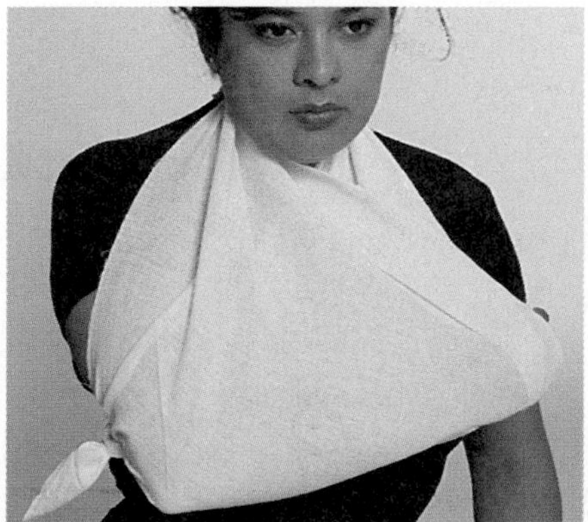

Figure 13.12 Sling.

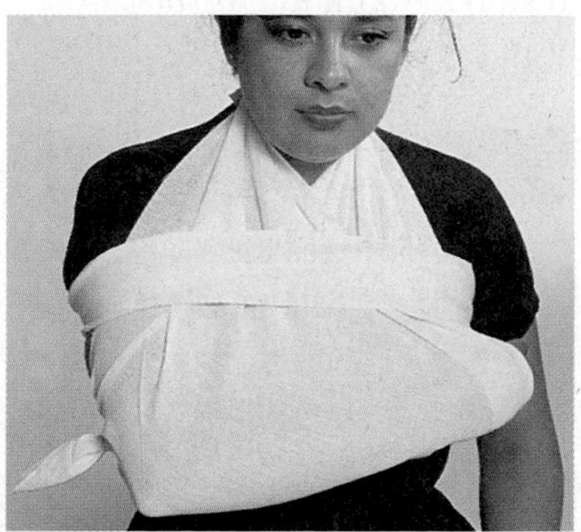

Figure 13.13 Sling and swathe.

Improvise

Improvised splints can be made from rolled newspapers, magazines, towels, or belts (**Figure 13.11**).

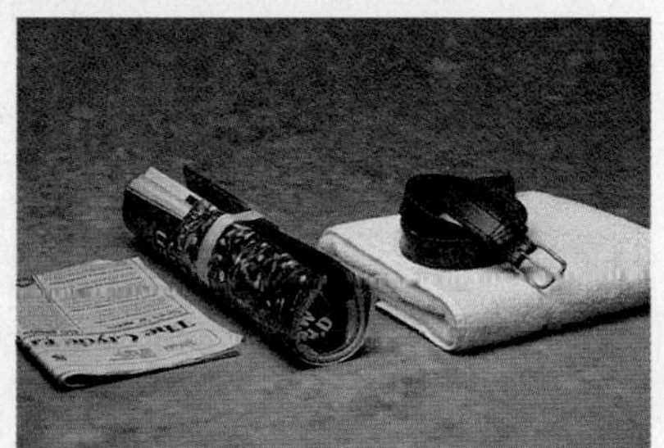

Figure 13.11 Improvised splints (magazines, newspapers, belt, towel).

Improvise

When triangular bandages are not available, loop a length of gauze (or even a belt) around the patient's wrist and suspend the limb from the neck (**Figure 13.14**). Secure the arm gently, but firmly, to the chest wall with another length of gauze or belt. If you haven't cut away the coat, you can also pin a coat sleeve to the front of the patient's coat as a temporary splint (**Figure 13.15**). This technique is less secure than a sling and swathe, but it may be of use in cold weather areas.

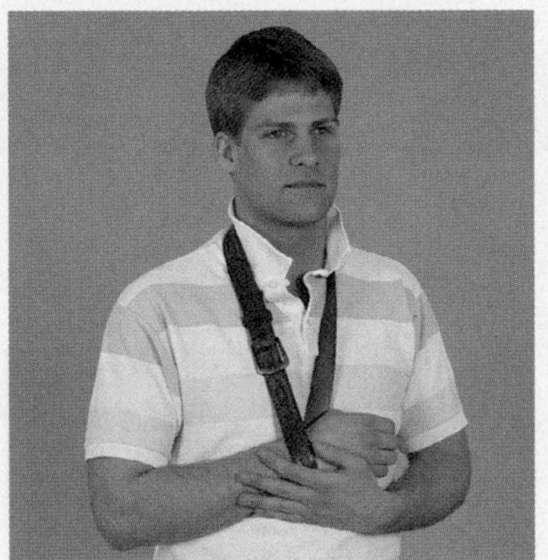

Figure 13.14 (above) Improvised sling using a belt.

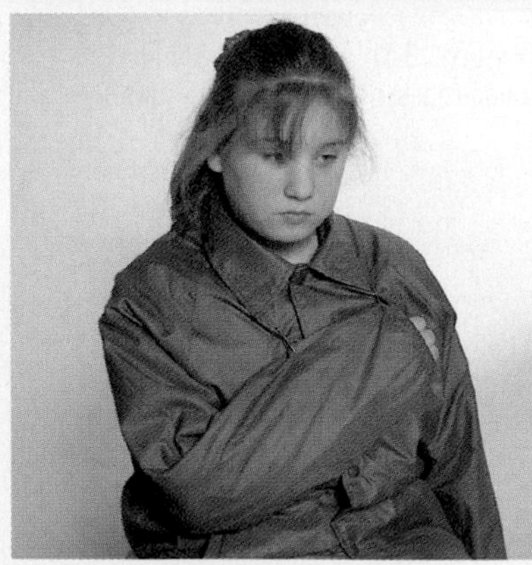

Figure 13.15 Improvised sling using safety pins.

Elbow Injuries

Do not move an injured elbow from the position in which you find it. The elbow must be splinted as it lies because any movement can cause nerve or blood vessel damage. If the elbow is straight, splint it straight. If the elbow is bent at an unusual angle, splint it in that position.

After splinting the injured elbow of a patient who does not have a significant shoulder injury (and only if it does not cause pain), gently move the splinted injury to the patient's side, for comfort and ease of transport.

An effective splint for an injured elbow is a pillow splint. Wrap the elbow in a pillow, add additional padding to keep the elbow in the position found, and secure the pillow as shown in **Figure 13.16**. The patient is usually transported in a sitting position with the splinted elbow resting on his or her lap. A padded wire ladder or SAM® splint is also effective for splinting elbows that are found in severely deformed positions.

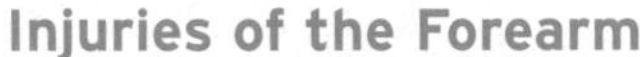

Figure 13.16 Pillow splint.

Injuries of the Forearm

Several splints can be used to stabilize the **forearm**: the air splint, the cardboard splint, the SAM® splint (**Figure 13.17**), even rolled newspapers and magazines. Be sure to pad all rigid splints adequately.

An air splint can be applied quickly and immobilizes the forearm quite well. Of the several types of air splints available, the one with a full-length zipper is easiest to use (**Figure 13.18**).

Unzip the air splint completely, keeping the air intake valve on the outside of the splint. Carefully support the injured forearm and slip the unzipped air splint under it. After the air splint is positioned to correctly support the injured site, connect the zipper, zip it shut, and inflate it by mouth until the plastic can be depressed slightly when you exert firm pressure with your fingers.

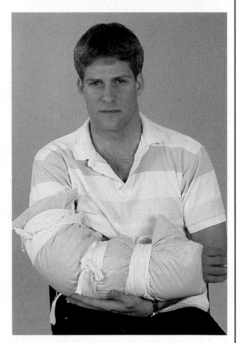

CAUTION

NEVER use anything but the air from your mouth to inflate air splints!

To apply an air splint without a zipper, place the air splint over your hand and lower arm and grasp the patient's hand. Have a second person support the patient's elbow and upper arm to prevent movement. Slip the air splint off your arm and onto the patient's injured forearm.

forearm The lower portion of the upper extremity; from the elbow to the wrist.

Skill Drill

Figure 13.17 Applying a SAM® Splint

1

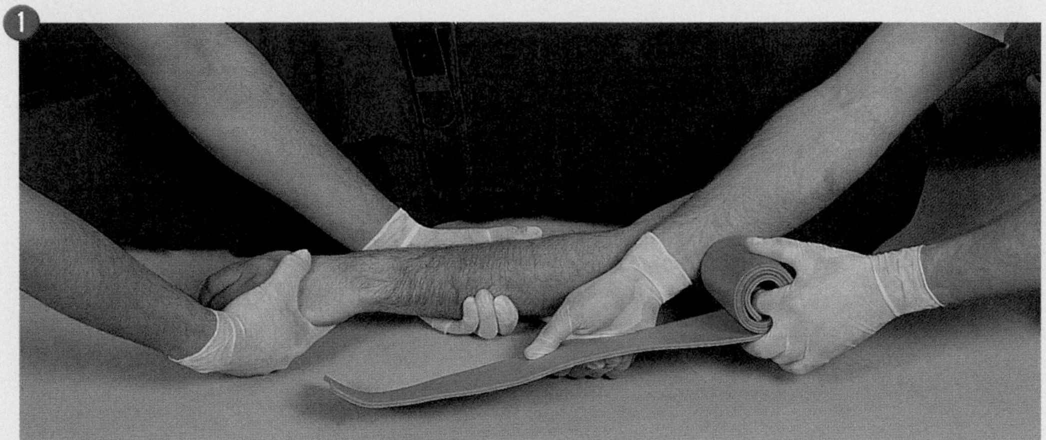

Stabilize injured limb. Form SAM® splint.

2

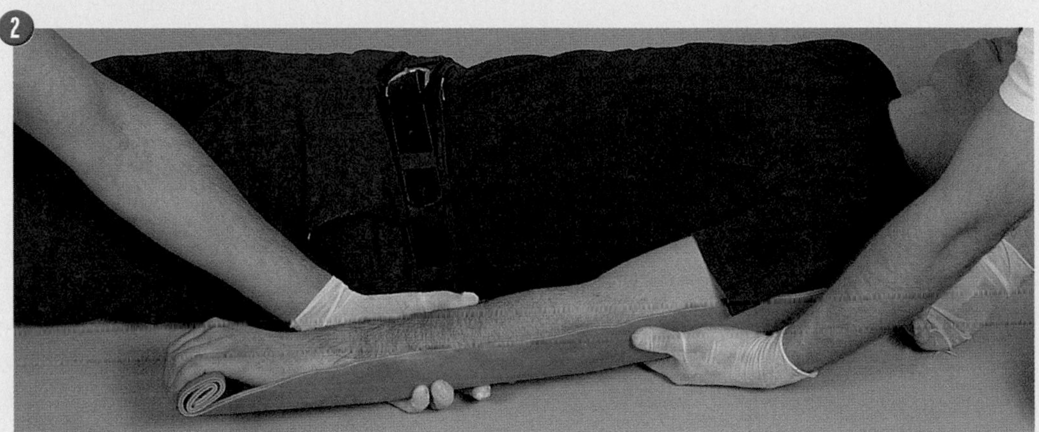

Place splint under injured limb.

3

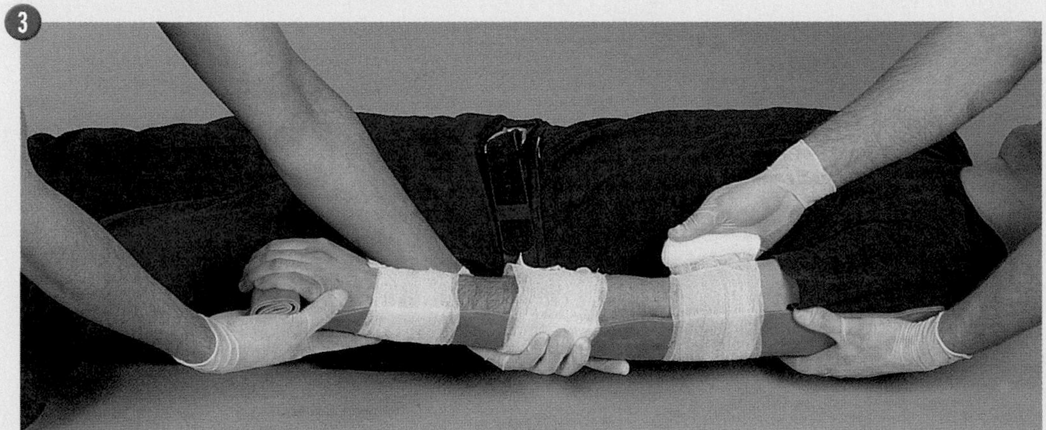

Secure with gauze.

Skill Drill

Figure 13.18 Applying an Air Splint

1

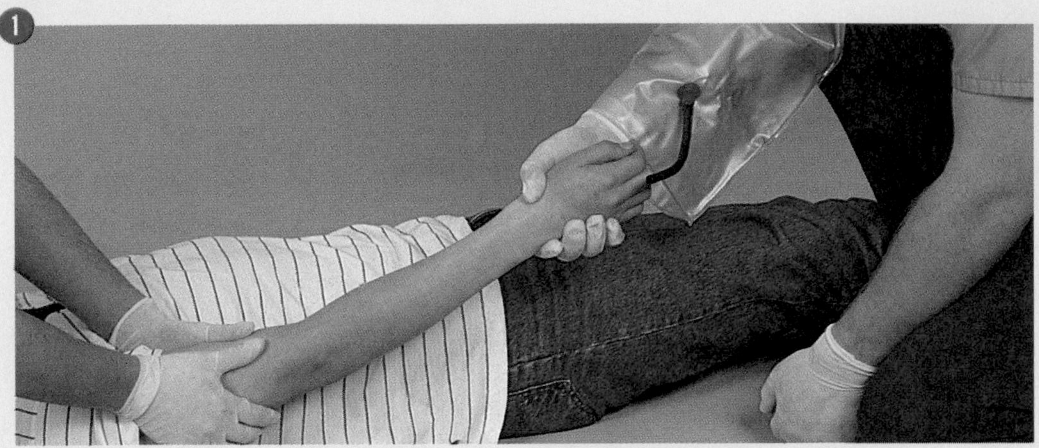

Stabilize injured forearm. Place air splint over your arm.

2

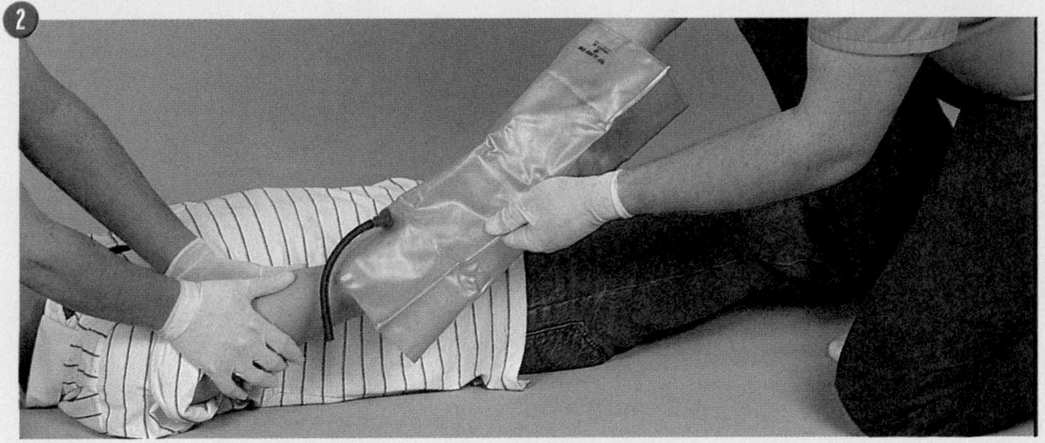

Slide air splint over injured arm.

3

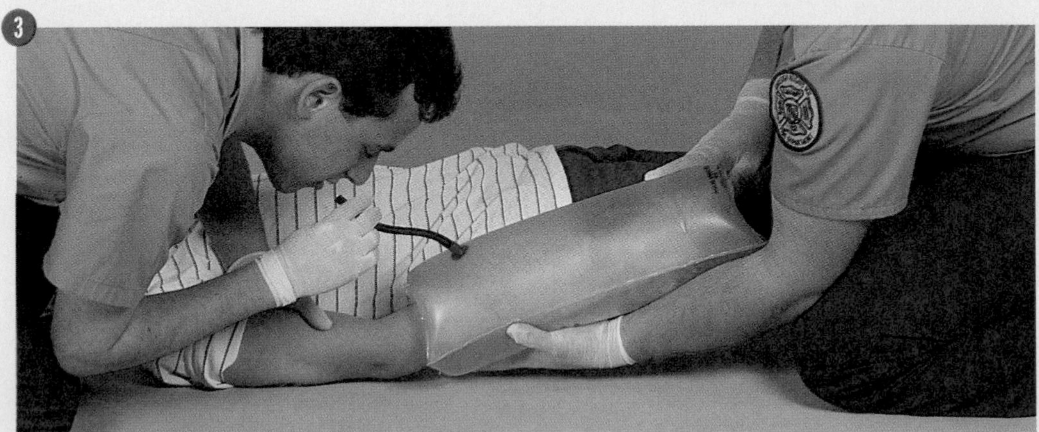

Inflate by mouth.

The air splint should extend over the patient's hand and wrist to prevent swelling. Inflate the splint, as described earlier.

Injuries of the Hand, Wrist, and Fingers

As a first responder, you will see a variety of hand injuries, all of which can be potentially serious. The functions of the fingers and hand are so complex that any injury, if poorly or inadequately treated, may result in permanent deformity and disability. Treat even seemingly simple lacerations carefully. Send any amputated parts to the hospital with the patient. You can use a bulky hand dressing and a short splint to immobilize all injuries of the wrist, hand, and fingers.

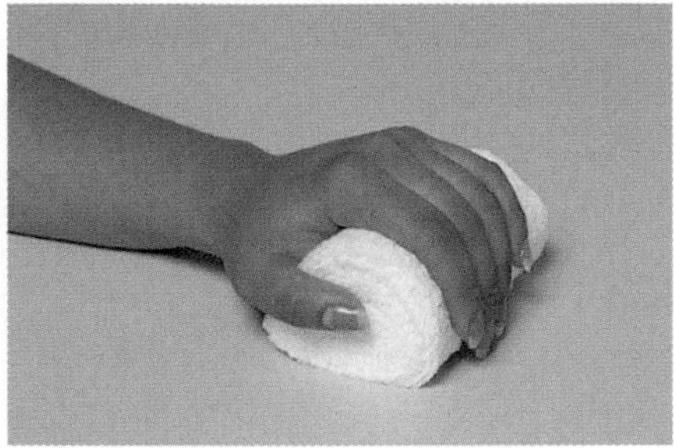

Figure 13.20 Position of function for hand and wrist.

First, cover all wounds with a dry, sterile dressing. Then place the injured hand and wrist into what is called the "position of function" (**Figure 13.20**). Place one or two soft roller dressings into the palm of the patient's hand. Apply a splint to hold the wrist, hand, and fingers in the position of function and secure the splint with a soft roller bandage.

Pelvic Fractures

Fractures of the pelvis often involve severe blood loss because the broken bones can easily lacerate the large blood vessels that run directly beside the pelvis. These vessels can release a great deal of blood into the pelvic area. Pelvic fractures commonly cause shock. Therefore, the first responder must always treat the patient for shock. However, do not raise the patient's legs until he or she is secured on a backboard.

The surest sign of pelvic fracture is tenderness when both your hands firmly compress the patient's pelvis (**Figure 13.21**). Immobilize fractures of the pelvis with a long backboard, as illustrated in **Figure 13.24**, page 304. EMTs may apply a pneumatic antishock garment (PASG) to stabilize the fracture and treat shock.

A
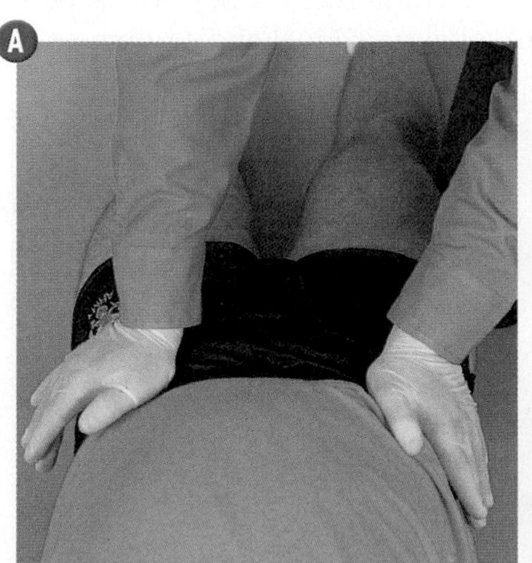

B
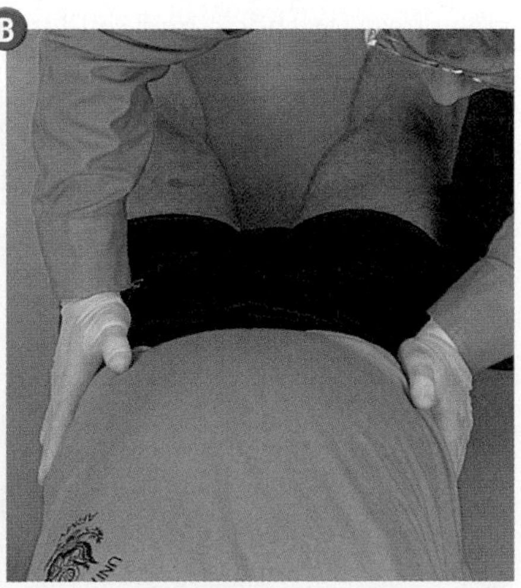

Figure 13.21 Examining the patient for pelvic fracture. **A.** Push down. **B.** Push in.

Improvise

If you have to improvise a splint for a forearm injury, **Figure 13.19** shows how to apply a splint made of magazines and newspapers.

1
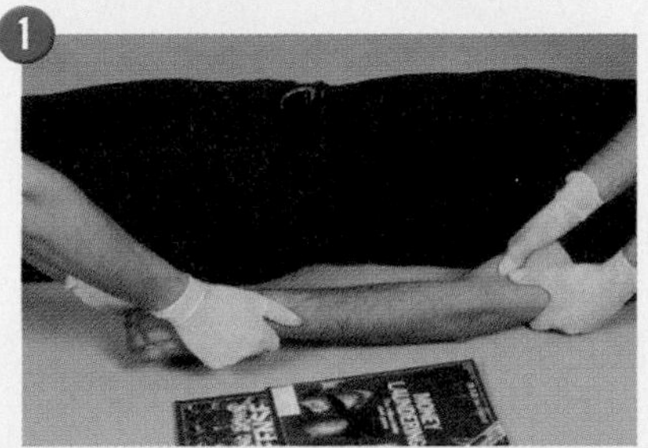

2
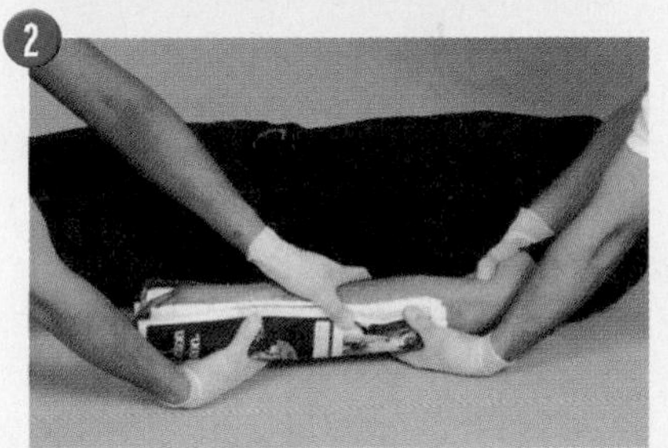

3
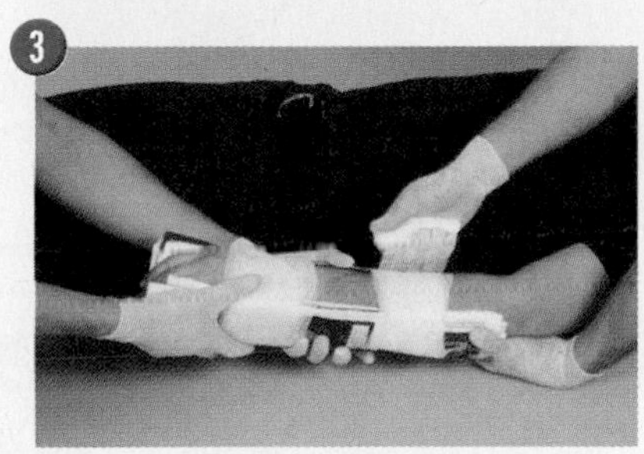

Figure 13.19 Applying an improvised splint using magazines. **1.** Stabilize injured limb. **2.** Place padded magazines under injured arm. **3.** Secure splint with gauze.

trauma A wound or injury, either physical or psychological.

osteoporosis Abnormal brittleness of the bones in older people caused by loss of calcium; affected bones fracture easily.

Hip Injuries

Two types of hip injuries are commonly seen: dislocations and fractures. Both injuries may result from high-energy **trauma**. When an unbelted automobile passenger is thrown forward in an accident and crashes against the dashboard, the impact of the knee against the dashboard is transmitted up the shaft of the thigh bone (femur), injuring the hip and often producing either a dislocation or a fracture (**Figure 13.22**).

Hip fractures actually occur at the upper end of the femur, rather than in the hip joint itself. Hip fractures do not occur only as a result of high-energy trauma; they can occur in elderly people, especially women, after only minimal trauma (such as falling down). These fractures in the elderly occur because bone weakens and become more fragile with advancing age, a condition called **osteoporosis**.

A dislocated hip is extremely painful, especially when any movement is attempted. The joint is usually locked with the thigh flexed and rotated inward across the midline of the body. The knee joint is often flexed as well. Fractures of the hip region usually cause the injured limb to become shortened and externally (outwardly) rotated (**Figure 13.23**).

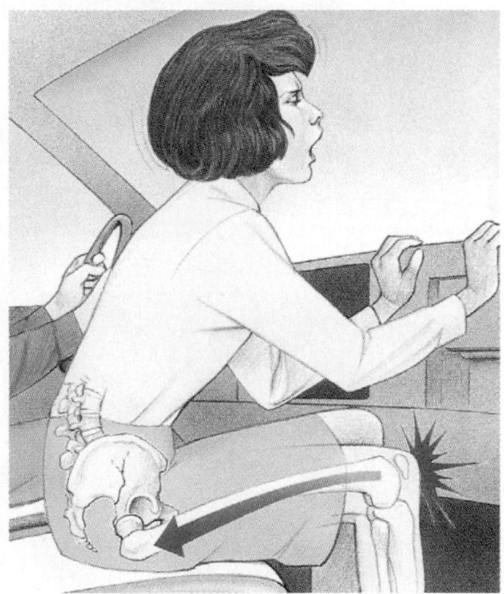

Figure 13.22 Posterior dislocation of hip can occur as a result of the knee hitting the dashboard in an automobile collision.

Treat all hip injuries by immobilizing the hip in the position found. Use several pillows and/or rolled blankets, especially under the flexed knee. The patient should be placed on a long backboard for transportation. The patient and the limb should be well stabilized to eliminate all motion in the hip region (**Figure 13.24**).

Because fractures of the upper end of the femur are so common in elderly patients, any elderly person who has fallen and complains of pain in the hip, thigh, or knee—even if there is no deformity—should be splinted and transported to the hospital for X-ray evaluation.

Injuries of the Thigh

Trauma to the thigh can bruise the muscles or fracture the shaft of the femur. A fractured femur is very unstable and usually produces significant thigh deformity. There is much bleeding and swelling.

The treatment of femur fractures (PSDE) requires skill and proper equipment. As a first responder, you can treat for shock and help prevent further injury. Place the patient in as comfortable a position as possible, treat for shock, and call for additional personnel and equipment.

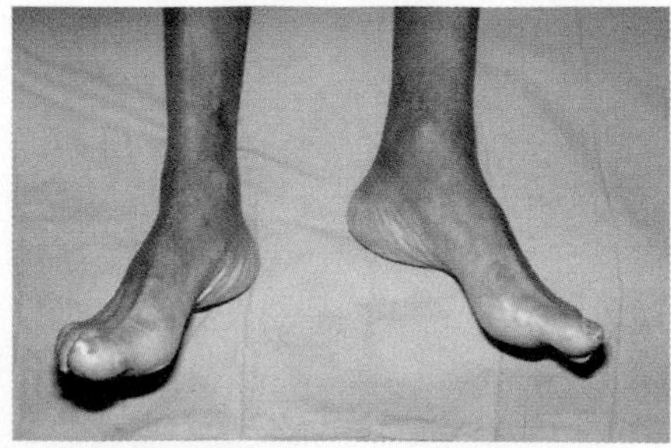

Figure 13.23 Signs of a hip fracture include external rotation and shortening of the injured leg.

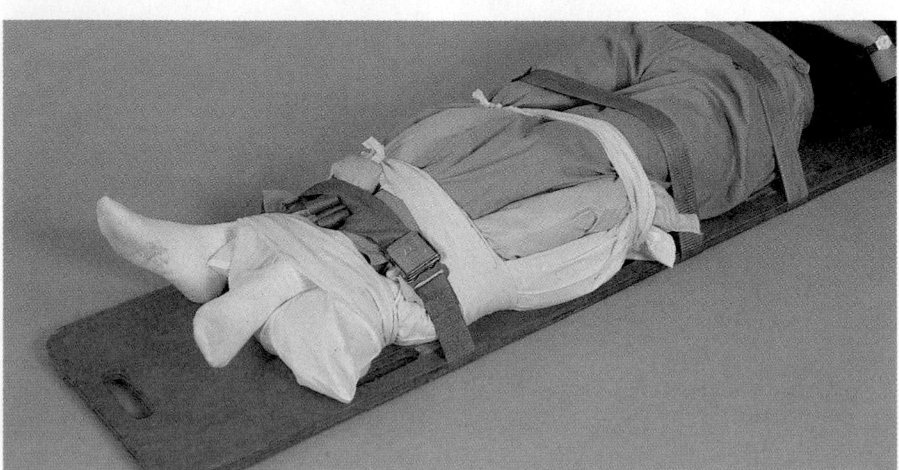

Figure 13.24 Immobilization of hip or pelvic injuries using a backboard.

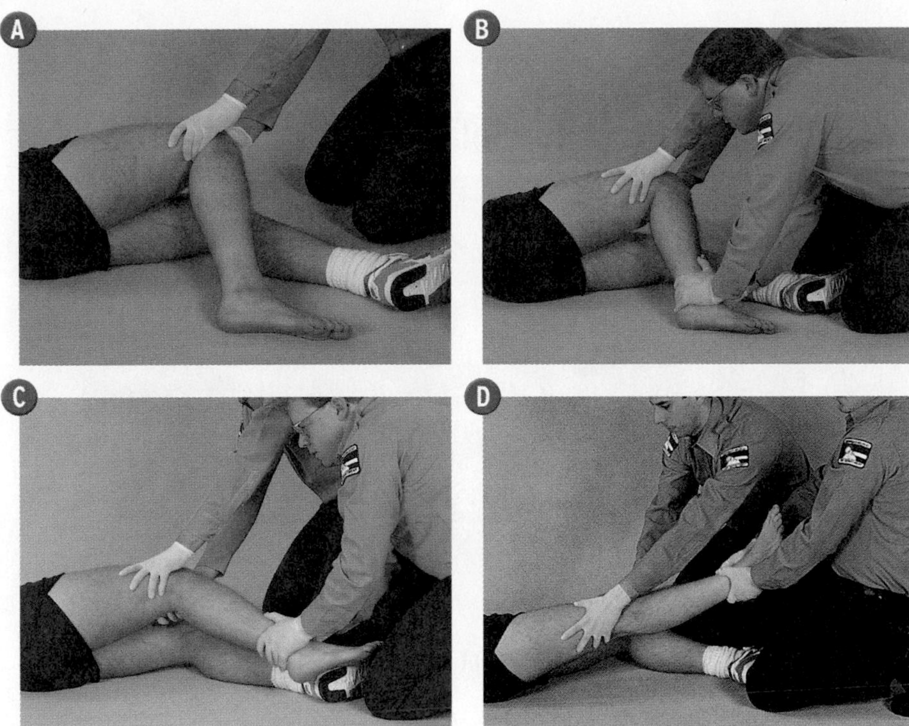

Figure 13.25 Straightening an injured leg for splinting. **A.** The first rescuer grasps the injured leg at the knee and applies traction in the long axis of the body. **B.** The second rescuer grasps the ankle. **C.** The second rescuer straightens the leg. **D.** The second rescuer maintains traction by leaning back.

CAUTION

DO NOT elevate the injured leg when treating for shock.

However, after a motor vehicle crash, you may have to move the patient quickly, even before proper equipment and additional personnel arrive. You should learn and practice emergency temporary splinting for lower extremity injuries. Secure both legs together with several swathes, cravats, or bandages so that the two lower extremities are immobilized as one unit. This technique allows you to remove the patient from a dangerous environment quickly.

A traction splint is the most effective way to splint a fractured femur. Traction splints are designed specifically for this purpose. Although you may not have a traction splint in your first responder life support kit, you should know how it works so that you can assist other EMS personnel, as needed.

Before applying a traction splint, trained EMTs align deformed fractures (PSDE) by applying manual longitudinal traction. Once manual traction is applied, it must be maintained until the traction splint is fully in place (**Figure 13.25**).

Many different types of traction splints are available. Most are applied basically using the same method (**Figure 13.26**, page 306):

1. An ankle hitch is placed around the ankle. Apply manual traction over the hitch.
2. (a) The traction splint is adjusted to the correct length by laying the splint beside the uninjured leg and extending it about 8 to 10 inches beyond the bottom of the patient's foot.

Skill Drill

Figure 13.26 Applying a Traction Splint

1

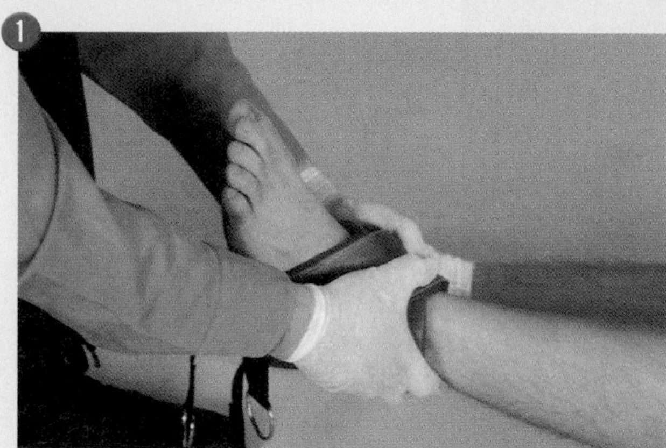

Apply manual traction over the ankle hitch.

2

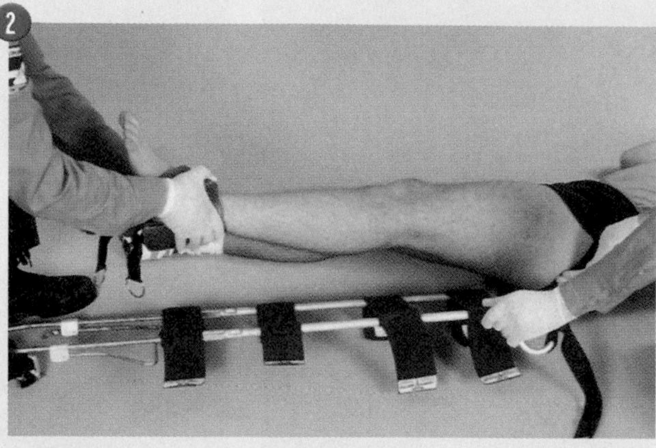

With the traction splint adjusted for length, place it under the injured limb.

3

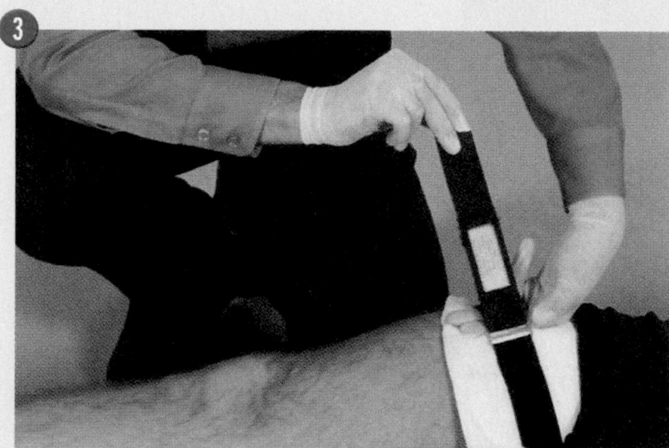

Pad the groin and fasten the strap.

4

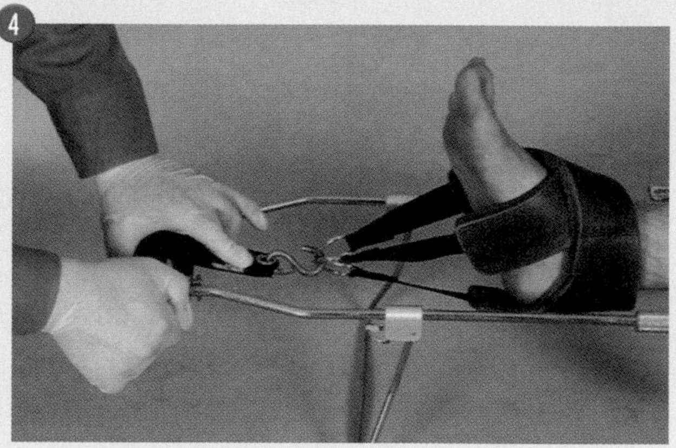

Apply traction.

5

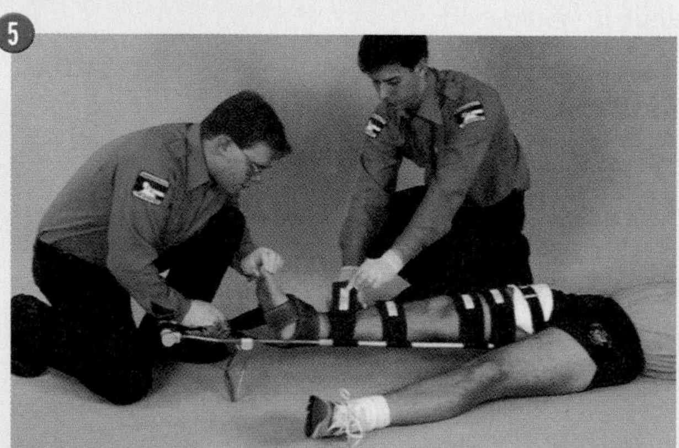

Secure and check support straps. Assess pulse, capillary refill, and nerve function.

(b) The splint is placed under the patient's injured leg and hip. Gently logroll the patient onto his or her uninjured side until you can place the splint under the injured limb, up to the level of the hip.

3. The splint is attached at the hip, using the strap provided for this purpose.
4. The ankle hitch is attached to the foot end of the splint and the mechanical traction device tightened until the mechanical traction force equals the manual force. The patient's pain will diminish when the correct amount of traction is applied.
5. Wide supporting straps are added to secure the limb to the splint. These supports are placed about every 8 inches along the limb. A support should not be placed directly on the injury site but there be one above and another below the site.

   To apply proper traction using this type of splint, it is essential that the foot end of the traction splint be elevated 6 to 8 inches off the ground. If the heel of the injured leg touches the ground, traction is lost and must be reapplied. Most traction splints include a foot stand that elevates the limb.

Check and recheck pulse, capillary refill, and nerve function before and after a splint is applied (**Figure 13.27**).

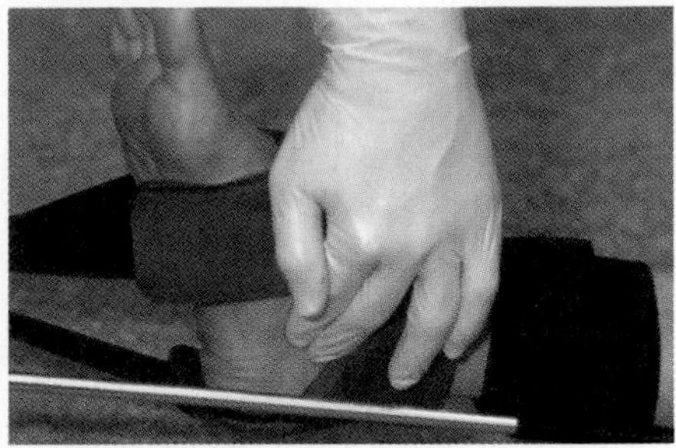

Figure 13.27 Checking the ankle pulse.

Knee Injuries

Always immobilize an injured knee in the same position that you find it. If it is straight, use long, padded board splints or a long-leg air splint. If there is a significant deformity, place pillows, blankets, or clothing beneath the knee, secure the splint materials to the leg with bandages, swathes, or cravats, and secure the injured leg to the uninjured leg (**Figure 13.28**). Then place the patient on a backboard.

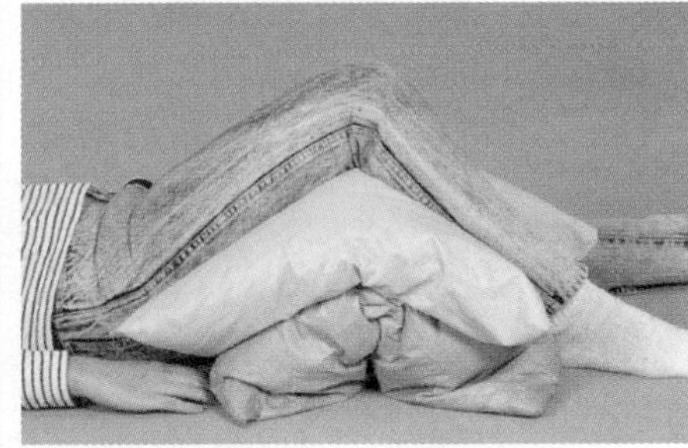

Figure 13.28 Immobilizing an injured knee.

Leg Injuries

Like fractures of the forearm, fractures of the leg can be splinted with air splints, cardboard splints, and even magazines and newspapers. **Figure 13.30** on page 308, shows how to apply an air splint to the leg.

It takes two trained people to splint an injured leg. One person supports the leg with both hands (above and below the injury site), while the other person applies the splint.

Injuries of the Ankle and Foot

Fractures of the ankle and foot can be splinted with either a pillow or an air splint. Place the pillow splint around the injured ankle and foot, and tie or pin it in place (**Figure 13.31**, page 309).

Additional Considerations

Remember that extremity injuries are not, in themselves, life threatening unless excessive bleeding is present.

You may not always have the equipment or help you need to manage all types of extremity injuries. You may not even have time to splint an injury before additional EMS personnel arrive. There will be times, however, when you are the only trained person at the scene of an accident. To prepare for such situations, practice splinting until you can apply the principles in any situation. Because you may find the patient in a variety of positions and locations, practice splinting both a sitting and a prone volunteer.

Remember

Pad all rigid splints to provide the best stabilization and pain relief. Do not apply any splint too tightly. Recheck pulse, capillary refill, and sensation after the splint is applied, to make sure that no damage has been done (**Figure 13.29**).

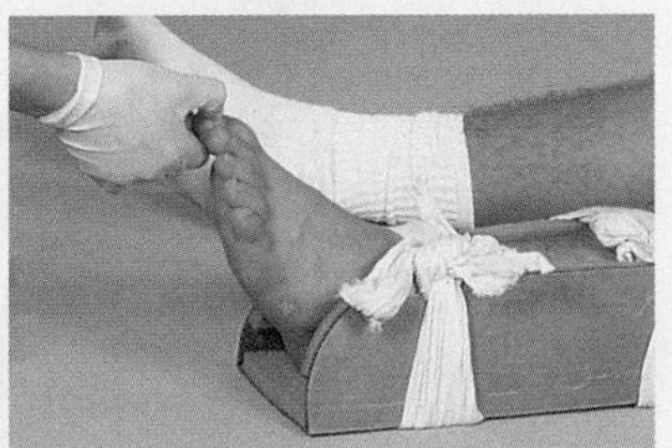

Figure 13.29 Checking capillary refill on splinted injured leg.

Skill Drill

Figure 13.30 Applying an Air Splint to the Leg

1

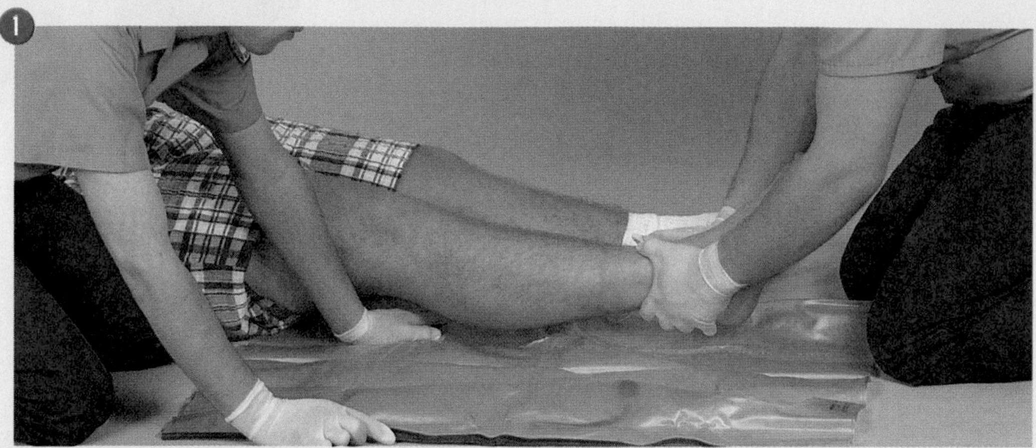

Support injured limb. Slide splint under limb.

2

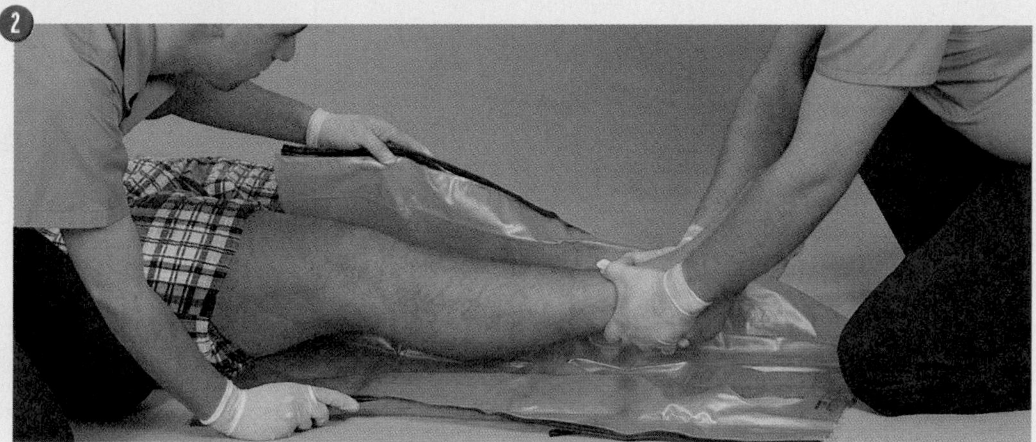

Place splint around limb.

3

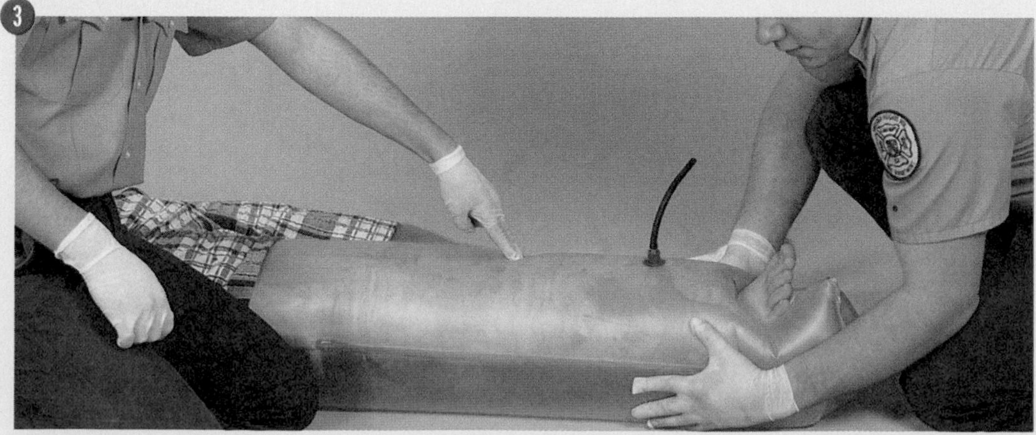

Inflate splint.

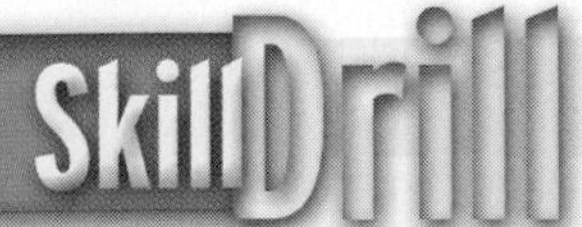

Figure 13.31 Applying a Pillow Splint for Ankle or Foot Injury

1

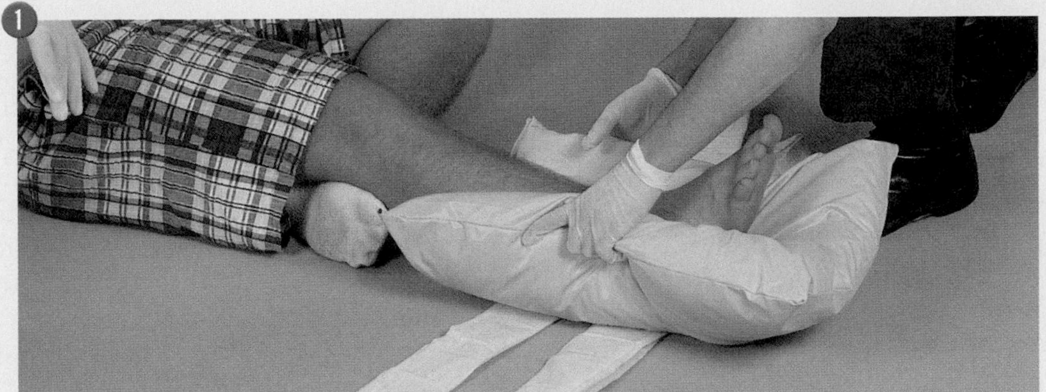

Place pillow under injured limb.

2

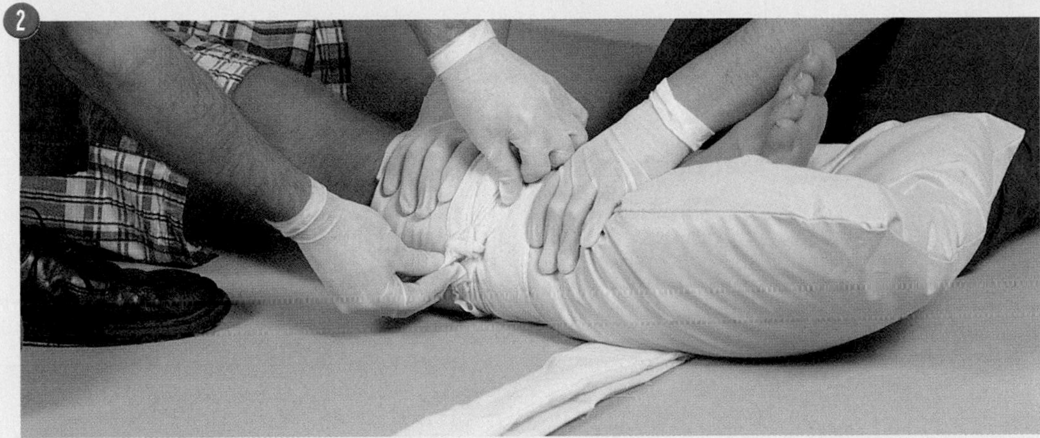

Secure with cravats, swathes or bandages.

3

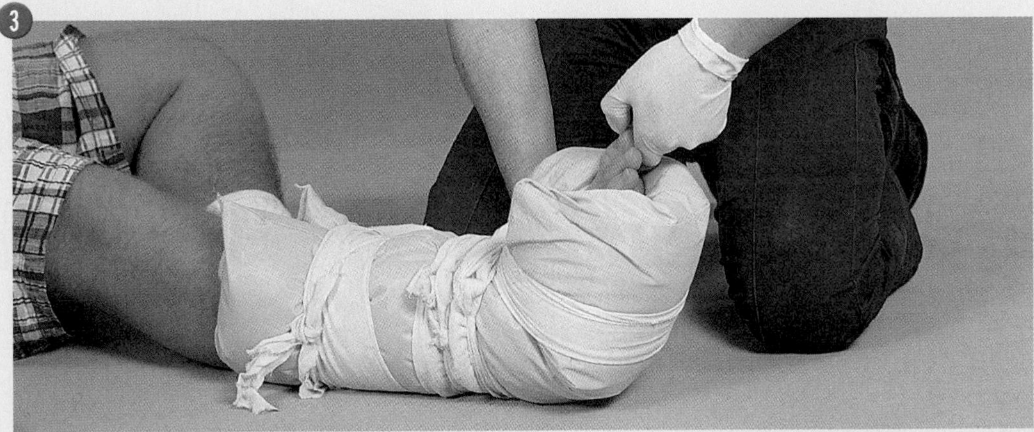

Recheck pulse, capillary refill and sensation.

It takes two people to adequately splint most limb injuries: one to stabilize and support the extremity and one to apply the splint. Most of the principles and techniques of splinting covered in this chapter require that you work with another member of the EMS team. Learn how the team functions as a unit during stressful situations and be prepared to work with any member of the EMS team who arrives to assist you.

Signs & Symptoms

HEAD INJURIES

- confusion
- unusual behavior
- unconsciousness
- nausea or vomiting
- blood from an ear
- decreasing consciousness
- unequal pupils
- paralysis
- seizures
- external head trauma: bleeding, bumps, and contusions

Injuries of the Head (Skull and Brain)

Severe head and spinal cord injuries can result from many different kinds of trauma. These injuries are common causes of death and can also lead to irreversible paralysis and permanent brain damage. Improperly handling a patient after an accident can cause further injury or death. Spinal injuries can be caused, for example, by well-intended citizens pulling a patient from a wrecked car, or by poor treatment from inadequately trained emergency personnel. As a first responder, you must know what to do to provide prompt treatment and avoid errors that may make the injury worse.

The human skull has two primary parts (**Figure 13.32**):

- The cranium, a tough four-bone shell that protects the brain
- The facial bones, which give form to the face and furnish frontal protection for the brain

seizures Sudden episodes of uncontrolled electrical activity in the brain.

Mechanisms of Injury

Head injuries are common with certain types of trauma. Of patients involved in automobile accidents, 70 percent suffer some degree of head injury.

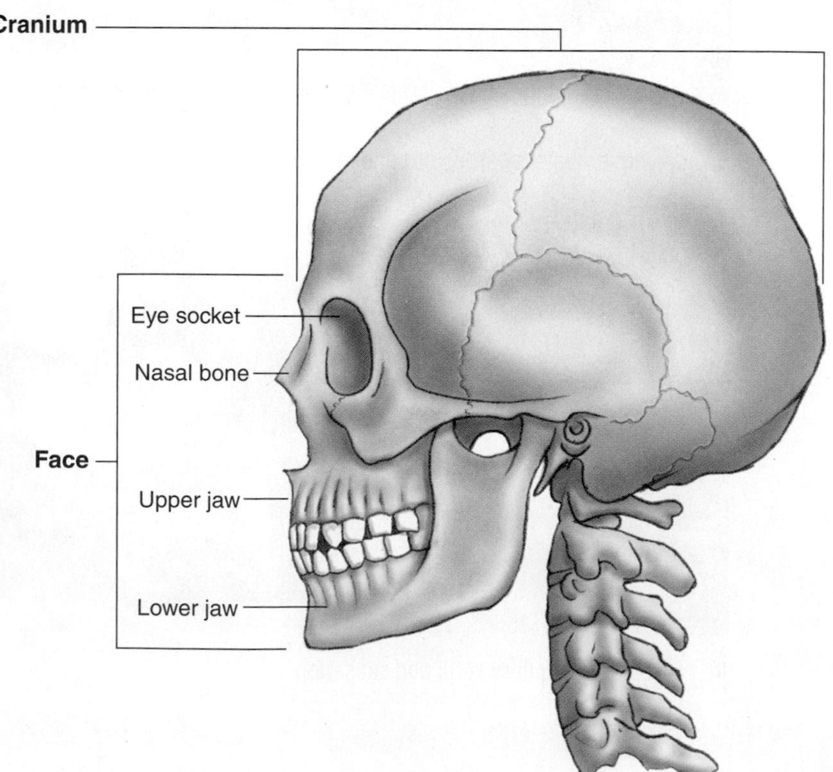

Figure 13.32 Cranium and face of the human skull.

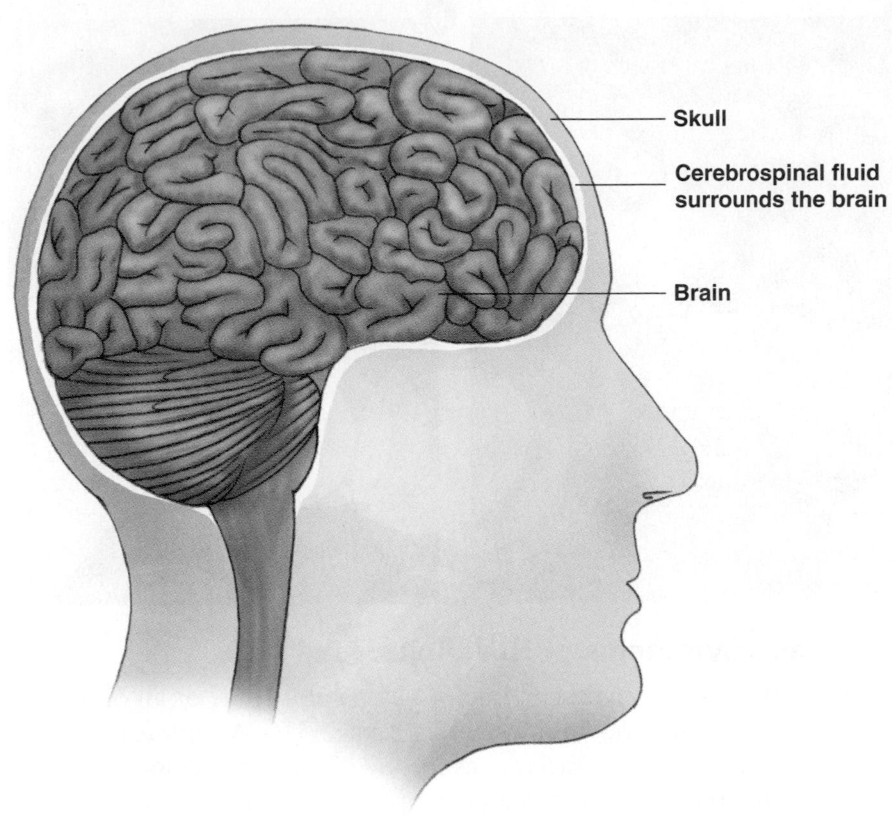

Figure 13.33 The brain.

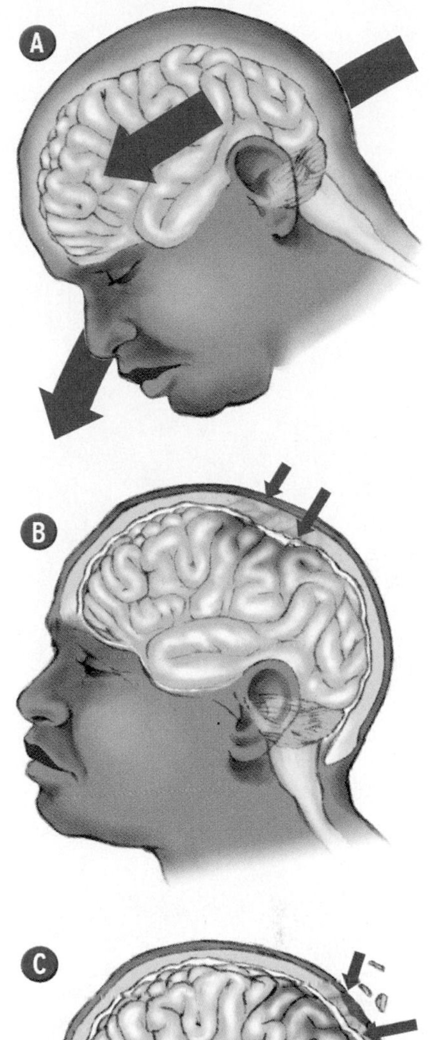

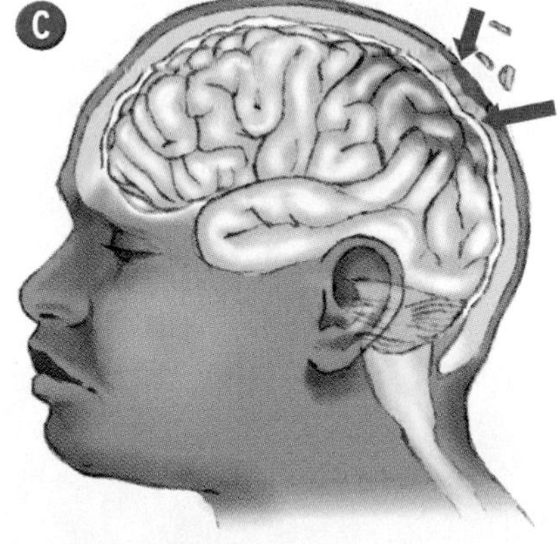

Figure 13.34 Open and closed head injuries. **A.** A head injury may cause a cervical spine injury. **B.** A closed head injury. **C.** An open head injury.

Imagine the cranium as a rigid bowl, containing the delicate brain (**Figure 13.33**). Between the skull and brain, a fluid called **cerebrospinal fluid (CSF)** cushions the brain from direct blows. A direct force such as a hammer blow can injure the skull and the brain inside. Indirect forces can also cause injury, as in an automobile accident when the head strikes the windshield (**Figure 13.5**, page 291) and causes the brain to bounce against the inside of the skull.

Spinal injury is often associated with head injury. The force of direct blows to the head is often transmitted to the spine, producing a fracture or dislocation. The injuries may damage the spinal cord or at least put it at risk for injury. Any time you suspect or identify an injury to the head or skull, you should also suspect injury to the neck and spinal cord. Therefore, all patients with head injuries must have the cervical spine splinted to protect the spinal cord.

Types of Head Injuries

Injuries of the head are classified as open or closed (**Figure 13.34**). In a **closed head injury**, bleeding and swelling within the skull may increase pressure on the brain, leading to irreversible brain damage and death if it is not relieved. An open injury of the head usually bleeds profusely. Severe open head injuries are serious but not always fatal.

Examine the nose, eyes, and the wound itself to see if any blood or cerebrospinal fluid (CSF) is seeping out. The CSF is clear, watery, and straw-colored. In severe cases of open head injury, brain tissue or bone may be visible.

cerebrospinal fluid (CSF) A clear, watery fluid that fills the space between the brain and spinal cord and their protective coverings.

closed head injury Injury where there is bleeding and/or swelling within the skull.

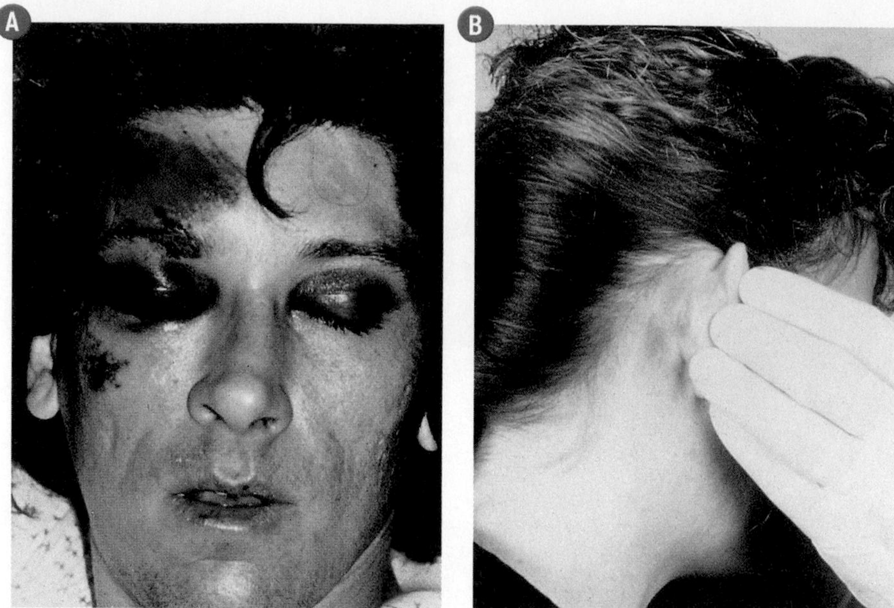

Figure 13.35 Signs of head injury. **A.** Raccoon eyes. **B.** Battle's sign.

Signs and Symptoms of Head Injuries

A patient suffering from a head injury may exhibit some or all of the signs and symptoms shown in the box on page 310. A serious head injury may also produce "raccoon eyes" and "Battle's sign." Raccoon eyes look like the black eyes that develop after a fist fight. Battle's sign appears as a bruise behind one or both ears (**Figure 13.35**).

Treatment of Head Injuries

When any one sign or symptom of head injury is present, proceed as follows:

1. Immobilize the head in a neutral position. Stabilize the patient's neck and prevent movement of the head.
2. Maintain an open airway. Use the jaw-thrust technique to open the airway (see Chapter 6). Avoid movement of the head and neck.
3. Support the patient's breathing. Be sure that the patient is breathing adequately on his or her own. If not, institute mouth-to-mask or mouth-to-barrier ventilation. As soon as oxygen becomes available, it should be administered to the patient. Oxygen helps minimize swelling of the brain.
4. Monitor circulation. Be prepared to support circulation by performing full CPR if the patient's heart stops.
5. Check to see if CSF or blood is seeping from a wound or from the nose or ears (**Figure 13.36**). CSF is clear, watery, and straw-colored. Do not try to stop leakage of CSF from a wound or any other opening because leakage from inside the skull relieves internal pressure.
6. Control bleeding from all head wounds with dry, sterile dressings. Use enough direct pressure to control the bleeding without disturbing the underlying tissue.
7. Examine and treat other serious injuries.
8. Arrange for T ***prompt transport*** to an appropriate medical facility.

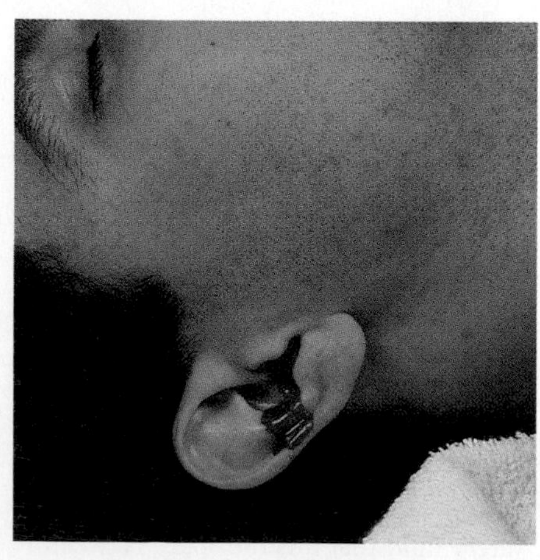

Figure 13.36 Blood or CSF from the ear indicates head injury.

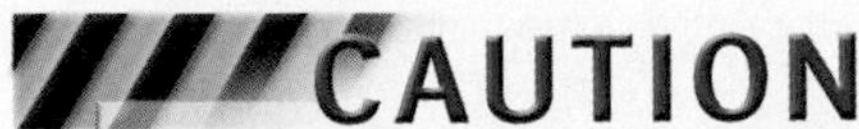

If a patient has a head injury, assume that an associated neck or spinal cord injury is also present. Do nothing that would cause undue movement of the head and spine. Always splint the entire spine before moving the patient.

Check point

- ○ List the steps for treating a patient with possible head injury.

Injuries of the Face

Facial injuries commonly result from:

- Motor vehicle crashes in which the patient's face hits the steering wheel or windshield
- Assaults
- Falls

Airway obstruction is the primary danger in severe facial injuries. Severe damage to the face and facial bones can cause bleeding and the collapse of the facial bones, leading to airway problems. If the patient has facial injuries, you should also suspect a spinal injury. Although facial injuries may bleed considerably, they are rarely life threatening unless the airway is obstructed.

Treatment of Facial Injuries

When facial injuries are present, proceed as follows:

1. Immobilize the head in a neutral position. Stabilize it to prevent further movement of the neck.
2. Maintain an open airway. Use the jaw-thrust technique to open the airway. Clear any blood or vomitus from the patient's mouth with your gloved fingers.
3. Support breathing. Be prepared to ventilate the patient, if necessary.
4. Monitor circulation.
5. Control bleeding by covering any wound with a dry, sterile dressing and applying direct pressure. Be sure to check for wounds inside the mouth. Try to prevent the patient from swallowing blood because this can cause vomiting.
6. Look for and stabilize other serious injuries.
7. Arrange for T ***prompt transport*** to an appropriate medical facility.

If these measures do not keep the airway clear, or if you are unable to control severe facial bleeding, logroll the patient onto his or her side, keeping the head and spine stable and rolling the whole body as a unit.

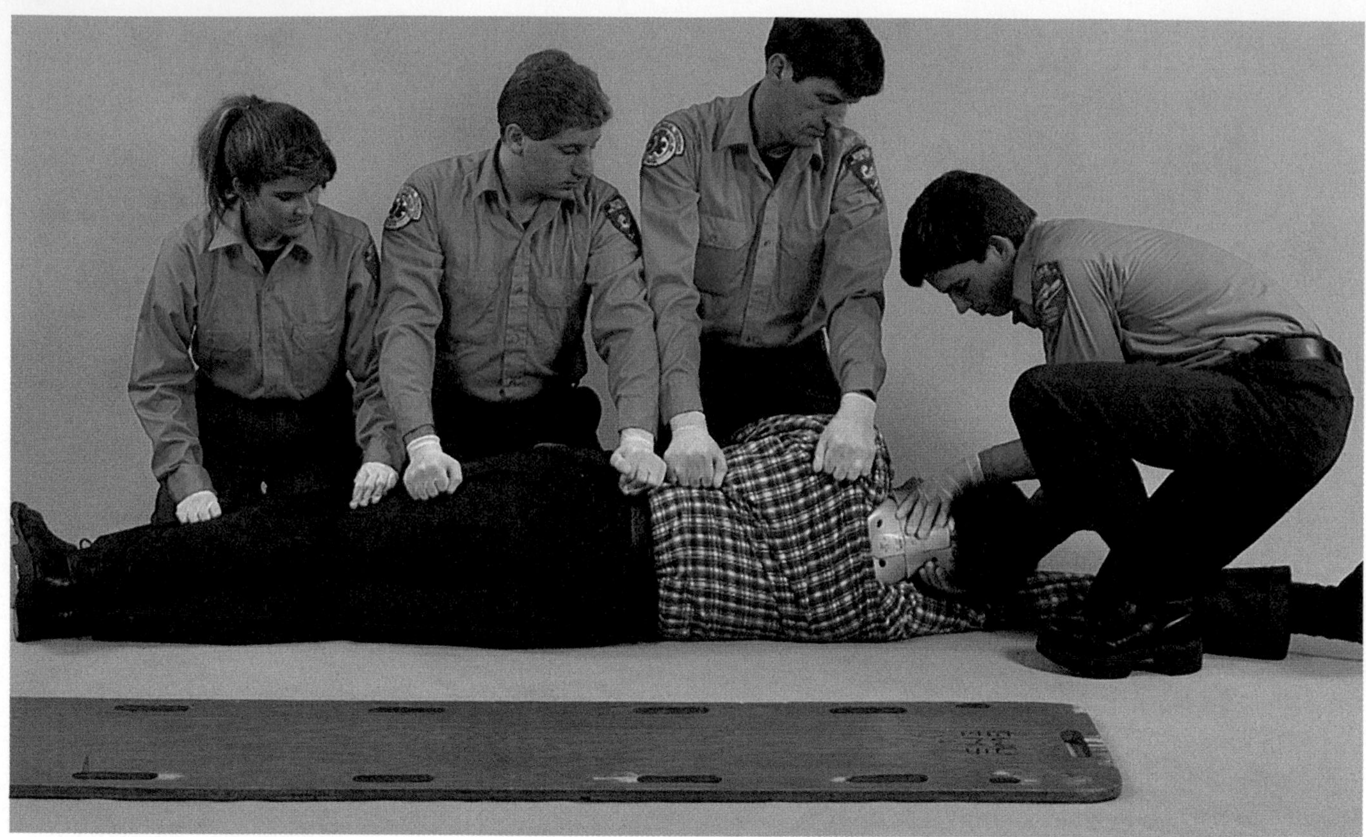

Figure 13.37 Keep the head and spine in alignment by using logroll technique.

Remember

The spine consists of 33 vertebrae stacked one upon the other and held together by ligaments. Each vertebra has a hollow center through which passes the great mass of nerves known as the spinal cord. The spinal cord is connected to the brain and can be compared to a large telephone trunk line in that it carries two-way communication to and from the brain.

Turn the head and body at the same time. The neck must not be allowed to twist (**Figure 13.37**).

CAUTION

If a patient has head or spine injuries, use a logroll to move the patient onto his or her side. Do not place these patients in the recovery position. Provide support for the head and neck.

Bandage facial injuries as described in Chapter 12. If possible, leave the patient's eyes clear of bandages so he or she can see what is happening. Being able to see reduces the patient's tendency to panic.

Injuries of the Spine

As mentioned earlier in this chapter, spinal injuries can cause irreversible **paralysis**. As a first responder, you must know how to properly handle a patient and provide prompt treatment. Errors may make the injury worse.

paralysis Inability of a conscious person to move voluntarily.

Mechanisms of Injury

If one or more vertebrae are injured, the spinal cord may also be injured. A displaced vertebra, swelling, or bleeding (**Figure 13.38**) may put pressure on the spinal cord and damage it. In severe cases, the cord may be

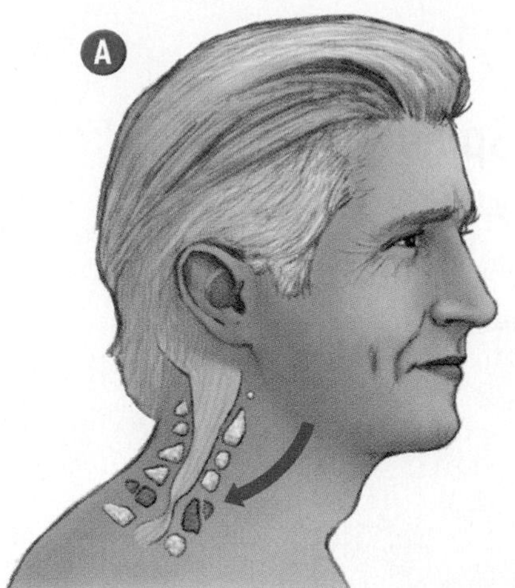
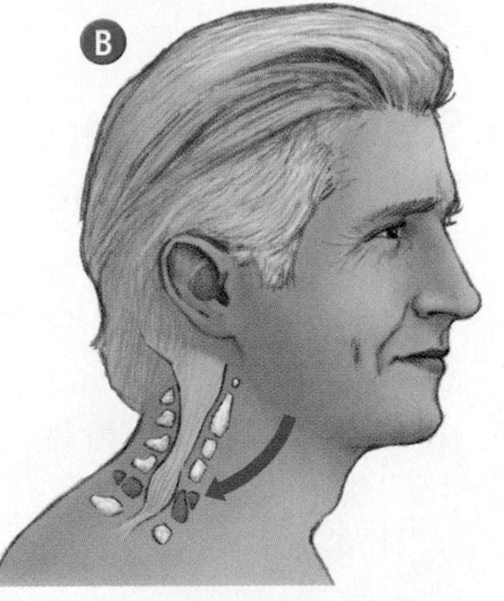
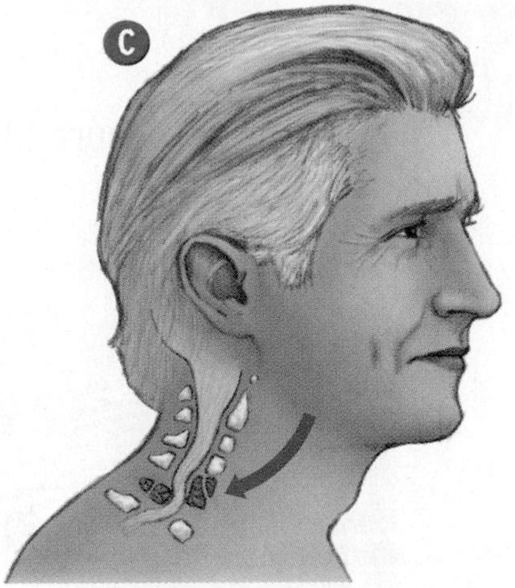

Figure 13.38 Types of spinal injuries. **A.** Pressure on the spinal cord from swelling or fracture. **B.** Bruising of the spinal cord by broken vertebrae. **C.** Injury by displacement and fractured vertebrae.

severed. If all or part of the spinal cord is cut, nerve impulses (which are like signals in the telephone cable) cannot travel to and from the brain. Then the patient is paralyzed below the point of injury. Injury to the spinal cord high in the neck paralyzes the diaphragm and results in death. Gunshot wounds to the chest or abdomen may produce spinal cord injury at that level.

Signs and Symptoms of Spinal Cord Injury

To determine if a patient has sustained an injury to the spinal cord, carefully examine and talk to the patient and attempt to determine the mechanism of injury. Gently conduct a hands-on examination, as described in Chapter 7, to detect paralysis or weakness. Ask the patient to describe any points of tenderness or pain. Do not move the patient during the examination. Further, do not allow the patient to move. The key signs and symptoms of a spinal injury are noted in the Signs and Symptoms box.

During your examination, be extremely careful. Take your time. Do not move patients unless they are in a hazardous area.

Signs & Symptoms

SPINAL INJURIES

- Laceration, bruise, or other sign of injury to the head, neck, or spine
- Tenderness over any point on the spine or neck
- Extremity weakness, paralysis, or loss of movement
- Loss of sensation or tingling in any part of the body below the neck

Treatment of Spinal Injuries

If any one sign or symptom of spinal injury is present, proceed as follows:

1. Place the head and neck in a neutral position (**Figure 13.39, step 1**, page 316). Avoid unnecessary movement of the head.
2. Stabilize the head and prevent movement of the neck (**Figure 13.39, step 2**).
3. Maintain an open airway. Use the jaw-thrust technique to open the airway to avoid movement of the head and neck (**Figure 13.39, step 3**). Clear any blood or vomitus from the mouth with your gloved fingers.
4. Support the patient's breathing. A spinal cord injury may paralyze some or all of the respiratory muscles, resulting in abnormal breathing patterns. In some cases, only the diaphragm may be working. Breathing using the diaphragm only is called **abdominal breathing**. The abdomen (not the lungs) swells and collapses with each breath. Help the patient breathe by administering oxygen (if available) and by keeping the airway open.
5. Monitor circulation.
6. Assess pulse, movement, and sensation in all extremities.

Remember

All head injuries indicate the possibility of spinal injuries.

abdominal breathing Breathing using only the diaphragm.

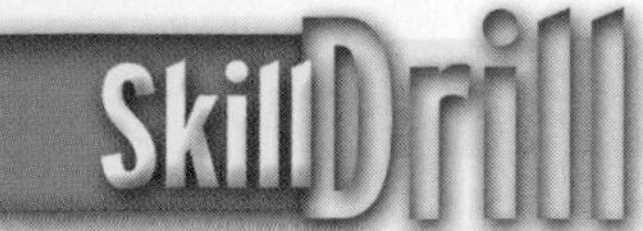

Figure 13.39 Stabilizing the Cervical Spine and Maintaining an Open Airway

1

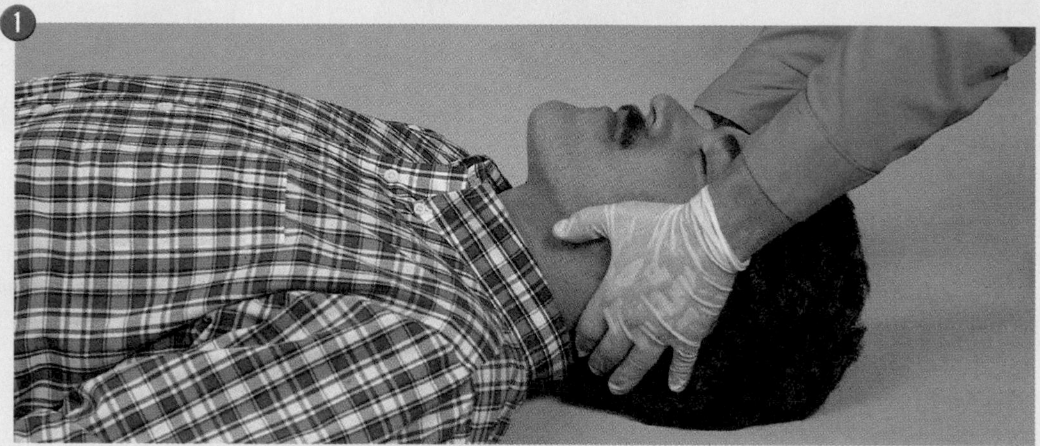

Stabilize the head and prevent movement of the neck. Place the head and neck in a neutral position.

2

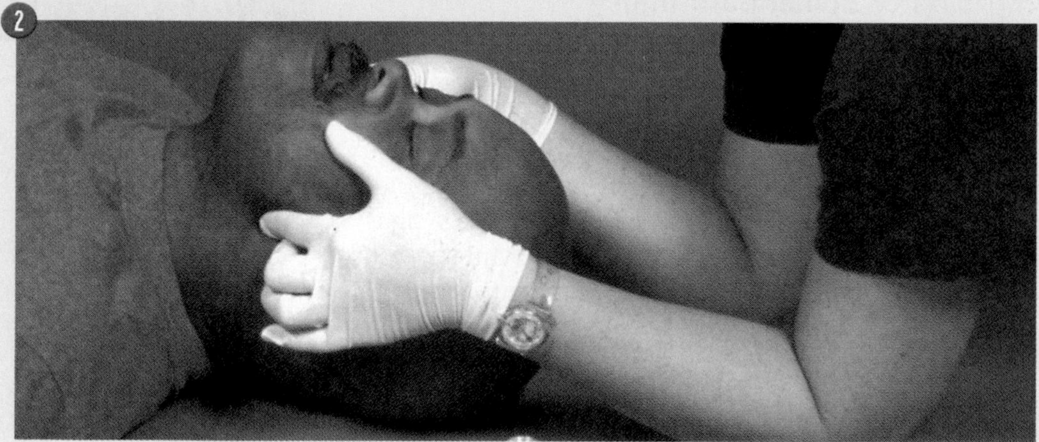

Use the jaw-thrust technique to open the airway and avoid head or neck movement.

7. Examine and treat other serious injuries.
8. Do not move the patient unless it is necessary to perform CPR or to remove him or her from a dangerous environment.
9. Assist in immobilizing the patient using a long or short backboard.
10. Arrange for **T** ***prompt transport*** to an appropriate medical facility.

Stabilizing the Cervical Spine

Stabilization of the cervical spine is initially accomplished manually, as shown in **Figure 13.39, step 2**. In this position, the rescuer can maintain an open airway with the jaw-thrust technique (**Figure 13.39, step 3**).

Stabilize the head and neck in a neutral position. (The neutral position was shown in **Figure 13.39, step 1**.) Do not manipulate or twist the head and neck. After you have manually stabilized the head and neck, you must maintain support until the entire spine is fully splinted. A rigid collar and a long or short backboard are used to splint the cervical spine.

Remember

If you suspect the presence of a spinal injury, it is absolutely essential that the injury be splinted and protected until hospital tests rule out a spinal cord injury.

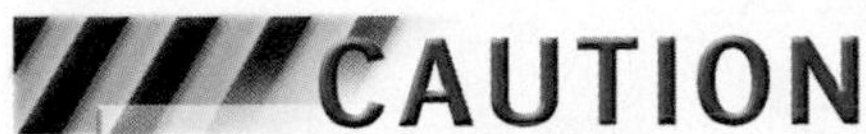

Do not move patients unless it is necessary to perform CPR or remove them from a dangerous environment.

Motorcycle and Football Helmets

Many patients with neck injuries are motorcyclists or football players who are wearing protective helmets. In almost all instances, helmets do not need to be removed. Indeed, they are frequently fitted so snugly to the head that they can be secured directly to the spinal immobilization device.

You should remove part, or all of a helmet only under two circumstances:

1. When the face mask or visor interferes with adequate ventilation, or with your ability to restore an adequate airway.
2. When the helmet is so loose that securing it to the spinal immobilization device will not provide adequate immobilization of the head.

When part of a motorcycle helmet interferes with ventilation, the visor should be lifted away from the face. In the case of a football helmet, the face guard should be removed. Most football face guards are fastened to the helmet by four plastic clips, which can be cut with a sharp knife or unscrewed with a screw driver to remove the face guard (**Figure 13.40**, page 318). Some newer football helmets have a tough plastic strap fixing the face guard to the mask. Trainers and coaches should have a special tool readily available that can remove the face guard. The chin strap should also be loosened to facilitate the jaw-thrust technique. In most instances, exposing the face and jaw allows you access to the airway to secure adequate ventilation.

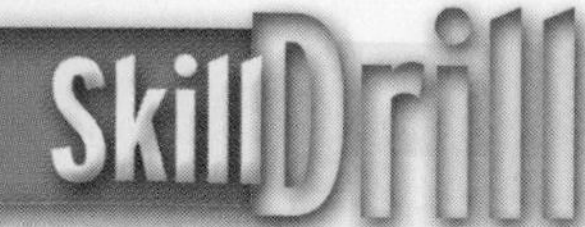

Figure 13.40 Removing the Mask on a Sports Helmet

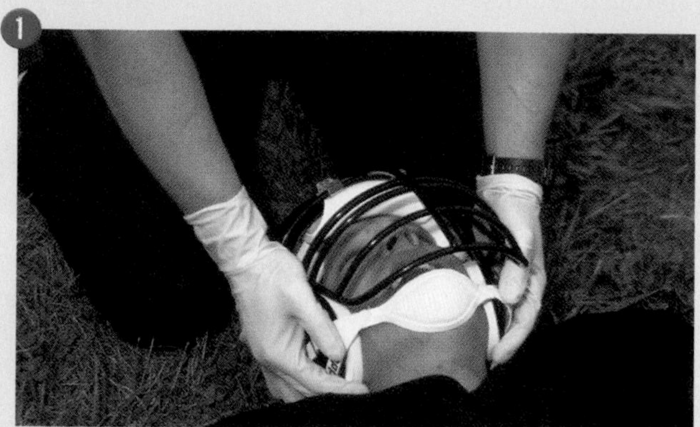

Stabilize the neck in a neutral, in-line position.

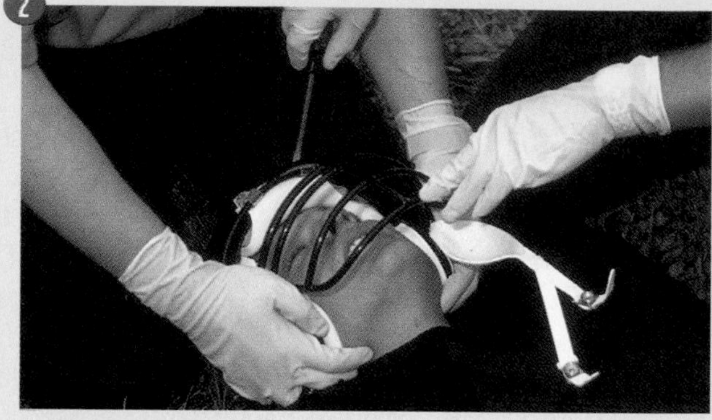

Unscrew or cut the straps that hold the mask to the helmet to access the airway.

The second indication for helmet removal is a loose helmet that will not ensure adequate immobilization of the head when secured to the spinal immobilization device. A loose helmet can be removed easily while the head and neck are being stabilized manually. The procedure for helmet removal in this circumstance is shown in **Figure 13.41**. Note that this procedure requires two experienced people.

Injuries of the Chest

The chest cavity contains the lungs, the heart, and several major blood vessels. The cavity is surrounded and protected by the chest wall, which is made up of the ribs, cartilage, and associated chest muscles. The most common chest injuries are fractures of the ribs, flail chest, and penetrating wounds.

Fractures of the Ribs

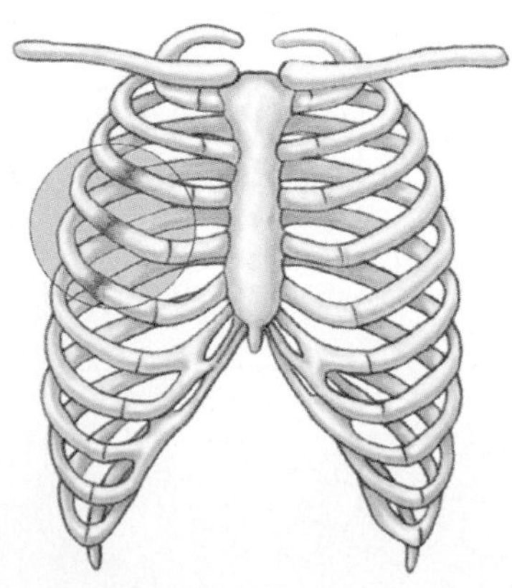

Figure 13.42 Broken or fractured ribs.

Injury may produce fracture of one or more ribs. Even a simple fracture of one rib produces pain at the site of the fracture and difficulty with breathing (**Figure 13.42**). Multiple rib fractures result in significant breathing difficulty. The pain may be so intense that the patient cannot breathe deeply enough to take in adequate amounts of oxygen. Rib fractures may be associated with injury to the underlying organs.

To tell if a rib is bruised or broken, apply some pressure to another part of the rib. Pain in the injured area indicates a bruise, crack or fracture.

If the injury is to the side of the chest, place one hand on the front of the chest and the other on the back and gently squeeze. To check an injury to the front or back of the rib cage, put your hands on either side of the chest and gently squeeze. If there is no pain, the rib is probably not broken.

In cases of rib fractures, be alert for signs and symptoms of internal injury, particularly shock.

Skill Drill

Figure 13.41 Removing a Helmet

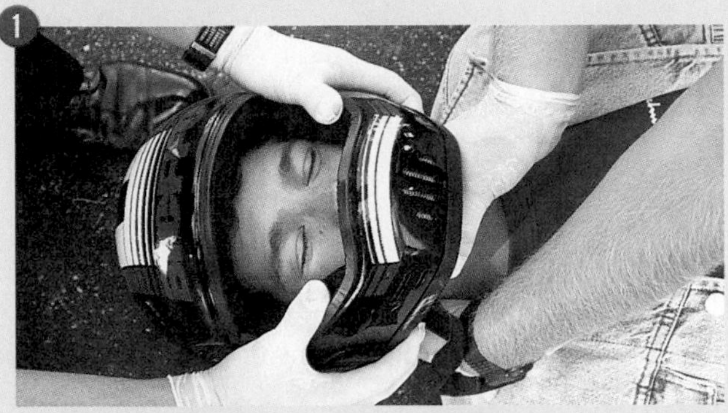

1 Kneel down at the patient's head, and open the face shield so that you can assess the airway and breathing. Remove eyeglasses if the patient is wearing them.

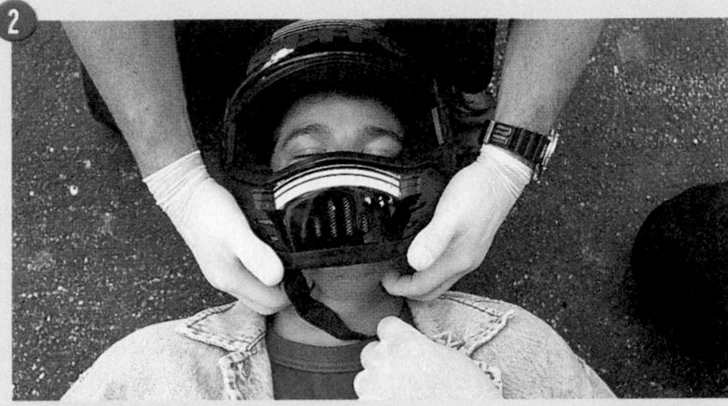

2 Stabilize the helmet by placing your hands on either side of it, ensuring that your fingers are on the patient's lower jaw to prevent movement of the head. Your partner can then loosen the strap.

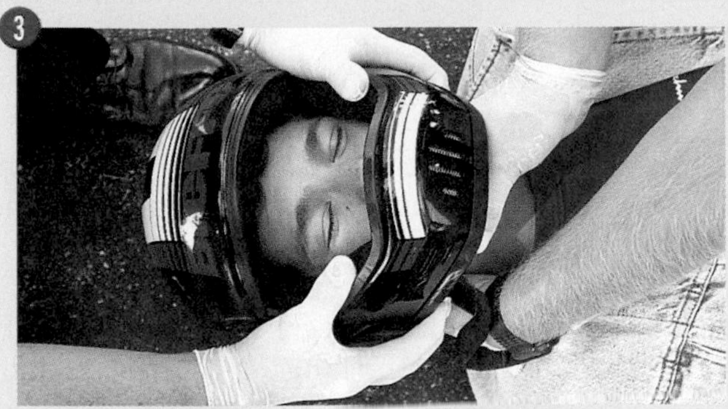

3 After the strap is loosened, your partner should place one hand on the patient's lower jaw and the other behind the head at the occiput.

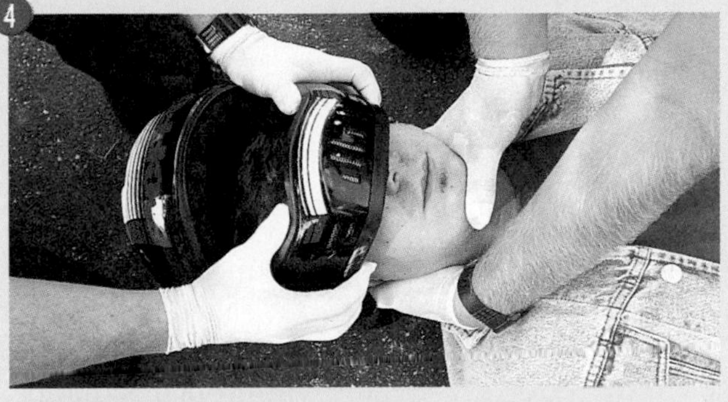

4 Once your partner's hands are in position, gently slip the helmet off about halfway, and then stop.

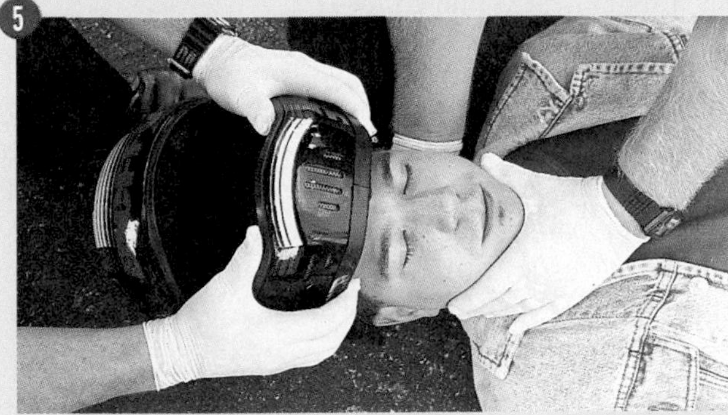

5 Have your partner slide his or her hand from the occiput to the back of the head to prevent the head from snapping back once the helmet is removed.

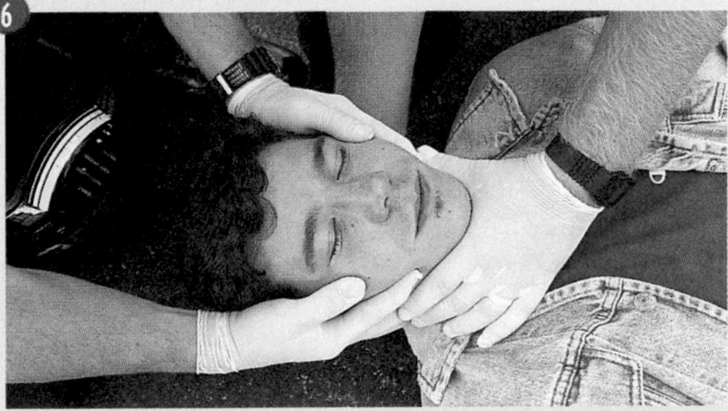

6 With your partner's hand in place, remove the helmet, and stabilize the cervical spine. Apply a cervical collar, and then secure the patient to a long backboard. Note: With large helmets or small patients, you may need to pad under the shoulders.

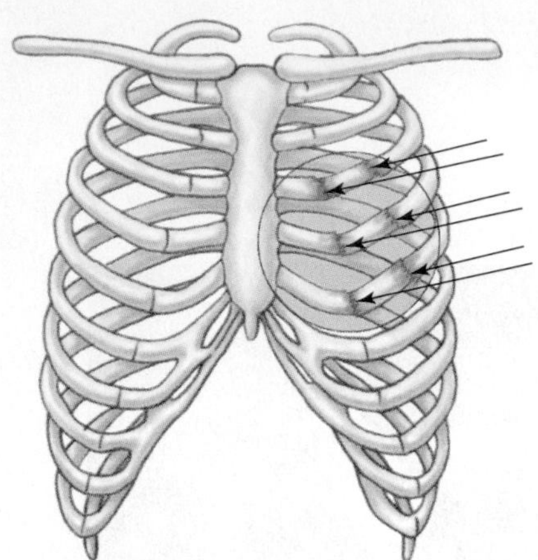

Figure 13.43 A flail chest occurs when three or more ribs are broken in at least two places.

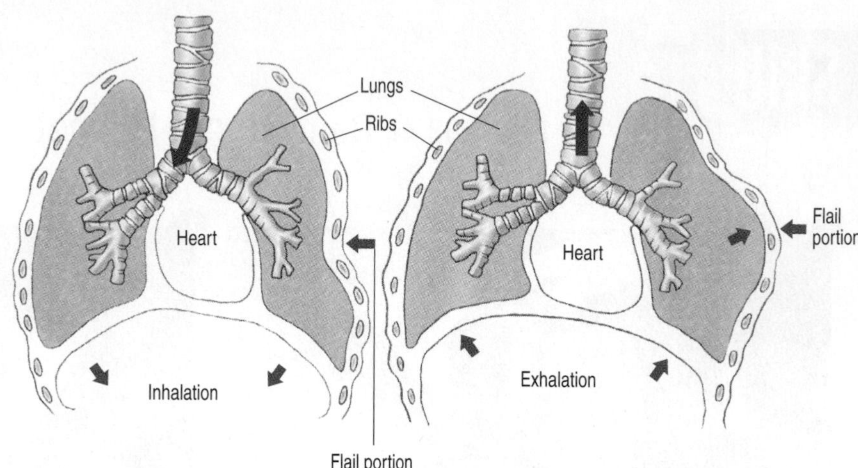

Figure 13.44 As the patient breathes, the flail portion of the chest moves in the opposite direction.

Treatment of Rib Fractures

Try to reassure and make a patient with rib fractures more comfortable by placing a pillow against the injured ribs to splint them. Prevent excessive movement of the patient as you prepare for transportation to an appropriate medical facility. Administer oxygen if it is available and you are trained to use it.

Flail Chest

If three or more ribs are broken in at least two places, the injured portion of the chest wall does not move at the same time as the rest of the chest. The injured part bulges outward when the patient exhales and moves inward when the patient inhales. This reversed movement is called a flail chest (**Figure 13.43**). A flail chest decreases the amount of oxygen and carbon dioxide exchanged in the lungs. It causes breathing problems that become progressively worse.

You can identify a flail chest by examining the chest wall and observing chest movements during breathing. If the injured portion of the chest moves inward as the rest of the chest moves outward (and vice versa), the patient has a flail chest (**Figure 13.44**).

Treatment of Flail Chest

If the patient is having difficulty breathing, firmly place a pillow (or even your hand) on the flail section of the chest to stabilize it. In severe cases of flail chest, it may be necessary to support the patient's breathing. This can be done by EMTs or paramedics with mouth-to-mask or bag-valve-mask resuscitation devices and by using supplemental oxygen. Monitor and support the patient's ABCs and arrange for T ***prompt transport*** to an appropriate medical facility.

Penetrating Chest Wounds

If an object (usually a knife or bullet) penetrates the chest wall, air and blood escape into the space between the lungs and the chest wall (**Figure 13.45**). The air and blood cause the lung to collapse. Lung collapse greatly reduces the amount of oxygen and carbon dioxide that is exchanged and can result in shock and death. Blood loss into the chest cavity can produce hemorrhagic shock.

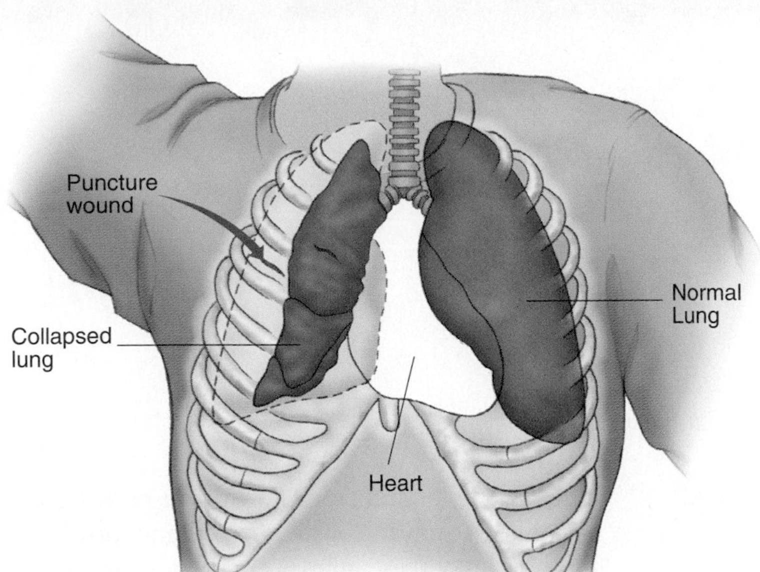

Figure 13.45 Penetrating chest wound may cause the patient's lung to collapse.

Treatment of Penetrating Chest Wounds

Quickly seal an open chest wound with something that will prevent more air from entering the chest cavity. (Occlusive dressings were discussed in Chapter 12, and are shown in **Figure 13.46.**) You can use petroleum jelly, gauze, aluminum foil, plastic wrap, or even cellophane.

In rare cases, sealing the wound may increase the patient's breathing difficulty. If it's harder for a patient to breath after you seal the wound, uncover one corner of the occlusive dressing to see if the breathing improves. Administer oxygen if it is available and you are trained to use it. If a knife or other object is impaled in the chest, do not remove it. Seal the wound around the object with a dressing to prevent air from entering the chest. Stabilize the impaled object with bulky dressings.

Any chest injury that results in air leakage and bleeding requires prompt attention. For these reasons, patients with severe chest injuries require T ***rapid transport*** to an appropriate medical facility.

A conscious patient with chest trauma may demand to be placed in a sitting position to ease breathing. Unless you must immobilize the spine or treat the patient for shock, help the patient assume whatever position eases breathing. If oxygen is available, administer it. If the patient's respirations are excessively slow or absent, perform mouth-to-mask breathing. A bag-valve-mask device may also be used by trained personnel. If the patient's heart stops, begin chest compressions, regardless of whether there are chest injuries.

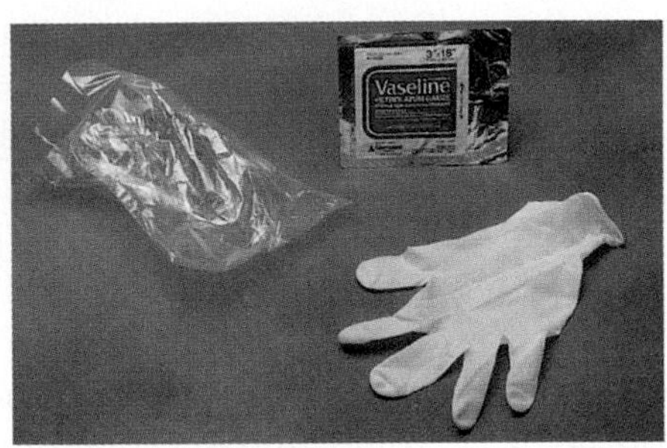

Figure 13.46 Occlusive dressings.

Checkpoint

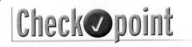

- ○ How would you examine and treat a patient with a penetrating chest wound caused by a gunshot?

13

Prep Kit

Ready for Review

Ready for Review thoroughly summarizes the chapter.

This chapter has covered the skills you need to handle musculoskeletal injuries of the extremities, head injuries, spine injuries, and injuries of the chest. Sometimes you will not have time to splint an extremity injury before additional EMS personnel arrive. There will be times, however, when you are the only trained person at the scene of an accident. To prepare for these situations and to be able to assist other EMS personnel with splinting procedures, you should practice splinting patients with extremity injuries. Many of these techniques can be accomplished with simple improvised materials.

This chapter has also outlined the major bones of the head, spine, and chest. Major injuries of the head, spine, and chest can result in permanent disability, paralysis, or death. Understanding the mechanism of these injuries and performing a thorough patient examination help you discover head, spine, and chest injuries. Proper treatment of these injuries consists of supporting the patient's ABCs, monitoring the patient's level of consciousness, bandaging open wounds, keeping the patient from moving the injured part, and arranging emergency medical transport to an appropriate medical facility. Remember that sometimes the best treatment you can give patients is the assurance that no further harm is done to them. Move patients with head or spine trauma only if you must remove them from a harmful environment or to perform CPR.

Vital Vocabulary

The Vital Vocabulary are the key terms for this chapter.

abdominal breathing—*page 315*
cerebrospinal fluid (CSF)—*page 311*
closed fracture—*page 292*
closed head injury—*page 311*
dislocation—*page 292*
forearm—*page 300*
joint—*page 289*
mechanism of injury—*page 291*
open fracture—*page 292*
osteoporosis—*page 304*
paralysis—*page 314*
rigid splints—*page 298*
seizures—*page 310*
sling—*page 299*
soft splint—*page 298*
sprain—*page 292*
traction splint—*page 299*
trauma—*page 304*

Practice Points

The Practice Points are the key skills you need to know.

1. Performing body substance isolation techniques on a patient with musculoskeletal injuries.
2. Examining a patient with musculoskeletal injuries.
3. Evaluating the circulation and sensation of a patient with an extremity injury.
4. Splinting the following musculoskeletal injuries
   A. Shoulder girdles
   B. Dislocation of the shoulder
   C. Elbow injuries
   D. Injuries of the forearm
   E. Injuries of the hand, wrist, and fingers
   F. Pelvic fractures
   G. Hip injuries
   H. Injuries of the thigh
   I. Knee injuries
   J. Leg injuries
   K. Injuries of the ankle and foot
5. Treating injuries of the face.
6. Stabilizing spine injuries.
7. Treating the following injuries of the chest:
   A. Fractured ribs
   B. Flail chest
   C. Penetrating chest wound

Skill Drills

The Skill Drills provide a visual summary of some of the more complex skills from the skills objectives.

13.8 Checking Circulation, Sensation, and Movement in an Injured Extremity—*page 296*

13.17 Applying a SAM® Splint—*page 301*

13.18 Applying an Air Splint—*page 302*

13.26 Applying a Traction Splint—*page 306*

13.30 Applying an Air Splint to the Leg—*page 308*

13.31 Applying a Pillow Splint for Ankle or Foot Injury—*page 309*

13.39 Stabilizing the Cervical Spine and Maintaining an Open Airway—*page 316*

13.40 Removing the Mask on a Sports Helmet—*page 318*

13.41 Removing a Helmet—*page 319*

Ready to Respond

Ready to Respond presents a fictitious scenario to help you review what you learned in this chapter.

You are called to the scene of a motorcycle collision. Upon your arrival you find a 32 year old man who lost control of his motorcycle and ended up lying on the road about forty feet from his motorcycle. No helmet is evident. As you examine the patient you find the following injuries: a large abrasion on his forehead, a deformed swollen left arm, and a deformed thigh.

1. Your first concern should be
   A. The injured thigh
   B. The injured arm
   C. The forehead laceration
   D. Scene safety
2. Based on the mechanism of injury you should be alert for
   1. Head injuries
   2. Internal injuries
   3. Allergies
   4. Past medical history
   A. 1 and 3
   B. 2,3,4
   C. 1 and 2
   D. All of the above
3. In treating this patient for a possible head injury
   A. Your first priority is the maintaining an airway.
   B. Your first priority is stabilizing the head and neck
   C. Both need to be done at the same time.
4. Which of the following could be signs and symptoms of a head injury?
   A. Battle's sign
   B. Warwick's sign
   C. Raccoon eyes
   D. Consciousness
   E. Vomiting
5. If this patient started to vomit what would you do?
6. Under what conditions would you choose to move this patient?
   A. To remove him from a dangerous situation
   B. To make him more comfortable
   C. To perform CPR
   D. To prevent traffic congestion

MODULE 5 Quick Quiz

Illness and Injury

1. A patient who moans when you pinch their earlobe should be classified as what level on the AVPU scale?

   A. "A" ______________________

   B. "V" ______________________

   C. "P" ______________________

   D. "U" ______________________

2. Which of the following is not a treatment for a patient suffering seizures

   A. Clear the area of harmful objects

   B. Place the patient in the recovery position after the seizure is stopped

   C. Restrain the patient

   D. Start rescue breathing after a seizure if the patient does not start breathing

3. Which of the following is not usually a sign of heatstroke

   A. High body temperature

   B. Sweating

   C. Dry skin

   D. Hot and red skin

4. Some seizures may been caused by stroke or diabetic emergencies

   A. True

   B. False

5. General treatment for a person who has ingested a poison includes all but which of the following:

   A. Try to get the patient to vomit

   B. Arrange for prompt transport to a hospital

   C. Call the poison control center for instructions

   D. Try to identify the poison

6. You respond to a residence for the report of an illness. When you arrive you find three family members suffering headache, nausea, and disorientation. The most likely cause of this illness is

   A. Food poisoning

   B. Flu

   C. Allergies

   D. Carbon monoxide poisoning

7. Which of the following is not a phase of a situational crisis?

   A. Remorse and grief

   B. Acceptance

   C. Denial

   D. Anger

8. What is the proper patient assessment for a patient with a behavioral emergency?

   A. ______________________________

   B. ______________________________

   C. ______________________________

   D. ______________________________

   E. ______________________________

9. Which of the following is not usually a sign or symptom of shock?

   A. thirst

   B. weakness or fainting

   C. weak rapid pulse

   D. damp, warm skin

   E. confusion or restlessness

10. Which position is best for the treatment of shock if there is no head injury?

    A. side lying

    B. supine with the legs elevated

    C. recovery position

    D. semi-sitting

11. Place the following treatments for external bleeding in the proper order:

    A. application of pressure at a pressure point

    B. elevation of the body part

    C. application of direct pressure

12. Match each type of burn with the appropriate signs or symptoms.

    1. Electrical burns ____
    2. Chemical burns ____
    3. Respiratory burns ____
    4. Thermal burns ____

    A. pain while breathing

    B. small external burn with major internal damage

    C. most common cause of burn

    D. powder on the skin

MODULE 5 QuickQuiz Continued

Illness and Injury

13. Four signs of injury you should look for during an examination of a limb

____

____

____

____

14. If a patient has no pulse or capillary refill in an injured limb, you should

A. ask the patient to try to move the limb

B. try to move the limb to a better position

C. arrange for immediate transportation to an appropriate medical facility

D. cool the limb to preserve it

15. Emergency care of a patient who has a painful, deformed femur should include

A. elevating the injured leg

B. treating the patient for shock

C. applying ice packs to injured leg

D. asking the patient to move the limb

1. C **2.** C **3.** B **4.** A **5.** A **6.** D **7.** B **8.** A. perform scene size-up, B. perform initial patient assessment, C. examine the patient head to toe, D. obtain SAMPLE medical history, E. obtain ongoing assessment **9.** D **10.** B **11.** C, B, A **12.** (1=B, 2=D, 3=A, 4=C) **13.** deformity, open wound, bruising or tenderness, swelling **14.** C **15.** B

Childbirth and Children

MODULE

6

Module CONTENTS

Chapter 14

Childbirth

TECHNOLOGY

www.FirstResponderTraining.com

- Online Chapter Pretest
- Web Links
- Online Glossary
- Anatomy Review
- Online Review Manual
- CyberClass
- Interactive First Responder

Chapter FEATURES

- Skill Drills
- Vital Vocabulary
- Voices of Experience
- Signs and Symptoms
- FYI
- Special Needs
- Safety Tips
- BSI Tips
- Caution
- Check Point
- Prep Kit

Objectives

Knowledge and Attitude Objectives

After studying this chapter, you will be expected to:

1. Identify the following structures:
   A. Birth canal
   B. Placenta
   C. Umbilical cord
   D. Amniotic sac
2. Define the following terms:
   A. Crowning
   B. Bloody show
   C. Labor
   D. Miscarriage (spontaneous abortion)
3. Explain the three stages of the labor and delivery process.
4. State the signs and symptoms that indicate that delivery is imminent.
5. State the steps you need to take to prepare a pregnant woman for delivery.
6. Explain the importance of body substance isolation in childbirth situations.

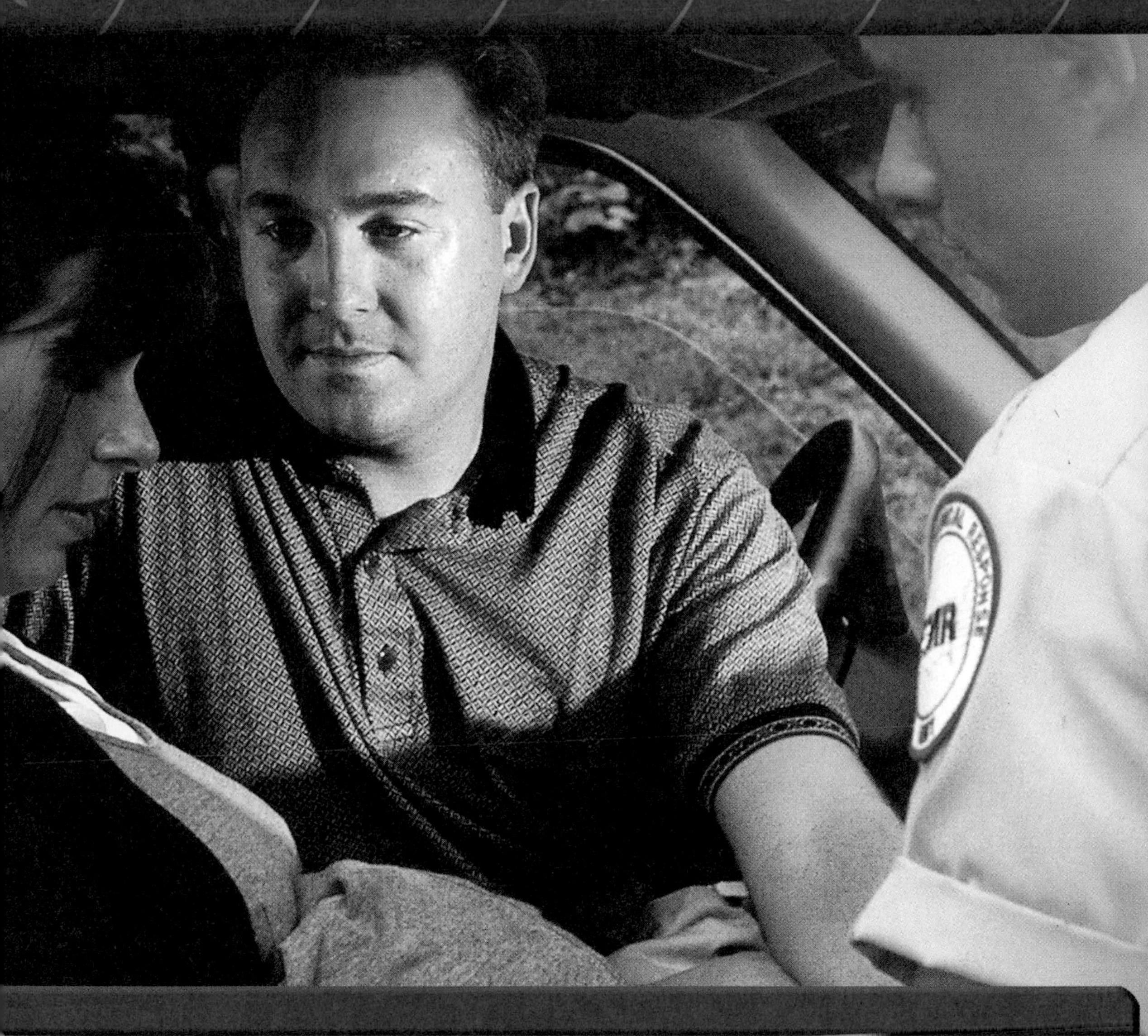

CHAPTER 14

7. Describe the equipment you should have for an emergency childbirth situation.
8. Describe the steps you should take to assist a pregnant woman in childbirth.
9. Describe the steps you should take to care for a newborn infant.
10. Discuss the steps in the delivery of the placenta.
11. List the steps you should take in caring for a mother after delivery.
12. Describe the steps in resuscitating a newborn infant.
13. Describe the steps you should take in caring for the following complications of childbirth:
    A. Unbroken bag of waters
    B. Breech birth
    C. Prolapse of the umbilical cord
    D. Excessive bleeding after delivery
    E. Miscarriage
    F. Stillborn
    G. Premature birth
    H. Multiple births

Skill Objectives

As a first responder, you should be able to:

1. Assist in the normal delivery of an infant.
2. Assist in the delivery of the placenta.
3. Provide care for a newborn infant.
4. Resuscitate a newborn infant.
5. Provide after-delivery care to a new mother.

As a first responder, you must sometimes assist in the birth of a child. A planned childbirth is an exciting, dramatic, and stressful event in itself. An unplanned childbirth, where you are called to assist, can be even more dramatic and stressful. However, if you remember some easy steps, you can effectively assist in the birth process and offer comfort and support to both mother and child.

Childbirth is a normal and natural part of life. If you are concerned about your ability to handle such a situation, just remember that thousands of deliveries occur each day and result in healthy babies. In many countries, medical assistance at childbirth is the exception, not the rule.

You may not have the time or necessary assistance to transport the expectant mother to the hospital. Therefore, you must be prepared to help the pregnant woman deliver the child wherever she is. In most cases, the pregnant woman is the one who delivers the child and you will only assist her as needed. During the birth process, the baby is literally pushed out of the pregnant woman. Your assistance involves "catching" the baby, helping it begin to breathe adequately, and keeping it warm.

Generally, pregnancy and the birth process are not a surprise for the mother, and she may be quite knowledgeable and well-prepared. However, the call to you may come because the timing of the childbirth caught everyone by surprise. In reviewing this chapter, you will find that the birth process has several stages. The two key indicators of an impending birth that concern you are the frequency of contractions and the crowning of the baby's head.

The Anatomy and Function of the Female Reproductive System

The major female reproductive organs are the ovaries, which produce eggs, and the **uterus**, which holds the fertilized egg as it develops during pregnancy. The ovaries and the uterus are connected by the fallopian tubes. The external opening of the female reproductive system is called the **birth canal**, or the **vagina**. The developing baby (**fetus**) is encased in an amniotic sac for support and floats in amniotic fluid. The **placenta**, or afterbirth, draws nutrients from the wall of the mother's uterus. These nutrients and oxygen are delivered to the fetus through the **umbilical cord**. **Figure 14.1** shows the anatomy of a pregnant female.

uterus (womb) Muscular organ that holds and nourishes the developing baby.

birth canal The vagina and the lower part of the uterus.

vagina The opening through which the baby emerges.

fetus A developing baby in the uterus or womb.

placenta Life-support system of the baby during its time inside the mother (commonly called the "afterbirth").

umbilical cord Rope-like attachment between the mother and baby; nourishment and waste products pass to and from the baby and the mother through this cord.

labor The process of delivering a baby.

Assessing the Birth Situation

Should you help deliver a baby away from the hospital or arrange to transport the mother to the hospital? To make this decision, you need to understand that normal **labor** consists of three distinct stages.

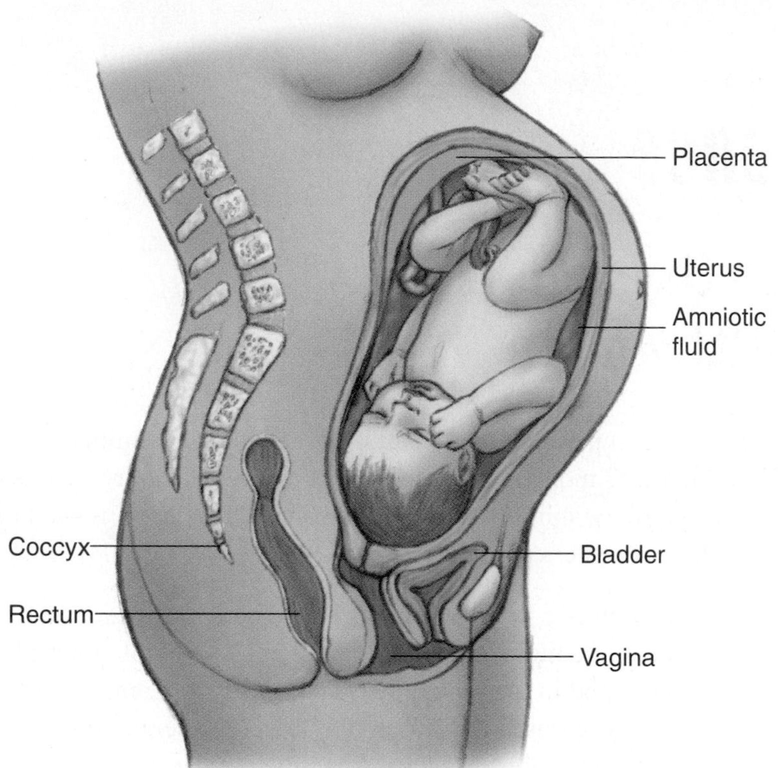

Figure 14.1 Anatomy of a pregnant woman.

Stages of Labor

1. ***Stage One*** is when the mother's body prepares for birth. This stage is characterized by the following conditions: initial **contractions** occur; the "water" breaks; the **bloody show** occurs, but the baby's head does not appear during the contractions. Carefully check the mother to determine whether the baby is **crowning**. Report your findings to the responding ambulance crew so that they can decide whether to transport the mother to the hospital during this stage of labor.
2. ***Stage Two*** involves the actual birth of the baby. You will see the baby's head crowning during contractions, at which time you must prepare to assist the mother in the delivery of the baby (**Figure 14.2**). No time for transport now!
3. ***Stage Three***, the final stage, involves delivery of the placenta (afterbirth). You must assist in stabilizing the mother and baby and delivering the placenta.

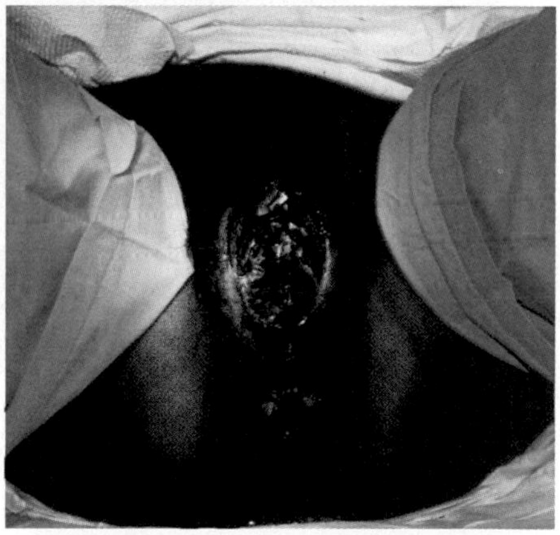

Figure 14.2 Crowning occurs when the infant's head appears at the vaginal opening.

Is There Time to Reach the Hospital?

The following questions will help you to determine how close the mother is to delivering her baby, and whether there is time to transport the mother to the hospital, or if you need to prepare for a delivery.

1. ***Has the woman had a baby before?*** The length of labor for a first-time mother is usually longer than for a woman who has had previous children. A woman who is experiencing her first labor will usually have more time to reach the hospital. It is also helpful to ask the woman when the baby is due, although labor can start before the baby's due date.

contractions Muscular movements of the uterus that push the baby out of the mother.

bloody show The bloody mucus plug that is discharged from the vagina when labor begins.

crowning Appearance of the baby's head during a contraction as it is pushed outward through the vagina.

Voices of Experience

Emergency Childbirth Produces Healthy Baby, Healthy Mom

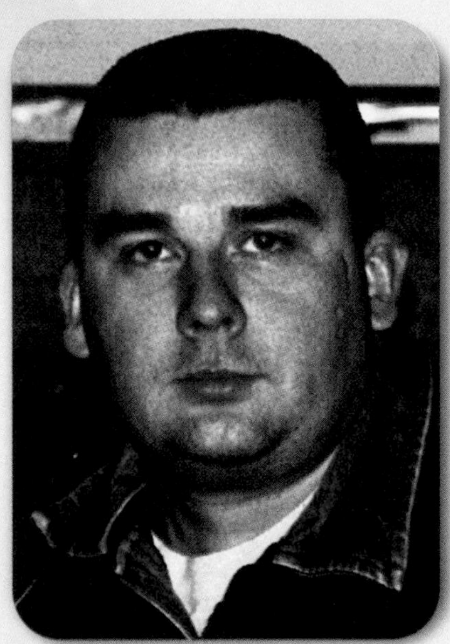

She woke up around 2:30 a.m. with incredible abdominal pain. She was 7 months pregnant, but it couldn't be labor – it was too soon. A few minutes later, she screamed. The father rushed to the bathroom and cried out, then called 911.

The call came in as a possible miscarriage. The police were the first to arrive. They found mom and a newly born baby boy still attached to the umbilical cord and in the toilet bowl. The officers remained calm and acted quickly. They used their shoelaces to tie off the umbilical cord and cut it so they could care for the baby and the mother. By the time the baby was removed from the toilet and wrapped in a blanket, the ambulance had arrived and the baby was passed off to the EMTs. When we arrived, the baby was being warmed and dried. He had a good strong cry with improving vital signs. Mother and son both did well thanks to the quick-thinking actions of the first responders and other members of the EMS team.

"She woke up around 2:30 a.m. with incredible abdominal pain. She was 7 months pregnant, but it couldn't be labor—it was too soon."

Childbirth emergencies create some form of anxiety in all of us. Our ability to overcome that anxiety, remain calm, and focus on the priorities of airway, breathing, and circulation, as these first responders did, makes all the difference in the care of this unique patient population. ❖

John J. Shea, MICP
Newark Beth Israel Medical Center
Resuscitation Services
Newark, NJ

2. ***Has the woman experienced a bloody show?*** As the baby starts its descent toward the birth canal, a plug of mucus, often mixed with blood, called the bloody show is expelled from the cervix and discharged from the vagina. This occurs as the first stage of labor is about to begin.
3. ***Has the bag of waters broken?*** The bag of waters is the amniotic sac and fluid in which the baby floats. The bag of waters usually breaks toward the end of the first stage of labor, and may give you some idea of the progress of the birth process. In a few cases, the bag of water may not break until the birth is actually occurring (see the section on complications of delivery).
4. ***How frequent are the contractions?*** If the contractions are more than five minutes apart, you can usually transport the woman to the hospital. Contractions less than two minutes apart usually indicate delivery will occur very soon and you need to prepare to deliver the baby. If the contractions are three to four minutes apart, then you should take the other factors listed here into account to make your decision.
5. ***Does the woman feel an urge to move her bowels?*** When the baby's head is in the birth canal, it presses against the rectum and the mother may feel the urge to move her bowels. DO NOT allow her to go to the toilet. This is an indication that delivery is imminent.
6. ***Is the baby's head crowning?*** Crowning is the appearance is the baby's head during a contraction. Crowning indicates that the baby will be born in the next few minutes, and you need to be ready to receive the baby.
7. ***Is transportation available?*** Find out not only if the ambulance is responding, but also how far it is to the hospital. Will bad weather, a natural disaster, or rush-hour traffic prevent prompt arrival of transportation?

bag of waters The amniotic fluid that surrounds the baby before birth.

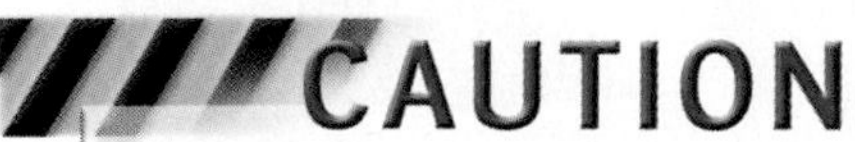

If the mother reports that she needs to move her bowels, do not allow her to go to the bathroom! This feeling is caused by the downward movement of the baby.

Timing Contraction Cycles

Time contraction cycles from the beginning of one contraction to the beginning of the next (**Figure 14.3**). Do not time the interval between contractions. If contractions are less than three minutes apart, delivery is close.

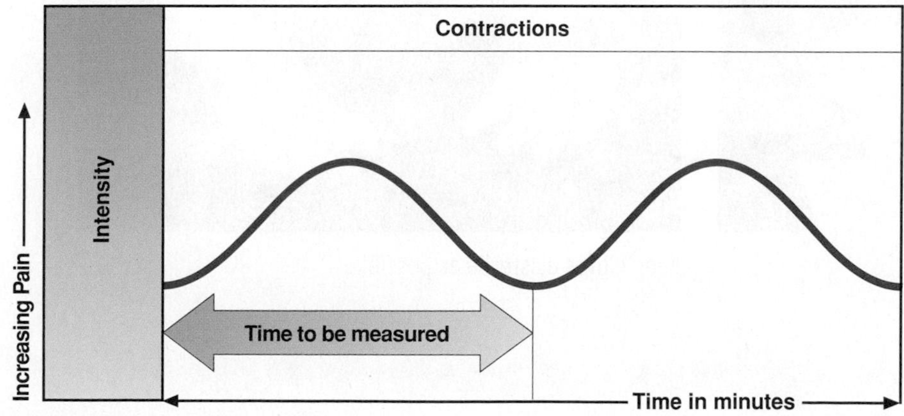

Figure 14.3 Time the contractions from the beginning of one to the beginning of the next.

Skill Drill

Figure 14.4 Putting on Sterile Gloves

1

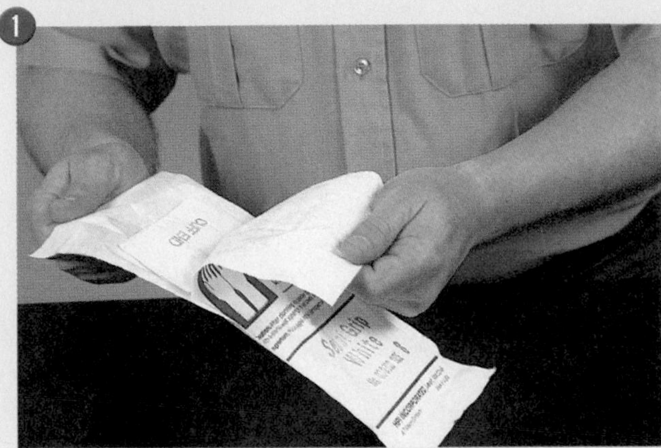

Open sterile glove package.

2

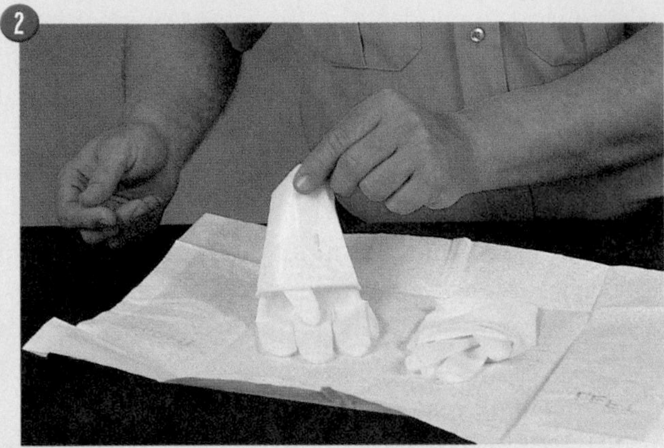

Pick up first glove by grasping it as shown.

3

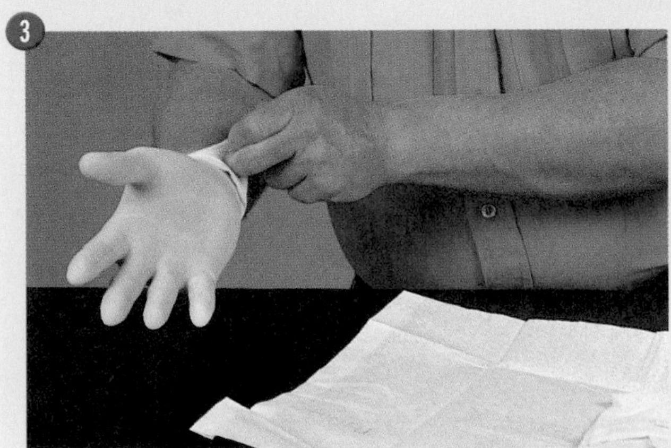

Put on first glove.

4

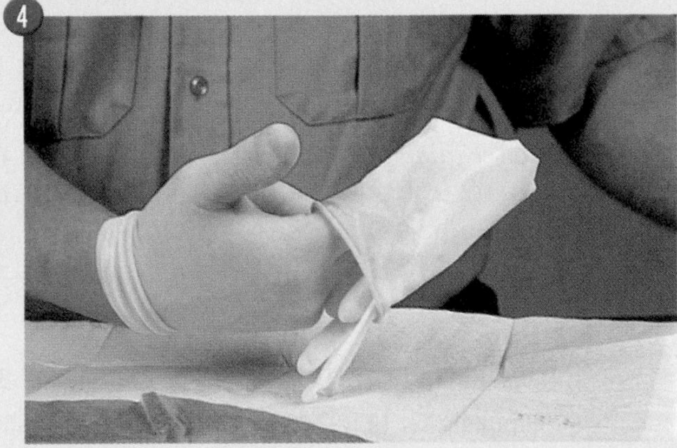

Grasp second glove as shown.

5

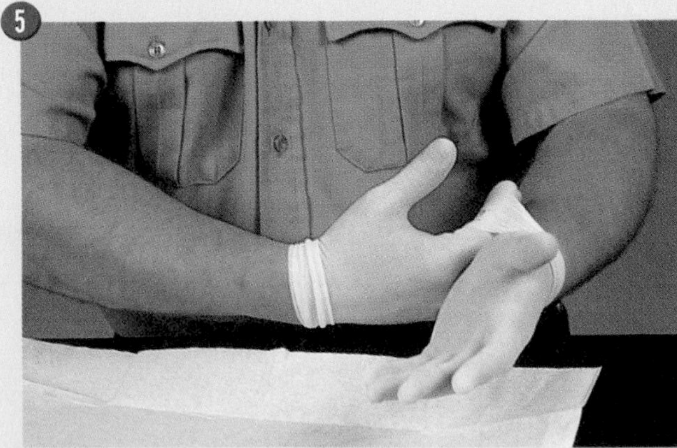

Put on second glove.

6

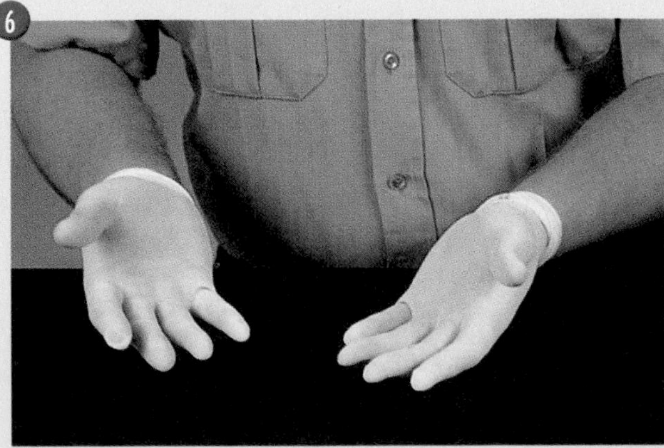

Keep gloves as sterile as possible.

Detecting Crowning

To determine whether the baby's head is crowning, you must observe the vagina during a contraction. If you see the baby's head crowning during the contraction, prepare for the delivery (**Figure 14.2**, page 331). Do not risk transporting the woman to the hospital.

Preparing for Delivery

As you prepare to assist in the delivery of a baby, keep these two things in mind:

1. Calm the woman. Delivery is a natural process.
2. Calm yourself. You are there to help.

Because you are not in a hospital, you will not be able to maintain sterile conditions. However, you must attempt to be as clean as possible. Wash your hands thoroughly. If you don't have a sterile delivery kit, use the gloves from your first responder life support kit (or even clean kitchen gloves, if they are available). If a shower curtain is available, place it on the bed for protection. Cover the shower curtain with clean newspapers, and then cover the newspapers with a clean sheet.

Have plenty of clean towels ready to cover the baby and to clean the mother after delivery has occurred. Childbirth is bloody and messy. Your practical and mental preparations to deal with the messiness can keep it from affecting your performance.

As the woman's contractions become more forceful, they push the baby down the vagina. The woman should be in a comfortable position. This is often on her back with knees bent and legs drawn up and apart.

Remember

Stay calm. You are going to assist in a natural occurrence. Think about all those cab drivers who deliver babies. If they can do it, so can you!

Body Substance Isolation and Childbirth

Because a woman in childbirth will expel both blood and bodily fluids, body substance isolation techniques should be used during the delivery. Try not to get any more blood or fluids on you than is absolutely necessary. Use sterile gloves during any delivery whenever possible. Sterile gloves not only protect the woman and infant from infection, they also protect you from any blood-borne diseases that the woman might have (**Figure 14.4**). Because you could get splattered on the face during the delivery process, wear face and eye protection to keep possible splatter out of your eyes, nose, and mouth. Wearing a surgical gown can help keep fluids off your body.

As a first responder, you will not have all the protective equipment that is available in a hospital. Do what you can to prevent unnecessary exposure to body fluids and report all direct exposures of blood or fluids to the emergency physician or to your medical director.

Equipment

You should have a prepackaged obstetrical (OB) delivery kit in your emergency care equipment (**Figure 14.5**).

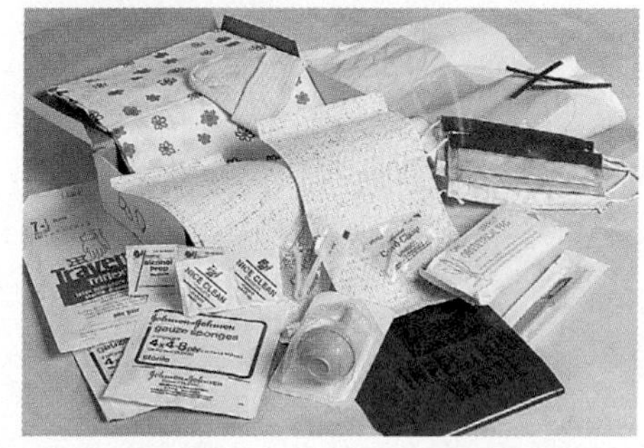

Figure 14.5 Commercial obstetrical (OB) kit.

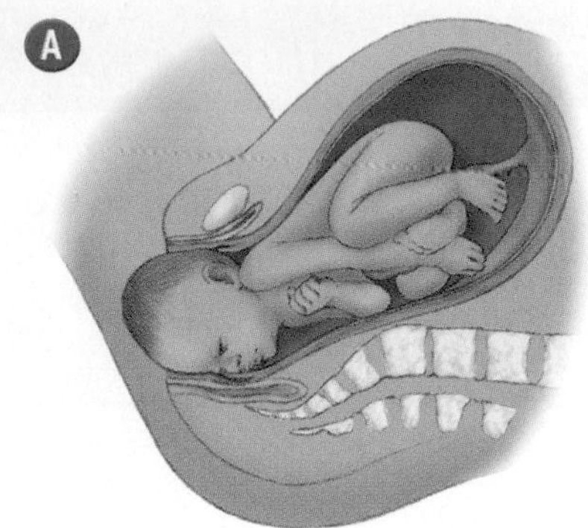

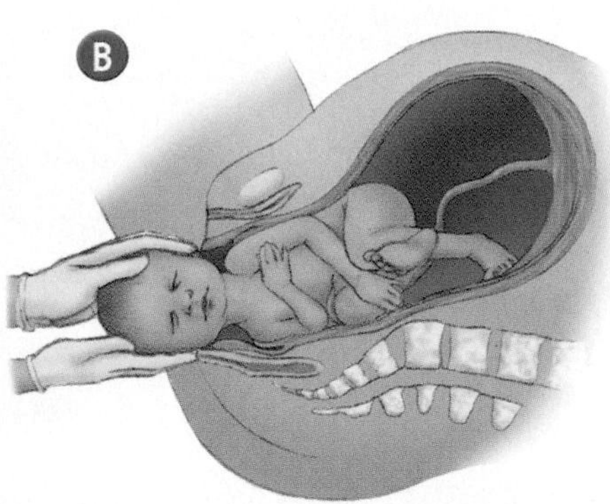

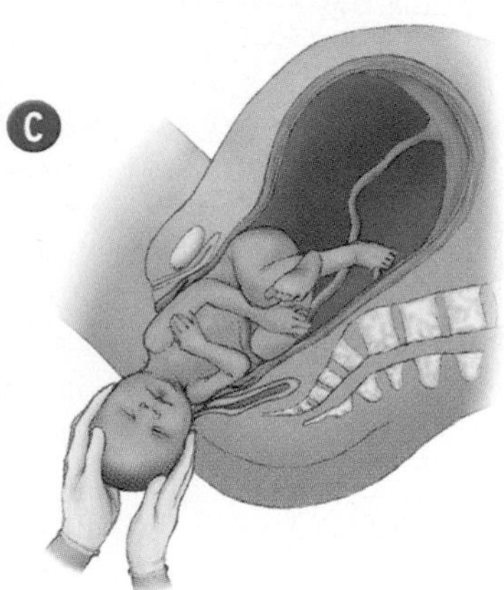

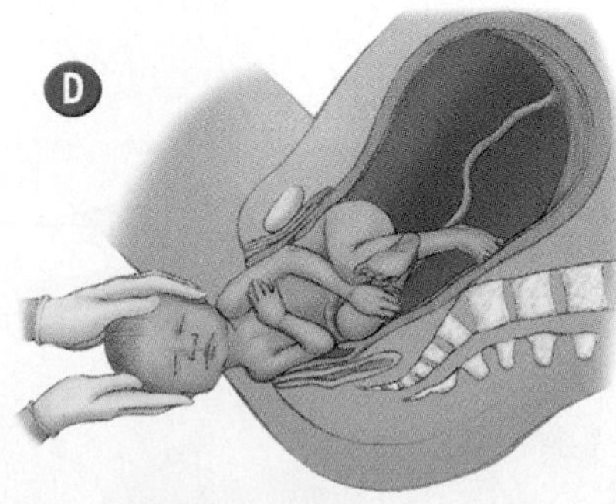

Figure 14.6 Phases of the second stage of labor. **A.** Head begins to deliver. **B.** Delivery of head. **C.** Delivery of upper shoulder. **D.** Delivery of lower shoulder.

The delivery kit includes:

- Sterile gloves
- Sterile drapes and towels
- 4- x 4-inch gauze pads
- Bulb syringe
- Umbilical cord clamp
- Sanitary pads
- A towel or blanket for the baby

In addition, you will need:

- Sheets or towels for the mother
- Oxygen (if available and if you're trained to use it)
- Suction (if available)
- Infant mask

If you do not have a delivery kit, look for appropriate substitute materials. You can probably find most of these items in your first responder life support kit or in most homes. Even if you do not have any equipment, remember that you can still assist in delivering a child with no more equipment than common sense and gloved hands.

Assisting with Delivery

Remember that your primary purpose is to assist in the delivery of the baby. The woman is going to feel pressure in the vaginal area, as if she has to move her bowels. This is a normal feeling during the delivery process. Do not let her go to the bathroom, and do not hold her legs together.

Be as clean as possible during the entire delivery process. Follow the BSI techniques described above. Do not touch the vaginal area except during the delivery. If you have a partner, have him or her stay with you during the delivery.

Have the woman lie on her back. If pillows or blankets are available, cover them with clean towels or sheets and place them under the mother's buttocks to elevate her hips slightly. Have the mother draw up her knees and spread her legs apart.

The baby's head should emerge slowly to prevent undue stress on the baby and tearing of the vagina. As the head emerges, support the baby's head and tell the mother to stop pushing. To help her stop, tell her to breathe rapidly. Some EMS systems advise their personnel to use the palm of the hand to provide slight counter-pressure over the baby's head to slow down the birth process. Be sure to check with your local medical authority on your EMS protocols for this situation.

Do not attempt to pull the baby during delivery. In a normal birth, the baby will turn to its side by itself after the head emerges, and the rest of the body will be delivered spontaneously (**Figure 14.6**). Continue to support the baby's head and be ready to catch the baby in a clean towel. Remember, the baby will be wet and slippery. As the torso and the legs are delivered, support the infant with both hands. Grasp the baby's feet as they are delivered. Keep the infant's head at about the level of the woman's vagina.

If the amniotic sac has not broken as the baby's head starts to deliver, tear it with your fingers and push it away from the infant's head and mouth. As the head emerges, check to make sure that the umbilical cord is not wrapped around the infant's neck. If it is, attempt to slip the

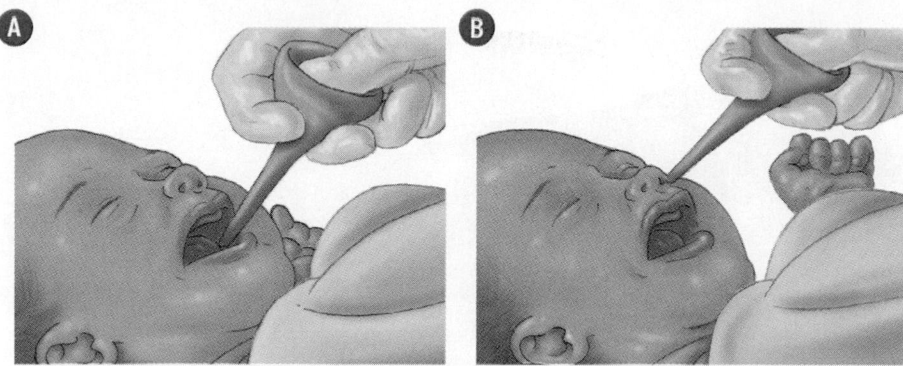

Figure 14.7 Suction the mouth and nose to clear the airway of mucus and amniotic fluid. **A.** Using a bulb syringe in a newborn's mouth. **B.** Using a bulb syring in a newborn's nose.

cord over the baby's shoulder. If you cannot do this, attempt to reduce the pressure on the cord. Never pull on the umbilical cord; it is extremely fragile and you do not want to tear or cut it until it is safe to do so.

Caring for the Newborn

As soon as you are holding the newborn baby in a clean towel, lay him or her down between the mother's legs and immediately clear the baby's mouth and nose. Suction the mouth and the nostrils two to three times. Use a **bulb syringe** from the delivery kit if one is available (**Figure 14.7**). Be careful not to reach all the way to the back of the baby's mouth. If a bulb syringe is not available, wipe the baby's mouth and nose with a gauze pad.

bulb syringe A rubber or plastic device used for gentle suction in newborns and small infants.

You can place the infant on the mother's abdomen. This will help to keep the baby from losing too much warmth. Wipe blood and mucus from the baby's mouth and nose with sterile gauze or with the cleanest object available. If the baby is not breathing, suction the baby's mouth and nose again. Rub the baby's back or flick the soles of the baby's feet to stimulate breathing (**Figure 14.8**). Use the towel to dry the infant and then wrap the child in a blanket to keep it warm. Place the infant on his or her side with the head slightly lower than the trunk. This will help to aid the drainage of secretions from the airway.

Note: Children can breathe with their mouths wide open but newborn babies can't. Newborns breathe only through their noses. Clean the newborn's nose carefully and completely.

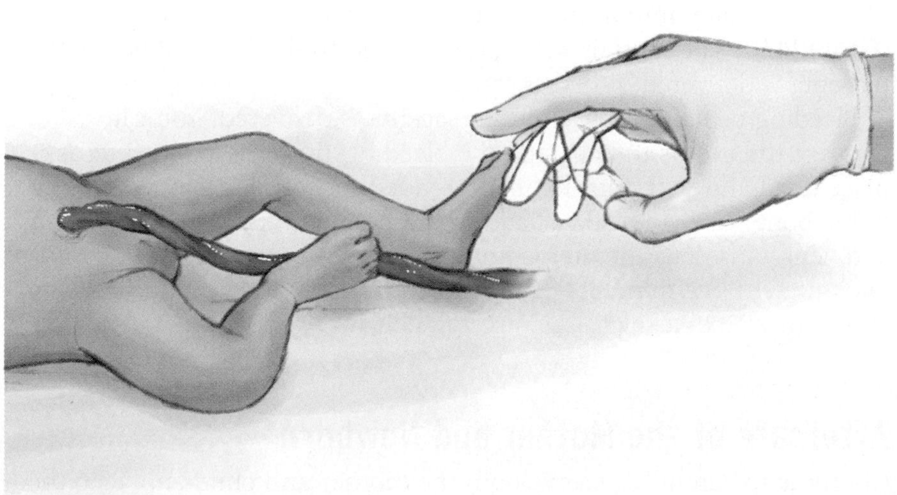

Figure 14.8 Gently snap your fingers against the soles of the feet to stimulate the baby.

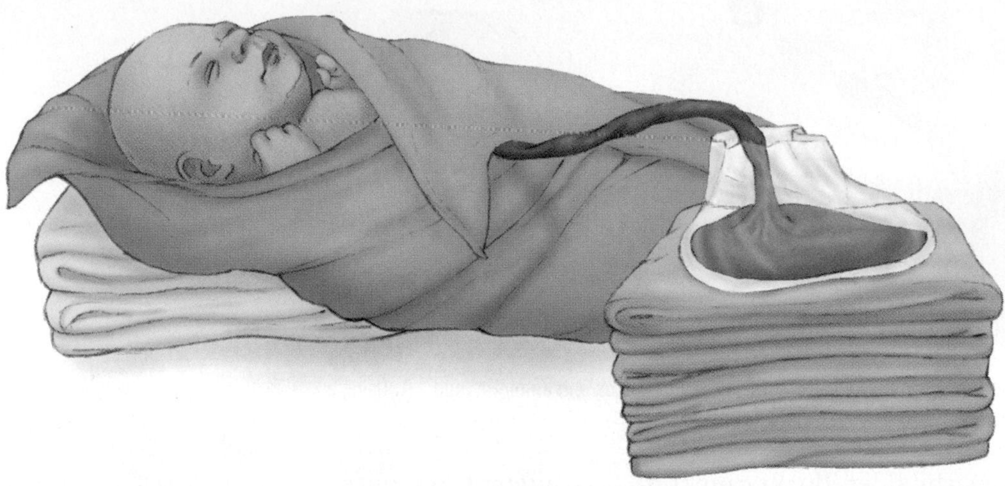

Figure 14.9 When sterile supplies are not available and you cannot cut the umbilical cord, keep the placenta, still attached to the cord, at the same level as the baby during transport to the hospital.

When the umbilical cord stops pulsating, tie it with gauze between the mother and the newborn. In a normal delivery there is no need for you to cut the umbilical cord. Keep the infant warm and wait until more highly trained EMS personnel arrive. They will have the proper equipment to clamp and cut the umbilical cord in an approved manner.

Note the time of the delivery so it can be properly reported on the baby's birth certificate. In the rare event that there may be multiple births, prepare for the second delivery.

Delivery of the Placenta

The placenta will deliver on its own, usually within 30 minutes of the baby's delivery. Never pull on the umbilical cord to help deliver the placenta!

The safest and best method for both mother and child is to leave the umbilical cord uncut and attached to both the placenta and the baby—at least until the transporting EMS unit arrives. After the placenta is delivered, wrap it in a towel or newspaper with three-quarters of the umbilical cord. Then, place it in a plastic bag and transport it to the hospital with the mother and child so it can be examined by a physician. Try to keep the placenta at the same level as the baby to help prevent any blood from the infant flowing back out into the placenta. This is especially important if you are unable to tie the umbilical cord (**Figure 14.9**). The mother can be transported to the hospital before the placenta is delivered, if necessary.

Bleeding usually stops after the placenta is delivered. You can massage the uterus to help stop the bleeding. To massage the uterus, place one hand with fingers fully extended just above the mother's pubic bone. Use your other hand to press down into the abdomen and gently massage the uterus until it becomes firm. This should take three to five minutes. As the uterus firms up, it should feel about the size of a softball or large grapefruit.

Aftercare of the Mother and Newborn

Continue to carefully observe both the mother and child and keep them both warm. Cover the baby's head and body to prevent loss of body heat.

About every three to five minutes, recheck the uterus for firmness. Also recheck the vagina to see if there is any excessive bleeding. In a normal delivery, the mother will lose about 300 to 500 mL (one to two cups) of blood. Continue to massage the uterus if it is not firm or if bleeding continues.

Clean the mother with clean, moist towels or cloths. Cover the vaginal opening with a clean sanitary pad or large dressing. Replace the sheets with clean ones, if possible. If the mother is thirsty, you can give her small amounts of water to drink.

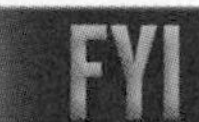

The newborn infant should:

- Breathe at a rate greater than 40 breaths per minute.
- Begin to cry right after birth.
- Have a pulse of greater than 100 beats per minute. (Check the pulse at the brachial pulse.)

Resuscitating the Newborn

If the infant does not breathe on its own within the first minute after birth, proceed with the following steps (**Figure 14.10**, page 340):

1. Tilt the infant's head down and to the side to encourage drainage of mucus.
2. Suction the mouth and nose with a bulb syringe (if available) after delivery of the shoulders. Drying and **suctioning** are usually enough stimulation to induce breathing. Other ways to stimulate breathing include gently snapping your fingers against the soles of the baby's feet and/or rubbing the infant's back. Rough handling is not needed. An infant responds best to simple, gentle techniques, but if the infant is still not breathing, proceed to the next step.
3. Begin mouth-to-mouth-and-nose or mouth-to-mask breathing by gently puffing twice into the infant's mouth and nose. If the infant begins breathing on its own, support and assist respirations and recheck the airway to be sure it remains clear (See Chapter 6).
4. If the infant is still not breathing, continue mouth-to-mouth-and-nose or mouth-to-mask breathing and check for a brachial pulse.
5. If you cannot feel a brachial pulse, or if the heart rate is less than 80 beats per minute, begin closed-chest cardiac compressions. Use your middle and ring fingers to depress the infant's chest. (See Chapter 8.)
6. Continue CPR until the infant begins breathing or until it is pronounced dead by a physician. Provide Ⓣ ***rapid transport*** to the hospital. Do not give up!

suctioning Aspirating (sucking out) fluid by mechanical means.

Automobile Crashes and the Pregnant Woman

Any pregnant woman involved in an automobile crash or suffering other trauma should be examined by a physician. The forces involved

BSI Tip

Report to the emergency physician if you did rescue breathing without a barrier device or if you may have been exposed to blood or fluids.

Skill Drill

Figure 14.10 Steps in Resuscitating a Newborn Infant

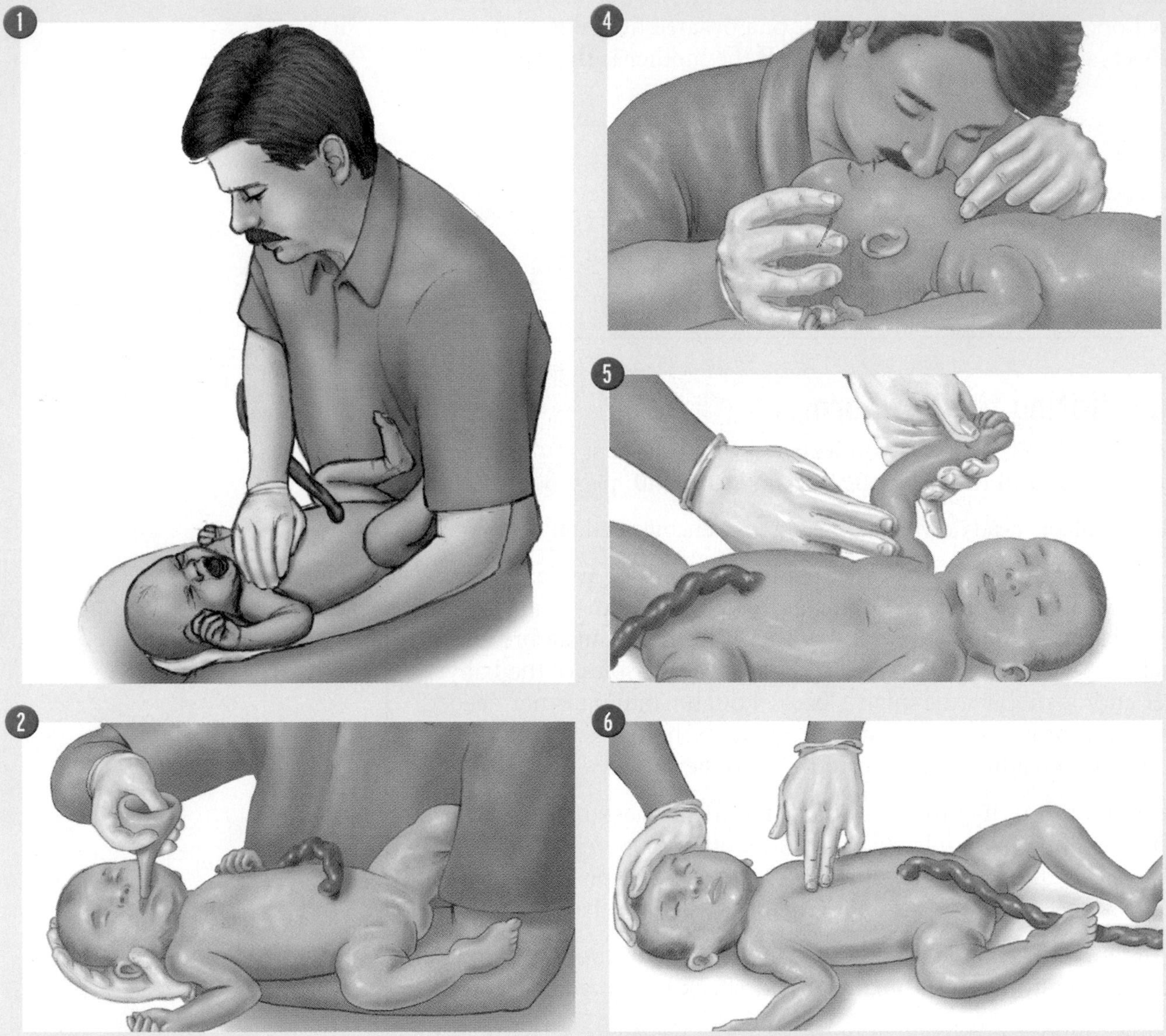

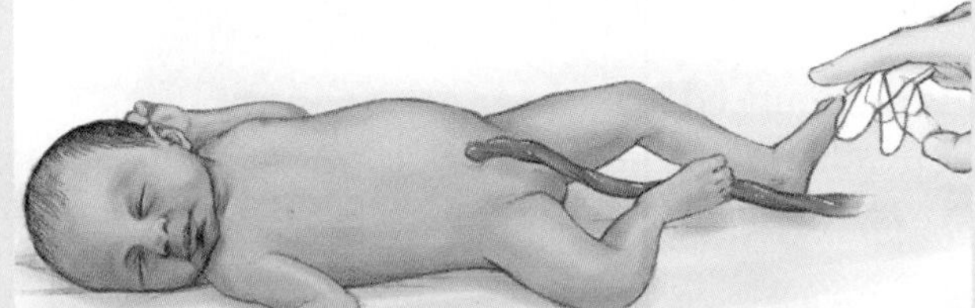

1. Tilt the infant so the head is down and to the side to clear the airway.
2. Suction the mouth and nose with a bulb syringe.
3. Gently snap your fingers on the soles of the infant's feet.
4. Begin rescue breathing.
5. Check for a brachial pulse.
6. Begin chest compressions using the middle and ring fingers.

in even minor crashes may be great enough to injure the mother or unborn child, even though the child is usually well protected in the uterus.

Promptly assess and transport a pregnant woman who has been involved in an auto crash to the hospital. If the woman exhibits signs or symptoms of shock, monitor the airway, breathing, and circulation. Arrange for administration of high-flow oxygen.

Have the mother lie on her left side rather than on her back. This will relieve pressure on the uterus and the abdominal organs and allow blood to return through the major veins in the abdomen.

CAUTION

Pregnant women showing signs and symptoms of shock should be transported while lying on the left side to prevent putting pressure on major abdominal organs and veins.

In rare circumstances, a crash can be severe enough to kill the mother, yet the unborn child can still be saved. Provide CPR to the mother while transporting her to the closest medical facility.

Complications of Childbirth

Although the vast majority of births are normal, you should be aware of possible complications.

Unbroken Bag of Waters

In rare instances, the bag of amniotic fluid that surrounds the baby does not break. If the baby is born surrounded by the bag of waters, carefully break the bag and push it away from the baby's nose and mouth so he or she can breathe. Be careful not to injure the baby in the process. Then suction the baby's nose and mouth to help him or her begin to breathe.

Breech Birth

In a breech birth, some part of the baby other than the top of its head comes down the birth canal first. In this abnormal delivery, the first thing you see may be the baby's leg, arm, shoulder, or buttocks. This type of delivery can result in injury to both the baby and the mother.

If, instead of the normal crowning, you see a **breech presentation**, make every attempt to arrange for ***prompt transport*** to a medical facility. A breech birth slows the labor, so there will be more time for transport to the emergency department. If you are stranded and cannot transport the mother to the emergency room, you will have to assist with the breech birth.

breech presentation A delivery in which the baby's buttocks, arm, shoulder, or leg appears first rather than the head.

Support the baby's legs and body as they are delivered; the head usually follows on its own. If the head does not deliver within three minutes, arrange for prompt transport to a hospital. Use your fingers to keep the baby's airway open.

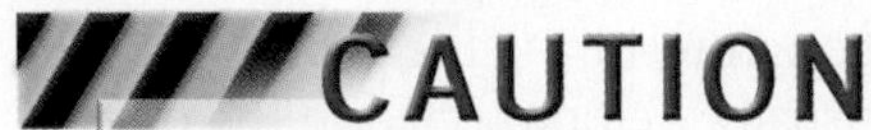

Do not attempt to pull a breech baby out of the vagina!

In very rare cases, the arm is the first part of the baby to appear in the birth canal. This circumstance is an extreme emergency that cannot be handled in the field. You must arrange for T *rapid transport* to the hospital by ambulance.

Prolapse of the Umbilical Cord

prolapse of the umbilical cord A delivery in which the umbilical cord appears before the baby does; the baby's head may compress the cord and cut off all circulation to the baby.

anus The distal or terminal ending of the gastrointestinal tract.

miscarriage Delivery of the fetus before it is mature enough to survive outside the womb (about 20 weeks), from either natural (spontaneous abortion) or induced causes.

On rare occasions, the umbilical cord comes out of the vagina before the baby is born. This is called **prolapse of the umbilical cord**. If this happens, the cord may be compressed between the baby and the mother's pelvis during contractions, cutting off the baby's blood supply. This is a serious emergency that requires immediate transport to a hospital.

Get the mother's hips up! Place the mother on her back and prop her hips and legs higher than the rest of her body with pillows, blankets, or articles of clothing. Keep the cord covered and moist and do not try to push it back into the vagina. Administer oxygen to the mother if it is available and you are trained to use it. Arrange for T *rapid transport* to the hospital.

Some EMS systems recommend placing the mother in a kneeling position (knee-chest position) to take the pressure off the cord. Check with your medical director regarding local procedures.

Excessive Bleeding after Delivery

In addition to the early bloody show that precedes birth, about one or two cups of blood are lost during normal childbirth. If the mother is bleeding severely, place one or more clean sanitary pads at the opening of the vagina, elevate her legs and hips, treat her for shock, and arrange for T *rapid transport* to the hospital by ambulance.

Encourage the baby to nurse at the mother's breast because nursing contracts the uterus and can often help stop the bleeding. Massage the uterus with your hand, as described earlier in this chapter.

If the area between the mother's vagina and **anus** is torn and bleeding, treat it as you would an open wound. Apply direct pressure, using sanitary pads or gauze dressings.

Miscarriage

A **miscarriage** (spontaneous abortion) is the delivery of an incomplete or underdeveloped fetus (baby). If a miscarriage occurs, you should save the fetus and all the tissues that pass from the vagina. Control the mother's bleeding by placing a sanitary pad or other large dressing at the vaginal opening. You should also treat her for shock. Arrange for T *prompt transport* to a hospital so that a physician can examine her and the fetal tissues and control any additional bleeding.

A mother who miscarries will be upset about losing the baby and will need your psychological support as well as your emergency medical care. Be sensitive to the needs and concerns of the mother and other members of the family.

Stillborn Delivery

Resuscitation should be started and continued on all newborns who are not breathing. However, sometimes a baby dies long before delivery. The baby will generally have an unpleasant odor and will not exhibit any signs of life. Such a lifeless fetus is referred to as a "stillborn." In a case like this, you should turn your attention to the mother in order to provide physical care and psychological support. Carefully wrap the stillborn in a blanket.

Premature Birth

Any baby weighing less than 5½ pounds or delivered before eight months of pregnancy is called premature. Premature infants are smaller, thinner, and usually redder than full-term babies.

You must keep **premature babies** warm because they lose body heat rapidly. Wrap the infant in a clean towel or sheet and cover its head. Wrapping the premature baby in an additional length of aluminum foil can also help maintain its temperature. Arrange for Ⓣ ***prompt transport*** to a medical facility.

premature baby A baby who delivers before eight months of gestation or who weighs less than 5½ pounds at birth.

Multiple Births

In the event of multiple births (such as twins), another set of labor contractions will begin shortly after the delivery of the first baby. A mother generally knows of a multiple birth in advance. However, occasionally everyone is surprised. Do not worry—just get ready to repeat the procedures you have completed for the first baby!

- ◯ After helping a mother deliver a normal, healthy baby, you notice excessive bleeding. What steps should you take?

14

Prep Kit

Ready for Review

Ready for Review thoroughly summarizes the chapter.

This chapter presents the skills and knowledge you need to assist in the delivery of an infant. It also covers the anatomy and function of the major structures of the female reproductive system. The key indicators in estimating how soon a delivery will occur are crowning and the time between contractions. By using these two factors, you can determine whether a woman should be transported to a medical facility or whether the baby will be born outside the hospital. The key steps in assisting with a normal delivery are also presented. You should remember to exercise good body substance isolation techniques when assisting with a delivery.

After the delivery, you have two patients to care for—the mother and the infant. You should have the skills needed to resuscitate a newborn. Careful delivery of the placenta is important. You should understand the complications that can occur during labor and delivery and know what to do if these complications arise. Finally, keep in mind that childbirth is normally a happy event. You are there to assist in the delivery, which in most cases has a happy, healthy outcome.

Vital Vocabulary

The Vital Vocabulary are the key terms for this chapter.

anus—*page 342*
bag of waters—*page 333*
birth canal—*page 330*
bloody show—*page 331*
breech presentation—*page 341*
bulb syringe—*page 337*
contractions—*page 331*
crowning—*page 331*
fetus—*page 330*
labor—*page 330*
miscarriage—*page 342*
placenta—*page 330*
premature baby—*page 343*
prolapse of the umbilical cord—*page 342*
suctioning—*page 339*
umbilical cord—*page 330*
uterus (womb)—*page 330*
vagina—*page 330*

Practice Points

The Practice Points are the key skills you need to know.

1. Assisting in the normal delivery of an infant or a manikin.
2. Assisting in the delivery of a real or simulated placenta.
3. Providing care for a newborn infant.
4. Resuscitating a newborn infant.
5. Providing after-delivery care to a new mother.

Skill Drills

The Skill Drills provide a visual summary of some of the more complex skills from the skills objectives.

14.4 Putting on Sterile Gloves—*page 334*

14.10 Steps in Resuscitating a Newborn Infant —*page 340*

Ready to Respond

Ready to Respond presents a fictitious scenario to help you review what you learned in this chapter.

You are dispatched to a house in the middle of a storm for an "unknown problem." Your assessment reveals a 28-year-old woman who reports that she is expecting a baby in ten days. Her bag of waters has broken and she has been experiencing labor pains for seven hours.

1. You should prepare to
   A. Ask about the discharge of bloody mucus, because delivery will be a long time off unless this has occurred.
   B. Transport her immediately to the nearest hospital because the length of her labor indicates a serious problem with the pregnancy.
   C. Time the contractions and check to see if the head is crowning before your decide whether there is time to transport the mother to a hospital before delivery.
   D. Deliver the baby, because birth will be imminent after eight hours of labor.

2. If the mother's contractions are four minutes apart, and the head has not yet crowned, what stage of labor is the mother experiencing?
   A. First
   B. Second
   C. Third
   D. Between second and third

3. If you do not have a delivery kit with you, what supplies might you obtain from her house?

4. The mother tells you that she feels she needs to move her bowels. You should
   A. Help her to the bathroom.
   B. Find a container to use as a bedpan.
   C. Ask her if she is sure it is not just the pressure of the baby that she is feeling.
   D. Tell her she is only feeling the pressure of the baby and should not try to go to the bathroom now.

5. After the baby has been delivered, you should immediately
   A. Try to get it to cry.
   B. Hold it up by the heels and spank it.
   C. Begin mouth-to-mouth resuscitation.
   D. Clear its nose and mouth of secretions.

Chapter 15

Infants and Children—Pediatric Emergencies

TECHNOLOGY

- Online Chapter Pretest
- Web Links
- Online Glossary
- Anatomy Review
- Online Review Manual
- CyberClass

www.FirstResponderTraining.com

- Interactive First Responder

Chapter FEATURES

- Skill Drills
- Vital Vocabulary
- Voices of Experience
- Signs and Symptoms
- FYI
- Special Needs
- Safety Tips
- BSI Tips
- Caution
- Check Point
- Prep Kit

Objectives

Knowledge and Attitude Objectives

After studying this chapter, you will be expected to:

1. Describe the differences between a child's and an adult's anatomy.
2. Describe the normal rates of respiration and pulse for a child.
3. Explain the differences between performing the following skills on a child and on an adult:
   A. Opening the airway
   B. Basic life support
   C. Suctioning
   D. Inserting an oral airway
4. Describe how to treat a child and an infant with:
   A. A partial airway obstruction
   B. A complete airway obstruction
   C. Respiratory distress
   D. Respiratory failure
   E. A swallowed object
   F. Circulatory failure

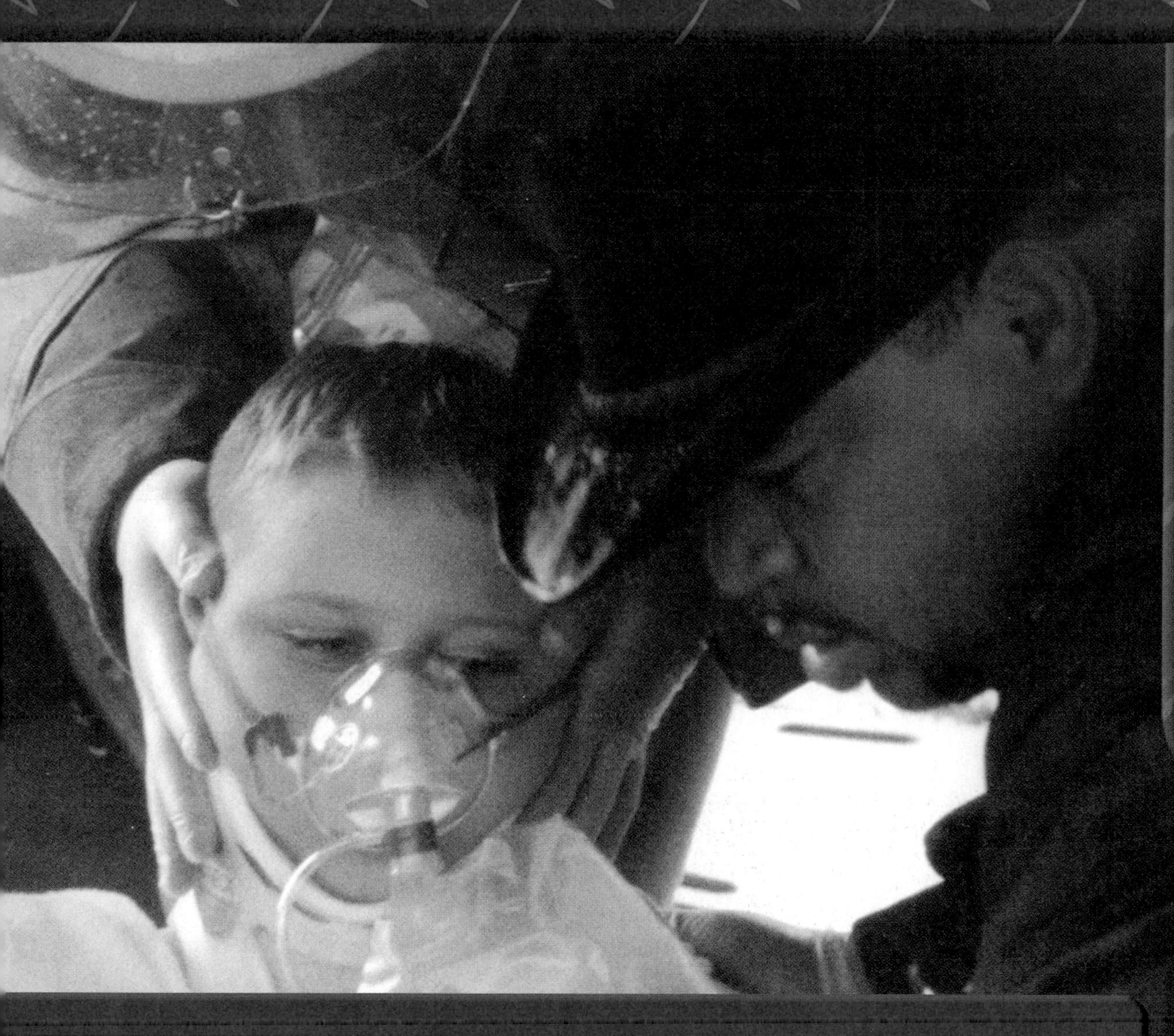

CHAPTER

15

5. Describe how to treat the following illnesses and medical emergencies:
   A. Altered mental status
   B. Asthma
   C. Croup
   D. Epiglottitis
   E. Near drowning
   F. Heat illnesses
   G. High fever
   H. Seizures
   I. Vomiting and diarrhea
   J. Abdominal pain
   K. Poisoning
   L. Sudden infant death syndrome
6. Describe the patterns of pediatric injury.
7. Describe the signs and symptoms of shock in pediatric patients.
8. Explain the steps you should take to care for a child who has signs of child abuse or sexual assault.
9. Describe the need for first responder critical incident stress debriefing.

Skill Objectives

As a first responder, you should be able to:

1. Determine a child's respiratory rate, pulse rate, and body temperature.
2. Perform the following respiratory skills on a child:
   A. Opening the airways
   B. Basic life support
   C. Suctioning
   D. Inserting an oral airway
3. Treat the following conditions:
   A. Partial airway obstruction in children and infants
   B. Complete airway obstruction in children and infants
4. Cool a child with a high fever.

Sudden illnesses and medical emergencies are common in children and infants. This chapter covers the special knowledge and skills you need to assess and treat children and infants.

This chapter covers the differences between the anatomy of an adult and a child and highlights the special considerations for examining pediatric patients. Respiratory care for children is very important. The chapter reviews the following respiratory skills: opening the airway, basic life support, suctioning, and relieving airway obstructions. The signs of respiratory distress, respiratory failure, and circulatory failure in children and infants are explained.

It is important that you learn some basic information and treatment for the following conditions: altered mental status, asthma, croup, epiglottitis, near drowning, heat illnesses, high fever, seizures, vomiting and diarrhea, abdominal pain, poisoning, and sudden infant death syndrome. Because trauma is the leading cause of death in children, this chapter covers patterns of injury and the signs of traumatic shock in children. Finally you should be able to recognize some of the signs and symptoms of child abuse and sexual abuse of children so you can take the proper steps to get help.

General Considerations

Managing a pediatric emergency can be one of the most stressful situations you face as a first responder. The child is frightened, anxious, and usually unable to communicate the problem to you clearly. The parents are anxious and frightened. In this atmosphere, where everyone else is tense, you must behave in a calm, controlled, and professional manner.

EMS personnel often have mixed feelings when treating a child. In some cases, the child reminds them of someone they know. Even the most experienced personnel respond emotionally to a seriously ill or injured child. Unless you are prepared, your anxiety and fear may interfere with your ability to deliver proper care.

The Parents

The child's parents or caregivers can be either allies or another problem. You must respond to them as much as to the child, although in a different way. Talk to both parents and to the child as much as possible. Parents are understandably concerned about their child's condition, especially if they don't clearly understand the situation or if they think the situation is more serious than it is. For instance, imagine a parent's reaction to a bleeding laceration of a child's forehead. You know that scalp wounds can bleed profusely, but that such bleeding can be easily controlled with direct pressure. However, most parents don't know that and may become emotional.

Children get many of their behavioral cues from their parents. Calm the parents, talk with them, and ask their assistance in calming

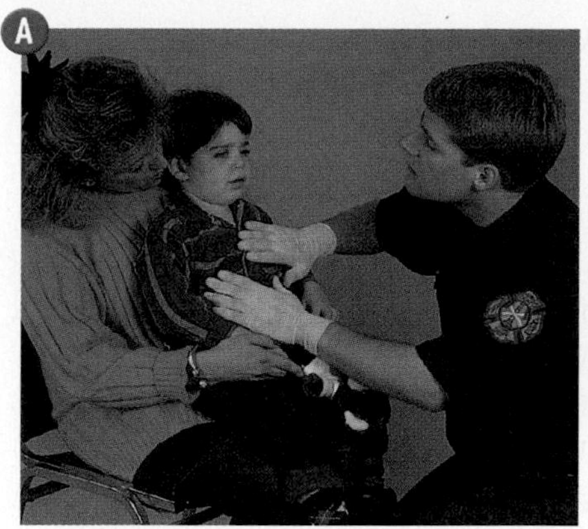

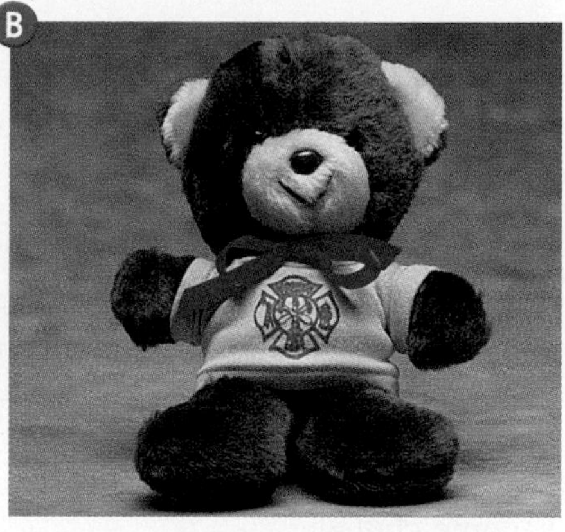

Figure 15.1 **A.** Allow the parent to hold the child if possible. **B.** The trauma teddy bear helps keep a child calm while being examined.

the child. It is a good idea to allow a parent to hold the child if the illness or injury permits (**Figure 15.1**). If the injury doesn't permit the parent to hold the child on a lap, let the parent hold the child's hand or keep the parents where the child can see them.

Quickly try to develop rapport with the child. Tell the child your first name, find out what the child's name is, and use the child's name as you explain what you are doing. Do not stand over the child. Squat, kneel, or sit down and establish eye contact. Ask the child simple questions about the pain, and ask the child to help you by pointing to (or touching) the painful area.

Be honest with the child. For instance, if you must move an arm or leg in order to splint it, tell the child what you are going to do and explain that the movement may hurt. Ask the child to help by being calm, lying still, or holding a bandage. The level of understanding and cooperation you can receive from an ill or injured child is often remarkable and may surprise you. Some emergency service agencies provide the child with a trauma teddy bear to hold while being examined.

Pediatric Anatomy and Function

Children and adults have the same body systems that perform the same functions, but there are certain differences, particularly in the airway, that you should know. A child's airway is smaller in relation to the rest of the body. Therefore, secretions or swelling from illnesses or trauma can more easily block the child's airway. Because a child's tongue is relatively larger than the tongue of an adult, a child's tongue can more easily block the airway if the child becomes unresponsive.

Because a child's upper airway anatomy is more flexible than that of an adult, you must remember to avoid hyperextending the neck of an infant or child when attempting to open the airway. Position the head in a neutral or slight sniffing position, but do not hyperextend the neck. Hyperextending a child's neck can occlude the airway. For at least the first six months of their lives, infants can breathe only through their noses. If an infant's nose becomes blocked by mucous secretions, the infant cannot breathe through the mouth. Therefore, it is important to clear the nose of an infant to enable breathing.

Children can quickly compensate as the demands on their respiratory system change. They can increase their breathing rate and their breathing efforts for a short period of time. However, they will "run out of steam" in a relatively short period of time. When this happens, the child may soon show signs of severe respiratory distress and rapidly progress into respiratory failure. Therefore, it is important to perform a complete and thorough assessment and to monitor the child's vital signs. Recheck the vital signs at least every five minutes when caring for seriously ill or injured pediatric patients.

Infants and children also have limited abilities to compensate for changes in temperature. Children have a greater surface area relative to the mass of their body. This means that they lose relatively more heat than adults do. Therefore, you need to keep the body temperature of children as close to normal as possible and warm them if they become chilled.

Examining a Child

Observe the child carefully when you first meet. Does the child appear to be ill or injured? Children often "look sick," or you may note an obvious injury (**Figure 15.2**).

The child who is unresponsive, lackluster, and appears ill should be evaluated carefully because lack of activity and interest can signal serious illness or injury. Infants and young children normally cry in response to fear or pain; a child who is not crying may have a decreased level of consciousness. If the child is crying, does the cry sound like a normal healthy cry or is it a subdued whimper?

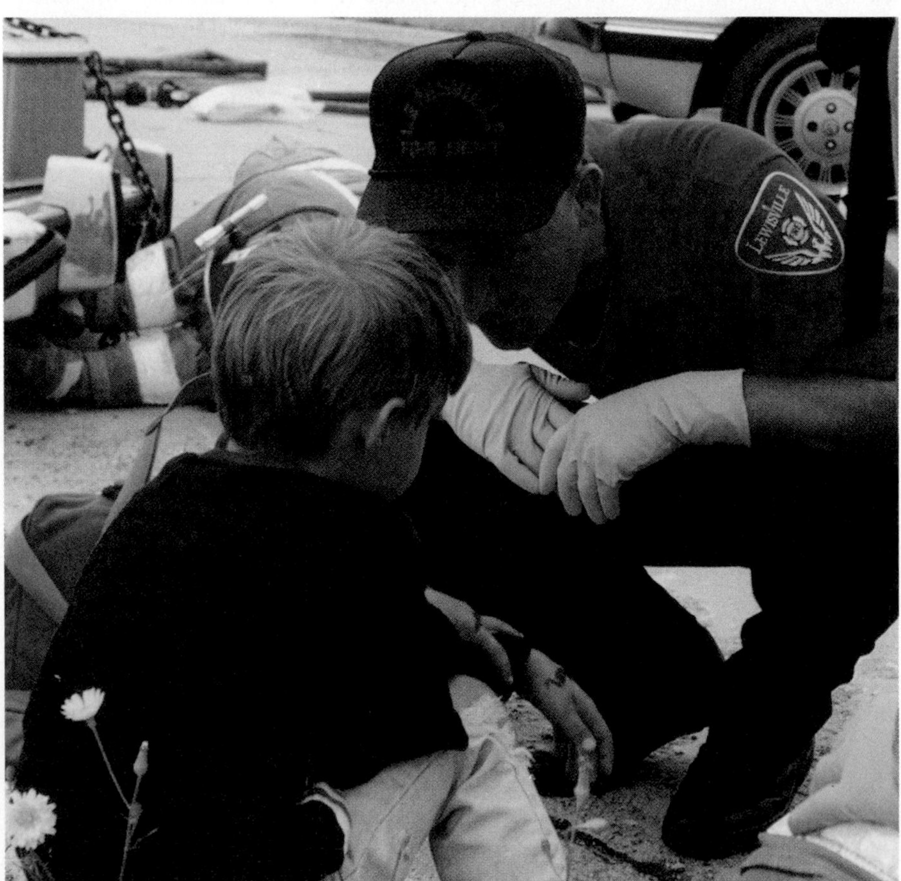

Figure 15.2 Observe the child carefully for signs of illness or injury.

Carry out the routine patient examination described in Chapter 7, paying special attention to mental awareness, activity level, respirations, pulse rate, body temperature, and color of the skin.

Respirations

You can calculate the respiratory rate of a child by counting respirations for 30 seconds and multiplying by two. Counting for less than 30 seconds can cause inaccurate results because children often have irregular breathing patterns.

As you examine a child, look for the following signs of respiratory distress: restlessness, noisy breathing, flaring of the nose, and retractions of the neck and chest. Respiratory distress is discussed under respiratory emergencies.

Pulse Rate

The normal pulse rate of a child—80 to 100 beats per minute—is faster than an adult's normal rate. For a child under one year of age take the brachial pulse, which is halfway between the shoulder and the elbow on the inside of the upper arm, or directly over the heart (**Figure 15.3**).

Table 15.1 describes the usual, normal vital signs for children at various ages.

High Body Temperature

High temperatures in children are often accompanied by flushed, red skin, sweating, and restlessness. You can often feel a high temperature just by touching the child's chest and head. A child's heart rate increases with each degree of temperature rise.

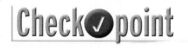

Checkpoint

- ◯ Describe the difference between examining a child and an adult.

Respiratory Care

Neither adults nor children can tolerate a lack of oxygen for more than a few minutes before permanent brain damage occurs. Therefore, the rules for applying basic life support are the same for both children and adults.

It is important for the first responder to open and maintain the airway and to ventilate adequately any child with respiratory problems.

Table 15.1

Normal Vital Signs in Children at Rest

Age	Heart Rate	Respirations
Newborn	140	40-60
1 year	130	22-30
3 years	80	20-26
10 years	75	18-22

Remember

From birth to about six months of age, children are "nose breathers." They have not yet learned to breathe through their mouths.

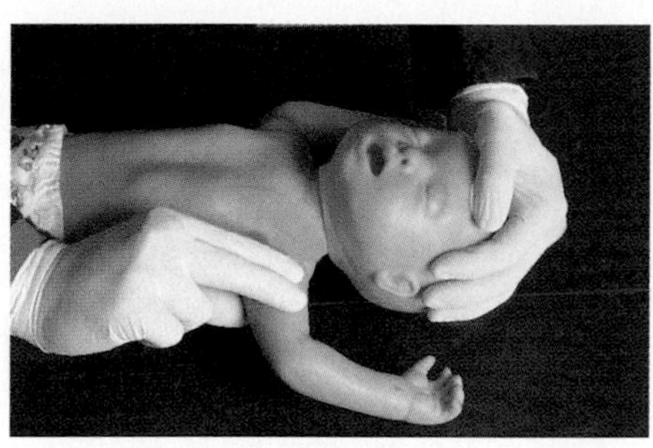

Figure 15.3 The best place to take the pulse in an infant is over the brachial artery or directly over the heart.

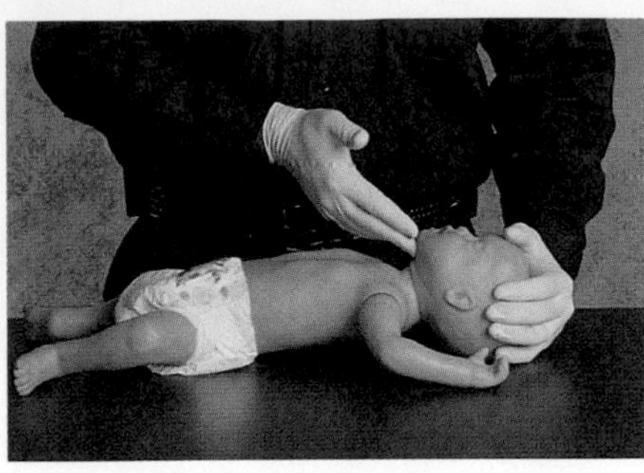

Figure 15.4 Open the infant's airway using the head tilt–chin lift technique.

Otherwise, the child may suffer respiratory arrest, followed by cardiac arrest because of the lack of oxygen to the heart. This is a different situation than adults, who usually suffer cardiopulmonary arrest as a result of a heart attack.

Some of the specific causes of cardiopulmonary arrest in children include suffocation caused by the aspiration of a foreign body, infections of the airway such as croup and acute epiglottitis, sudden infant death syndrome (SIDS), accidental poisonings, and injuries around the head and neck. This chapter covers each problem in detail.

Treating Respiratory Emergencies in Infants and Children

Opening the Airway

Use the same general techniques to open the airway of a child or an infant that you use for an adult patient. The head tilt–chin lift technique can be used for children who have not suffered an injury to the neck or head (**Figure 15.4**). When using the head tilt–chin lift technique on a child, be sure that you do not hyperextend (overextend) the neck when you tilt the head back. Hyperextending a child's neck can occlude the airway. Use a neutral or slight sniffing position. You can place a folded towel under the child's shoulders to help maintain this position. If the possibility of injury to the head or neck exists, do not use the head tilt–chin lift technique. Instead use the jaw-thrust technique as you keep the head and neck stabilized.

Remember

Essential Skills

- Opening the airway
- Basic life support
- Suctioning
- Using airway adjuncts

Basic Life Support

Because children are smaller than adults, you must use specific techniques when you perform CPR on children. There are special procedures for hand placement, compression pressure, and airway positioning.

CPR for children (1 to 8 years old) is different from adult CPR in four ways:

1. If you are alone, without help, and EMS has not been called, you should perform one minute of CPR before activating the EMS system.
2. Use the heel of one hand to perform chest compressions rather than both hands (**Figure 15.5**).
3. Depress the sternum about 1 to 1½ inches.
4. Provide 100 compressions per minute, giving one rescue breath after every five chest compressions.

CPR for infants (less than 1 year old) has six differences from adult CPR:

1. Check for responsiveness by tapping the foot or gently shaking the shoulder.
2. Give gentle rescue breaths, using mouth-to-mouth-and-nose ventilations.
3. Check the pulse by using the brachial pulse as shown in **Figure 15.3**, page 351.
4. Use your middle and ring fingers to compress the sternum.
5. Compress the sternum approximately ½ to 1 inch.
6. Perform chest compressions at least 100 times per minute.

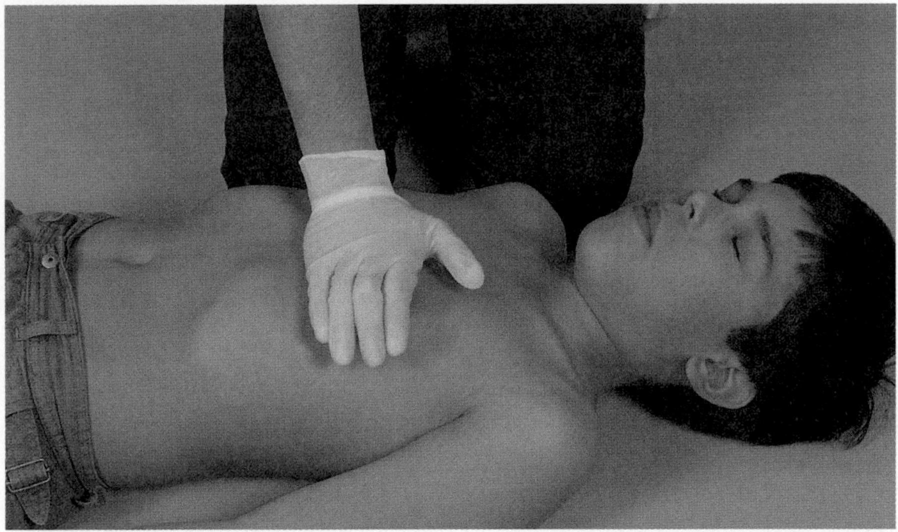

Figure 15.5 Place one hand two fingers above the bottom of the sternum.

Suctioning

Airways that are blocked by secretions, vomitus, or blood should be cleared initially by turning the patient on the side and using gloved fingers to scoop out as much of the substance as possible. You can use suctioning to remove the foreign substances that cannot be removed with your gloved fingers. Suctioning to open a blocked airway can be a lifesaving procedure.

Note: CPR for infants and children is described in detail in Chapters 6 and 8. To review these techniques, see these chapters.

The procedure used for suctioning infants and children is generally the same as for adults, with the following exceptions:

1. Use a tonsil sucker to suction the mouth. Do not insert the tip any farther than you can see.
2. Use a flexible catheter to suction the nose of a child; set the suction on low or medium.
3. Use a bulb syringe to suction the nose of an infant. Remember that an infant can only breathe through the nose.
4. Never suction for more than five seconds at one time.
5. Try to ventilate and reoxygenate the patient before repeating the suctioning.

For a complete description of how to use suctioning, review the material presented in Chapters 6 and 14.

Airway Adjuncts

Oral airways can maintain an open airway after you have opened the patient's airway by manual means.

Use the following steps to insert an oral airway in a child or an infant:

1. Select the proper sized oral airway by measuring from the patient's earlobe to the corner of the mouth.
2. Open the patient's mouth with one hand using the jaw-thrust technique.
3. Depress the patient's tongue with two or three stacked tongue blades. Press the tongue forward and away from the roof of the mouth.

Remember

You must be careful not to overextend the neck. In infants and some small children, the overextension may actually obstruct the airway because of the flexibility of the child's neck. Smaller children may breathe easier if the neck is held in a neutral position rather than overextended. To maintain the neutral position, you can use your hands to support the shoulders.

4. Follow the anatomic curve of the roof of the patient's mouth to slide the airway into place.
5. Be gentle. The mouths of children and infants are fragile.

First responders usually do not use nasal airways for children. If you have questions about using nasal airways in pediatric patients, check with your medical director.

Partial Airway Obstruction

You can usually relieve a partial airway obstruction by placing the child on his or her back (supine), tilting the head, and lifting the chin (**Figure 15.6**) in the usual manner (the head tilt–chin lift technique).

A blocked airway from an aspirated foreign object (small toy, piece of candy, or balloon) is a common problem in young children, particularly in children who are crawling. If the foreign object is only partially blocking the airway, the child will probably be able to pass some air around the object. You can remove the object if it is clearly visible in the mouth and can be removed easily.

However, if you cannot see the object, or if you do not think it can be removed easily, you should not attempt to remove it as long as the child can still breathe air around the object. Sometimes trying to remove an object that is partially blocking the airway can result in a complete airway blockage, which is an extremely serious situation.

CAUTION

The American Heart Association specifically states that "blind" finger sweeps should not be performed on infants and children because they might move the object and completely block the airway.

Children with a partial airway obstruction should be *transported* to the hospital. You should talk constantly to a child with a partially obstructed airway about what you are doing. Talking also comforts the child and reduces the terror of having something "stuck in the throat."

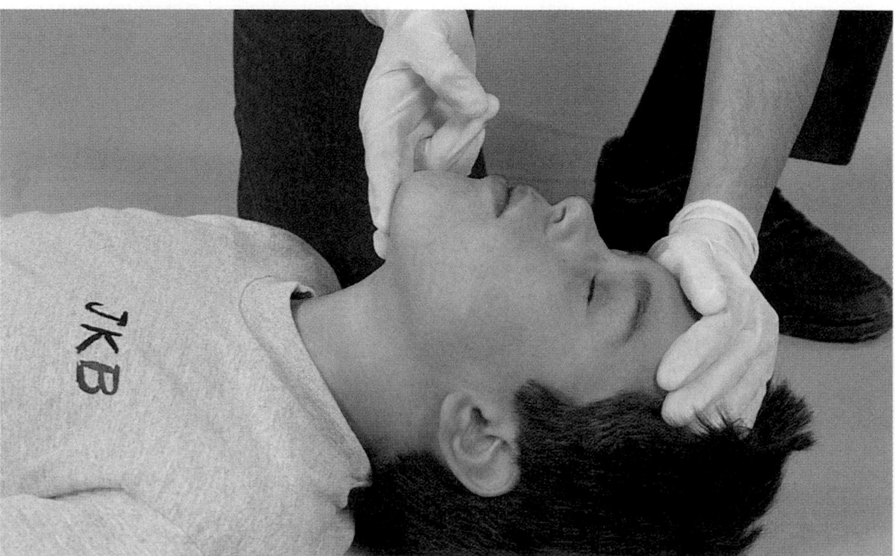

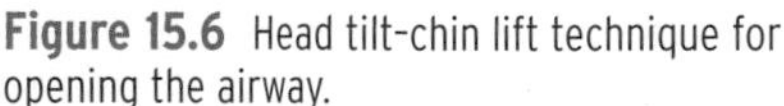

Figure 15.6 Head tilt-chin lift technique for opening the airway.

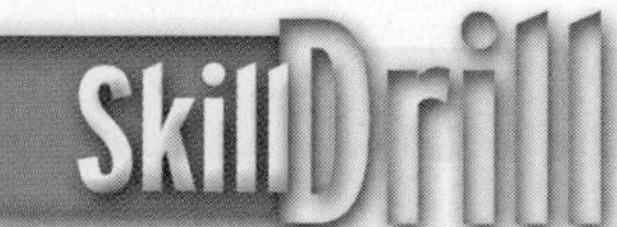

Figure 15.7 Performing Abdominal Thrusts on a Child

1

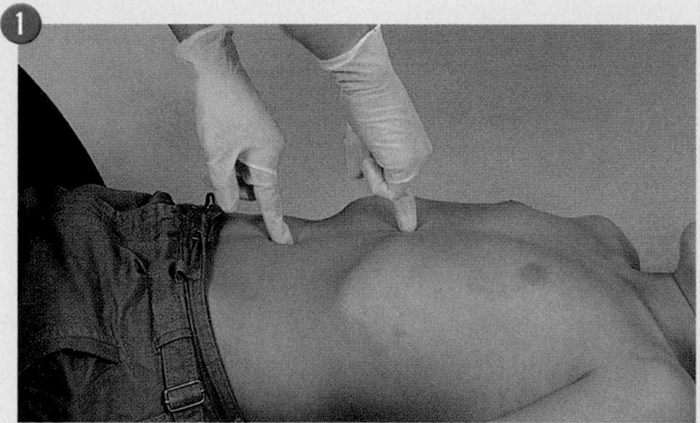

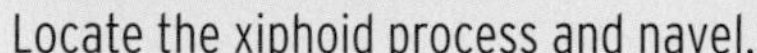
Locate the xiphoid process and navel.

2

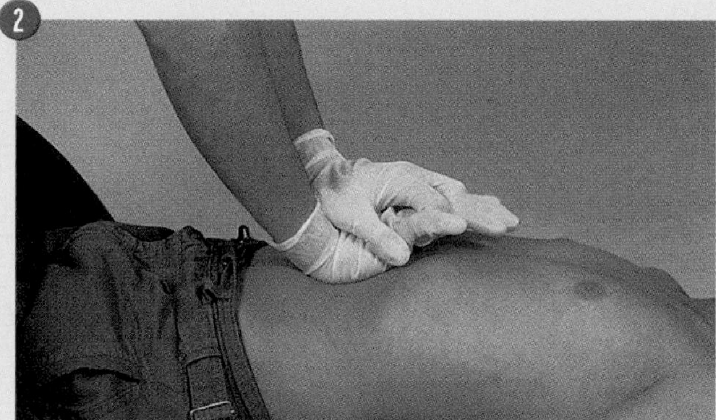

Perform the abdominal thrust.

The presence of a parent during transport can provide psychological support to both the parent and the child. The parent's presence can often reassure and calm the child. You should judge each situation carefully. Not all parents can remain calm themselves during such a serious situation. However, most of the time, when the parents realize the seriousness of the situation, they are able to redirect their emotions and work with you to reassure and calm the child.

If you have oxygen available and are trained in its use, administer it by gently placing the oxygen mask over the child's mouth and nose. Don't try to get an airtight seal on the mask; hold it 1 or 2 inches away from the child's face. If you tell the child what you are doing with the oxygen and how it will make breathing easier, you may be able to calm and relax the child. Carefully monitor this critical situation to ensure that the partial obstruction does not become a complete obstruction!

Complete Airway Obstruction in Children

A complete airway obstruction is a serious emergency because no air is able to pass the foreign object. You have only a few minutes to act before permanent brain damage occurs. Use the abdominal-thrust maneuver (**Figure 15.7**) because it provides enough energy to expel most foreign objects that could completely block a child's airway.

Airway Obstruction in a Conscious Child

Remove an airway obstruction in a conscious child (1 to 8 years old) using the same steps as for an adult patient, but do not perform blind finger sweeps. Instead, perform the tongue-jaw lift, look down into the airway, and use your fingers to sweep the airway only if you can actually see the obstruction.

A skill performance sheet titled "Foreign Body Airway Obstruction—Conscious Child" is included for your review and practice (**Figure 15.8**, page 356).

Figure 15.8 Skill Performance Sheet

Foreign Body Airway Obstruction—Conscious Child

Steps	Adequately Performed
1. Ask "Are you choking?"	
2. Give abdominal thrusts.	
3. Repeat thrusts until effective or victim becomes unconscious.	
Child Foreign Body Airway Obstruction—Victim Becomes Unconscious	
4. If second rescuer is available, have him or her activate the EMS system.	
5. Perform a tongue-jaw lift, and if you see the object, perform a finger sweep to remove it.	
6. Open airway and try to ventilate; if obstructed, reposition head and try to ventilate again.	
7. Give up to five abdominal thrusts.	
8. Repeat steps 5 through 7 until effective.*	
9. If airway obstruction is not relieved after about 1 minute, activate the EMS system.	

** If victim is unresponsive but breathing, place in recovery position.* *Based on the latest CPR guidelines.*

Airway Obstruction in an Unconscious Child

If the child is unconscious, follow basically the same steps for relieving a complete airway obstruction in an an unconscious adult patient. However, do not perform a finger sweep on an unconscious child unless you can actually see the object that is obstructing the airway. Because the child's airway is so much smaller than an adult's, it is important that you do not push the foreign object farther down into the child's airway. If you are alone, you should attempt to remove the foreign body obstruction for one minute before stopping to activate the EMS system.

A skill performance sheet titled "Foreign Body Airway Obstruction—Unconscious Child" is included for your review and practice (**Figure 15.9**).

Complete Airway Obstruction in Infants

An infant (under one year of age) is very fragile. Infants' airway structures are very small, and they are more easily injured than those of an adult. If you suspect an airway obstruction, first assess the baby to determine if there is any air exchange. If the baby is crying, the airway is not completely obstructed. If no air is moving in or out of the baby's mouth and nose, suspect an obstructed airway. Find out what was happening when the baby stopped breathing. Someone may have seen the baby put a foreign body into the mouth. To relieve an airway obstruction in an infant, use a combination of back blows and the **chest-thrust maneuver**.

chest-thrust maneuver A series of manual thrusts to the chest to relieve upper airway obstruction; used in the treatment of infants, pregnant women, or extremely obese people.

Figure 15.9 Skill Performance Sheet

Foreign Body Airway Obstruction–Unconscious Child

Steps	Adequately Performed
1. Establish unresponsiveness. If second rescuer is available, have him or her activate the EMS system.	
2. Open airway, check breathing (look, listen, and feel), try to ventilate; if obstructed, reposition head and try to ventilate again.	
3. Give up to five abdominal thrusts.	
4. Perform a tongue-jaw lift and if you see the object, perform a finger sweep to remove it.	
5. Try to ventilate; if still obstructed reposition the head and try to ventilate again.	
6. Repeat steps 3 through 5 until effective.*	
7. If airway obstruction is not relieved after about 1 minute, activate the EMS system.	

** If victim is unresponsive but breathing, place in recovery position.*

Based on the latest CPR guidelines.

Be sure you are holding the infant securely as you alternate the back blows and the chest thrusts (**Figure 15.10**, page 358).

Airway Obstruction in a Conscious Infant

To assist a conscious infant who has a complete airway obstruction, you must proceed with the following steps:

1. Assess the infant's airway and breathing status. Determine that there is no airway exchange.
2. Place the infant in a face down position over one arm and deliver five back blows. Support the infant's head and neck with one hand and place the infant in a face down position with the head lower than the trunk. Support the infant over your forearm and rest your forearm on your thigh. Use the heel of your hand to deliver up to five back blows forcefully between the infant's shoulder blades.
3. Turn the infant face up by sandwiching the head between your hands and arms to provide support, and turning the infant on the back with the head lower than the trunk.
4. Deliver up to five chest thrusts in the middle of the sternum. Use two fingers to deliver the chest thrusts in a firm manner.
5. Repeat the series of back blows and chest thrusts until the foreign object is expelled or until the infant becomes unconscious.

A skill performance sheet titled "Foreign Body Airway Obstruction – Conscious Infant" is included for your review and practice (**Figure 15.11**, page 358).

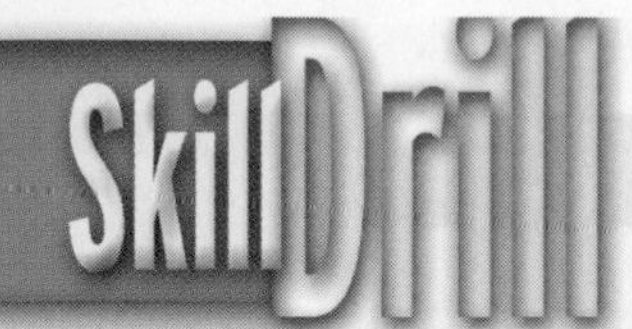

Figure 15.10 Administering Back Blows and Chest Thrusts in an Infant

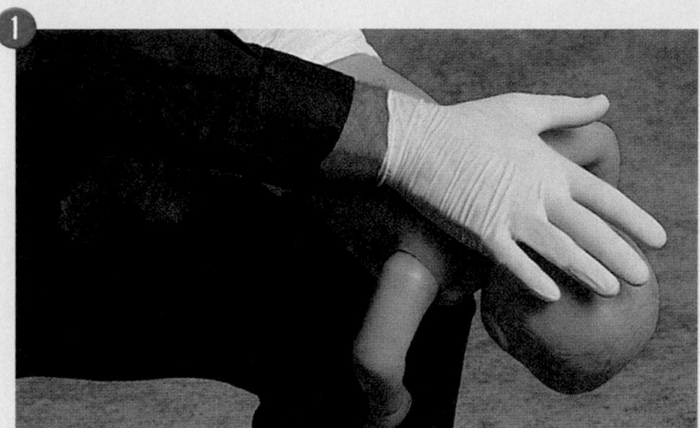

1 Administer five back blows.

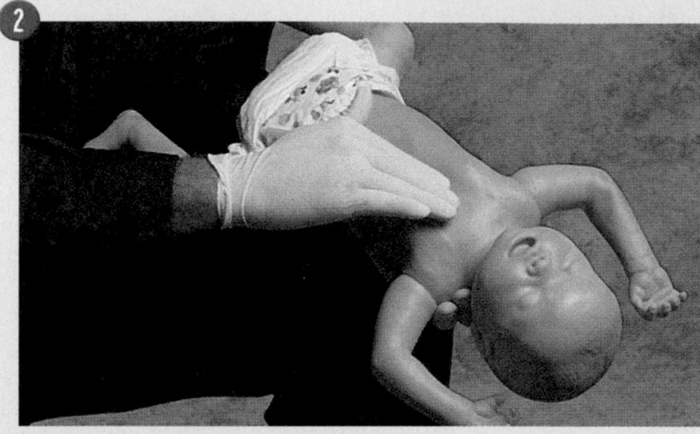

2 Followed by five chest thrusts.

Figure 15.11 Skill Performance Sheet

Foreign Body Airway Obstruction—Conscious Infant

Steps	Adequately Performed
1. Confirm complete airway obstruction. Check for serious breathing difficulty, ineffective cough, no strong cry.	
2. Give up to five back blows and chest thrusts.	
3. Repeat step 2 until effective or victim becomes unconscious.	
Infant Foreign Body Airway Obstruction—Victim Becomes Unconscious	
4. If second rescuer is available, have him or her activate the EMS system.	
5. Perform a tongue-jaw lift, and if you see the object, perform a finger sweep to remove it.	
6. Open airway and try to ventilate; if obstructed, reposition head and try to ventilate again.	
7. Give up to five back blows and chest thrusts.	
8. Repeat steps 5 through 7 until effective.*	
9. If airway obstruction is not relieved after about 1 minute, activate the EMS system.	

** If victim is unresponsive but breathing, place in recovery position.*

Based on the latest CPR guidelines.

Airway Obstruction in an Unconscious Infant

Use the same sequence of back blows and chest thrusts relieve an airway obstruction in an unconscious infant as you used for a conscious infant. However, you must first take steps to determine unconsciousness and the presence of an airway obstruction.

Practice the following steps until you can do them automatically. To assist an unconscious infant with a complete airway obstruction, follow these steps:

1. Determine unresponsiveness by gently shaking the shoulder or by gently tapping the bottom of the foot.
2. Position the infant on a firm, hard surface and support the head and neck.
3. Open the airway using the head tilt–chin lift technique. Be careful not to tilt the infant's head too far back.
4. Determine breathlessness by placing your ear close to the infant's mouth and nose. Listen and feel for the infant's breathing.
5. Attempt rescue breathing. If unsuccessful, continue to Step 6.
6. Reposition the airway and reattempt rescue breathing.
   Note: Steps 1 through 6 are the same sequence used for infant rescue breathing.
7. Deliver up to five back blows using the same technique as for a conscious infant.
8. Deliver up to five chest thrusts using the same technique as for a conscious infant.
9. Perform tongue-jaw lift and remove any foreign object that you can see.
10. Repeat the sequence of back blows and chest thrusts until the foreign body is expelled.

A skill performance sheet titled "Foreign Body Airway Obstruction—Unconscious Infant" is included for your review and practice **(Figure 15.12**, page 360).

Swallowed Objects

Children often swallow small, round objects like marbles, beads, buttons, and coins. If they do not become airway obstructions, they usually pass uneventfully through the child and are eliminated in a bowel movement. However, sharp or straight objects such as open safety pins, bobby pins, and bones are dangerous if swallowed. Arrange for Ⓣ ***transport*** to an appropriate medical facility because special instruments and techniques are required to locate and remove the object from the stomach and intestinal tract.

Respiratory Distress

Respiratory distress indicates that a child has a serious problem that requires immediate medical attention. Often respiratory distress quickly leads to respiratory failure.

You must be able to recognize the following signs of respiratory distress:

1. A breathing rate of more than 60 breaths per minute in infants.
2. A breathing rate of more than 30 to 40 breaths per minute in children.

Figure 15.12 Skill Performance Sheet

Foreign Body Airway Obstruction—Unconscious Infant

Steps	Adequately Performed
1. Establish unresponsiveness. If second rescuer is available, have him or her activate the EMS system.	
2. Open airway, check breathing (look, listen, and feel), try to ventilate; if obstructed, reposition head and try to ventilate again.	
3. Give up to five back blows and five chest thrusts.	
4. Perform a tongue-jaw lift and if you see the object, perform a finger sweep to remove it.	
5. Try to ventilate; if still obstructed, reposition the head and try to ventilate again.	
6. Repeat steps 3 through 5 until effective.*	
7. If airway obstruction is not relieved after about 1 minute, activate the EMS system.	

** If victim is unresponsive but breathing, place in recovery position.* *Based on the latest CPR guidelines.*

3. Nasal flaring on each breath.
4. Retraction of the skin between the ribs and around the neck muscles.
5. Stridor, a high-pitched sound on inspiration.
6. Cyanosis of the skin.
7. Altered mental status.
8. Combativeness or restlessness.

If any of the listed signs is present, try to determine the cause. Support the child's respirations by placing the child in a comfortable position, usually sitting. Keep the child as calm as possible by letting a parent hold the child if practical. Prepare to administer oxygen if it is available and you are trained in its use. Monitor the child's vital signs and arrange for T ***prompt transport*** to an appropriate medical facility.

Respiratory Failure/Arrest

Respiratory failure often results as respiratory distress proceeds. It can be caused by many of the same factors that cause respiratory distress.

Respiratory failure is characterized by the following conditions:

1. A breathing rate of fewer than 20 breaths per minute in an infant.
2. A breathing rate of fewer than 10 breaths per minute in a child.
3. Limp muscle tone.
4. Unresponsiveness.
5. Decreased or absent heart rate.
6. Weak or absent distal pulses.

A child in respiratory failure is on the verge of respiratory and cardiac arrest. You must immediately assess the child and take whatever steps are appropriate to support the patient. Support respirations by performing mouth-to-mask ventilations. Administer oxygen if it is available and if you have been trained to use it. Begin chest compressions if the heart rate is slow or absent. Arrange for T ***prompt transportation*** to an appropriate medical facility. Continue to monitor the patient's vital signs and support the airway, breathing, and circulation functions as well as you can.

Circulatory Failure

The most common cause of circulatory failure in children is respiratory failure. Uncorrected respiratory failure in children can lead to circulatory failure, and uncorrected circulatory failure can lead to cardiac arrest. That is why it is so important to correct respiratory failure before it progresses to circulatory failure. But this is not always possible, so you should learn the signs of circulatory failure and its treatment.

An increased heart rate, pale or bluish skin, and changes in mental status indicate circulatory failure. Your treatment consists of completing the patient assessment sequence, supporting ventilations, administering oxygen if available, and observing vital signs for any changes.

Checkpoint

- ○ Describe the difference between the respiratory care of an adult and a child.

Sudden Illness and Medical Emergencies

Not many illnesses occur suddenly in young children, but most of the medical calls for children will involve these sudden illnesses. It is important that you be able to recognize and treat these key pediatric illnesses.

Treating Altered Mental Status

Altered mental status in children can be caused by a variety of conditions, including low blood sugar, poisoning, postseizure state, infection, head trauma, and decreased oxygen levels. Sometimes you will be able to determine the cause of the altered mental status and take steps to correct the problem. For example, if the parent tells you that the child is diabetic and suffering from insulin shock, you can give sugar to increase the patient's blood sugar. But in many cases, you will not be able to determine the cause and will have to treat the patient's symptoms.

Complete your patient assessment, paying particular attention to any clues at the scene. Question any bystanders or family about the situation and try to get as much medical history as possible. Pay particular attention to the patient's initial vital signs. Recheck vital signs regularly to monitor any changes. Calm the patient and the patient's family. Be prepared to support the patient's airway, breathing, and circulation if needed. Place unconscious patients in the recovery position to help keep an open airway and to aid them in handling their secretions.

KEY PEDIATRIC ILLNESSES

- *Altered mental status*
- *Respiratory emergencies*
  - *Asthma*
  - *Croup*
  - *Epiglottitis*
- *Near drowning*
- *Heat illness*
- *High fever*
- *Seizures*
- *Vomiting and diarrhea*
- *Abdominal pain*
- *Poisoning*
- *Sudden infant death syndrome (SIDS)*

Treating Respiratory Emergencies

A respiratory problem in an infant or child can range from a minor cold to complete blockage of the airway. Because infants breathe primarily through their noses, even a minor cold can cause breathing difficulties. The excessive mucus in the nose resulting from a cold makes it more difficult for an infant to breathe than for an older child who can breathe through both the nose and mouth. Although most common respiratory problems in children are caused by colds, you should also be able to recognize and treat the three more serious conditions listed in the box on the left.

> **RESPIRATORY EMERGENCIES**
> - *asthma*
> - *croup*
> - *epiglottitis*

Asthma

A child who has **asthma** is usually already being treated for the condition by a physician and is taking a prescribed medicine. The parents call for assistance or transport only if the child experiences unusual breathing difficulty.

asthma An acute spasm of the smaller air passages marked by labored breathing and wheezing.

croup Inflammation and narrowing of the air passages in young children causing a barking cough, hoarseness, and a harsh, high-pitched breathing sound.

Asthma can occur at any age. It is caused by a spasm or constriction (narrowing) of the smaller airways in the lungs that produces a characteristic wheezing sound. Asthma attacks can range from mild to severe and can be triggered by many factors, including feathers, animal fur, tobacco smoke, pollen, and even emotional situations.

A child who is having an asthma attack is in obvious respiratory distress. During a severe attack, you can clearly hear the characteristic wheezing on exhalation—even without a stethoscope. The child can inhale air without difficulty but must labor to exhale. The effort to exhale is both frightening and tiring for the child.

Your primary treatment consists of calming and reassuring both the parents and the child. Tell them everything possible is being done and encourage them to relax.

Place the child in a sitting position to make breathing more comfortable. Ask the child to purse his or her lips, as if blowing up a balloon. Tell the child to blow out with force while doing this. Pursed-lip breathing helps in two ways: both parents and the child feel that "something is being done," and this type of breathing relieves some of the internal lung pressures that cause the asthma attack (**Figure 15.13**).

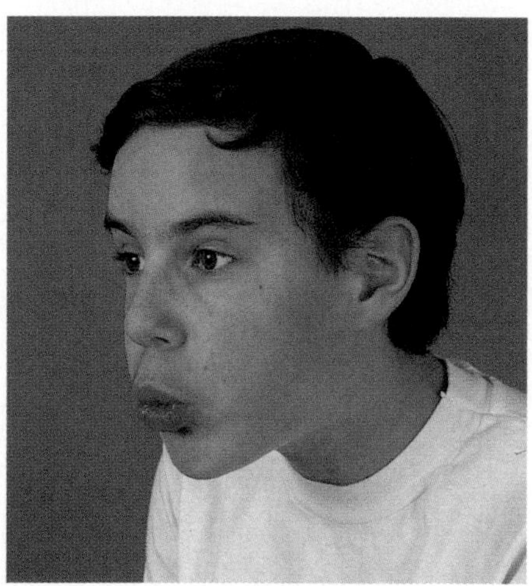

Figure 15.13 Pursed-lip breathing can help relieve an asthma attack.

If a child has asthma medication but has not yet taken it, help the parent administer the medication. The parents should contact the child's physician for further advice. If the child's physician is not available, arrange for *prompt transport* to a hospital emergency department.

Croup

Croup is an infection of the upper airway that usually occurs in children from 6 months to 4 years of age. The lower throat swells and compresses (narrows) the airway, resulting in a characteristic hoarse, whooping noise during inhalation and a seal-like barking cough.

Croup occurs often in colder climates (during fall and winter) and is frequently accompanied by a cold. The child usually has a moderate fever and a croupy noise that has developed over time. The worst attacks of croup usually occur in the middle of the night.

> **Signs & Symptoms**
> **CROUP**
> - Noisy, whooping inhalations
> - Barking seal-like cough
> - History of a recent or current cold
> - Lack of fright or anxiety
> - Willingness to lie down

The last two signs, lack of fright or anxiety and a willingness to lie down, are important because they help you distinguish croup from epiglottitis. Epiglottitis is a more serious condition discussed in the next section.

Although croup is frightening for parents, it may not frighten children. As with many childhood emergencies, you must respond to the psychological needs and concerns of the parents as well as the medical needs of the child. Do not assume that noisy breathing is caused by croup! Look to see if the child is choking on a toy, food, or foreign object caught in the airway.

If the EMS unit is delayed, ask the parents to turn on the hot water in the shower and close the bathroom door. When the bathroom steams up, ask the parent to wait there with the child until the EMS unit arrives. This effectively treats the child and reassures the parent. The moist, warm air relaxes the vocal cords and lessens the croupy noise. Contact the child's physician for further instructions or arrange for Ⓣ *transport* to an appropriate medical facility.

Epiglottitis

The third, and most severe, major respiratory problem is **epiglottitis**. Epiglottitis is a severe inflammation of the epiglottis, the small flap that covers the trachea during swallowing. In this condition, the flap is so inflamed and swollen that air movement into the trachea is completely blocked. Epiglottitis usually occurs in children from 3 to 6 years of age.

At first examination, you may think the child has croup. However, because epiglottitis poses an immediate threat to life, you must be able to recognize the differences and know the signs and symptoms of epiglottitis.

CAUTION

Do not examine a child's throat if you suspect epiglottitis! An examination can cause more swelling of the epiglottis, resulting in a complete airway blockage.

If you encounter a child with these signs and symptoms, you need to recognize it as a serious respiratory emergency. There is little else you can do except to make the child comfortable, with as little handling as possible, keep everyone calm, administer oxygen (if you have it available and have been trained to use it), and arrange for Ⓣ *prompt transport* to an appropriate medical facility. You may consider letting a parent hold the child during transport if the emotional attitudes of the child and parent are appropriate.

Signs & Symptoms

EPIGLOTTITIS

- The child is usually sitting upright (he or she does not want to lie down).
- The child cannot swallow.
- The child is not coughing.
- The child is drooling (**Figure 15.14**).
- The child is anxious and frightened (he or she knows that something is seriously wrong).
- The child's chin is thrust forward.

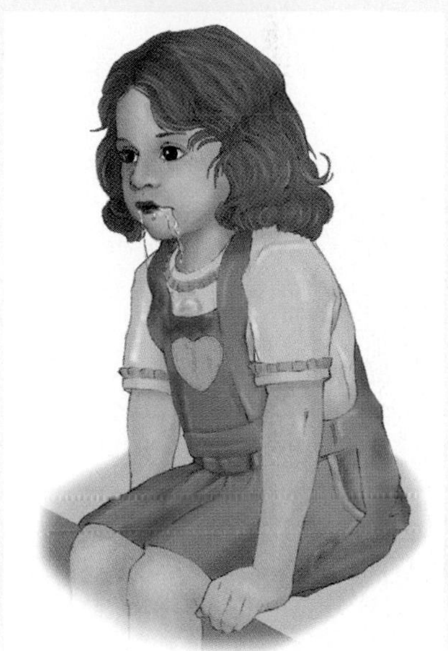

Figure 15.14 A key sign of epiglottitis is drooling.

Near Drowning

Drowning is the second most common cause of accidental death among children 5 years of age or younger in the United States. Although swimming pools, lakes, streams, and oceans present significant risks of drowning, ordinary water sources around the home increase the risk of drowning for young children. Children left unattended in wash bowls or bath tubs for even a few minutes can drown. Buckets of water and toilet bowls also pose threats to young children who put their heads down to look into the water, lose their balance, fall in, and are unable to get out.

Victims of **near drowning** are people who survive the experience of suffocation under water. The many sources of water around a home increase the chance that you, as a first responder, may encounter a near-drowning situation in responding to a medical emergency involving a child.

FYI

Note: The child with epiglottitis must have medical attention to ensure an open airway.

epiglottitis Severe inflammation and swelling of the epiglottis; a life-threatening situation.

drowning Death from suffocation after submersion in water.

near drowning Survival, at least temporarily, after suffocation in water.

If you respond to a near-drowning situation, make sure that you do not put yourself in danger as you attempt a rescue. (See Chapter 18 for more information on water rescues.) After the child is removed from the water, begin assessment and treating. Signs and symptoms of near drowning may include lack of breathing and no pulse.

Begin by assessing the airway, breathing, and circulation. Make sure the airway is clear of water. Turn the child to one side and allow the water to drain out. Use suction if it is available, start rescue breathing if necessary, and administer supplemental oxygen if it is available. If no pulse is present, start chest compressions. Because there is a chance that the cervical spine was injured, stabilize the neck. To reduce the risk of hypothermia, dry the child with towels and cover with dry blankets or jackets. Arrange for T ***prompt transport*** of the patient to an appropriate medical facility. All patients who have experienced submersion need to be evaluated by a physician.

Heat Illnesses

Heat illnesses may range from relatively minor muscle cramps to vomiting, heat exhaustion, and heatstroke.

The most dangerous heat illness in children is heatstroke. Any child who is in a closed, parked car on a hot day or in a poorly ventilated room and who has hot, dry skin may be suffering from heatstroke. This is a serious and potentially fatal condition that requires rapid treatment from you to cool the child and reduce body temperature.

Undress and sponge or immerse the child with water and fan him or her to help lower body temperature quickly. You may wrap the child in wet sheets (if they are available) to speed up the evaporation and cooling process, but do not let the child become chilled. Finally, be sure that you have arranged for T ***rapid transport*** to an appropriate medical facility. (See Chapter 9 for a more detailed description of heatstroke.)

Treating High Fevers

Fevers are quite common in children and can be caused by many different infections, especially ear and gastrointestinal infections. Because the temperature-regulating mechanism in young children has not fully developed, a very high temperature (104°F to 106°F, or 40°C to 41°C) can develop even with a relatively minor infection. Most children can tolerate temperatures as high as 104°F (40°C), but a high fever may require that the child be hospitalized so that the underlying cause can be discovered and treated.

Your first step in treating a child with a high fever is to uncover the child so that body heat can escape. Layers of clothing or blankets retain body heat, and can increase body temperature high enough to cause convulsions. About 10 percent of children between 1 and 6 years of age are susceptible to seizures brought on by high fevers. Remember that in attempting to reduce high fever, you are only treating the symptom and not the source. The child must be seen by a physician as soon as possible to determine the cause of the fever.

If you encounter a child with a high fever above 104°F (40°C), take these steps to treat the fever symptoms:

1. Make certain the child is not wrapped in too much clothing or too many blankets.
2. Attempt to reduce high temperature by undressing the child.
3. Fan the child to cool him or her down.
4. Protect the child during any seizure (do not restrain the child's motion) and make certain that normal breathing resumes after each seizure.

Treating Seizures

Seizures (convulsions) can result from high fever or from disorders such as **epilepsy** (see Chapter 9). Seizures can vary in intensity from simple, momentary staring spells (without body movements) to generalized seizures in which the entire body stiffens and shakes severely.

epilepsy A disease manifested by seizures, caused by an abnormal focus of electrical activity in the brain

Although seizures can be frightening to parents, bystanders, and rescuers, they are not usually dangerous. During a seizure, a child loses consciousness, the eyes roll back, the teeth become clenched, and the body shakes with severe jerking movements. Often, the child's skin becomes pale or turns blue. Sometimes the child loses bladder and bowel control, and soils his or her clothing. Seizures caused by high fever usually last about 20 seconds.

If a seizure occurs, place the child on a soft surface (sofa, bed, or rug) to protect the child from injury during the seizure. Reassure the child's parents, who may be frightened by the seizure. If they become too emotional, ask them to leave the room. Carefully monitor the child's airway during and after the seizure.

As a first responder, you can provide the following treatment for seizures:
1. Place the patient on the floor or bed to prevent injury.
2. Maintain an adequate airway after the seizure ends.
3. Provide supplemental oxygen after the seizure if it is available and if you are trained to use it.
4. Arrange for T ***prompt transport*** to an appropriate medical facility.
5. Continue to monitor the patient's vital signs and support the ABCs if necessary.
6. After the seizure is over, cool the patient if the patient has a high fever.

FYI

Vomiting and Diarrhea

Children are very susceptible to vomiting and diarrhea, which are usually caused by gastrointestinal infections. Prolonged vomiting and diarrhea may produce severe dehydration. The dehydrated child is lethargic and has very dry skin, which can be especially noticeable around the mouth and nose. Hospitalization may be required to replace fluids through the veins. If you suspect that a child may be dehydrated, arrange for T ***transport*** to an appropriate medical facility.

Abdominal Pain

One of the most serious causes of abdominal pain in children is appendicitis. Although it can occur at any age, appendicitis is often seen in people who are between 10 and 25 years old. A cramping pain usually starts in the belly button area of the stomach. Within a matter of hours, the pain moves to the right lower quadrant of the abdomen becoming steady and more severe. Usually the child is nauseated, has no appetite, and occasionally will vomit.

Because there are several potential causes of abdominal pain, including appendicitis, do not try to make a diagnosis in the field. Even physicians may find it difficult to diagnose the cause of abdominal pain. A good rule to follow is to treat every child with a sore or tender abdomen as an emergency and arrange for T ***transport*** to an appropriate medical facility for an appropriate diagnosis.

Poisoning

Little children are curious and often like to sample the contents of brightly colored bottles or cans looking for something good to eat or drink. However, many common household items contain poisonous substances. The two most common types of poisonings in children are caused by ingestion and absorption.

Ingestion

An ingested poison is taken by mouth. A child who has ingested a poison may have chemical burns, odors, or stains around the mouth and be suffering from nausea, vomiting, abdominal pain, or diarrhea. Later symptoms may include abnormal or decreased respirations, unconsciousness, or seizures.

If you believe a child has ingested a poisonous substance, you should:

1. Try to identify what the child has swallowed, attempt to estimate the amount ingested, and send the bottle or container along with the child to the emergency department.
2. Gather any spilled tablets if the child swallowed tablets from a medicine bottle and replace them in the bottle so they can be counted. The emergency physician may then be able to determine how many tablets the child has taken.
3. Contact your local poison control center if transportation to an appropriate medical facility is delayed. The poison control center will need to know:
   - Age of the patient
   - Weight of the patient
   - Identification of the poison
   - Estimated quantity of the poison taken
4. Follow the directions provided by the poison control center. You may need to:
   a. Dilute the poison by giving the child large amounts of water;
   b. Administer activated charcoal if it is available and you have been trained in its use (the usual dose for pediatric patients is 12.5 to 25 grams);
   c. Induce vomiting using syrup of ipecac if you have been trained in its use and have permission from your medical director or poison control center (the usual dose for pediatric patients is 1 tablespoon).
5. Monitor the child's breathing and pulse closely. This is a critical step and you must be prepared to give emergency care, including rescue breathing and CPR.
6. Arrange T ***transport*** to an appropriate medical facility for examination by a physician.

See Chapter 10 for additional information on the emergency treatment for various poisons.

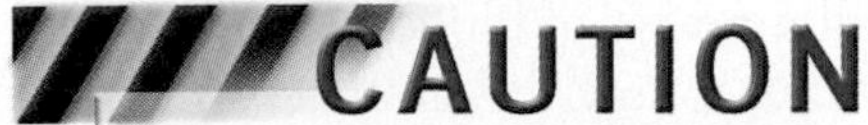

Do not attempt to give liquids or induce vomiting in an unconscious or partially conscious child because of the danger of aspiration of the vomitus.

Absorption

Poisoning by absorption occurs when a poisonous substance enters the body through the skin. A child who has absorbed poison may have localized symptoms, such as skin irritation or burning, or may have systemic signs and symptoms of the poisoning, such as nausea, vomiting, dizziness, and shock.

If you believe a child has absorbed a poisonous substance, you should:

1. Ensure that the child is no longer in contact with the poisonous substance.
2. Remove the child's clothing if you think it is contaminated.
3. Brush off any dry chemical. After you have removed all dry chemical, wash the child with water for at least 20 minutes.
4. Wash off any liquid poisons by flushing with water for at least 20 minutes.
5. Try to identify the poison, and send any containers with the child to the emergency department.
6. Monitor the child for any changes in respiration and pulse. Be prepared to administer rescue breathing or CPR if needed.
7. Arrange Ⓣ ***transport*** to an appropriate medical facility for examination by a physician.

See Chapter 10 for additional information on emergency treatment of poisoning.

Safety Tips

Be careful not to get any chemical onto your skin.

Note: Chemical burns to the eyes cause extreme pain and injury. Gently flush the affected eye or eyes with water for at least 20 minutes. Hold the eye open to allow water to flow over its entire surface. Direct the water from the inner corner of the eye to the outward edge of the eye. After flushing the eyes for 20 minutes, loosely cover both eyes with gauze bandages and arrange for Ⓣ ***prompt transport*** to an appropriate medical facility.

Sudden Infant Death Syndrome

A condition that is frequently mistaken for child abuse is sudden infant death syndrome (SIDS), also called crib death. It is the sudden and unexpected death of an apparently healthy infant. SIDS usually occurs in infants between the ages of 3 weeks and 7 months. The babies are usually found dead in their cribs.

There is currently no adequate scientific explanation of SIDS. These deaths are not the result of smothering, choking, or strangulation. SIDS deaths often remain unexplained, even after a complete and thorough autopsy.

You can imagine the shock and grief felt by parents who find their apparently healthy babies dead in bed. Your actions and words can help relieve their feelings of remorse and guilt.

If the infant is still warm, begin CPR and continue until help arrives (infant CPR is described in Chapter 6). In many cases, the infant has been dead several hours, and the body is cold and lifeless. Do not mistake the large, bruise-like blotches on the baby's body for signs of child abuse. The blotches are caused by the pooling of the baby's blood after death. Sometimes you may find a small amount of bloody foam on the infant's lips. If the child is obviously dead, follow the protocol in you community for dealing with dead patients.

Know your local guidelines for the management of SIDS. Remember that the parents could do nothing to prevent the death. Be compassionate and supportive during this tragic situation.

Pediatric Trauma

Trauma remains the number one killer of children. Each year, many young lives are lost because of accidental injury, particularly automobile crashes.

Treat an injured child as you would treat an injured adult, but remember the following differences:

1. A child cannot communicate symptoms as well as an adult.
2. A child may be shy and overwhelmed by adult rescuers (especially those in uniform), so it is important to develop a good relationship quickly to reduce the child's fear and anxiety
3. You may have to adapt materials and equipment to the child's size.
4. A child does not show signs of shock as early as an adult but can progress into severe shock quickly.

Patterns of Injury

The patterns of injuries suffered by children will be related to the type of trauma they experience, the type of activity causing the injury, and the child's anatomy. Motor vehicle crashes produce different patterns of injuries depending on whether the patient was using a seat belt, whether the patient was strapped in a car seat, or whether an air bag inflated in the crash. Unrestrained patients tend to have more head and neck injuries. Restrained passengers often suffer head injuries, spinal injuries, and abdominal injuries. Children struck while riding a bicycle often have head injuries, spinal injuries, abdominal injuries, and extremity injuries. The use of bicycle helmets greatly reduces the number and severity of head injuries. Pedestrians who are struck by a vehicle often suffer chest and abdominal injuries with internal bleeding, injured thighs, and head injuries. Falls from a height or diving accidents tend to cause head and spinal injuries and extremity injuries. Burns are a major cause of injuries to children. Injuries from sports activities cause a wide variety of injuries depending on the type of sports activity. By learning some of the basic patterns of injury, you can anticipate the injuries you may find when carefully examining pediatric patients.

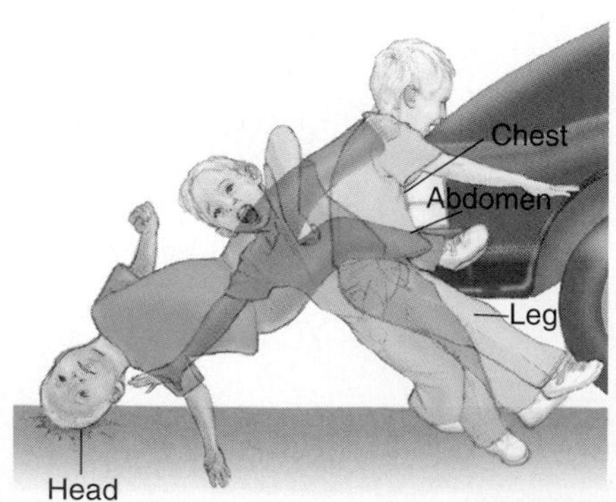

Figure 15.15 Look for these typical injuries when a child has been hit by a car.

If the child has been hit by a car, look for the common types of injuries shown in **Figure 15.15**. Major trauma in children usually results in multiple system injuries. No matter what the cause of injury, your first priority is always to check the patient's ABCs. Stop severe bleeding, treat the patient for shock, and proceed with the head-to-toe examina-

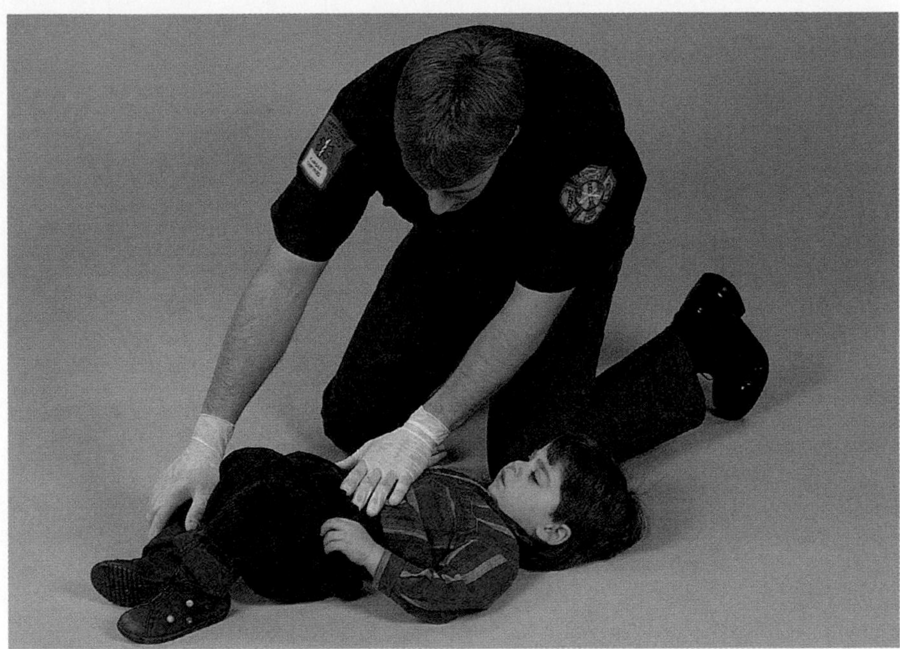

Figure 15.16 Examine every child from head to toe.

tion described in Chapter 7 to determine the extent of any other injuries (**Figure 15.16**). The head-to-toe examination is a hands-on procedure. A complete examination is especially important because a child cannot always communicate symptoms.

Involve the child in the physical examination as much as possible. Ask the child simple questions. Complete the head-to-toe examination even if the patient is too young to understand what is happening. Then stabilize all injuries you find. Splint suspected fractures, bandage wounds, and immobilize suspected spinal injuries.

If you are dealing with head lacerations, remember that the generous blood supply to the scalp can result in severe bleeding. These wounds can be treated with direct pressure and appropriate bandaging techniques. See Chapter 12 for a review of effective bandaging techniques.

Traumatic Shock in Children

Children show shock symptoms much more slowly than adults, but they progress through the stages of shock quickly. An injured child displaying obvious shock symptoms such as cool, clammy skin, a rapid, weak pulse, or rapid or shallow respirations is already suffering from severe shock. It is vital that you learn to recognize and treat of shock quickly. Review the signs and symptoms of shock in Chapter 12. Immediate treatment for an injured child suffering from shock includes controlling external bleeding, elevating the feet and legs, keeping the child warm, and administering oxygen if it is available. Children who show signs of shock should be transported as soon as possible to an emergency department. Seizures are relatively common in children who have sustained a serious head injury. Be prepared to manage this problem by maintaining the airway and protecting the child from further injury.

The greatest dangers to any patient who has suffered trauma are airway obstruction and hemorrhage. The most important things you can do for the injured child are to:

Note: Children under 9 years of age who are in seatbelts without a booster seat are at risk for sliding out of the lap belt during the crash. Rapid, jackknife bending increases the chances of intra-abdominal, spinal cord, and brain injuries.

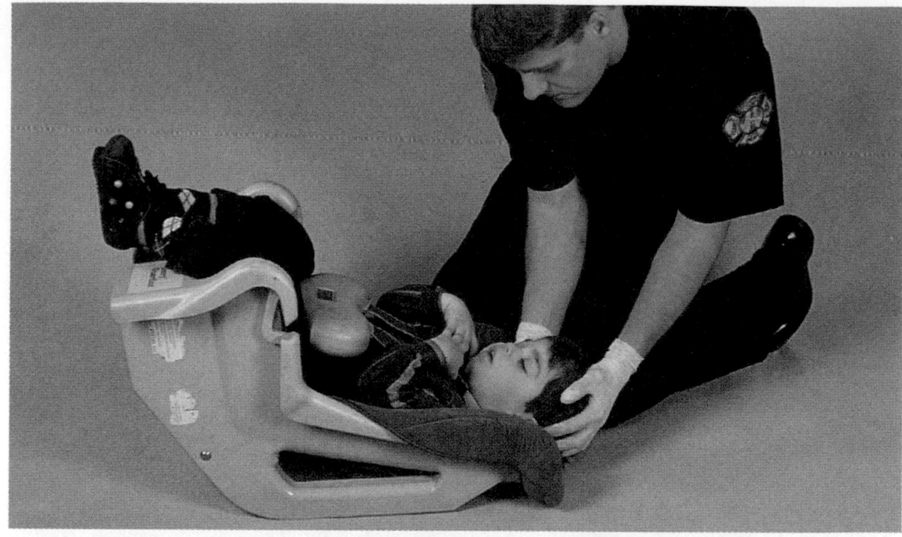

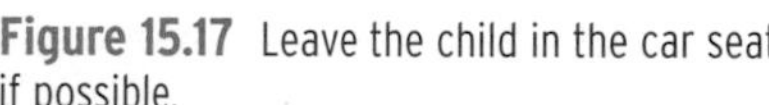

Figure 15.17 Leave the child in the car seat if possible.

- Open and maintain the airway.
- Control bleeding.
- Arrange for Ⓣ ***prompt transport*** to an appropriate medical facility.

Car Seats and Children

FYI

The impact of mandatory child restraint laws means that first responders are finding more children still strapped into car seats after crashes. You should become familiar with child restraint seats and understand how to gain access to children restrained in them.

If you find a child properly restrained in a car seat, leave the child in the car seat until the ambulance arrives (**Figure 15.17**). In many cases, a child can be secured in the seat, the seat removed from the vehicle, and both the seat and the child transported together (**Figure 15.18**) to the hospital.

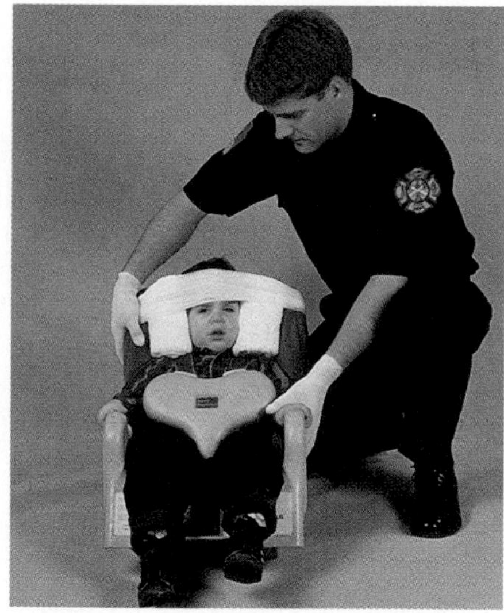

Figure 15.18 A child can be immobilized in the car seat.

Checkpoint

- ◯ Describe the differences between adult and child injury patterns.

Signs & Symptoms

NEGLECT

- Lack of adult supervision
- Malnourished-appearing child
- Unsafe living environment
- Untreated chronic illness

Child Abuse

Child abuse is not limited to any ethnic, social, or economic group or to families with any particular level of education. Suspect child abuse if the child's injuries do not match the story you are told about how the injuries occurred. Child abuse is often masked as an accident.

The abused or battered child may have many visible injuries—all at different stages of healing. The child may appear to be withdrawn, fearful, or even hostile. You should be concerned if the child refuses to discuss how an injury occurred. Occasionally the child's parents or caretaker will reveal a history of several "accidents" in the past. Treat the child's injuries and, if you think you are dealing with a case of child abuse, ensure the safety of the child.

Make sure that the child receives Ⓣ *transport* to an appropriate medical facility. If the parents object to having the child examined by a physician, summon law enforcement personnel and explain your concerns to them. The safety of the child is your foremost concern in these situations.

Neglect is also a form of child abuse. Children who are neglected are often dirty or too thin or appear developmentally delayed because of lack of stimulation. You may observe such children when you are making calls for unrelated problems.

The parents of an abused child need help, and the child may need protection from the parents' future actions. Handle each situation in a nonjudgmental manner. Know whom you need to contact (usually the emergency department staff or law enforcement personnel), and report any instances of suspected child abuse.

Sexual Assault of Children

Sexual abuse occurs in children as well as adults. It may occur in both male and female infants, young children, and adolescents. In addition to sexual assault, the child may have been beaten and may have other serious injuries.

If you suspect sexual assault has occurred, obtain as much information as possible from the child and any witnesses. Realize that the child may be hysterical or unwilling to talk, especially if the abuser is a brother or sister, parent, or family friend. A caring approach to these children is very important, and they should be shielded from onlookers.

All victims of sexual assault should receive Ⓣ *transport* to an appropriate medical facility. Sexual assault is a crime, and you should cooperate with law enforcement officials during their investigation.

First Responder Debriefing

As a first responder, you will respond to many calls that involve children. These calls tend to produce strong emotional reactions. At times you may experience a feeling of helplessness when an innocent child is seriously injured or gravely ill. You may be reminded of your own children when you see an ill or injured child. You may feel especially angry or helpless when you suspect neglect or abuse of a child.

After you have completed your treatment and transferred the responsibility for care to other EMS personnel, you may need to talk about your frustrations with a counselor or with another member of your department. After a major incident or an especially emotional incident involving children, it may be helpful to set up a critical incident stress debriefing (CISD) session. Although you cannot change the types of traumatic events you see, but you can use your department's resources to work through your feelings about these events. By debriefing you can maintain a healthy approach to future calls.

Signs & Symptoms

CHILD ABUSE

- Multiple fractures
- Bruises in various stages of healing (especially those clustered on the torso and buttocks) (**Figure 15.19A**)
- Human bites (**Figure 15.19B**)
- Burns (particularly cigarette burns and scalds from hot water) (**Figure 15.19C**)
- Reports of bizarre accidents that do not seem to have a logical explanation

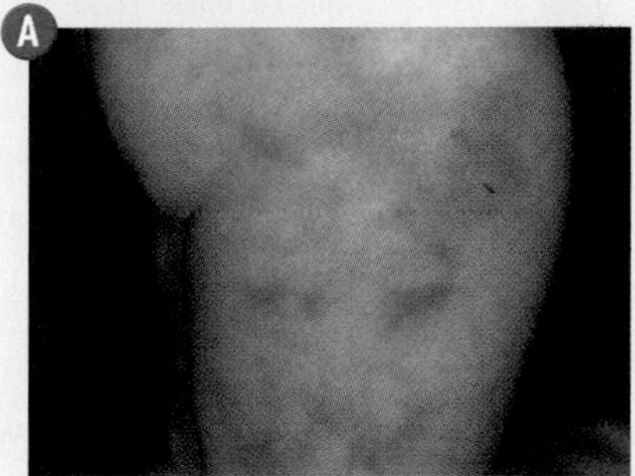

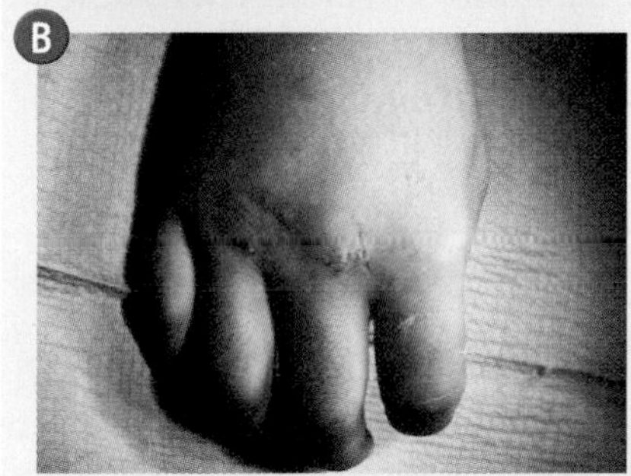

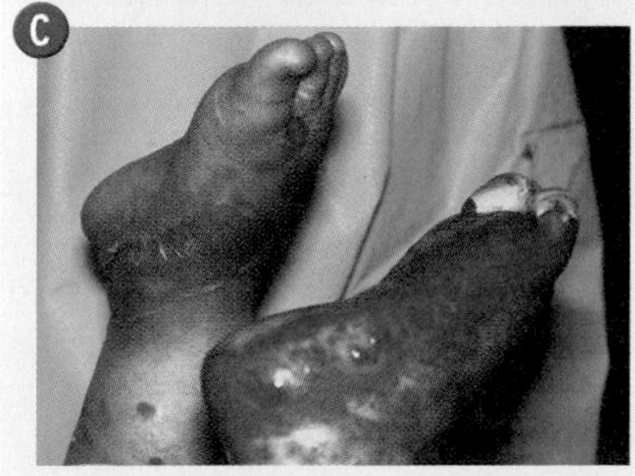

Figure 15.19 **A.** Bruises of different ages suggest physical maltreatment. New bruises are red or pink; over time, bruises turn blue, green, yellow-brown, and faded. **B.** A human bite wound has a characteristic appearance. **C.** Stocking/glove burns of the hands and feet in the infant or toddler are almost always inflicted injuries.

15 Prep Kit

Ready for Review

Ready for Review thoroughly summarizes the chapter.

This chapter describes the unique illnesses and considerations that you must know to treat children effectively. Children are young and helpless, and they have long lives ahead. You may find that you respond with your best efforts when you are called to treat illness or injury in a child.

First responders and other rescue personnel frequently underestimate the severity of a child's injuries and may not provide adequate treatment. The chapter covers the factors that make caring for a pediatric patient different from treating an adult patient, common child illnesses and injuries, and special assessment and treatment considerations. By learning some special approaches to caring for pediatric patients, you will be able to give more effective care to these patients and will not have to wonder how to treat them.

Treating and handling an ill or injured child can be extremely difficult, and it is almost always an emotional experience. The first responder must approach every child in a calm, professional manner, with personal feelings kept in check. Although helping ill or injured children may not be easy, it can have great rewards.

Vital Vocabulary

The Vital Vocabulary are the key terms for this chapter.

asthma—*page 362*
chest-thrust maneuver—*page 356*
croup—*page 362*
drowning—*page 363*
epiglottitis—*page 363*
epilepsy—*page 365*
near drowning—*page 363*

Practice Points

The Practice Points are the key skills you need to know.

1. Determining the respiratory rate, pulse rate, and body temperature in a child.
2. Performing the following respiratory skills
   A. Opening the airway
   B. Basic life support
   C. Suctioning
   D. Inserting an oral airway
3. Treating the following conditions
   A. Partial airway obstruction in children and infants
   B. Complete airway obstruction in children and infants
4. Cooling a child with a high fever.

Skill Drills

The Skill Drills provide a visual summary of some of the more complex skills from the skills objectives.

15.7 Performing Abdominal Thrusts on a Child —page 355

15.10 Administering Back Blows and Chest Thrusts on an Infant—page 358

Ready to Respond

Ready to Respond presents a fictitious scenario to help you review what you learned in this chapter.

You are called to a home where a 4-year-old girl is sitting in her mother's lap. The mother says that her daughter seemed hot and did not eat or drink much all day. She says that the child vomited once. You notice that the girl's forehead seems hot.

1. In what order should you examine this child?
   1. Level of consciousness
   2. Head to toe
   3. Airway, breathing and circulation
   4. Depends on the history of the illness

   A. 3, 4, 2, 1
   B. 3, 1, 4
   C. 1, 3, 2
   D. 4, 2, 3, 1
2. Based on the history and assessment of this child, which of the following conditions would be of concern to you?
   A. Possibility of seizures
   B. Possibility of gastrointestinal illness
   C. Dehydration
   D. All of the above
3. The best place to examine this child is
   A. Lying on a table
   B. Lying on the floor
   C. In the mother's lap
   D. With the child on her back
4. If this child started to seize, you should do all of the following except
   A. Place the child on a soft surface
   B. Monitor the airway after the seizure ends
   C. Cool the patient after the seizure is over
   D. Keep the child on her back
5. Your first responder treatment in this case is to
   A. Cancel any EMS units that have been dispatched to this address
   B. Help arrange for transportation to an appropriate medical facility
   C. Tell the mother to call her physician in the morning
   D. Advise the mother that her child needs to drink some fluids

MODULE 6 QuickQuiz

Childbirth and Children

1. Describe the function of each of the following structures of the female reproductive system
   A. uterus
   B. ovaries
   C. placenta
   D. umbilical cord

2. Crowning is determined by
   A. asking the mother how many children she has had before
   B. asking the mother if she feels like she has to move her bowels
   C. waiting until the contraction is over and then look at the vagina
   D. examining the vagina during a contraction

3. You should check which pulse in a newborn infant?
   A. femoral
   B. radial
   C. brachial
   D. carotid

4. A newborn infant should breathe at a rate of
   A. 10 to 20 breaths per minute
   B. 20 to 30 breaths per minute
   C. 30 to 40 breaths per minute
   D. over 40 breaths per minute

5. Immediately after the baby has been delivered you should
   A. try to get it to cry
   B. clear its nose, mouth, and throat of secretions
   C. begin rescue breathing
   D. lower its head

6. Which of the following complications requires immediate transportation to the hospital?
   A. prolapse of the umbilical cord
   B. stillborn delivery
   C. miscarriage
   D. unbroken bag of waters

7. Premature infants lose heat rapidly and must be keep warm.

   A. true

   B. false

8. When performing chest compressions on an infant you should

   1. avoid hyperextending the neck
   2. press on the lower half of the sternum
   3. use the heel of one hand
   4. use two fingers

   A. 1, 2, 3

   B. 1, 3

   C. 1, 2, 4

   D. 1, 2, 3, 4

9. To relieve a foreign body airway obstruction in an infant you should use

   1. abdominal thrusts
   2. back blows
   3. chest thrusts
   4. Heimlich maneuver

   A. 1 and 2

   B. 3 and 4

   C. 1 and 4

   D. 2 and 3

10. Which of the following are signs of respiratory distress?

    A. A respiratory rate of greater than 30 to 40 breaths per minute in children

    B. A high-pitched sound on inspiration

    C. A respiratory rate of less than 10 breaths per minute in infants

    D. A decreased heart rate

11. Which of the following is not a sign of croup

    A. noisy whooping inhalations

    B. child cannot swallow

    C. willingness to lie down

    D. barking seal-like cough

12. Seizures in children are most commonly caused by

    A. drug overdose

    B. epilepsy

    C. head injuries

    D. high fever

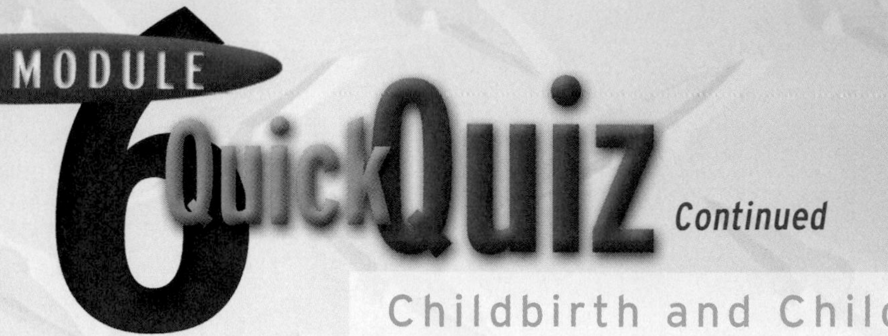

Continued

Childbirth and Children

13. A weak, rapid pulse and shallow breathing are signs of

A. a coma

B. a seizure

C. shock

D. asthma

14. If you need to remove a child from a car after a motor vehicle collision, you should

A. leave him in the car seat if possible

B. place him on a backboard

C. use a clothes drag

D. wait until other EMS personnel arrive

15. List five signs that could indicate child abuse

____

____

____

____

____

1. A. muscular organ that holds and nourishes the developing baby, B. organ that produces the eggs, C. life-support system of the baby during its time inside the mother, D. rope-like attachment between the baby and mother; nourishment and waste products pass to and from the baby and mother through this cord **2.** D **3.** C **4.** D **5.** B **6.** A **7.** A **8.** C **9.** D **10.** A & B **11.** B **12.** D **13.** C **14.** A **15.** bruises, human bites, cigarette burns, scalds from hot water, bizarre accidents without logical explanations

EMS Operations

MODULE

Module CONTENTS

Chapter 16

EMS Operations

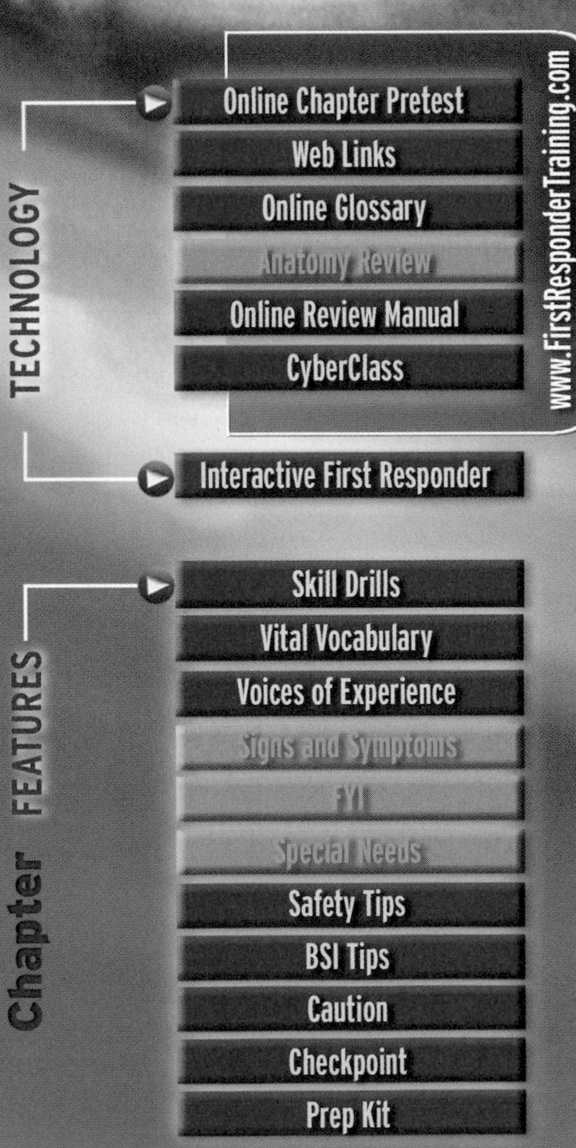

TECHNOLOGY
Online Chapter Pretest
Web Links
Online Glossary
Anatomy Review
Online Review Manual
CyberClass
www.FirstResponderTraining.com
Interactive First Responder
Chapter FEATURES
Skill Drills
Vital Vocabulary
Voices of Experience
Signs and Symptoms
FYI
Special Needs
Safety Tips
BSI Tips
Caution
Checkpoint
Prep Kit

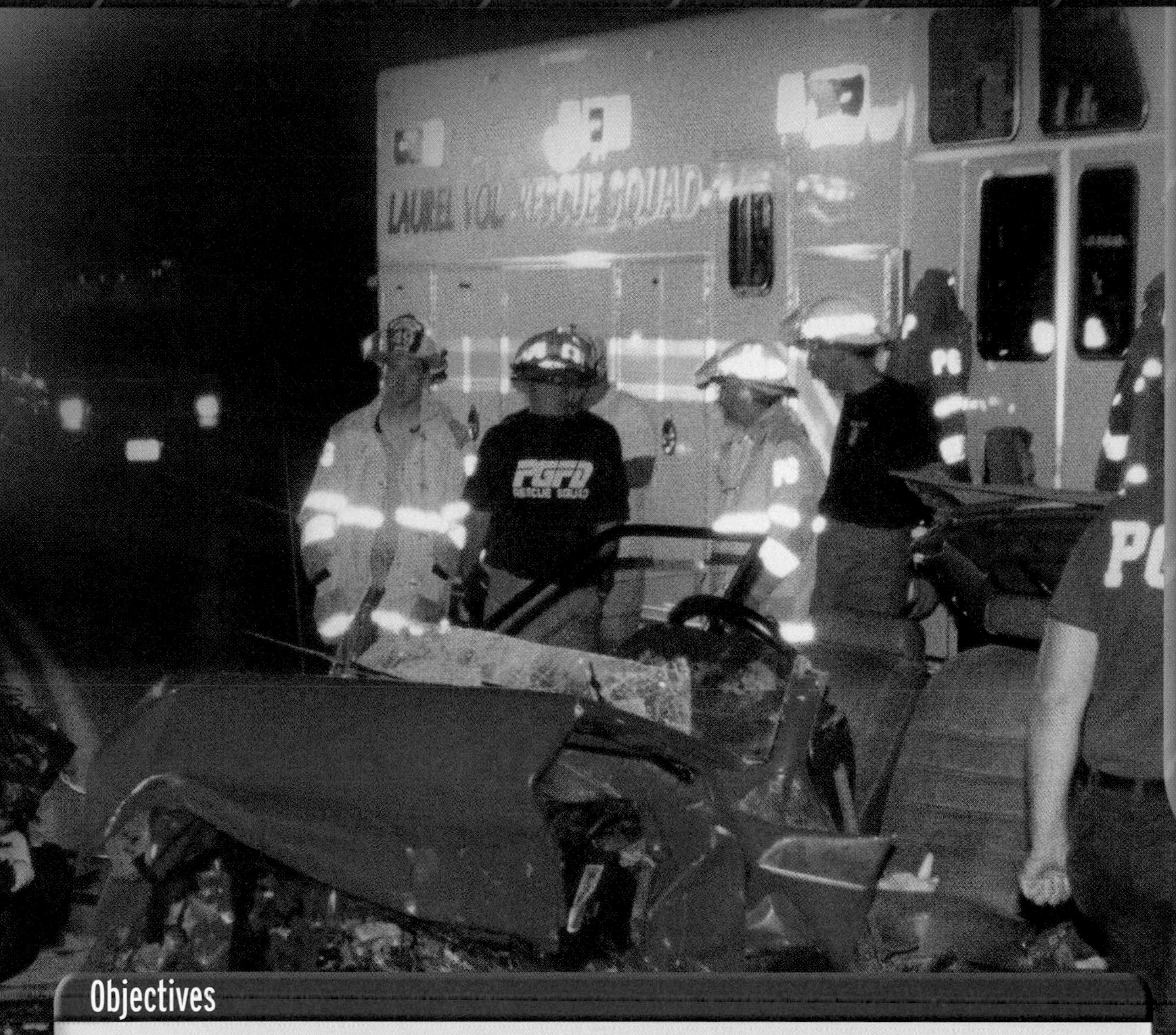

CHAPTER

16

Objectives

Knowledge and Attitude Objectives

After studying this chapter, you will be expected to:

1. Explain the medical and nonmedical equipment needed to respond to a call.
2. List the five phases of an emergency call for a first responder.
3. Discuss the role of a first responder in extrication.
4. List the seven steps in the extrication process.
5. List the various methods of gaining access to a patient.
6. Describe the simple extrication procedures that a first responder can perform.
7. List the complex extrication procedures that require specially trained personnel.
8. State the responsibilities of the first responder in incidents where hazardous materials are present.
9. Describe the actions that a first responder should take in hazardous materials incidents before the arrival of specially trained personnel.
10. Define a multiple-casualty incident.
11. Describe the role of a first responder in a multiple-casualty incident.
12. Describe the steps in the START triage system.

Skill Objectives

As a first responder, you should be able to:

1. Perform simple procedures for gaining access to a wrecked vehicle.
2. Triage a simulated multiple-casualty incident using the START triage system.

As a first responder in an EMS operation, you must take several steps to render care to an ill or injured patient. You must be prepared to respond when the call comes in. You must respond in a safe and timely manner and must have the proper equipment to render care. In addition, you must be able to perform simple extrication procedures and assist other responders with patient extrication. Because many first responders work with air medical EMS providers, this chapter covers basic information on that aspect of EMS operations as well. First responders should also be able to identify the signs of a hazardous materials incident and to prevent injury to themselves and to others in the first minutes of a hazardous materials incident. Because you may be dispatched to a multiple-casualty incident, you must understand the purpose of basic triage and be able to perform the steps involved in the START triage system.

Preparing for a Call

In your primary role as a law enforcement officer, a firefighter, or other worker, you are also on call as a medical first responder. In preparing yourself for a call, you must understand your role as a member of the emergency medical system. You may respond using a fire department vehicle, a law enforcement vehicle, your private vehicle, or on foot. You must be prepared to respond promptly, using the most direct route available. You must have the proper equipment to perform your job, including the medical equipment in your first responder life support kit, your personal safety equipment, and equipment to safeguard the accident scene. A recommended equipment list is shown in **Figure 16.1** and **Table 16.1**. This equipment must be stocked and maintained on a regular basis according to the schedule specified by your agency.

Response

Response to an emergency call involves five different phases.

The sequence of actions in an emergency call was covered in Chapter 1, and you may find it helpful to review this material.

> **THE FIVE PHASES OF RESPONSE**
>
> - *Dispatch*
> - *Response to the scene*
> - *Arrival at the scene*
> - *Transferring the care of the patient to other EMS personnel*
> - *Post-run activities*

Dispatch

The dispatch facility is a center citizens can call to request emergency medical care. Most centers are part of a 9-1-1 system that is responsible for dispatching fire, police, and EMS. You should understand how the

Table 16.1

Suggested Contents of a First Responder Life Support Kit

Patient Examination Equipment	1 flashlight
Personal Safety Equipment	5 sets gloves 5 face masks
Resuscitation Equipment	1 mouth-to-mask resuscitation device 1 portable hand-powered suction device 1 set oral airways 1 set nasal airways
Bandaging and Dressing Equipment	10 gauze-adhesive strips 1" 10 gauze pads 4" x 4" 5 gauze pads 5" x 9" 2 universal trauma dressings 10" x 30" 1 occlusive dressing for sealing chest wounds 4 conforming gauze rolls 3" x 5 yd 4 conforming gauze rolls 4½" x 5 yd 6 triangular bandages 1 adhesive tape 2" 1 burn sheet
Patient Immobilization Equipment	2 (each) cervical collars: small, medium, large or 2 adjustable cervical collars 3 rigid conforming splints (SAM™ splints) OR 1 set air splints for arm and leg OR 2 (each) cardboard splints 18" and 24"
Extrication Equipment	1 spring-loaded center punch 1 pair heavy leather gloves
Miscellaneous Equipment	2 blankets (disposable) 2 cold packs 1 bandage 1 pair of scissors 1 obstetrical kit

Other Equipment:

1 set personal protective clothing (helmet, eye protection, EMS jacket)
1 reflective vest
1 fire extinguisher (5 lb ABC dry chemical)
1 *Emergency Response Guidebook*
6 fusees
1 pair of binoculars

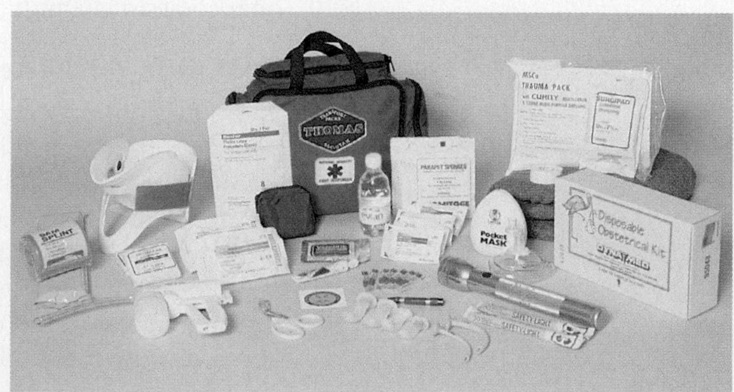

Figure 16.1 Suggested contents of a first responder life support kit.

dispatch facility used by your department operates. Your job will be easier if the dispatcher obtains the proper information from the caller. Dispatchers should also be able to instruct callers on how to perform lifesaving techniques such as CPR until you arrive.

You may receive your dispatch information by telephone, radio, pager, computer terminal, or written printout. Regardless of the transmission method, the information should include: the nature of the call, the name and location of the patient, the number of patients, and any special problems. The dispatcher should also obtain a call-back number in case you need more information from the caller. Without good dispatch information, you will not be able to respond properly.

Response to the Scene

Your first priority in responding to the scene is to get there quickly and safely. Consider traffic patterns and the time of day before you select the best route to the scene. Follow the safety procedures outlined by your department, including the use of safety belts and the proper use of vehicle warning devices. Above all else, drive so you are not involved in an accident.

Arrival at the Scene

When you arrive at the scene, remember to place your vehicle in a safe location to minimize the chance of injury. Consider how best to use your vehicle warning lights. Remember to overview the scene as outlined in the patient assessment sequence (Chapter 7), and to consider scene safety.

Take into account the number of patients and determine if you need additional help. Follow the patient assessment sequence you learned in Chapter 7. Practice being as efficient and as organized as you can.

BSI Tip

Always follow BSI procedures. Do not forget to take appropriate precautions to prevent contamination by the patient's body fluids.

Transferring the Care of the Patient to Other EMS Personnel

As more highly trained EMS personnel arrive on the scene, you will have to transfer care of the patient to them. Give them a brief report of the situation as you initially observed it and tell them what care you have provided. Ask them if they have any questions for you. Finally, offer to assist them in caring for the patient.

Post-Run Activities

You may think you are done with a call after you have cared for the patient and provided assistance to other EMS personnel. But your job is not done until you have completed the paperwork. Documentation is important, as emphasized in Chapter 1. In addition to completing paperwork, you must also clean your equipment and replace needed supplies. Only after you have completed these activities, should you resume regular duties or notify your dispatcher or supervisor that you are ready for another call.

Checkpoint

- ○ Describe the five phases of response to an EMS incident.

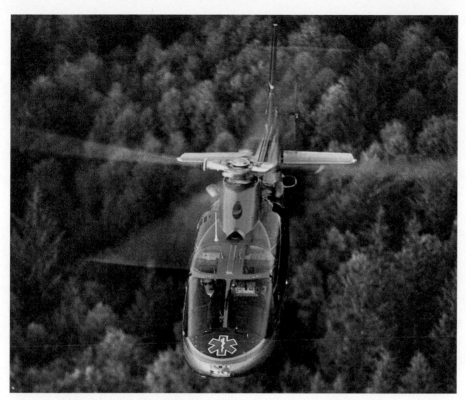

Figure 16.2 An EMS helicopter.

Helicopter Operations

Helicopters are used by EMS systems to reach patients, transport patients to medical facilities, or remove patients from inaccessible areas (**Figure 16.2**). If your EMS system uses a helicopter, obtain a copy of the ground operations procedures, or schedule an orientation session with helicopter personnel. As a first responder, you may be responsible for making the initial call for helicopter assistance or for setting up and preparing a landing site in the field.

Helicopter Safety Guidelines

Helicopters can provide life-saving transport for patients with serious injuries to an appropriate medical facility. But helicopters are also dangerous to untrained personnel. The main rotor of the helicopter spins at more than 300 revolutions per minute (rpm), and may be just 4 feet above the ground. The tail rotor spins at more than 3,000 rpm, and may be invisible to an unwary person. Additionally, the rotors can generate a "wash" equivalent to winds of 60 to 80 miles per hour (mph). Because a rescuer who approaches without caution may be severely injured by walking upright or by raising an arm above the head, it is important to understand safe helicopter operations.

Setting Up Landing Zones

When choosing a landing site, remember that pilots usually land and take off into the wind. The size of a landing zone will vary and depends on the size of the helicopter. Most civilian helicopters need a landing zone of at least 100 feet x 100 feet (10,000 square feet). Military aircraft may need a larger area. The landing zone should be as flat as possible and free of debris that could become airborne in the 60 mph winds generated by the helicopter. Check carefully for any nearby wires.

Safety Tips

1. Be alert for electrical wires when identifying a landing zone for a helicopter.
2. Always approach helicopters from the front so the pilot can see you. Approaching a helicopter from the rear is dangerous because the tail rotor is nearly invisible when spinning.
3. Do not approach the helicopter until the pilot signals that it is safe to do so.
4. Keep low when you approach the helicopter to avoid the spinning main rotor blades. Helicopters are very noisy, and you may not be able to hear a shouted warning. Maintain eye contact with the pilot.
5. Follow the directions of the helicopter crew.

Wires that you can see may be invisible to the pilot. If the site slopes or has any obstacles, notify the pilot.

Check with your helicopter service to see how you should secure and mark the perimeter of the site. Avoid using traffic cones, flags, or other objects that can be blown away by the force of the helicopter rotor wash. Fusees (red signal flares) create a fire hazard and should not be used. Turn off unnecessary white lights and avoid flashing emergency lights because they interfere with the pilot's vision during landing and take-off. Keep vehicles clear of the landing zone. Close the windows and doors of any nearby vehicles, and remove any loose objects on the vehicles that could become airborne. Some helicopter services request that a charged hose line be available for fire emergencies.

Loading Patients into Helicopters

Certain safety precautions must be followed during the loading of a helicopter patient. Secure all loose clothing, sheets, and instruments such as stethoscopes. Use eye protection to prevent debris from getting into your eyes. Approach a helicopter from the front, and only after the pilot or a crew member signals that it is safe (**Figure 16.3**).

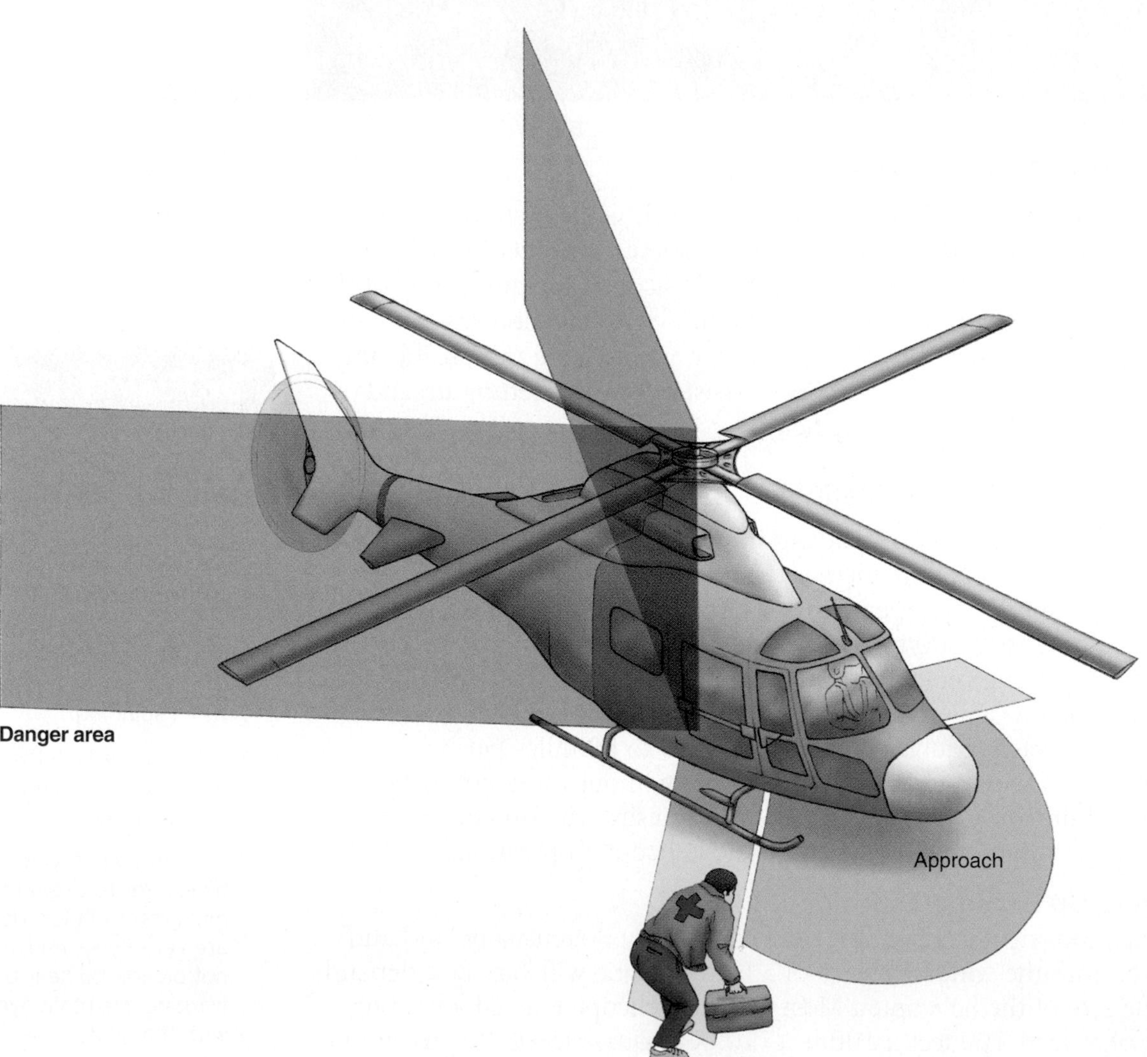

Figure 16.3 Approach helicopters from the front so the pilot can see you.

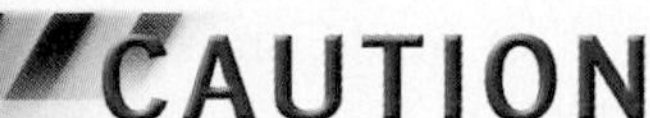

Several "DO NOTs" are important. DO NOT approach the helicopter landing zone unless necessary. DO NOT approach a helicopter from the up side if it is on a slope. DO NOT run near a helicopter. DO NOT raise your hand when approaching a helicopter.

The helicopter crew may need help carrying equipment to the patient. Follow their instructions. Give your patient report to the crew, away from the helicopter's noise, and offer your assistance. It is harder to load a helicopter stretcher than an ambulance stretcher. Because loose sheets or blankets can blow off the stretcher, patients need to be packaged properly and securely.

As a first responder, you can provide ground support and assistance during helicopter ambulance operations, provided that you take proper safety precautions. If you will be working with a helicopter ambulance, arrange an orientation with helicopter personnel so you will be prepared in an emergency.

Extrication

This section describes simple techniques you can use to access, treat, and extricate patients who are trapped inside wrecked vehicles. The ability to think quickly and use the principles and guidelines that are presented here are essential for the first responder. You will also need several hours of practical exercises to become skilled in the process of **extrication**.

extrication Removal from a difficult situation or position; removal of a patient from a wrecked car or other place of entrapment.

Your first responder course should include a demonstration of the entire extrication operation. You should be familiar with extrication equipment, its use, and the hazards involved in the extrication operation. You should know what equipment is available in your community and what to do to summon this equipment.

First responders usually use extrication techniques for automobile accidents, but many of the same principles apply to other situations. Resourcefulness, common sense, and knowledge gained through training are key attributes of the first responder, which underlie every act of patient care.

The safety of both rescuers and patients is an important consideration during the extrication process. Ideally, rescuers would wear protective equipment similar to a fire fighter's outfit: full bunker gear consisting of coat, pants, boots, helmet with face shield, and gloves. Minimally, a helmet with face shield or goggles and gloves should be worn.

A situation in which patients are trapped in an automobile can be complex enough to tax the skills and resources of even the most highly trained and well-equipped EMS system. To ensure the best care, many different agencies may need to cooperate: law enforcement personnel, the fire department, EMS personnel, and sometimes the utility company, the gas company, and a wrecker operator. Achieving the cooperation and mutual understanding that is needed for a safe, smooth extrication effort requires prior coordination and practice.

As you read this section, keep in mind these basic guidelines:

- Know the limitations of your training, equipment, and skill.
- Identify any hazards (gasoline, power lines or wires, or hazardous materials).
- Control those hazards for which you are trained and equipped.
- Gain access to the patients.
- Provide patient care and stabilization.
- Move the patients only if absolutely necessary.

STEPS IN THE EXTRICATION PROCESS

1. *Conduct an overview of the scene.*
2. *Stabilize the scene, control any hazards, and stabilize the vehicle.*
3. *Gain access to patients.*
4. *Provide initial emergency care.*
5. *Help disentangle patients.*
6. *Help prepare patients for removal.*
7. *Help remove patients.*

As a first responder, you have two primary extrication goals: to obtain safe access to the patients and to ensure patient stabilization. To achieve these goals, your role in the extrication process can be divided into the seven steps listed in the box at left.

As a first responder, you will usually be responsible only for the first four steps of the extrication process. However, you will often have to assist other EMS personnel in completing the remaining steps. You cannot give this assistance unless you fully understand what must be done and how it is accomplished. Think safety so that you do not become injured. An injured rescuer becomes a second patient.

The actions you take as the first trained person on the scene can make the difference between an organized and a disorganized rescue effort, perhaps even the difference between life and death! You set the stage, and you have an essential role in the extrication process. Remember this as you review the example of an automobile crash described in this section.

Step One: Overview of the Scene

As soon as the dispatcher tells you of the incident, begin to anticipate and plan for what you are likely to find upon arrival. You may, for instance, know that a certain type of accident frequently occurs at a particular intersection or along a specific stretch of highway. Do not, however, become complacent about responding to the "same old thing." Use your knowledge, but be flexible in planning.

If the dispatch information is complete, you will know the types of vehicles involved (for example, two cars, a car and motorcycle, a truck and car, or a train and truck) and whether there are injured or trapped people, burning vehicles, or hazardous materials present.

As you approach the accident scene and before you exit your vehicle, get an overview of the entire incident (**Figure 16.4**). Remember that you must locate the patients before you can treat them! Rapidly determine the extent of the accident or incident, try to estimate the number of patients, and try to locate any hazards that may be present. Then call for whatever assistance you may need to manage the accident.

Step Two: Stabilization of the Scene and Any Hazards

It is especially important to keep a sharp lookout for hazards that can result in injury, disability, or death to a patient, yourself, other

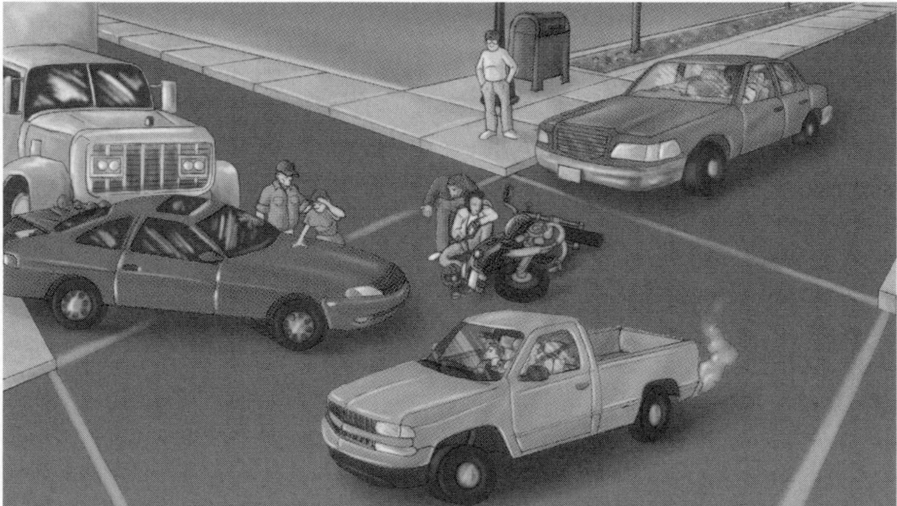

Figure 16.4 As you approach an accident, look over the entire scene.

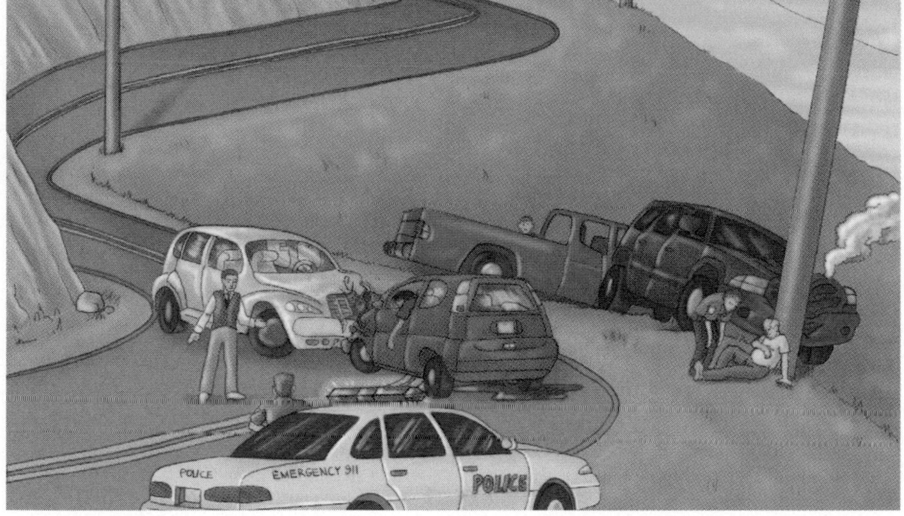

Figure 16.5 A single accident scene may contain many hazards.

emergency personnel, or bystanders. Some of the most common hazards found at automobile crash scenes include infectious diseases, traffic, bystanders, spilled gasoline or other hazardous materials, automobile batteries, downed electrical wires, unstable vehicles, and vehicle fires (**Figure 16.5**).

Infectious Diseases

Many patients involved in motor vehicle crashes will have soft-tissue injuries and active bleeding from open wounds or from their mouth or nose. Follow standard body substance isolation (BSI) precautions at all motor vehicle crash scenes. If sharp glass or metal is present, you should wear heavy-duty rescue type gloves; otherwise, vinyl or latex gloves should be sufficient. If there is the danger of splattering blood, you should consider using face protection.

Traffic Hazards

First, park your vehicle and other emergency vehicles so that they protect the scene and warn oncoming traffic to avoid the crash site. In most situations, park in a location that does not obstruct open traffic lanes, but do not hesitate to use your vehicle to block traffic to protect you, your patients, and other rescuers.

If other emergency personnel are already on the scene, ask them where you should park your vehicle. Consider the design of your vehicle's warning lights and park so you can use them to their best advantage. Do not leave your trunk lid open after removing your emergency equipment; the lid may block your warning lights!

fusee A warning device or flare that burns with a red color; usually used in scene protection at motor vehicle crash sites.

Another way to protect the scene is to ignite **fusees** (red signal flares) or warning flares as soon as possible. Place the flares or fusees up and down the road to warn oncoming traffic and give other drivers time to slow down safely. After you've taken these traffic-protective measures, survey the scene for other hazards.

CAUTION

Always keep fusees and flares away from flammable liquids.

Bystanders

Keep bystanders away from the crash scene to minimize the danger to themselves and patients. It is not usually enough to ask everyone to move back. You should give specific directions such as, "Move back to the other side of the road" or "Move back onto the sidewalk." You can also pick out one or two bystanders and ask them to assist you in keeping others away from the scene.

A rope or police/fire barrier tape is very effective if it is available. People respond appropriately to such "barriers" and usually will not cross them once they are set up.

Spilled Gasoline

Gasoline spills are common during automobile crashes. Expect to find a fuel spill if an automobile has been hit near the rear, is on its side, or is upside down. If there are fuel spills (or if the car is in a position that suggests there will be), call the fire department to minimize the fire hazard and to clean up any spilled fuel.

If patients are in a car with a fuel spill and the fire department has not arrived, consider covering the fuel with dirt. This reduces the amount of vapor coming from the spill, which, in turn, reduces the danger of fire. Fuel vapors tend to stay close to the ground and will travel with the wind. In any event, be sure to call the fire department whenever you suspect a fuel spill.

CAUTION

Keep all sources of ignition such as cigarettes and flares well away from a fuel spill.

Automobile Batteries

Automobile batteries are hazardous, and you must avoid contact with them. In a front-end collision, the battery may already be broken open and acid will be leaking. Reduce the possibility of an electrical short circuit by turning off the automobile's ignition. Do not attempt to

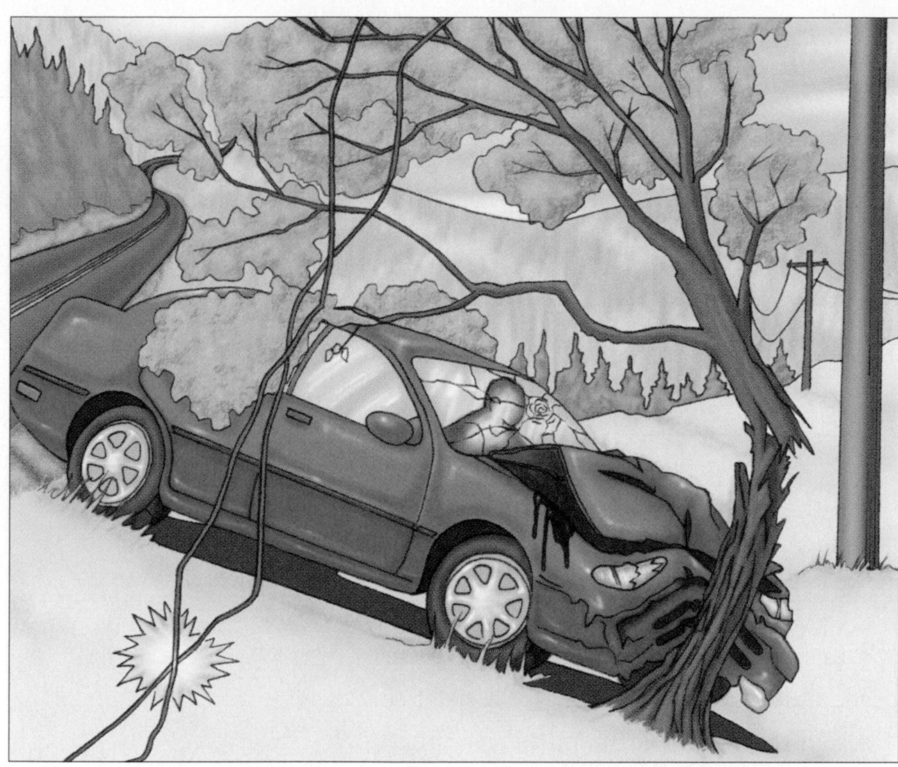

Figure 16.6 Be alert for downed electrical wires.

disconnect the battery because you could be injured by a short circuit, explosion, or contact with battery acid.

Downed Electrical Wires

Downed electrical wires may be caused by weather problems or by a vehicle hitting a utility pole. Sometimes, downed electrical wires explode in arcs of spectacular flashes and sparks; other times, they simply lay across the vehicle, fully charged with electricity and capable of causing injury or death to the unwary (**Figure 16.6**).

Locate the wires but avoid contact! If a vehicle has a downed wire across it and passengers are trapped inside, immediately instruct them to stay inside the car. Then summon the utility company and fire department. Move bystanders back in all directions, to at least the distance between two power poles.

Do not forget that electrical hazards can come from other sources as well, including traffic light control boxes and underground power feeds. Be sure to check everywhere, including under the vehicles, for electrical hazards. However, you should not attempt to deal with electrical hazards at accident scenes.

CAUTION

Treat all downed wires as if they are charged (live) until you receive specific clearance from the electric company. Even if the lights are out along the street where the wires are down, never assume that the wires are dead. Be especially alert for downed wires after a storm that has blown down trees and tree limbs.

chocking A piece of wood or metal placed in front of or behind a wheel to prevent vehicle movement.

wooden cribbing Wooden 2- x 4-inch or 4- x 4-inch boards used for stabilization or bracing.

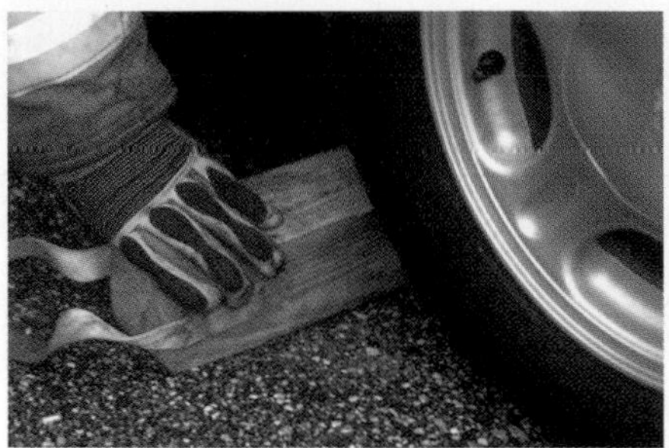

Figure 16.7 Chock the wheels.

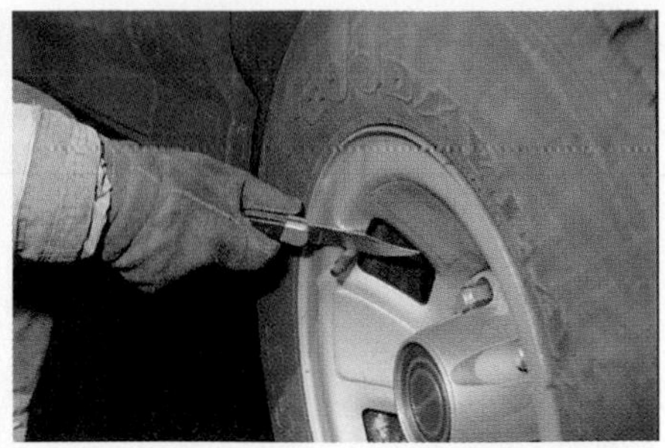

Figure 16.8 Deflating the tires will help to stabilize the vehicle.

Safety Tips

Even vehicles that are positioned upright on all four wheels should be stabilized.

Response Guidelines: Automobile in Contact with Electric Wire

- If the wire is draped over the car, instruct trapped persons to remain inside the car. Any attempt to remove either the wire or the passengers may result in serious injury or death to yourself as well as the passengers.
- Keep all bystanders away from the car.
- Call the utility company for assistance.
- Call the fire department for assistance.

Unstable Vehicles

Assume that every vehicle involved in a crash is unstable, unless you have manually stabilized it. Vehicles on a hill, on their sides, upside down, or teetering over the edge of an embankment or bridge are obviously unstable. But no matter how stable the vehicle appears to be, it may suddenly roll away or topple over. Be sure to check and ensure the stability of every vehicle before you attempt to enter it or treat the passengers inside.

Vehicles on Their Wheels If the car is upright and on its wheels, you can ensure stability by **chocking** the front or back of each wheel with hubcaps or pieces of wood (**Figure 16.7**). You can also deflate the tires by safely cutting or pulling the valve stems (**Figure 16.8**).

Vehicles on Their Sides or Upside Down A vehicle on its side is extremely unstable. Fortunately, this position is fairly unusual. Stabilizing these vehicles is beyond the range of skills and equipment for many first responders and should be handled by rescue squads or fire departments. Many fire departments and rescue squads carry **wooden cribbing** and "step-chocks" to deal with this problem.

If you must enter a vehicle on its side to respond to a life-threatening situation, do not climb up on the vehicle. Carefully break the rear window glass and enter through the back of the vehicle. Bend over or crouch down to stay close to the ground. This will help prevent upsetting the car's center of gravity.

An upside-down vehicle is relatively stable. The primary hazard in this situation is spilled gasoline, which must be handled by the fire department.

Improvise

If wooden blocks or hubcaps are not available, improvise by using materials found at the scene.

Safety Tips

Your purpose is to keep the vehicle in the position found. Do not move it. Any movement could cause the vehicle to tip over.

Vehicle Fires

Even though fires happen infrequently at automobile crash sites, they are a cause of great concern among EMS personnel. There are two types of fires related to automobile crashes: impact fires and postimpact fires.

Impact fires occur when the gas tank ruptures during the collision. The vehicle is usually rapidly engulfed in flames, and it soon becomes impossible to approach it for a rescue attempt. Passengers rescued from this type of fire are usually saved by bystanders and witnesses to the accident who act immediately to remove them.

Postimpact fires are often caused by electrical short circuits, and can be prevented by turning off the ignition. These fires usually do not develop into major fires if prompt action is taken. Should one occur, first turn off the ignition. Then extinguish the fire with a portable fire extinguisher. Remove the passengers from the vehicle as soon as possible.

Emergency Actions for Automobile Fires If you arrive at a crash scene and find a car on fire with people trapped inside, remember the following procedures:

- Use your dry chemical fire extinguisher (**Figure 16.9**). Most dry chemical fire extinguishers can be used on ordinary combustibles, flammable liquids, or electrical fires. Be sure you know how to use the extinguisher in your vehicle.

Did You Know?

According to Insurance Institute for Highway Safety statistics, only one of every 1,100 automobile accidents results in an automobile fire

A

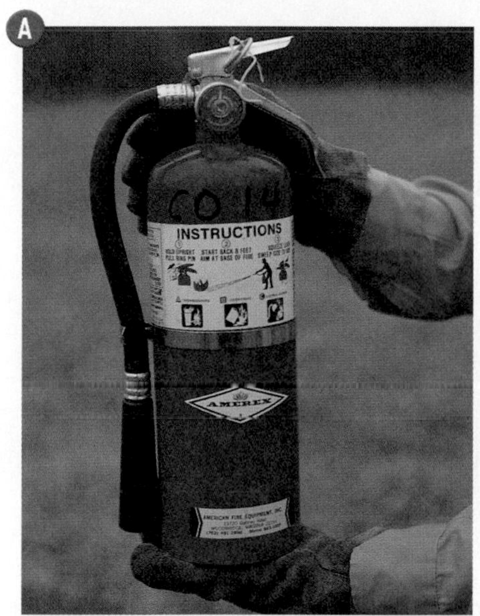

B

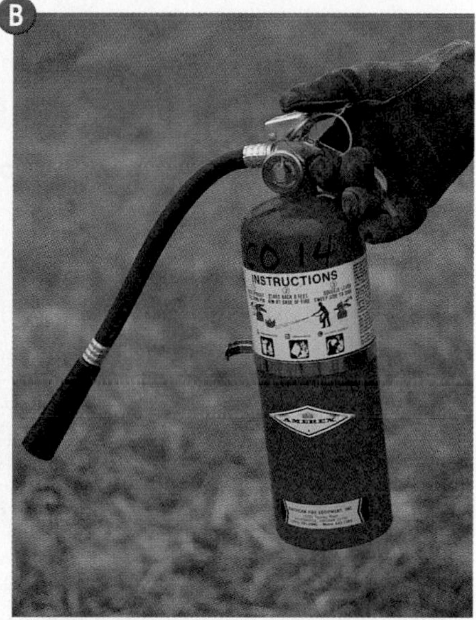

C

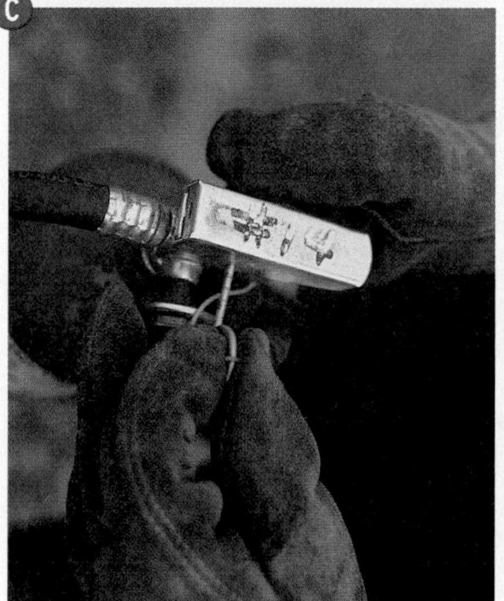

D

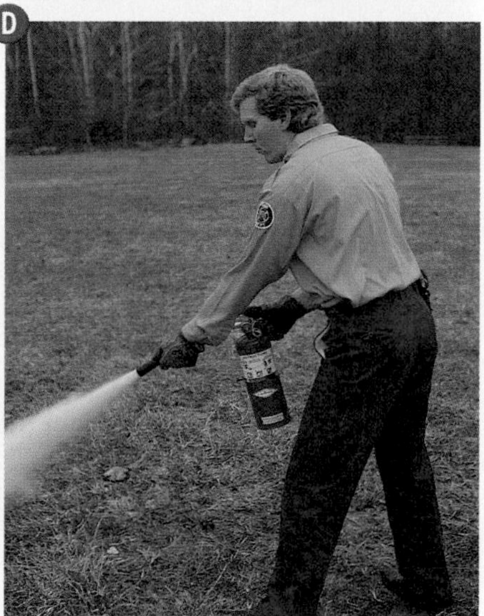

Figure 16.9 Use of a dry chemical fire extinguisher. **A.** Check pressure gauge. **B.** Release hose. **C.** Pull locking pin. **D.** Discharge at base of fire.

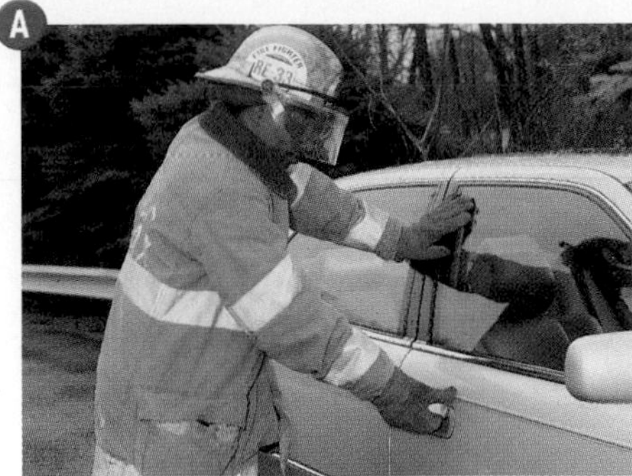
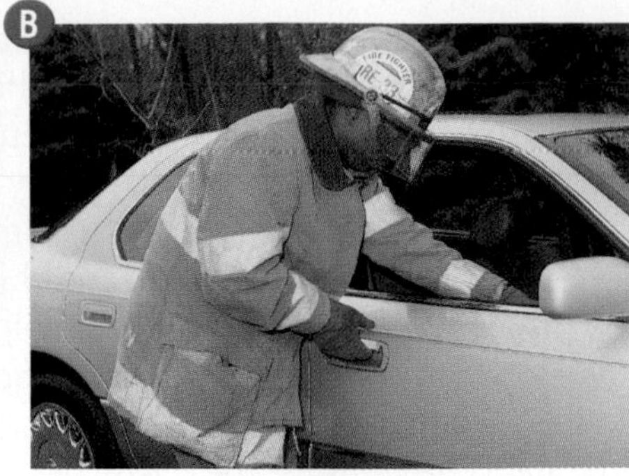

Figure 16.10 Access the vehicle through the doors, if possible. **A.** Try all doors first. **B.** Try inside and outside handles at the same time.

Note: Do not mistake hot water vapor from a damaged radiator for smoke from an engine compartment fire. If the smoke disappears rapidly (10 feet to 15 feet away from the car), it is probably steam and not smoke.

- Use your extinguisher to keep flames out of the passenger compartment. Direct the extinguisher to the base of the fire—not at the passenger compartment.
- Do not worry about discharging the extinguisher onto the passengers. The dry chemical powder is nontoxic.
- Immediately have someone else gather fire extinguishers from other vehicles on the scene. Do not wait until your extinguisher runs out!
- Remove patients as quickly as possible. Be careful because they may be injured.
- Move everyone at least 50 feet away from any vehicle that is on fire.

Step Three: Gain Access to Patients

Access through Doors

Before you can provide patient care, you must gain access to the patient. Between 85 percent and 90 percent of all motor vehicle patients can be reached simply by stabilizing the vehicle and then opening a door or rolling down a window. Try all the doors first—even if they appear to be badly damaged. It is an embarrassing waste of time and energy to open a jammed door with heavy rescue equipment when another door can be opened easily and without any equipment.

Attempt to unlock and open the least damaged door first. Make sure that the locking mechanism is released. Then try the outside and inside handles at the same time (**Figure 16.10**).

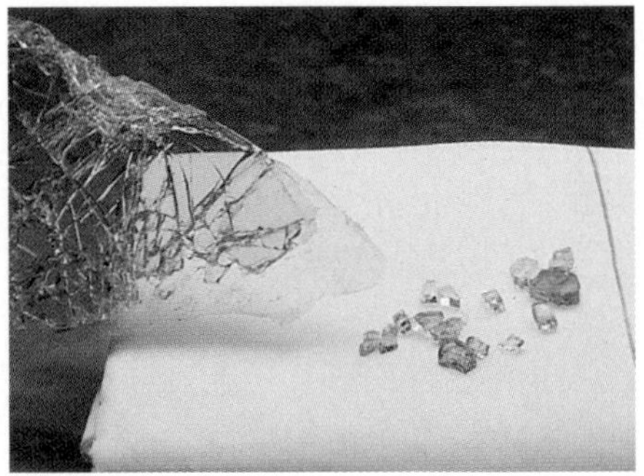

Figure 16.11 The two types of glass in vehicles: laminated glass (left) and tempered glass (right).

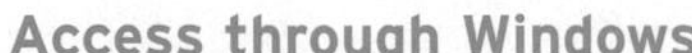

Access through Windows

If you believe that any passenger's condition is serious enough to require immediate care (for example, if the passengers are not sitting up and talking) and you cannot enter through a door, you should break a window.

Do not try to break and enter through the windshield because it is made of plastic-laminated glass (**Figure 16.11**). The side and rear windows are made of **tempered glass**, and will break easily into small pieces when hit with a sharp, pointed object such as a tire iron, spring-loaded center punch, or fire ax. Because these windows do not pose a safety threat, they should be your primary access route.

tempered glass Safety glass that breaks into small pieces when hit with a sharp, pointed object.

A spring-loaded center punch (available from many hardware stores) should be carried in your first responder's life support kit (**Figure 16.12**). It can be used rapidly, takes up little room in the kit, and is nearly always successful in breaking the side and rear windows on the first try (**Figure 16.13, steps 1 and 2**).

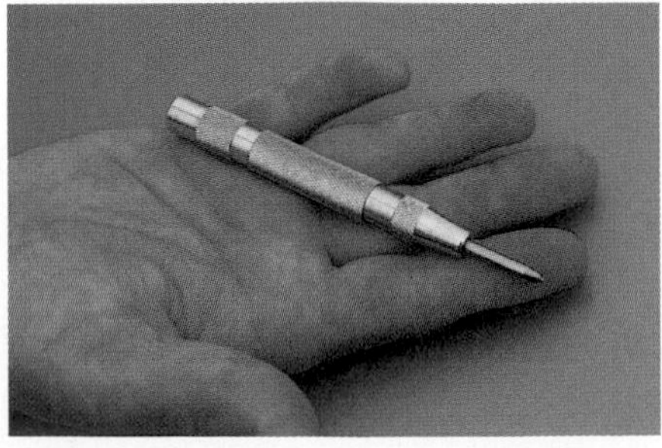

Figure 16.12 Spring-loaded center punch for breaking tempered glass.

Skill Drill

Figure 16.13 Accessing the Vehicle Through the Window

1

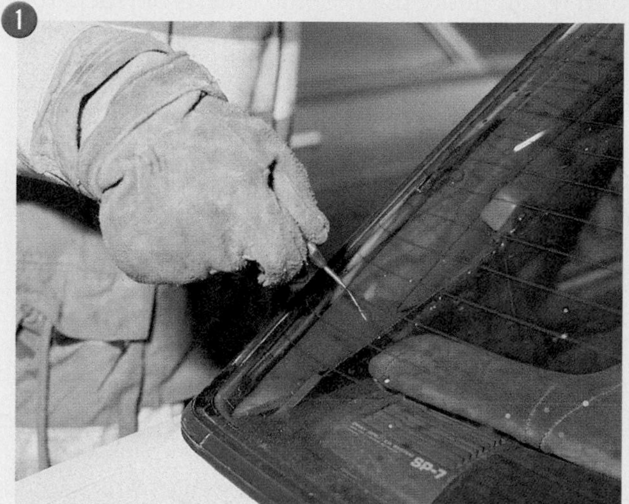

Place spring-loaded center punch at the lower corner of the window.

2

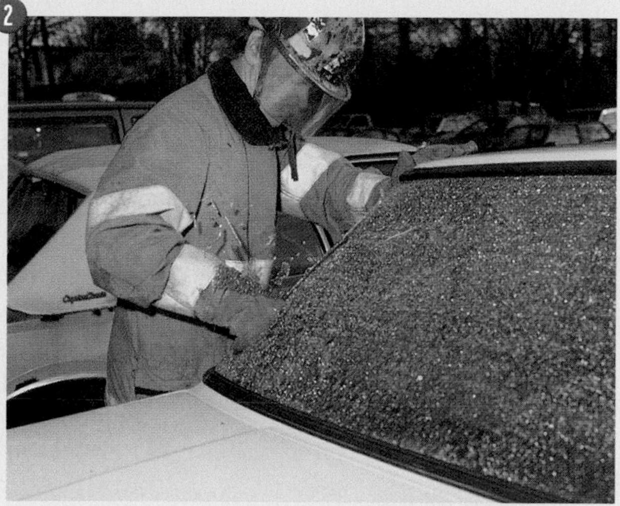

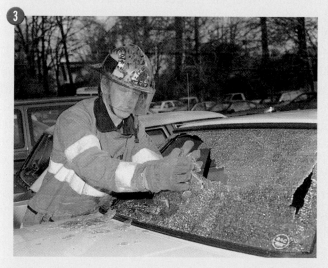

Press on center punch to break window.

3

Remove the glass to the outside.

4

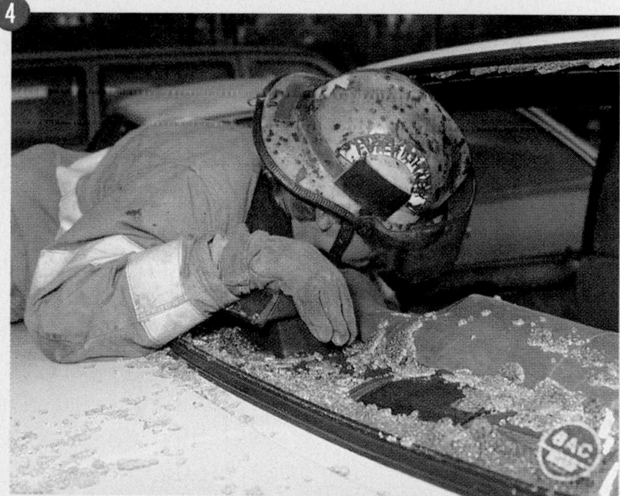

Enter the vehicle through the rear window.

Note: Always warn trapped car passengers that you are going to break the glass.

Safety Tips

Most cars and pickup trucks have driver side and passenger side airbags. Some newer vehicles have supplemental side-mounted airbags. Airbags that do not activate during a collision present a danger to rescuers until they are deactivated.

Note: Check the trunk. This is especially important in border areas where significant numbers of illegal aliens are transported in automobile trunks to avoid detection (**Figure 16.14**).

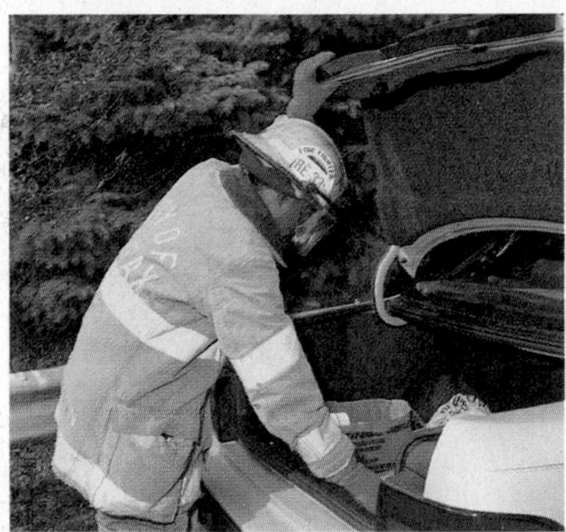

Figure 16.14 Check the trunk for "hidden" patients.

Golden Hour A concept of emergency patient care that attempts to place a trauma patient into definitive medical care within one hour of injury.

If you must break a window to open a door or gain access, try to break one that is far from the patient. But if the patient's condition warrants your immediate entry, do not hesitate to break the closest side or rear window, even if the glass will fall onto a patient.

Tempered pieces of glass do not usually pose a danger to people trapped in cars. Advise ambulance personnel if a passenger is covered with broken glass so they can notify the hospital emergency department. If there is glass on a passenger, pick it off—don't brush it off.

After breaking the window, use your gloved hands to pull the remaining glass out of the window frame so it does not fall onto any passengers or injure any rescuers (**Figure 16.13, steps 3 and 4**).

If you are using something other than a spring-loaded center punch to break the window, always aim for a lower corner. That way, the window frame will help prevent the tool (such as a tire iron, fire ax, or large screwdriver) from sailing into the car and hitting the person inside.

Once you have broken the glass and removed the pieces from the frame, try to unlock the door again. Release the locking mechanism, and then use both inside and outside door handles at the same time. This will often enable you to force a jammed locking mechanism, even in a door that appears to be badly damaged.

Using the simple techniques described and illustrated in this section, you should be able to gain access to nearly all automobile crash victims, even those in an upside-down car. If you cannot gain access, you must do what you can to assist the patients. This means stabilizing the vehicle and protecting the scene until the proper equipment arrives.

Step Four: Provide Initial Emergency Care

After you gain access to passengers, immediately begin initial emergency medical care. Conduct a patient assessment on every patient. After you determine the status of each patient, you should monitor ABCs, control bleeding, treat for shock, stabilize the cervical spine, and provide psychological reassurance. Don't forget to maintain the patient's body temperature. If you have time, you can now perform a patient examination. **Figure 16.15** shows you how to perform initial airway management when the patient is in a vehicle.

Leave patients in the vehicle unless it is on fire or they are otherwise in immediate danger. Keep the patients stabilized and immobilized until they are properly packaged and can be removed from the vehicle by other rescuers.

Step Five: Help Disentangle Patients

Extrication operates on the principle of "removing the vehicle from around the patient." This process usually requires tools and specialized equipment, such as air chisels, manual or powered hydraulic rescue equipment, and air bags. In some serious extrication situations, disentanglement can take up to 30 minutes and requires advanced training (**Figure 16.16**).

Modern rescue crews use the concept of the **Golden Hour** when dealing with serious trauma situations. The Golden Hour concept

Skill Drill

Figure 16.15 Airway Management in a Vehicle

1

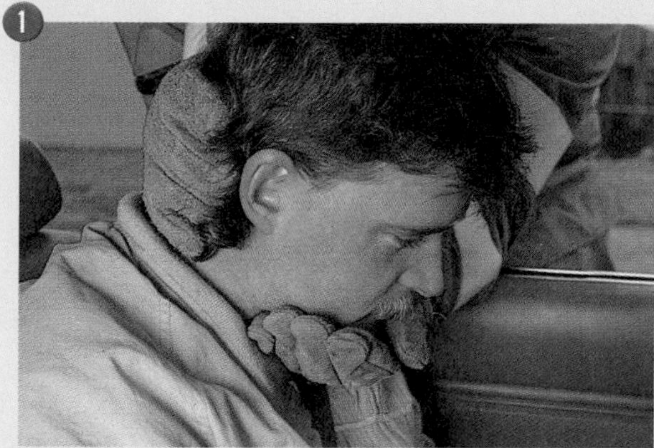

To open the airway, place one hand under the chin and the other hand on the back of the patient's head.

2

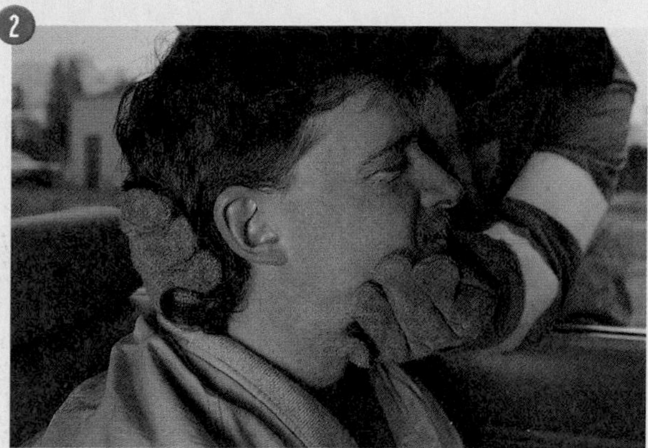

Raise the head to neutral position to open the airway.

means that the less time spent on the scene with a seriously injured patient, the better. The patient's chances for survival increase if rescuers can get the patient to a trauma center within one hour of the injury.

Your familiarity with the phases of the extrication effort may enable you to assist the rescue and extrication crews. You can do many things to help, and you should take the time to find out about the rescue and extrication resources in your community. Ask the crews how you can assist them; they will probably be delighted to have your help and support.

Remember

Access and patient stabilization are the two primary goals of first responders.

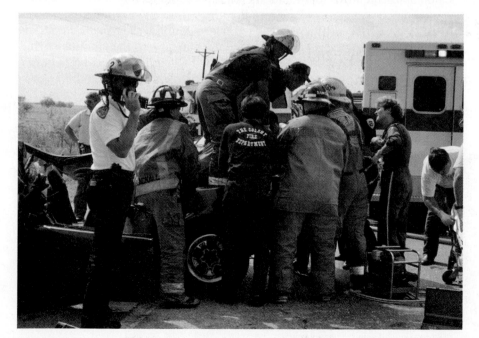

Figure 16.16 A serious extrication situation requires teamwork from all responders.

Voices of Experience

Quick Action Prevents Paralysis in Spinal Injury Patient

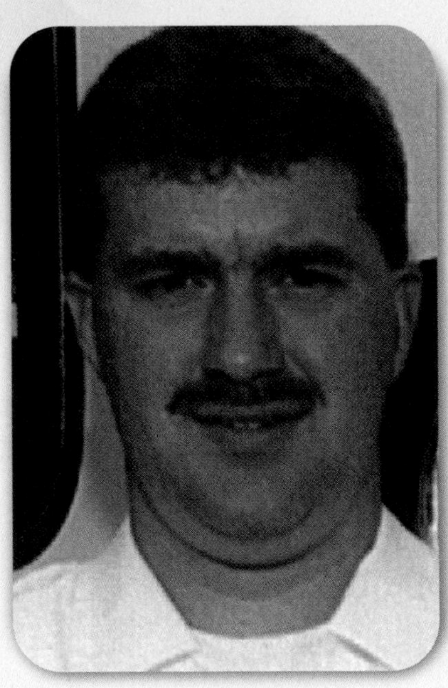

On November 22, 1996, my partner and I were called to a motor vehicle crash in a rural area of our county. There was a lengthy drive about fifteen minutes or so from our location to the crash. While en route we received a report called in by a nearby neighbor who said that the victim of the crash had been ejected and was lying in the field in very bad shape.

The first responder fire department arrived on the scene five minutes before we did, and was treating the young male patient who indeed had been ejected and thrown several feet from the vehicle. Upon our arrival, we made our way to the victim and took a glimpse of the car. It was destroyed in the crash. I asked the first responder at the head, "What do we have?" He responded with, " I am not sure, but I am doing what I was taught." This was indeed true—he was holding c-spine and talking to the victim, telling him not to move and assuring him that everything was being done to help him.

The situation we had was a male in his early twenties who had left school where he was a coach. He was on his way home when he lost control of his car and rolled over several times before being ejected. Upon assessment we found that the victim had no feeling or movement from the nipple line down. Immediately we realized our situation was critical. We rapidly loaded the patient into the ambulance and en route to the hospital started a large bore IV, high-flow oxygen, and checked for other signs of trauma. This was all being done while the patient was still conscious and asking why he couldn't move his lower body. Once we arrived at the local emergency department, we turned care over to an orthopaedic physician.

> **"The first responder was holding c-spine and talking to the victim, telling him not to move and assuring him that everything was being done to help him."**

We later found out that he had received an injury to his thoracic spinal cord and was going to need several weeks of rehabilitation. This is an excellent example of how first responders fit into EMS operations, and can have a major impact on how a scene of this magnitude can be resolved in an effective manner. ❖

Kevin Sargent
Lt. Firefighter/ Paramedic
Shift Training Officer
Mt. Vernon Fire Department
Mt. Vernon, Illinois

Lead Paramedic Instructor
Rend Lake College
Ina, Illinois

Step Six: Help Prepare Patients for Removal

As disentanglement proceeds, the patient is prepared (packaged) for removal. Dressings, bandages, and splints are applied and the head and spine are immobilized. If you are familiar with the procedures and equipment, you may be able to assist in this effort. For example, extra trained hands are useful to help move and secure the patient onto a long backboard for removal. (See Chapter 5.)

It is important to realize that the access route to the patient may not be adequate as an extrication route. The extrication route must be large enough to permit the safe removal of the packaged patient, whereas the access route may be a relatively small entry hole.

Step Seven: Help Remove Patients

Once packaged, the patient is removed from the automobile and placed onto the stretcher of the transporting ambulance.

Although a first responder is directly involved in only the first four of the seven extrication steps, you should be aware of the entire operation. Your actions or inaction can have a vital impact on the entire operation.

Review of the Extrication Process

Remember these steps when you arrive on the scene of a vehicle crash with trapped passengers:

- Call for extrication help.
- Specify the types of vehicles involved.
- Do not stand idly by while waiting for help:
  - Identify and contain hazards.
  - Park your vehicle so that its headlights and warning lights can be used to protect and light the scene.
  - Clear a working area around the accident before you or rescue personnel attempt to stabilize the vehicle(s).
  - Use your head! Think and use what tools you already have.
  - Remember to try opening the doors first, rather than breaking windows.
  - Once you gain access to the patients, assess and monitor their conditions.
  - Above all, keep your cool!

Checkpoint

- ◯ List seven hazards you may find at the scene of an emergency and describe what actions you can take to minimize or control each of these hazards.

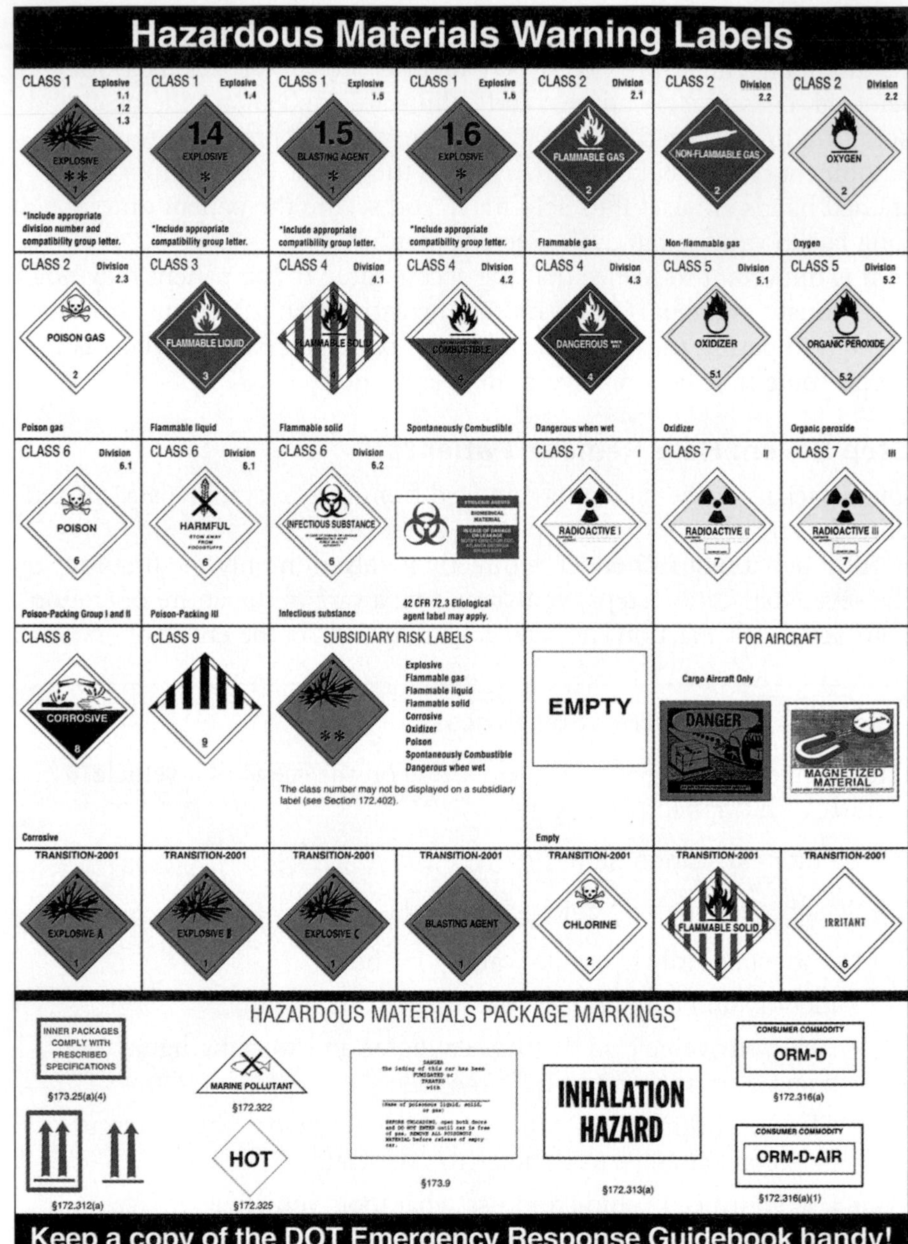

Figure 16.17 Hazardous materials warning labels.

Hazardous Materials Incidents

HazMat Hazardous material or chemical.

Hazardous materials (**HazMat**) incidents involving chemicals occur every day and expose many people to injury or contamination. During a hazardous materials incident, first responders must protect themselves from injury and contamination.

The single most important step when handling any hazardous materials incident is to identify the substance(s) involved. Federal law requires that all vehicles containing certain quantities of hazardous materials display a hazardous materials placard. When you see a hazardous materials placard, you know that a potential problem exists. You will have to find the proper response to the problem before beginning patient treatment (**Figures 16.17** and **16.18**). The placard should also have a four-digit identification number, which can be used to identify the substance and to obtain emergency information.

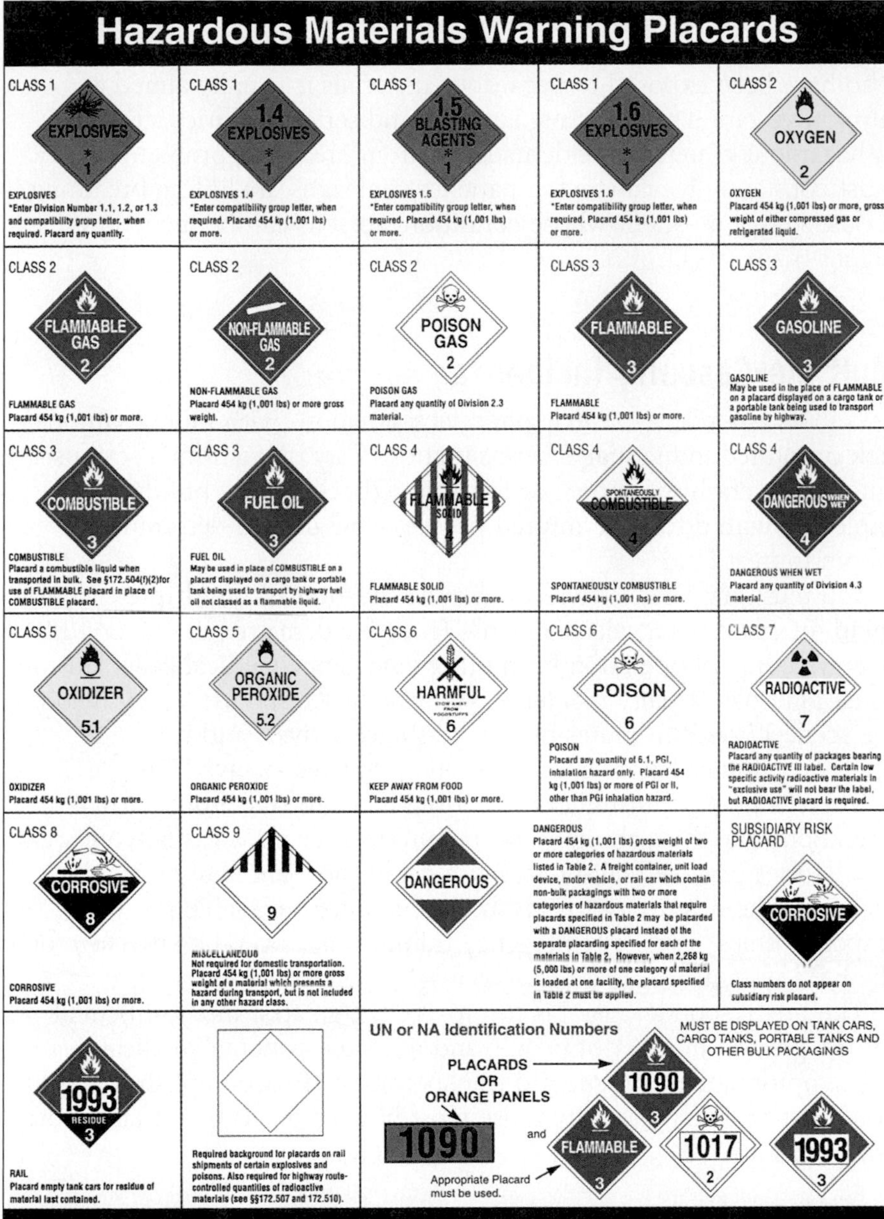

Figure 16.18 Hazardous materials warning placards.

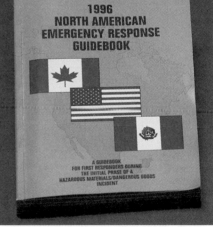

Figure 16.19 *Emergency Response Guidebook.*

The *Emergency Response Guidebook*, published by the U.S. Department of Transportation, lists the most common hazardous materials, their four-digit identification numbers, and the proper emergency actions to control the scene. It also describes the emergency care of patients who become ill or injured after exposure to these substances (**Figure 16.19**).

Unless you have received training in handling hazardous materials and can take the necessary precautions to protect yourself, you should keep away from the contaminated area, or **hot zone**.

hot zone A contaminated area.

Once the rescuers have been properly protected, the next step in hazardous materials incidents is to identify victims who have sustained an acute injury as a result of exposure to hazardous materials. These patients should be removed from the contaminated area, decontaminated by trained personnel, given any necessary emergency care, and transported to a hospital.

Safety Tips

Contaminated patients will contaminate unprotected rescuers!

There are very few specific antidotes or treatments for most hazardous materials injuries. Consequently, the emergency treatment of patients who have been exposed to hazardous materials is usually aimed at supportive care. Because most fatalities and serious injuries sustained in hazardous materials incidents result from breathing problems, you must constantly reevaluate the patient's vital signs, including breathing status, so that a patient whose condition worsens can be moved to a higher triage level.

Multiple-Casualty Incidents

As a first responder, you may often face situations with more than one sick or injured individual. These situations may range from a serious automobile crash with three or four injured people to a building explosion with dozens of injured people. How do you determine whom to treat first?

multiple-casualty incident An accident or situation involving more patients than you can handle with the initial resources available.

triage The sorting of patients into groups according to the severity of their injuries; used to determine priorities for treatment and transport.

casualty sorting The sorting of patients for treatment and transportation.

You must first be able to recognize the situation as a **multiple-casualty incident** or mass-casualty incident. These incidents require a very different method of operation from other emergency medical calls. During some multiple-casualty incidents, you (the first responder) may be on the scene 15 to 20 minutes before assistance arrives, and it may be 45 to 60 minutes before enough rescue resources are available.

There is no easy formula for deciding when to shift from normal operations into the techniques of the multiple- or mass-casualty incident. Simulations provide realistic situations, but there are many variables, including the severity of the crash, access routes, available resources, response times, levels of emergency training, and overall experience of the EMS system.

The first responder's goal is to provide the greatest medical benefit for the greatest number of people and to match patients' medical needs with appropriate treatment and transportation. To accomplish this goal, you must be able to identify those most in need of treatment and those who can wait.

Casualty Sorting: Creating Order Out of Chaos

The sorting of patients into groups according to their need for treatment is called **triage**. Triage is a French word that has come to mean **casualty sorting** in the emergency care field. The purpose of casualty sorting is to determine the order in which patients should be treated so that the most good can be done for the most people.

Ideally, your casualty-sorting system should be simple and fast, based on the skills and knowledge you already have. Do not worry about making a specific diagnosis before categorizing patients; a casualty-sorting system is meant to provide the basis for a system of rapid, lifesaving actions.

A casualty-sorting system focuses your activities in the middle of a chaotic and confusing environment. You must identify and separate patients rapidly, according to the severity of their injuries and their need for treatment.

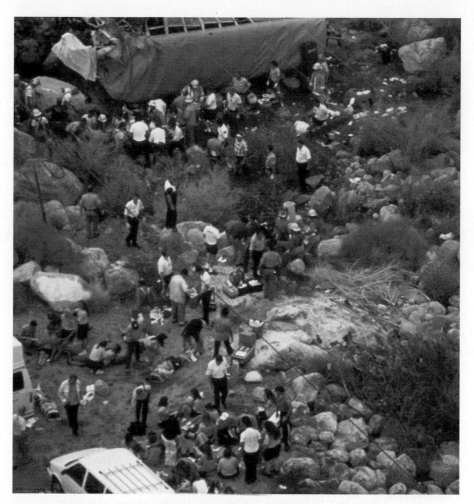

Figure 16.20 An incident requiring triage.

The Visual Survey: The Eye Sees It All

As you are on the way to the scene, you should be preparing yourself mentally for what you may find (**Figure 16.20**). Perhaps you've responded to other accidents at the same location. Where will additional help come from? How long will it take for help to arrive?

When you arrive at the scene of a major incident, force yourself to stay as calm as possible. Make a visual assessment of the entire accident scene. This visual survey gives you an initial impression of the overall situation, including the potential number of patients involved and, possibly, the severity of their injuries. The visual survey should enable you to estimate how much and what kind of help you will need to handle the situation.

Your Initial Radio Report: Creating a Verbal Image

The initial radio report is often the most important radio message of a disaster because it sets the emotional and operational stage for everything that follows. As you prepare to key the microphone for that first vital report, use clear language, be concise, be calm, and do not shout into the microphone.

Try to give the communications center a concise verbal picture of the scene.

The key points to communicate are:

- Location of the incident
- Type of incident
- Any hazards
- Approximate number of victims
- Type of assistance required

Be as specific with your requests as possible. A good rule of thumb in multiple- or mass-casualty situations is to request one ambulance for every five patients. For example, for 35 patients, request seven ambulances; for 23 patients, request five ambulances; and so forth.

After taking several deep breaths (to give yourself time to absorb what you've seen and to try to calm your voice), you might give the following radio report about a commercial bus crash: "This is a major accident involving a truck and a commercial bus on Highway 233, about 2 miles west of Route 510. There are approximately 35 victims. There are people trapped. Repeat: This is a major crash. I am requesting the fire department, rescue squad, and seven ambulances at this time. Dispatch additional police units to assist."

CAUTION

Recent studies show that the failure to provide adequate traffic control at the emergency scene is a common and often fatal error in multiple-casualty incidents. Immediately after radioing for help, establish a traffic control plan. This process should only take a couple of minutes.

1. **Determine the perimeters for emergency vehicles only and exclude all other vehicles.**
2. **Establish a one-way route for emergency traffic to approach the scene and a separate one-way route for emergency traffic to exit the scene.**
3. **Allow adequate room for emergency vehicles that need to be close to the scene.**
4. **Keep vehicles and personnel that are not needed at a given time in a staging area.**

Sorting the Patients

It is important not to become involved with treating the first or second patient whom you see. Remember that your job is to get to each patient as quickly as possible, conduct a rapid assessment, and assign patients to broad categories based on their need for treatment.

You cannot stop during this survey, except to correct airway and severe bleeding problems quickly. Your job is to sort (triage) the patients. Other rescuers will provide follow-up treatment.

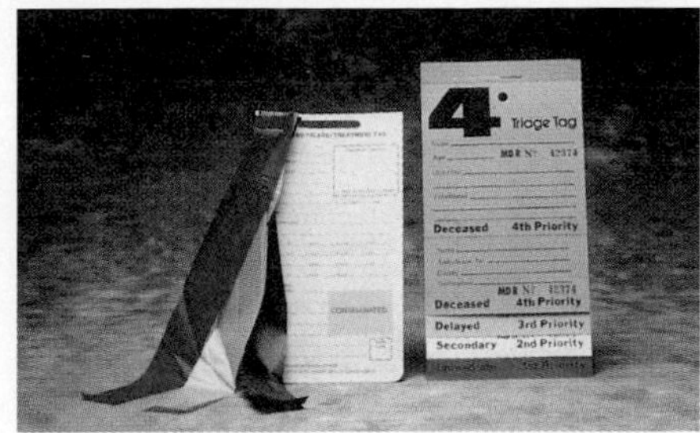

Figure 16.21 Triage tags.

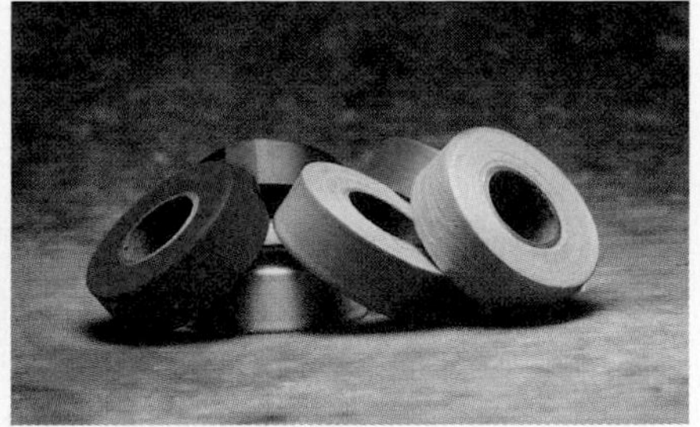

Figure 16.22 Triage tape.

The START System: It Really Works!

Different communities use many variations of triage systems, and you will need to learn the specific role that you have in your community's triage plan. Many EMS systems rely on the **START system** because it is simple and easy to remember and implement.

START system A system of casualty sorting using Simple Triage And Rapid Treatment.

The Simple Triage And Rapid Treatment (START) system lets first responders triage each patient in 60 seconds or less, based on three primary observations: breathing, circulation, and mental status (BCM).

The START system is designed to help rescuers find the most seriously injured patients. As more rescue personnel arrive, patients can be re-triaged for further evaluation, treatment, stabilization, and transportation. This system also allows first responders to open blocked airways and stop severe bleeding quickly.

Triage Tagging: Telling Others What You've Found

Patients are tagged so that other rescuers arriving on the scene can easily recognize their triage level. Tagging uses colored surveyor's tape or colored paper tags (**Figures 16.21** and **16.22**), and is based on the method determined by your local EMS system.

The Four Colors of Triage

The START system consists of four levels of triage, each with its own color code:

- Priority One (red tag): Immediate care/life threatening.
- Priority Two (yellow tag): Urgent care/can delay up to 1 hour.
- Priority Three (green tag): Delayed care (walking wounded)/can delay up to 3 hours.
- Priority Four (gray or black tag): Patient is dead/no care required.

The First Step in START: Get Up and Walk!

The first step in START is to tell all the people who can get up and walk to move to a specific area. If patients can get up and walk, they rarely have life-threatening injuries.

To make the situation more manageable, ask those victims who can walk to move away from the immediate rescue scene to a designated safe area. These patients are the "walking wounded" designated as Priority Three (green tag/delayed care). A patient who complains of pain when

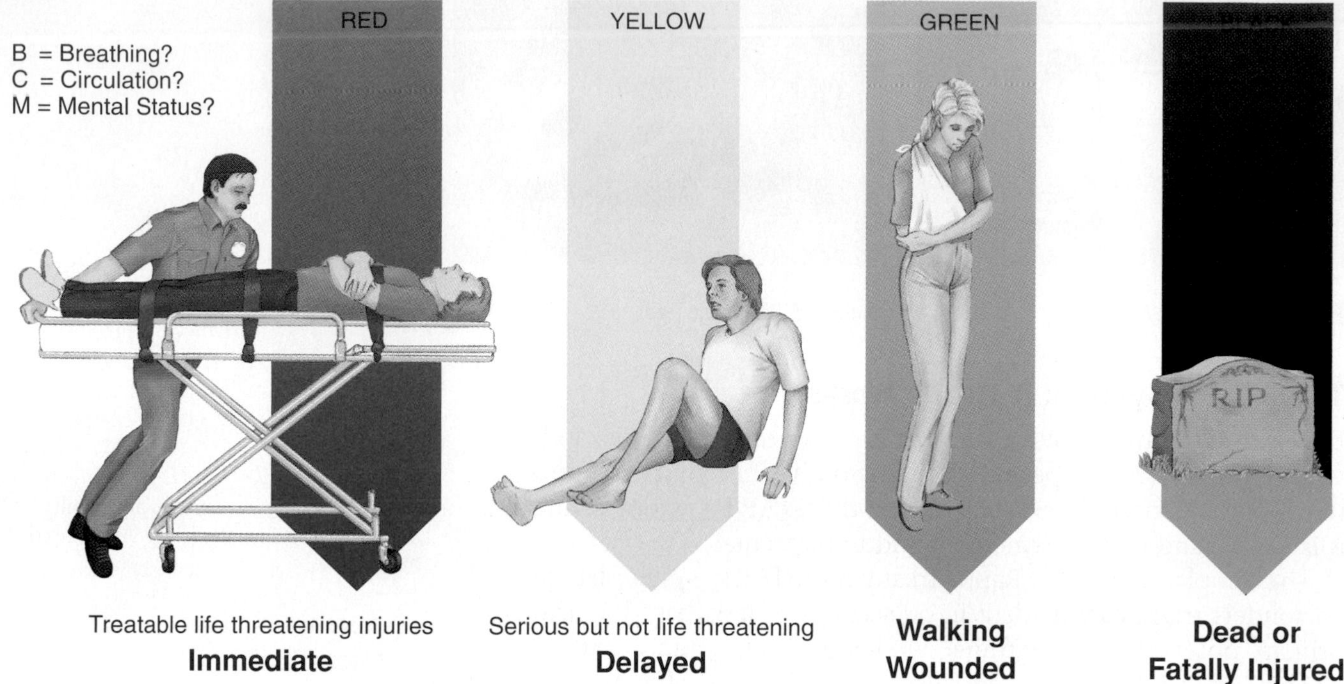

Figure 16.23 Use START to sort patients into appropriate groups for treatment.

he or she attempts to walk or move should not be forced to move. Now you can concentrate on the patients who are left in the rescue scene.

The Second Step in START: Begin Where You Stand

Begin the second step of START by moving from where you stand. Move in an orderly and systematic manner through the remaining victims, stopping at each person for a quick assessment and tagging. The stop at each patient should never take more than one minute.

Your job is to find and tag the Priority One patients—those who require immediate attention. Examine these patients, correct life-threatening airway and breathing problems, tag the patients with a red tag, and move on!

How to Evaluate Patients Using BCM

The START system is based on three observations: breathing, circulation, and mental status (BCM). Each patient must be evaluated quickly, in a systematic manner, starting with breathing (**Figure 16.23**).

Breathing: It All Starts Here

If the patient is breathing, you need to determine the breathing rate. Patients with breathing rates greater than 30 per minute are tagged Priority One (red tags). These patients are showing one of the primary signs of shock and need immediate care as soon as it is available.

If the patient is breathing at a rate less than 30 per minute, move on to the circulation and mental status observations in order to complete your 60-second survey.

If the patient is not breathing, quickly clear the mouth of foreign matter. Use the head-tilt technique to open the airway. In a multiple- or mass-casualty situation, you may have to ignore the usual cervical spine guidelines when you are opening airways during the triage process. This is the only time in emergency care when you may not have time to properly stabilize every injured patient's spine.

Open the airway, position the patient to maintain the airway, and—if the patient breathes—tag the patient Priority One (red tag). Patients who need help maintaining an open airway are Priority One (red tags). If you are in doubt as to the patient's ability to breathe, tag the patient as Priority One (red tag). If the patient is not breathing and does not start to breathe with simple airway maneuvers, tag the patient Priority Four (gray/black tag).

Circulation: Is Oxygen Getting Around?

The second BCM triage test is the patient's circulation. The best field method for checking circulation (to see if the heart is able to circulate blood adequately) is to check the carotid pulse.

The carotid pulse is close to the heart. It is large and easily felt in the neck. To check the carotid pulse, place your index and middle fingers on the larynx and slide your fingers into the groove between the larynx and the muscles at the side of the neck. You must keep your fingers there for 5 to 10 seconds to find and measure the pulse rate. (See Chapter 7.) If the carotid pulse is weak or irregular, tag the patient Priority One (red tag). If the carotid pulse is strong, move on to the mental status observation, the third step of the BCM series.

Treat patients with a weak carotid pulse for shock by elevating the legs to return as much blood as possible to the brain, lungs, and heart. Then try to stop any severe bleeding. Do not spend time controlling the bleeding yourself. Get the patient to assist or ask one of the walking wounded Priority Three (green tag) patients to help. These patients are often eager to assist with emergency treatment.

If the pulse is absent, tag the patient with a Priority Four (gray/black tag).

Mental Status: Open Your Eyes!

The last BCM triage test is the mental status of the patient. This observation is done on patients who have adequate breathing and adequate circulation.

First determine whether the patient responds to verbal stimuli. Tell the patient to follow a simple command: "Open your eyes," "Close your eyes," "Squeeze my hand." Patients who can follow these simple commands and have adequate breathing and adequate circulation are tagged Priority Two (yellow tag). According to the AVPU scale, which is described in Chapter 7, such patients are considered to be "alert" and "responsive" to verbal stimuli.

A patient who cannot follow this type of simple command is "unresponsive" to verbal stimuli, according to the AVPU scale. Tag these patients as Priority One (red tag).

START Is Just the Beginning

In every situation involving casualty sorting, the goal is to find, stabilize, and move Priority One patients first. The START system is designed to help rescuers find the most seriously injured patients. As more rescue personnel arrive on the scene, the patients will be re-triaged for further evaluation, treatment, stabilization, and transportation.

Remember that injured patients do not stay in the same condition. The process of shock may continue and some conditions will become more serious as time goes by. As time and resources permit, go back and recheck the condition of Priority Two and Priority Three patients to catch changes in condition that may require upgrading to Priority One (red tag) attention (**Figure 16.24**).

Working at a Multiple- or Mass-Casualty Incident

You may or may not be the first person to arrive on the scene of a multiple- or mass-casualty incident. If other rescuers are already at the scene when you arrive, be sure to report to the incident commander before going to work. Because many activities are going on at the same time, the incident commander will assign you to an area where your help and skills can best be used. The incident commander, based on training and local protocols, is in charge of the rescue operation. An effective incident command system depends upon integrated, agreed-upon protocols and procedures involving fire, law enforcement, and emergency medical services personnel. You should learn the incident command system (ICS) that is used in your community.

If you are the first on the scene, you will have to make the initial overview, clearly and accurately report the situation, and conduct the initial START triage. In addition, you will probably also be called on to participate in many other ways during multiple- and mass-casualty incidents.

As more highly trained rescue and emergency personnel arrive on the scene, accurately report your findings to the person in charge by using a format similar to that used in the initial arrival report. Note the following information:

- Approximate number of patients
- Number of patients that you have triaged into the four levels
- Additional assistance required
- Other important information

After you have reported this information, you may be assigned to provide emergency care to patients, to help move patients, or to assist with ambulance or helicopter transportation. You may also be asked to assist with traffic control or help provide fire protection.

Checkpoint

- ◯ Describe your role as the first person arriving on the scene of a multiple-casualty incident.

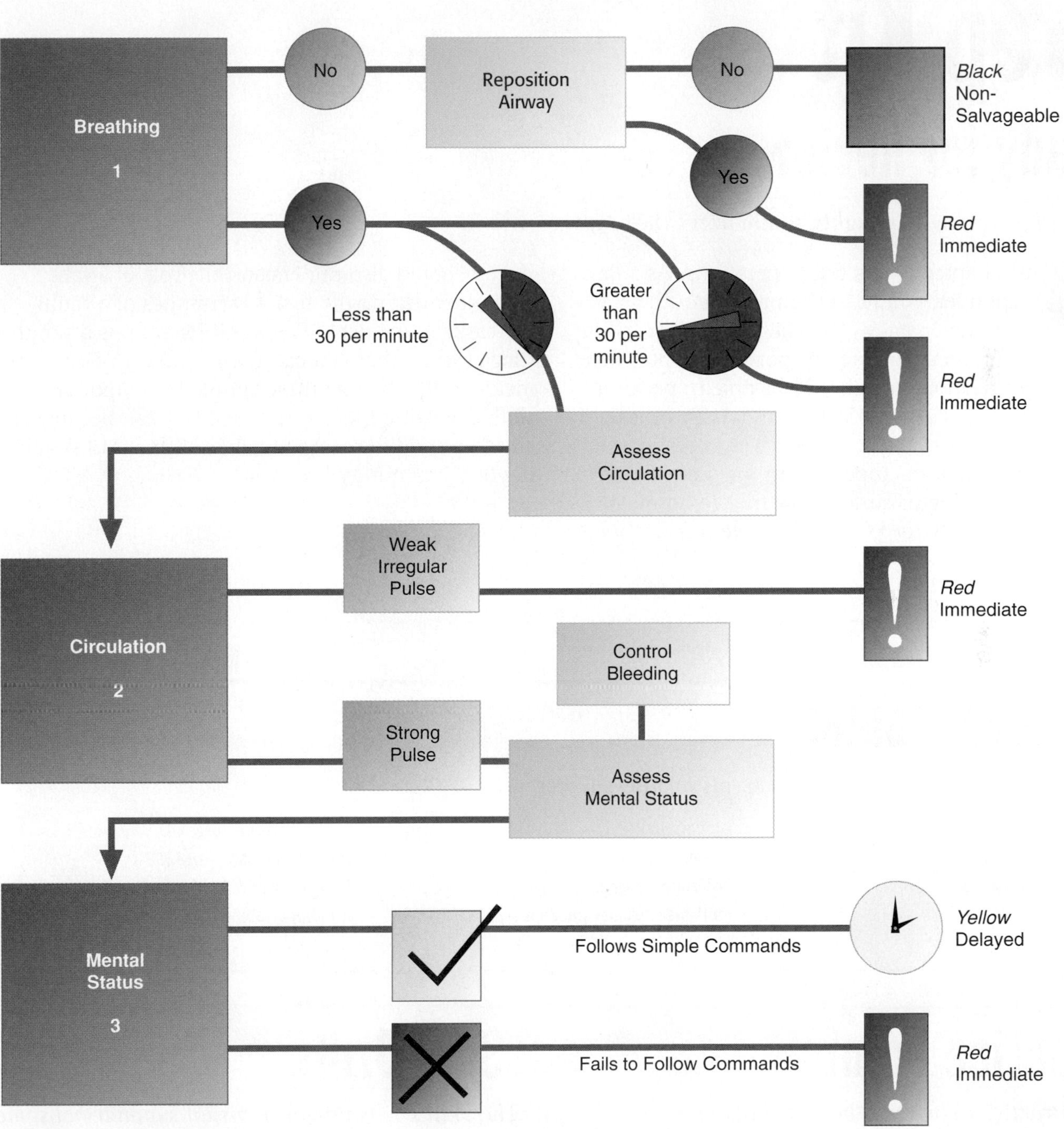

Figure 16.24 START algorithm.

16

Prep Kit

Ready for Review

Ready for Review thoroughly summarizes the chapter.

This chapter covers EMS operations. As a first responder, you need the proper equipment on an emergency call. The chapter covers the five phases of an emergency response and the seven steps of extrication. You should be able to perform the first four steps of extrication and assist other rescuers with steps five through seven. Because you may be the first trained person on the scene of an incident involving hazardous materials, you must be able to identify the potential problem and respond appropriately.

You should also understand the role of a first responder during the first few minutes of a multiple-casualty incident. The START system is a simple triage system that you can use at a multiple-casualty incident. By learning these simple but important skills involving EMS operations, you can become an effective and life-saving member of the EMS system in your community.

Vital Vocabulary

The Vital Vocabulary are the key terms for this chapter.

casualty sorting—*page 400*
chocking—*page 390*
extrication—*page 385*
fusee—*page 388*
Golden Hour—*page 394*
HazMat—*page 398*
hot zone—*page 399*
multiple-casualty incident—*page 400*
START system—*page 403*
tempered glass—*page 392*
triage—*page 400*
wooden cribbing—*page 390*

Practice Points

The Practice Points are the key skills you need to know.

1. Performing simple procedures for gaining access to a patient in a wrecked vehicle.
2. Using the START system during simulated multiple- or mass-casualty incidents.

Skill Drills

The Skill Drills provide a visual summary of some of the more complex skills from the skills objectives.

16.13 Accessing the Vehicle Through the Window—*page 393*

16.15 Airway Management in a Vehicle—*page 395*

Ready to Respond

Ready to Respond presents a fictitious scenario to help you review what you learned in this chapter.

You are dispatched to a motor vehicle collision at the corner of Oak Street and Norwood Avenue at 5:47 PM. The temperature is 57°F (14°C) and the sky is cloudy.

1. Your first responsibility after receiving this call is
   A. Quick response to the scene
   B. Fastening your seat belt
   C. Rapid and safe response to the scene
   D. Stopping at each intersection

As you arrive, you observe a sport utility vehicle that hit a utility pole. The second vehicle is a van resting on its side in the middle of the intersection.

2. What is the first step you should take when you arrive at this scene?
   A. Gain access to the patients
   B. Provide initial patient care
   C. Help remove patients
   D. Conduct an overview of the scene

3. What agencies are most likely to be needed at this scene?
   A. Gas utility
   B. Electric utility
   C. Fire department
   D. Law enforcement

4. You should be especially alert for which hazard when you approach the van?
   A. Battery acid
   B. Spilled fuel
   C. Wild animals
   D. Transmission fluid

5. Your first step in gaining access to the patients in the van would be
   A. Through a window
   B. Through a door
   C. Through the windshield
   D. Through the top of the van

You notice that two electrical wires are broken and are resting on the hood and top of the sport utility vehicle. You should:

1. Set up a safety perimeter around the vehicle

2. Tell the occupants to jump away from the vehicle

3. Call the power company

4. Talk to the occupants of the vehicle and tell them not to move

   A. 2, 3, 4
   B. 1, 3. 4
   C 1, 2, 3
   D. All of the above

MODULE 7 QuickQuiz

EMS Operations

1. Place the following steps of response in the correct order

A. post-run activities

B. arrival at the scene

C. response to the scene

D. dispatch

E. transferring care of the patient to other EMS personnel

2. As a minimum, what protective clothing should a first responder have for extrication?

A. ______________________________

B. ______________________________

C. ______________________________

3. You should make an overview of a vehicle collision scene before you leave your vehicle?

A. true

B. false

4. The first step in the START system is to

A. begin tagging patients

B. walk among the injured patients

C. instruct patients who can walk to move to a specified area

D. ask each patient if he or she can walk to a different area

5. Match each of the colors below with the appropriate level of triage in the START system.

__ Immediate care/life threatening

__ Urgent care can be delayed up to one hour

__ Patient is dead—no care is required

__ Care can be delayed up to 3 hours

A. green

B. black

C. red

D. yellow

1. D, C, B, E, A **2.** helmet, heavy gloves, eye protection **3.** A **4.** C **5.** C, D, B, A

Supplemental Skills

MODULE

8

Module CONTENTS

Chapter 17

Special Patients and Considerations

TECHNOLOGY

- Online Chapter Pretest
- Web Links
- Online Glossary
- Anatomy Review
- Online Review Manual
- CyberClass

www.FirstResponderTraining.com

- Interactive First Responder

Chapter FEATURES

- Skill Drills
- Vital Vocabulary
- Voices of Experience
- Signs and Symptoms
- FYI
- Special Needs
- Safety Tips
- BSI Tips
- Caution
- Checkpoint
- Prep Kit

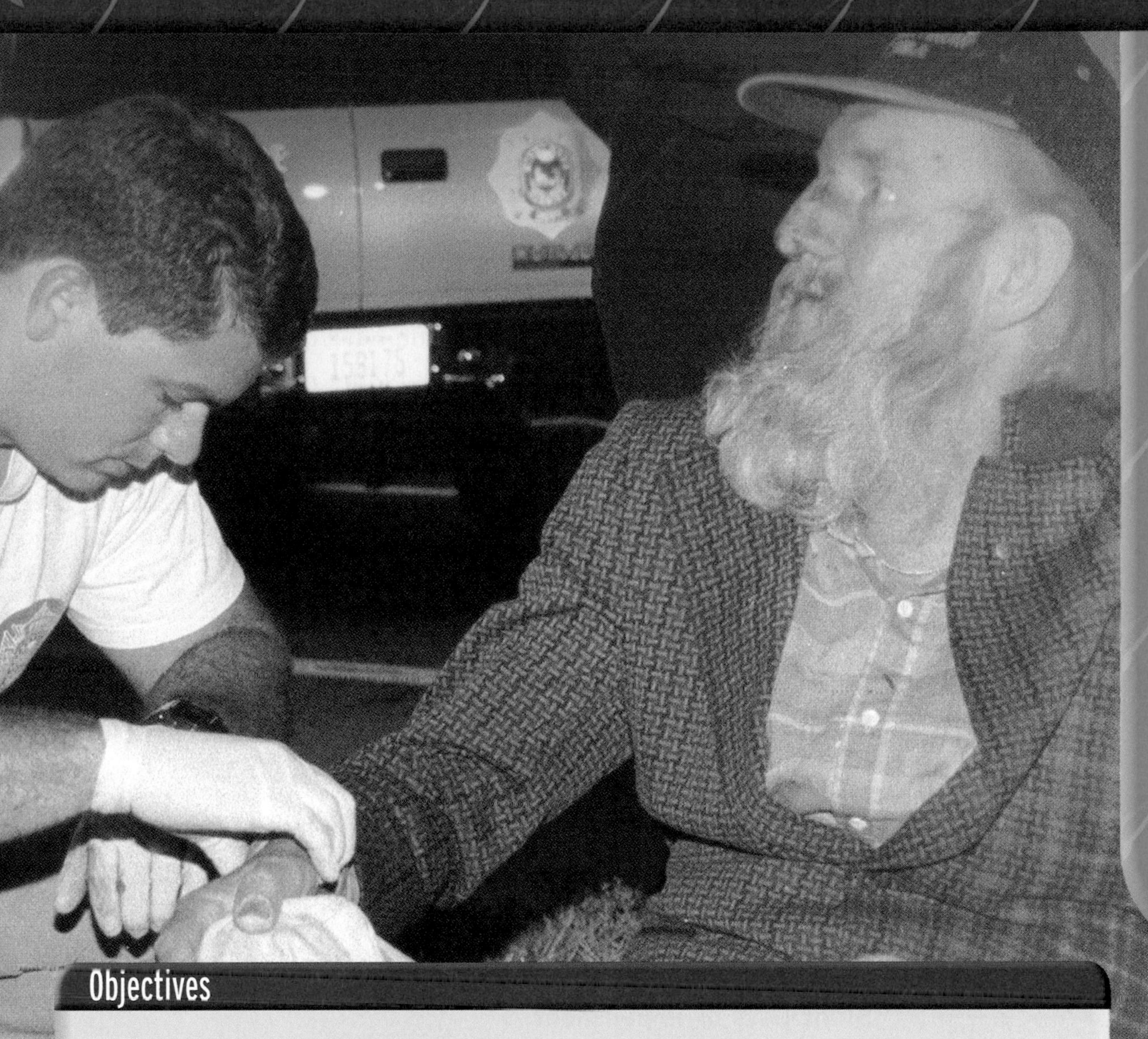

CHAPTER 17

Objectives

Knowledge and Attitude Objectives

After studying this chapter, you will be expected to:

1. Describe the approach you should use when dealing with elderly patients.
2. Describe the approach you should use when dealing with chronic-care patients.
3. Describe the approach you should use when dealing with hearing-impaired patients.
4. Describe the approach you should use when dealing with visually-impaired patients.
5. Describe the approach you should use when dealing with non–English-speaking patients.
6. Describe the approach you should use when dealing with developmentally disabled patients.
7. Describe the approach you should use when dealing with patients who display disruptive behavior.

Skill Objectives

After studying this chapter, you should be able to:

1. Communicate with elderly patients.
2. Communicate with hearing-impaired patients.
3. Communicate with visually-impaired patients.
4. Communicate with non–English-speaking patients.
5. Communicate with developmentally disabled patients.
6. Communicate with patients who display disruptive behavior.

As a first responder, you will encounter patients who have special needs and deserve special consideration. These patients include elderly patients, chronic-care patients, patients who are visually- or hearing-impaired, patients who do not speak your language and developmentally disabled patients. By better understanding these conditions and learning some simple communications techniques, you will be able to work more effectively with these patients.

DISABILITIES THAT MAY OCCUR WITH AGE

- *Hearing loss or impairment*
- *Sight loss or impairment*
- *Slowed movements*
- *Fractures*
- *Senility*
- *Loss of bowel and bladder control*

Elderly Patients

The population of older people is the fastest growing segment of our society. Today's seniors are often active, vital people who do not fit older stereotypes. You will reach greater rapport with older patients if you deal with each as an individual, not as a member of some arbitrary group defined by age (**Figure 17.1**).

Hearing Loss or Impairment

Hearing loss is an invisible disability. Be sure an elderly patient can hear and understand what you say. Speak slowly and clearly. If you think the patient has difficulty hearing you, do not shout. Speak directly into the patient's ear, or talk while facing the patient and maintaining eye contact. Many elderly patients read lips to help compensate for hearing loss.

Sight Loss or Impairment

If an elderly patient wears eyeglasses, keep them with the patient if at all possible. If the eyeglasses are lost during a medical emergency,

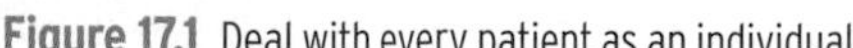

Figure 17.1 Deal with every patient as an individual.

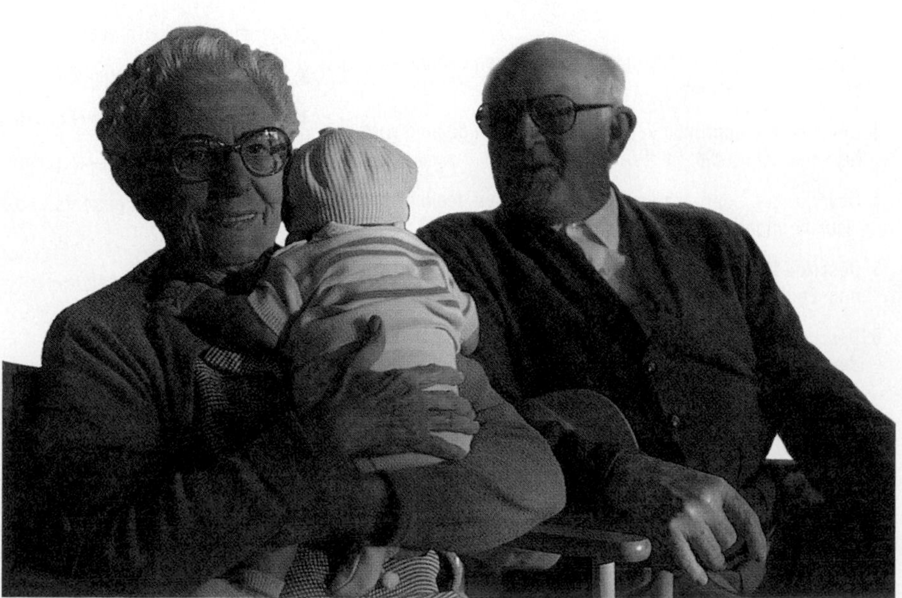

search everywhere to try and find them! The patient may be severely handicapped and anxious without his or her glasses; knowing that the glasses are close and not lost will be a great relief. Imagine how you would feel if you were in an emergency situation and could not see; bring that understanding and empathy to your dealings with patients.

Slowed Movements

When you assist an elderly patient, remember that as a person ages, movements become slower. Lend a helping hand or supporting arm. Most elderly patients are afraid of falling, and your support will help them overcome this fear.

Fractures

Fractures occur often in the elderly because, as we age, our bones lose calcium and become quite brittle. The condition, called **osteoporosis**, affects both women and men. Fractures of the wrist, spine, and hip are particularly common.

osteoporosis Abnormal brittleness of the bones in older people caused by loss of calcium; affected bones fracture easily.

externally rotated Rotated outward, as in a fractured hip.

Hip fractures usually result from a fall and occur mostly in elderly women. As you do your initial assessment, remember that other conditions may have contributed to the fall. Patients may have experienced a minor stroke, heart attack, or confusion before the fall; they may not have seen an obstacle.

In a hip fracture, the injured leg is usually (but not always) shortened as compared to the other leg. The toes of the injured leg are pointed outward (**externally rotated**), and there may be so much pain that the patient cannot move the leg. Every elderly patient who complains of pain after a fall must be X-rayed for possible fractures.

Splint the patient as described in Chapter 13 and arrange for T ***prompt transport*** to an appropriate medical facility.

Senility

Old age sometimes brings senility. This can include the loss of short-term and/or long-term memory, confusion, inability to follow directions, and even hostile behavior. Despite your best efforts to help some elderly patients, effective communication and interaction may be impossible. Senile patients or patients with Alzheimer's disease are a challenge for even the most highly trained medical personnel. You must remain calm and keep talking with them. Senile patients often respond to your gentle and caring approach even if they can not understand your actual words. Remember that the patient needs help, and you are there to provide it (**Figure 17.2**).

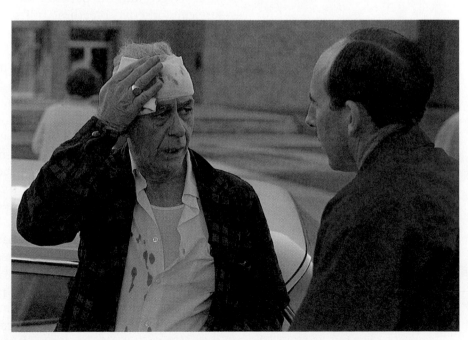

Figure 17.2 Treat elderly patients with consideration and respect.

Elderly people often wear more clothing than other people, even during the middle of the summer. Do not use the presence of extra clothes as a reason to do a less-than-complete physical examination. Conduct a complete head-to-toe examination.

Loss of Bowel and Bladder Control

The loss of bowel and bladder control occurs frequently in the elderly. This situation can be distressing and embarrassing to both you and the patient. Do not let this problem interfere with appropriate patient care.

Additional Considerations for Elderly Patients

If the elderly patient is at home and needs to be taken to a hospital, gather all medications and send them to the hospital with the patient.

Often the elderly patient's spouse needs your attention, too. It is frightening to see your loved one injured or seriously ill and then be separated as he or she is transported in an ambulance. Take a few minutes to speak with the patient's spouse or family and tell them what is being done and why these actions are being taken.

Chronic-Care Patients

Modern medical science has made great advances in treating patients with chronic conditions. In the past, most patients with serious chronic medical conditions were treated in hospitals or rehabilitation facilities; many died shortly after their conditions were diagnosed. Today, many patients are treated at home by nurses or family members, and their lifespan has increased.

A variety of complex medical devices is used with chronic-care patients. Devices that help patients breathe include ventilators that push oxygen into the patients' lungs, oxygen-enrichment devices, surgically-inserted breathing tubes, and monitors that sound an alarm if a patient stops breathing. Patients with certain heart conditions may have pacemakers and automatic defibrillators under their skin. Tubes inserted into a patient's arm, neck or stomach provide fluids or food. Catheters drain urine from the patient's bladder. To make matters even more complex, chronic-care patients must often take a wide variety of medications.

As a first responder, you may be called to assist with these patients for a variety of reasons, ranging from trauma or illness to mechanical failures or transport needs. What may be a minor illness for a healthy person can be life threatening for a patient with a chronic condition. Some patients fall and suffer musculoskeletal trauma, while others may only need help getting back to bed. Medical equipment may stop working because the power or backup batteries failed. Patients may need transport to a hospital for assessment and treatment.

When you receive such a call, remember your role as a first responder. Your job is to assess the immediate problem and use your training to take the appropriate steps in caring for the patient. Do not get overwhelmed or distracted by the complex equipment. You are not expected to understand how all these complex medical devices work. The people caring for the patient are familiar with the equipment they use each day. Do not be afraid to ask them about the equipment and condition of the patient.

Do not hesitate to question the patient and the patient's caregivers about the problem. They can probably tell you what the problem is and how you can help. Keep in mind the principles of your training. These patients need open airways and adequate breathing and circulation. In most situations, you need to help stabilize the patient for only a few minutes, until more highly trained EMS providers arrive to provide care.

Hearing-Impaired or Deaf Persons

A major challenge faced by first responders is communicating with a deaf person. Most people have few skills for dealing with deaf persons and feel uncomfortable when asked to do so.

A patient of any age may be unable to hear you for a variety of reasons: **hereditary deafness,** long-term deafness caused by illness, ear infections or injury, or **temporary deafness** caused by an explosion or other loud noise. A patient who has been deaf for a long time usually develops skills to help compensate for the deafness. A patient who is temporarily deaf (such as from an explosion) does not have such skills.

hereditary deafness Deafness present at birth.

temporary deafness Deafness that is usually caused by an explosion or loud noise; hearing usually returns after a short time.

In either case, your job is to address the medical needs of the patient. Ask, "Can you hear me?" A patient who is used to being deaf will probably respond by pointing at his or her ear and shaking his or her head to indicate deafness.

The temporarily deaf person may feel anxious and panicky because he or she suddenly cannot hear. Help him or her focus on the problem by pointing at your ear and shaking your head to indicate deafness, or write out the question, "Can you hear?" on a piece of paper and show it to the patient.

After you determine that the patient is deaf, do not continue to rely on verbal communication; use other methods. It is difficult to read lips, and someone who is temporarily deaf will not have that skill anyway. A patient with long-term deafness may attempt to communicate with you by signing (using the hands and fingers to communicate). If you cannot sign, rely on writing and gestures to communicate.

As you examine the patient for injury or pain, use your own body to show the patient how to indicate whether there is pain in a particular location. Touch a place on your body and make a face to indicate pain. Then look at the patient and repeat the procedure on the patient's body. Most people will understand what you are trying to do. Do a complete patient assessment on every patient, whether or not they can communicate with you.

Keep the patient informed by making gestures to indicate that certain things are happening (for example, when the ambulance is arriving). Touching is an important part of communication and reassurance for both deaf and hearing patients. Hold the patient's hand so that he or she knows you are there to help.

When working with deaf patients:

- Identify yourself by showing the patient your patch or badge.
- Touch the patient; a deaf patient needs human contact just as much as a hearing patient.
- Face the patient when you speak so he or she can see your lips and facial expressions.
- Speak slowly and distinctly; do not shout.
- Watch the patient's face for expressions of understanding or uncertainty.
- Repeat or rephrase your comments in clear, simple language.
- If all this fails, write down your questions and offer paper and pencil to the patient to respond.
- Some people are both deaf and blind. This double loss may make these patients difficult to treat. Take your time, be patient, and use touch as a way of communicating.

Children and the Deaf

If the patient is a hearing child of deaf parents, be sure to communicate with the parents about the child's condition and your actions. Like all other parents in similar circumstances, deaf parents must give their consent for you to treat their child. They have a right to know what is being done and are probably just as upset as hearing parents would be.

If the patient is a deaf child of hearing parents, you need to involve the parents even more than usual. They can assist you in communicating with the child.

If the patient is a deaf parent with a hearing child, resist the urge to use the child as an interpreter unless the child is obviously mature and capable. Young children cannot understand medical terminology, and misinterpretation can have very serious results. Communicate directly with the deaf patient, using whatever methods you can.

Visually-Impaired or Blind Patients

During your initial overview of the scene, look for signs that indicate the patient may be visually impaired. These may include the presence of eye glasses, a white cane, or a seeing-eye dog (**Figure 17.3**). Then, as you approach and introduce yourself to the patient. If you think the patient is blind, ask, "Can you see?"

A visually-impaired patient may feel vulnerable, especially during the chaos of an accident scene. The patient may have learned to use other senses such as hearing, touch, and smell, to compensate for the loss of sight. The sounds and smells of an accident may be disorienting. The patient may rely on you to make sense of everything. Tell the patient what is happening, identify noises, and describe the situation and surroundings, particularly if you must move the patient.

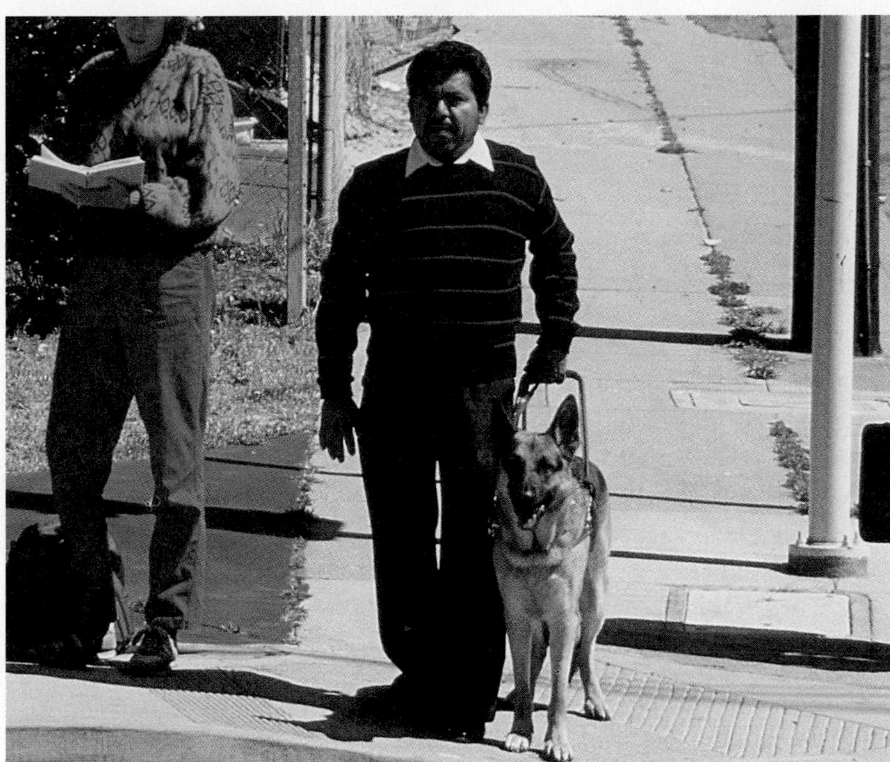

Figure 17.3 Blind patients may have a seeing-eye dog.

Find out what the patient's name is and use it throughout your examination and treatment, just as you would with a sighted patient. Touch the patient to provide psychological support. If the patient has a guide dog, he or she may initially be more concerned about the dog than about their own injuries. Recognize that the dog and the patient are a unique team who depend on each other. Let the patient direct the dog or tell you how to handle the dog. Use the techniques of restatement and redirection to focus the patient's attention on the problem at hand. Remember that guide dogs are usually not aggressive and try to keep the patient and the dog together.

Note: Always lead a blind patient—never push!

If a blind patient must be moved and can walk, ask the patient to hold onto your elbow and stand slightly to your side and rear. Tell the patient about obstructions, steps, and curbs as you lead the way.

Non-English-Speaking Patients

In many areas of the country and in many urban areas, there are communities where English is not the first or even the most common language. If your patient speaks a language other than English and you cannot understand each other, you must find ways to communicate so that you can meet your responsibility as a first responder to provide the appropriate standard of care. You may be able to adapt some of the techniques recommended for communicating with a deaf patient. Determine how much English the patient speaks. Seek out a family member or friend to be your interpreter.

Voices of Experience

Human Touch and Compassion Bridge the Gap

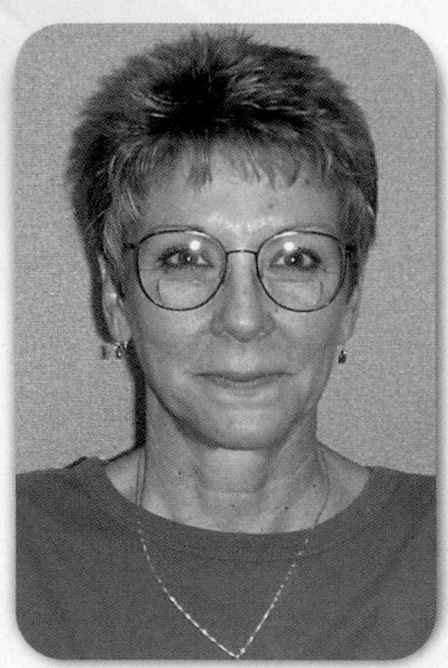

I have had the opportunity to work in emergency medicine and emergency medical services for more than 15 years. My jobs as an instructor, bedside nurse, and EMS program coordinator have allowed me to encounter a variety of patients as well as many illnesses and injuries. Every day I am challenged by what I encounter and often stand in awe of the strength that individuals exhibit. Every patient encounter over the years has served to strengthen my belief in the power of human touch.

Imagine being alone, in pain, and unable to get up from the floor. Imagine being unable to communicate with or see those around you. Imagine being confused and scared by all the lights and people surrounding you in an emergency situation. These are just some of the issues faced by the special patients you will encounter. Whenever I am caring for someone challenged by their environment or by physical limitations, I feel frustrated and, despite my best attempts, unprepared. While I search for a way to bridge our gap, I am able to convey my concern, compassion, and willingness to keep trying by placing my hand on their arm.

“Every patient encounter over the years has served to strengthen my belief in the power of human touch.”

Remember, one day we will all be old and in need of a gentle helping hand, or perhaps in a crisis in a foreign land and in need of help. One day we will hope that those around us will take time, show concern, and demonstrate compassion. Never forget the power of human touch.

Liz Criss, RN, CEN, MEd
Clinical Educator
Emergency Services
University Medical Center
Tucson, AZ

Supplement your questions with hand gestures, finger pointing, and facial expressions. If your jurisdiction has a large non–English-speaking population, you should make a serious attempt to learn common phrases and questions so that you can use them when treating these patients.

Developmentally Disabled Patients

You may find it difficult to communicate with developmentally disabled patients. Ask the family about the patient's typical level of communication. Speak slowly, using short sentences and simple words. You may need to repeat statements several times, or to rephrase them until the patient understands what you want.

Again, offer support by taking time to touch your patients. Because the commotion surrounding an accident may confuse these patients or make them afraid, use extra care in dealing with developmentally disabled patients. You may be able to adapt many of the techniques that you use when treating children to your work with developmentally disabled patients.

Persons Displaying Disruptive Behavior

Disruptive behavior can present a danger to the patient or others, and can cause delays in treatment. At some time in your career, you will encounter a person who challenges your patience and communication skills.

In managing any patient who is exhibiting disruptive behavior, take the following steps:

1. Assess the situation. Try to determine the cause of the patient's disruptive behavior.
2. Protect the patient and yourself.
3. Do not take your eyes off the patient or turn your back.
4. If the patient has a weapon, stay clear and wait for law enforcement personnel—no matter how badly injured the patient seems to be.
5. As soon as your personal safety is assured, carry out the appropriate emergency medical care.

There may be times when you are unable to approach a patient; the person will not allow anyone to come near, despite all efforts to help. Sometimes family or friends of the disruptive patient may insist that you take the person to the hospital. But you cannot take the patient to the hospital against his or her wishes (unless you are a law enforcement officer).

Frightened, agitated, drugged, or disruptive patients can cause serious injury to the first responder, bystanders, or themselves. It is best to wait for additional assistance in these cases.

17

Prep Kit

Ready for Review

Ready for Review thoroughly summarizes the chapter.

This chapter describes special considerations and skills needed when working with elderly patients, chronic-care patients, hearing-impaired patients, visually impaired patients, non–English-speaking patients, developmentally disabled patients, and patients displaying disruptive behavior.

Elderly people often need specific instructions and more time. They may move more slowly and need more assistance. Chronic-care patients may be dependent on complex medical equipment and you may need to rely on assistance from caregivers to deal with these calls.

Deaf patients may be able to read your lips. Or you can write out your questions and instructions. Be aware of clues that can indicate a visually impaired patient and recognize the special partnership between a blind patient and his or her guide dog.

If you live in an area with a large population of non–English-speaking patients, learn some simple phrases in their language. Use bystanders or family as translators to communicate with these patients. Developmentally disabled patients can often understand you if you speak slowly and use simple words. Patients displaying disruptive behavior will often react positively if you maintain a calm approach. You need to keep your safety in mind when dealing with these patients.

Vital Vocabulary

The Vital Vocabulary are the key terms for this chapter.

externally rotated—*page 415*
hereditary deafness—*page 417*
osteoporosis—*page 415*
temporary deafness—*page 417*

Practice Points

The Practice Points are the key skills you need to know.

1. Communicating with elderly or chronic-care patients.
2. Communicating with hearing-impaired patients.
3. Communicating with visually impaired patients.
4. Communicating with non–English-speaking patients.
5. Communicating with developmentally disabled patients.
6. Communicating with patients displaying disruptive behavior.

Ready to Respond

Ready to Respond presents a fictitious scenario to help you review what you learned in this chapter.

You are dispatched to a residence for the report of an elderly person with an unknown medical problem. Your dispatcher indicates that she does not have any further information because a neighbor made the call. When you arrive at the house, you are met by the neighbor, who states that Mrs. Jones "does not seem to be herself" today.

1. As you begin to talk to your patient, she shakes her head "no." She may be trying to tell you
   A. You should not speak to her
   B. She wants you to repeat what you said
   C. She is senile
   D. She is deaf
2. During your examination of Mrs. Jones, you notice that she is dressed in several layers of clothing, even though it is about 80°F (26°C) outside. You should
   A. Take her vital signs only
   B. Remove her clothing only if she stays in a warm place
   C. Remove as much of her clothing as you need to examine her properly
   D. Do a less-than-complete physical exam
3. There is an increased chance that Mrs. Jones may have a broken bone because of
   A. Diabetes
   B. Senility
   C. Arthritis
   D. Osteoporosis
4. If it becomes necessary to transport Mrs. Jones to a medical facility, you should make sure that the EMS crew also takes along her
   A. Medical insurance policy
   B. Coat
   C. Address book
   D. Medications

Chapter 18

Special Rescue Situations

TECHNOLOGY

- Online Chapter Pretest
- Web Links
- Online Glossary
- Anatomy Review
- Online Review Manual
- CyberClass

www.FirstResponderTraining.com

- Interactive First Responder

Chapter FEATURES

- Skill Drills
- Vital Vocabulary
- Voices of Experience
- Signs and Symptoms
- FYI
- Special Needs
- Safety Tips
- BSI Tips
- Caution
- Checkpoint
- Prep Kit

CHAPTER

18

Objectives

Knowledge and Attitude Objectives

After studying this chapter, you will be expected to:

1. Describe the steps you can take in assisting with a water rescue.
2. Describe the initial treatment of a patient in the water.
3. Describe the initial treatment of a patient with diving problems.
4. Describe the steps you can take in assisting with an ice rescue.
5. Describe your role in assisting with a confined space rescue.
6. Describe your role in responding to terrorism.

Skill Objectives

After studying this chapter, you should be able to:

1. Assist with a water rescue.
2. Provide initial treatment for a patient in the water.
3. Assist with an ice rescue.
4. Assist with a confined space rescue.

This chapter covers special rescue situations that are life threatening to both the rescuer and the victim. These situations include water rescue, ice rescue, and confined space rescue. This chapter also provides you with guidelines for dealing with them. In each situation, your first objective is to maintain your personal safety. In addition, there are basic rescue procedures you can perform without endangering yourself or the victim.

Water and Ice Rescue

You may encounter situations in which a person needs to be rescued from the water. The person may be fatigued, may have suffered a diving injury, or may have fallen through the ice in the winter. A book of this scope cannot teach you the skills of a certified lifesaver. It does describe some simple techniques you can use to perform a water or ice rescue without endangering your own safety.

FOUR STEPS FOR WATER RESCUE

1. <u>Reach</u>
2. <u>Throw</u>
3. <u>Row</u>
4. <u>Go</u>

Water Rescue

When you see a person struggling in the water, your first impulse may be to jump in to assist. However, that action may not result in a successful rescue and can endanger your own life. If you are faced with a water rescue situation, remember the steps listed and illustrated in **Figure 18.1**.

If you follow these steps, you may be able to perform a successful water rescue without ever entering the water. It may even be possible for someone who cannot swim to rescue a struggling person.

Reach

Use any readily available object to reach the threatened person. If the victim is close to shore, a branch, pole, oar, or paddle may be long enough. If you are at a swimming pool, there may be a specially designed pole available for this purpose. Use it.

Throw

If you cannot reach the person, throw something. At a swimming pool, dock, or supervised beach, a **flotation device** (such as a ring buoy) may be available. If a life buoy is available, throw it to the person in distress.

If no buoy is handy, then improvise. Throw a rope, plastic milk jug, or sealed Styrofoam™ cooler. Even a car's spare tire can support several people in the water. Think before you act!

Note: If you are using something like a plastic milk jug or picnic jug, fill the container with about 1 inch of water to add weight before you seal it and throw it to the victim.

Row

If you cannot reach the person by throwing something that floats, you may be able to row out to the drowning person if a small boat or canoe is available. It is important that you know how to operate or propel the craft properly. Protect yourself by wearing an approved personal flotation device.

reach-throw-row-go A four-step reminder of the sequence of actions that should be taken in water rescue situations.

flotation device A life ring, life buoy, or other floating device used in water rescue.

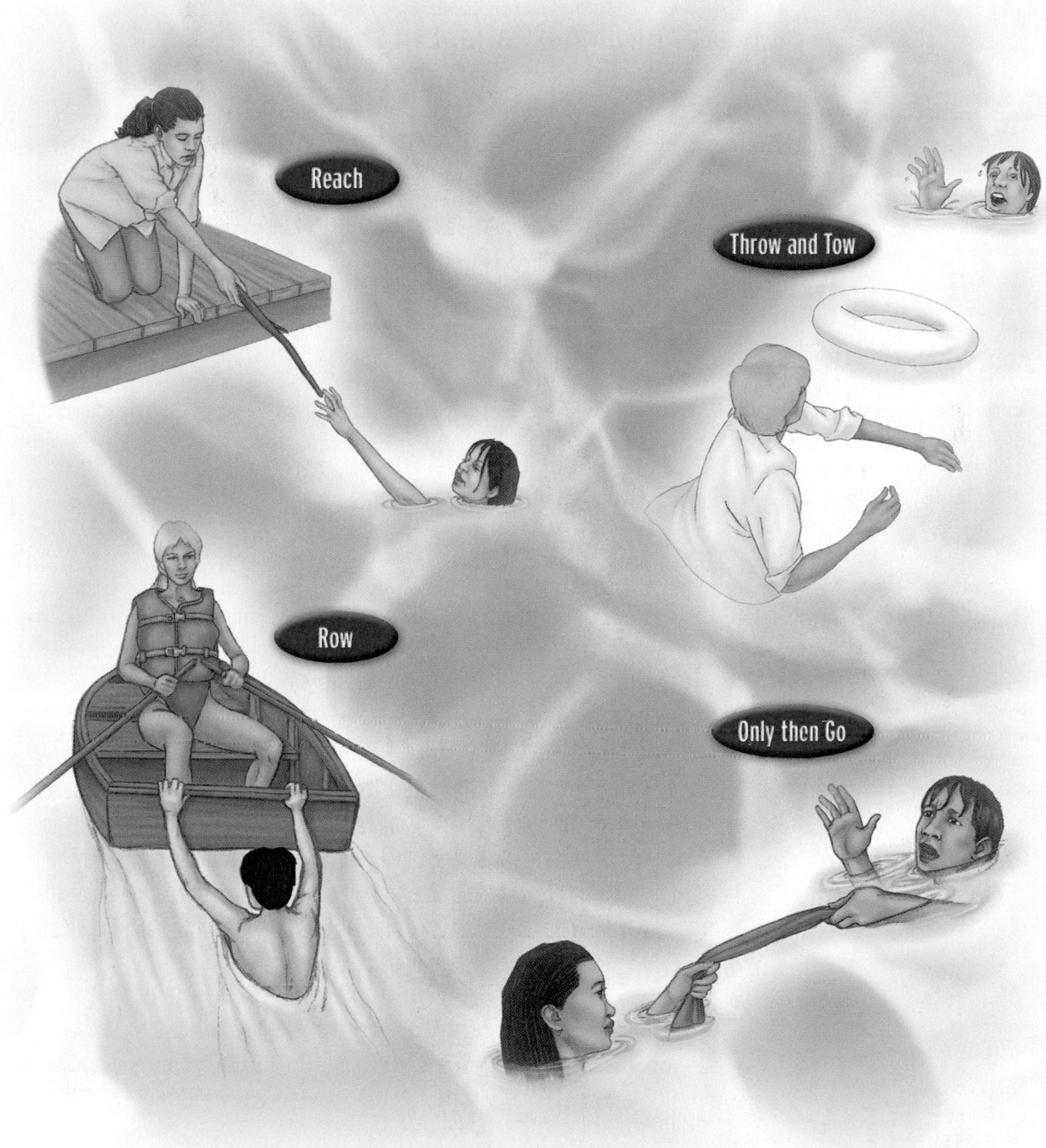

Figure 18.1 Water rescue rules: reach-throw-row-go.

Skill Drill

Figure 18.2 Turning a Patient in the Water

1

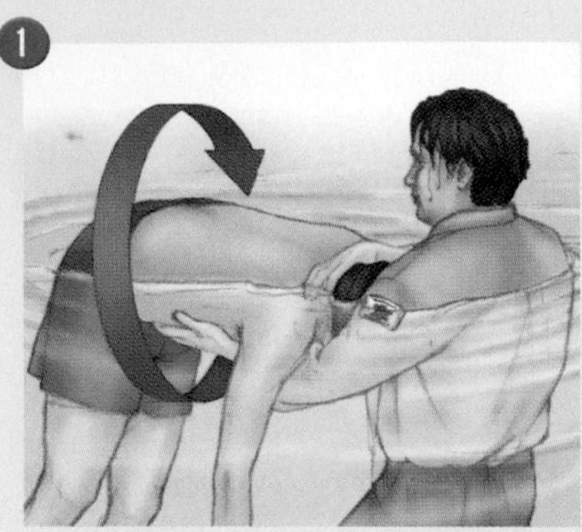

Support the back and head with one hand. Place other hand on the front of the patient.

2

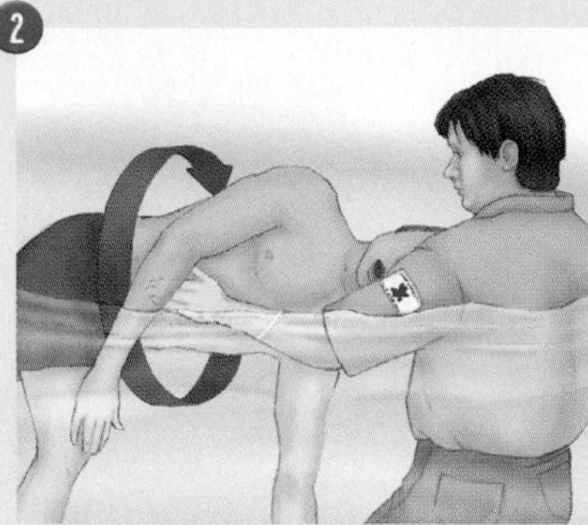

Carefully turn the patient as a unit.

3

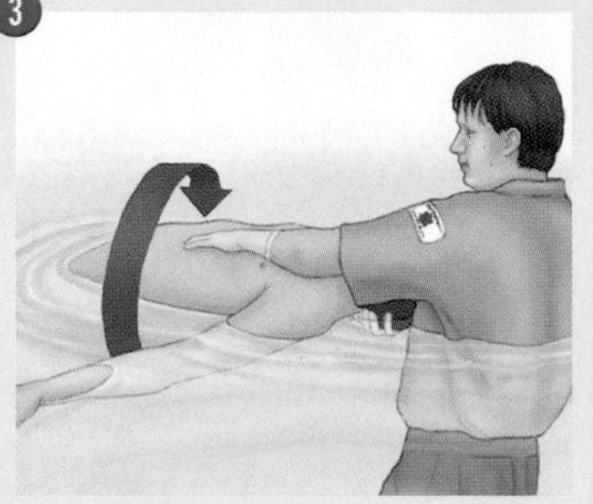

Stabilize the patient's head and neck.

Go

As a last resort, you may have to go into the water to save the victim. Enter the water only if you are a capable swimmer trained in lifesaving techniques. Remove encumbering clothing before entering the water. Take a flotation device with you if one is available.

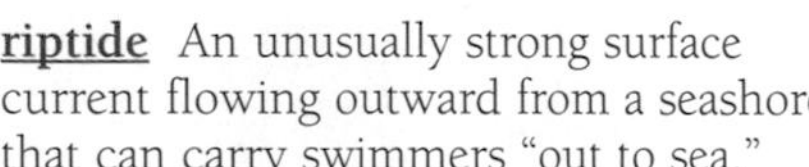

riptide An unusually strong surface current flowing outward from a seashore that can carry swimmers "out to sea."

CAUTION

Currents in streams or strong currents (riptides) at ocean beaches can pull both victim and rescuer rapidly away from shore. In an area below a dam, rapids, or waterfall, deadly currents may be present. An untrained rescuer should never attempt to enter the water under these conditions. If you do, both you and the victim will probably need to be rescued.

Initial Treatment of a Person in the Water

If you are in a water rescue situation, your primary concerns must be to open an airway, establish breathing and circulation, and stabilize spinal cord injuries.

Turn patients who are face down in the water face up. Support the back and neck with one hand and use the other hand to turn the patient face up, keeping the neck stabilized. Keep the head in the neutral position (**Figure 18.2**).

Use the jaw-thrust technique to open the airway. Do not hyperextend the neck because of the high risk of associated spinal cord injuries.

Look, listen, and feel for signs of breathing. If the patient is not breathing, start rescue breathing while the patient is still in the water (**Figure 18.3**). Ventilation will be much easier if you can stand on the bottom.

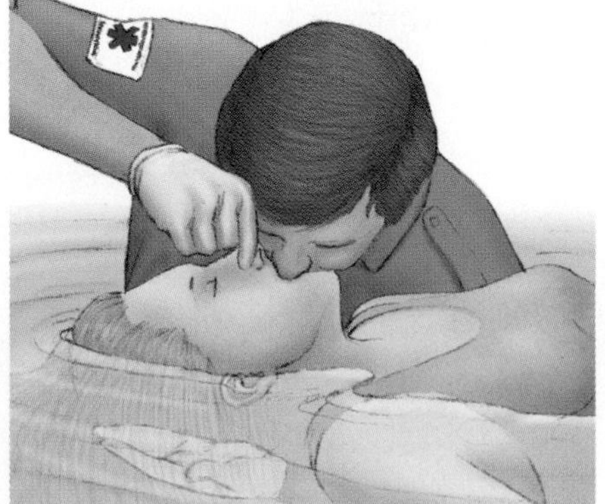

Figure 18.3 Begin rescue breathing in the water.

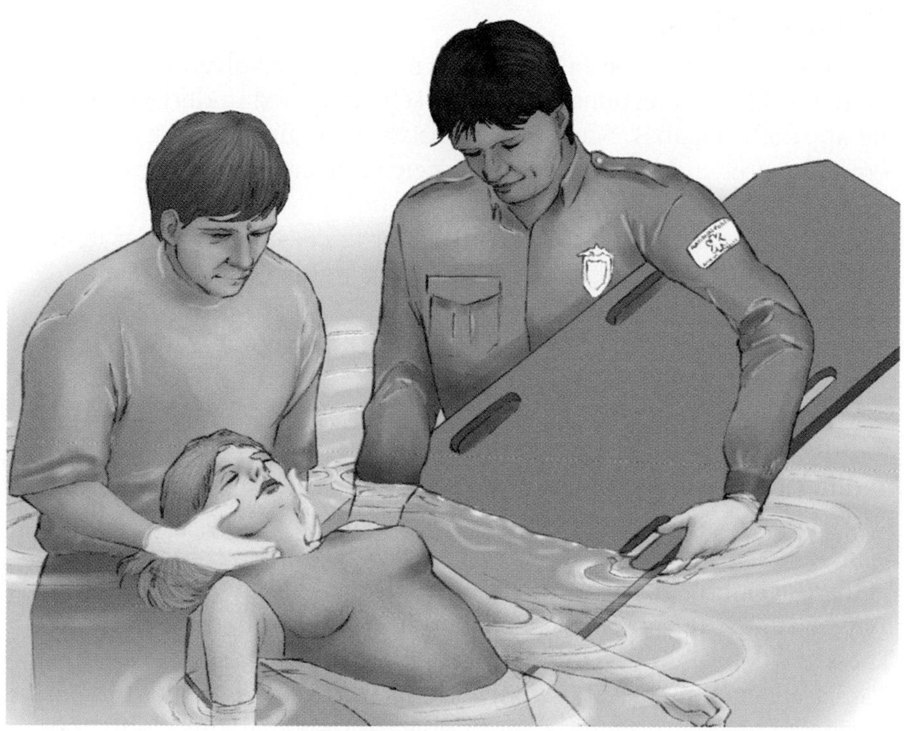

Figure 18.4 Apply the backboard while the patient is still in the water.

If the patient has suffered cardiac arrest, quickly stabilize the head and neck and remove the patient from the water. Place the patient on a hard surface before you begin CPR (see Chapter 8).

Treat a patient who is unconscious in the water as if a spinal cord injury were present. Also assume the presence of a spinal cord injury if a conscious patient in the water complains of numbness or tingling in the arms or legs, inability to move the extremities, or neck pain. Support the patient by floating a backboard in the water under the patient (**Figure 18.4**).

Strap the patient to the backboard, stabilize the head and neck, and remove the patient from the water.

If no rigid device is available and the patient must be removed from the water before EMS personnel arrive, six people, using their hands, can lift and support the patient (**Figure 18.5**).

Improvise

If no backboard is available, you can use a chaise lounge, door, or piece of plywood to provide rigid support under the patient.

Remember

One rescuer should give the commands to lift, move, and set the patient down.

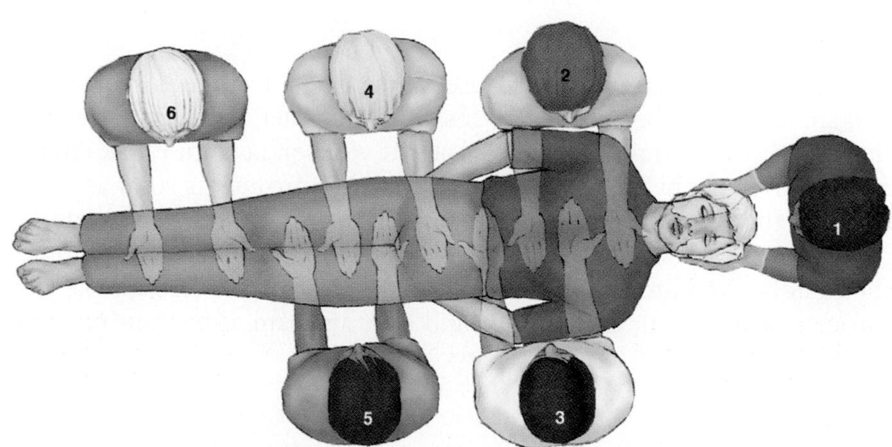

Figure 18.5 In emergency situations, a patient can be removed from the water using six people.

Diving Problems

First responders may be called to care for people involved in diving accidents. Most recreational divers use self-contained underwater breathing apparatus (scuba). Scuba gear consists of an air tank, a regulator, a mouthpiece, and a facemask. Commercial divers use either scuba gear or equipment that supplies air through a hose.

Most underwater diving accidents occur in coastal regions or in areas with large lakes. Diving accidents can cause trauma, near drowning, or specialized injuries. In cases involving trauma or near drowning, remove the patient from the water and treat the patient using information and skills you have already learned.

air embolism A bubble of air obstructing a blood vessel.

decompression sickness (the bends) A condition seen in divers in which gas, especially nitrogen, forms bubbles in blood vessels obstructing them.

There are two specialized injuries associated with diving, **air embolism** and **decompression sickness.** Usually it will not be possible for you to differentiate between these two conditions. Both are caused by air bubbles being released in the body as a result of the changes in pressure while diving.

If an air bubble affects the brain or spinal cord, the signs and symptoms may be similar to those of a stroke or cerebral vascular accident (CVA). These include dizziness, difficulty speaking, difficulty seeing, and decreased level of consciousness. Patients may have difficulty in maintaining an open airway. If the air bubble causes a collapsed lung, the signs and symptoms will include chest pain, shortness of breath, and pink or bloody froth coming from the mouth or nose. If the air bubble obstructs blood flow to the abdomen, the patient will experience severe abdominal pain and may be bent over. If the air bubble involves a joint, there will be severe pain in that joint.

To treat a patient with a suspected air embolism or decompression sickness, you must maintain the patient's airway, breathing, circulation, and normal body temperature. Oxygen should be administered as soon as it is available. Some physicians recommend placing the patient on their left side with the head of the patient slightly lowered. This may help to prevent further damage if there is an air bubble in the central nervous system. Patients with diving injuries may need to be transported to a hospital that is equipped with a hyperbaric (recompression) chamber. If you live in an area where diving injuries occur, you should receive specialized training and be familiar with the protocols of your local EMS system.

Ice Rescue

Ice rescue is very hazardous because no ice is safe ice! Ice is changeable and should always be considered unsafe. Think safety first; do not exceed the limits of your training and do not put yourself at undue risk. You cannot save anyone if you go through the ice yourself. As soon as you arrive at the scene of an ice rescue, visually mark the location where the person was last seen. This will enable other rescuers to concentrate their efforts on a limited area. You should know who is responsible for ice rescue in your community, and call this team as soon as possible.

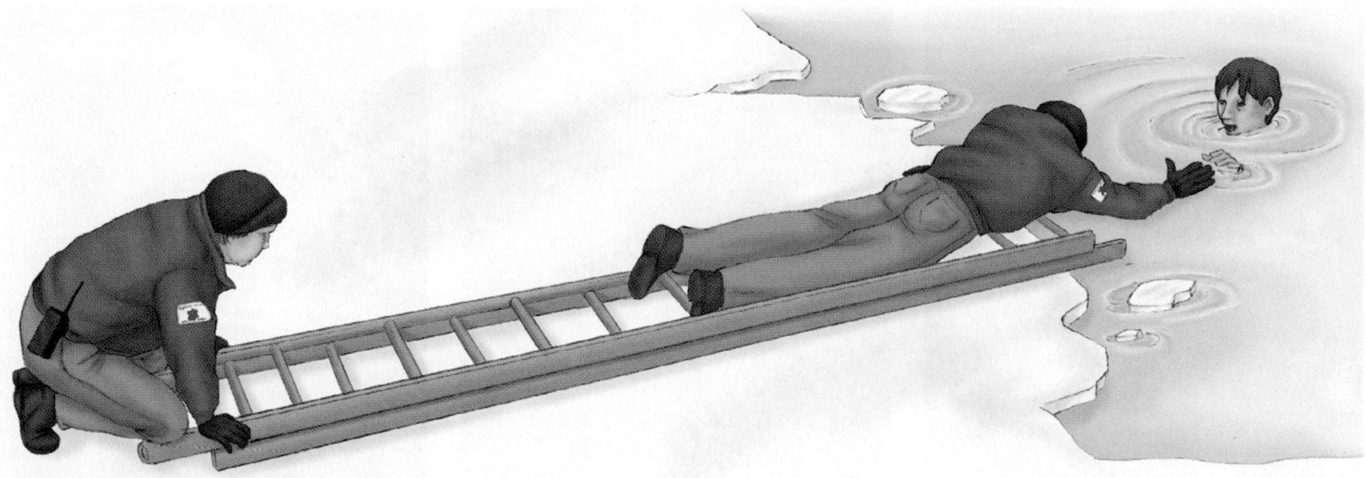

The basic rules of ice rescue are the same as water rescue: reach-throw-row-go. Reach for the victim using anything that will extend your natural stretch, such as a ladder, a pike pole, a tree branch, or a backboard. Next, throw a flotation device, rope, or anything that floats to pull in the victim. Third, row or propel a small boat to the victim, if you can break through the ice, or use a toboggan to get across the ice. Using a toboggan will spread your weight over a wider area and reduce your chances of falling through the ice. Be sure that you have a rope and that the boat or toboggan is secured to the shore as well. Finally, if you must go, secure yourself to shore with a rope around your waist, lie on your stomach, and proceed across the ice. Spreading your weight over a wider area reduces your chances of falling through the ice (**Figure 18.6**). Be sure you have good communication with other rescuers.

Figure 18.6 Ice rescue. The ladder distributes the rescuer's weight over a larger area, making it less likely that he or she will also fall into the water.

A car on the ice presents a risky situation. Instruct the car's occupants to avoid unnecessary movement. If the car has not gone through the ice, instruct the occupants to open the car doors. This may help to slow the sinking of the car if the ice breaks. If the doors cannot be opened, instruct the occupants to roll down the windows so they have a better escape route. If you must approach the car, remember that the added weight of rescuers can cause movement of the car. Do not place your head inside the car. If the car sinks, you may be unable to get out.

During ice rescues, both victims and rescuers are at risk for hypothermia. Keep all rescuers as warm as possible. Rescue personnel who are not directly involved in the rescue operation should remain in a warm vehicle until they are needed. Victims should be dried and warmed as soon as they are removed from the water. Remember that people can survive for a long time in cold water. If the patient has no pulse, start CPR and continue until the patient has been transported to a hospital and warmed. See Chapter 9 for more information on treating hypothermia.

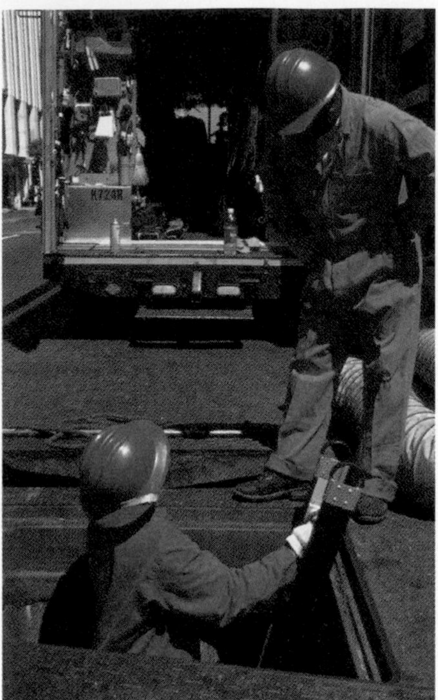

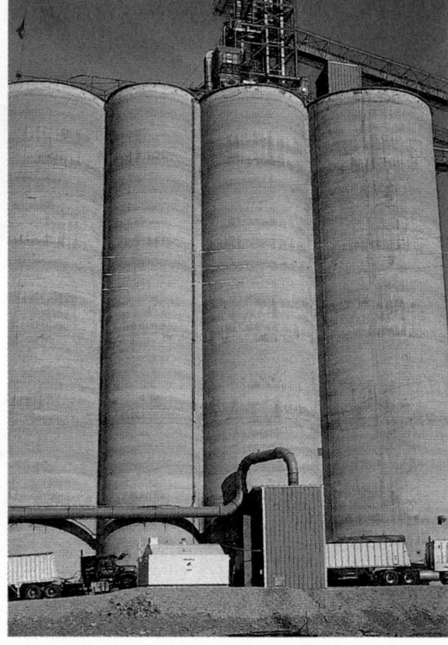

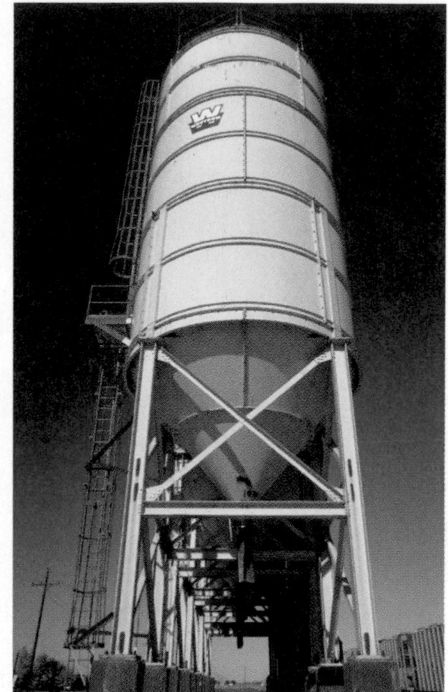

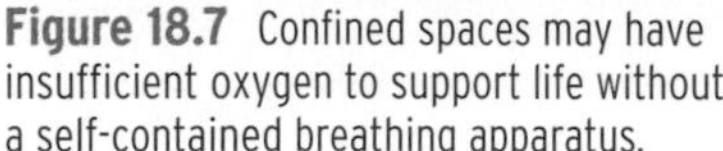

Figure 18.7 Confined spaces may have insufficient oxygen to support life without a self-contained breathing apparatus.

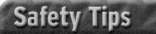

Confined Space Rescue

Confined spaces are structures designed to keep something in or out. Confined spaces may be below ground, ground level, or elevated structures. Below-ground confined spaces include manholes, below-ground utility vaults, storage tanks, old mines, cisterns, and wells. Ground-level confined spaces include industrial tanks and farm storage silos. Elevated confined spaces include water towers and storage tanks (**Figure 18.7**).

Rescue situations involving confined spaces have two deadly hazards. The first hazard is respiratory. There may be insufficient oxygen to support life, or a poisonous gas may be present. Rescuers must never enter a confined space without the proper respiratory protection. Anyone entering a confined space without proper respiratory protection stands a high chance of becoming a second victim.

The second hazard is the danger of collapse. In a mine, for example, rescuers may need to shore up the confined space before they can safely enter. Confined space rescue requires a specially trained team. As soon as you determine there is a confined space situation, call for additional assistance and do not enter the space until help arrives.

Safety Tips

More rescuers die in confined space incidents than victims! Of all deaths in confined space rescue incidents, 60 percent are rescuers. Do NOT enter a confined space without proper breathing apparatus and special training.

Response to Terrorism

Terrorism is the systematic use of violence by groups to intimidate a population or government and achieve a goal. Terrorism receives a lot of attention and is a high-profile crime. Although many more people in the United States are injured or killed by auto crashes than by terrorists, you need to be aware of the steps you can take to respond to a terrorist event.

Terrorists may use biologic or chemical agents, as well as explosive or nuclear devices. Each has different implications for first responders. During a biologic attack, your role would be very limited. Hospitals and public health agencies would be responsible for identifying the problem and treating infected patients. A chemical attack would be similar to a hazardous materials incident. If you arrive at an emergency scene and find multiple patients suffering similar signs and symptoms, suspect a chemical agent. Stay at a safe location upwind, and request a hazardous materials team for investigation and rescue.

Explosives are a favorite tool of terrorists because they are easy to make or obtain and are often deadly. However, whether the explosion is accidental or the work of terrorists, the injuries suffered by victims are the same. Emergency response to an explosion requires close teamwork between fire, rescue, and law enforcement personnel. The most extreme explosive is a nuclear weapon. Although a nuclear attack is unlikely, you should be aware that a small nuclear device could be anywhere in your community. Know where radioactive materials are stored in your community, such as nuclear power plants or research facilities.

Terrorism is no longer something that happens "somewhere else," as the bombings in Oklahoma City and at the World Trade Centers in New York proved. As a first responder, you should be aware of the possibility of a terrorist event. Realize that a major incident may be dispatched as a routine call. Your skill in assessing scene safety could be vital in saving lives. Be especially alert for clues that point toward special hazards and take advantage of training offered in your local community.

18

Prep Kit

Ready for Review

Ready for Review thoroughly summarizes the chapter.

Ice, water, undersea diving, confined space, and terrorist response rescue situations require extensive skills and special training. It is important to help the victims, but not at the expense of your own safety. In water and ice rescue situations, there are some simple steps you can take to help the victim without endangering yourself. You may not be able to distinguish between the two major medical emergencies created by underwater diving incidents, but you can provide basic care and summon appropriate assistance. In confined space rescue, your primary goals are to call for additional assistance and prevent other people, including yourself, from becoming victims. If you are the first responder after a terrorist attack, you must be alert to scene safety and work within your EMS protocols to assist fire, rescue, and law enforcement personnel.

Vital Vocabulary

The Vital Vocabulary are the key terms for this chapter.

air embolism—*page 430*
decompression sickness (the bends)—*page 430*
flotation device—*page 426*
reach-throw-row-go—*page 426*
riptide—*page 428*

Practice Points

The Practice Points are the key skills you need to know.

1. Assisting with a water rescue.
2. Providing initial treatment for a patient in the water.
3. Assisting with an ice rescue.
4. Assisting with a confined space rescue.

Skill Drills

The Skill Drills provide a visual summary of some of the more complex skills from the skills objectives.

18.2 Turning a Patient in the Water—*page 428*

Ready to Respond

Ready to Respond presents a fictitious scenario to help you review what you learned in this chapter.

Late one night as you drive past a small lake at the edge of town, you are flagged down by an excited teenager who tells you that his buddy was swimming and disappeared under the water. He admits that they had been drinking "a few beers" before the friend decided to start swimming. The friend swam across the lake and was heading back when he disappeared.

1. Your first action should be to

A. Swim out to find him.

B. Determine where he was last seen.

C. Call for assistance.

D. Find a boat to use.

2. The first step you should consider to rescue this person is

A. Go

B. Throw

C. Row

D. Reach

3. If this patient is in shallow water close to shore and is floating on his stomach, how would you turn him over?

A. Lift up on the patient's chest with both hands.

B. Hold the patient by both shoulders, and then push up on one shoulder and down on the other.

C. Support the patient's head and neck with one hand, and then lift the patient's head out of the water with the other hand.

D. Support the patient's head and neck with one hand while rolling the patient over with the other.

4. To open the airway on this patient you should use

A. Head tilt–chin lift maneuver

B. Head-tilt back

C. Jaw-thrust maneuver

D. Rescue breathing

Chapter 19

Supplemental Skills

TECHNOLOGY

- Online Chapter Pretest
- Web Links
- Online Glossary
- Anatomy Review
- Online Review Manual
- CyberClass

www.FirstResponderTraining.com

- Interactive First Responder

Chapter FEATURES

- Skill Drills
- Vital Vocabulary
- Voices of Experience
- Signs and Symptoms
- FYI
- Special Needs
- Safety Tips
- BSI Tips
- Caution
- Checkpoint
- Prep Kit

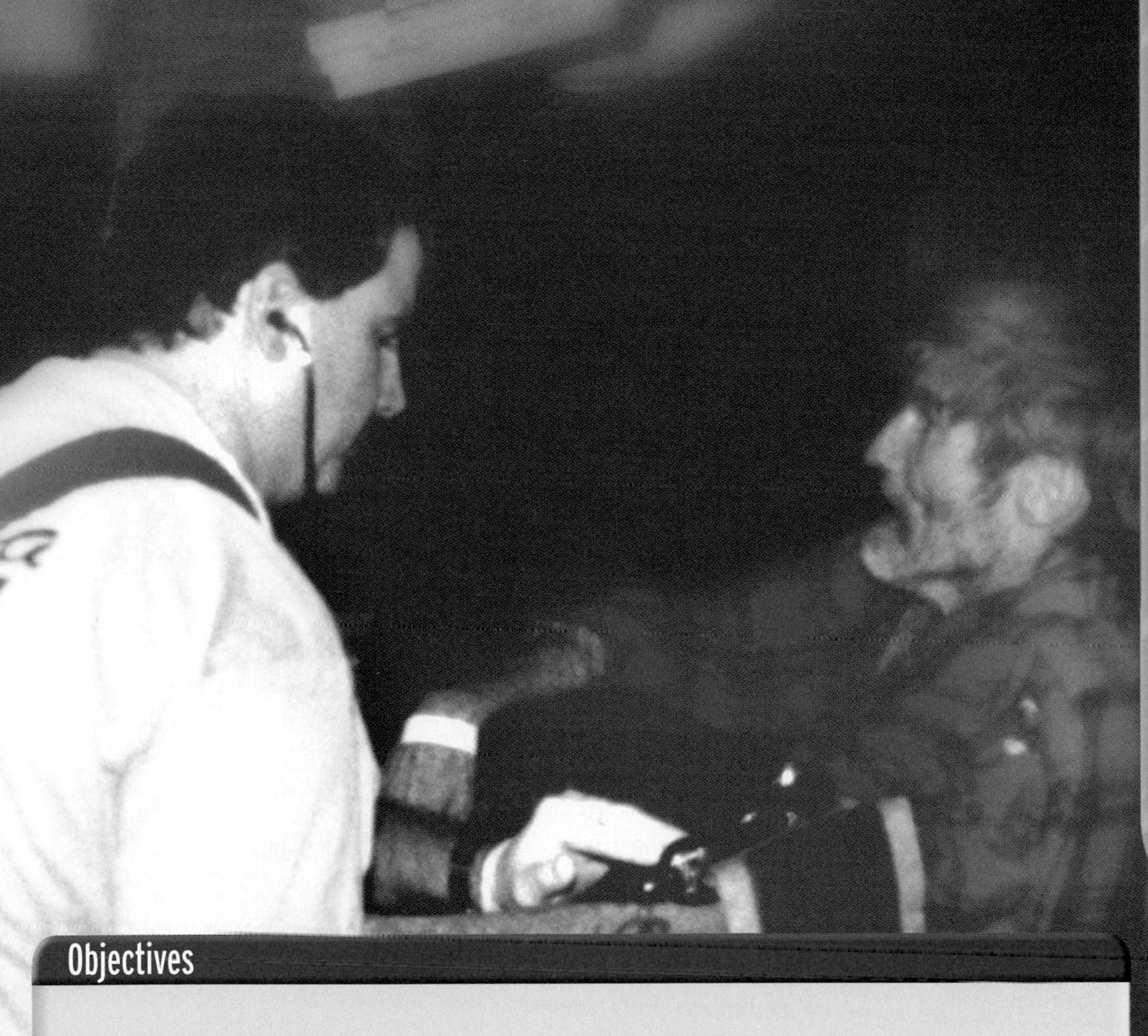

CHAPTER

19

Objectives

Knowledge and Attitude Objectives

After completing this chapter, you will be expected to:

1. Describe how to measure blood pressure by palpation.
2. Describe how to measure blood pressure by auscultation.
3. Describe the indications for using supplemental oxygen.
4. Describe the equipment used to administer oxygen.
5. Describe the safety considerations and hazards of oxygen administration.
6. Explain the benefit of automated external defibrillation in the cardiac chain of survival.
7. Describe the indications and use of a bag-valve-mask device.
8. Describe the indications for the use of automated external defibrillation.
9. Describe the steps in using automated external defibrillation.

Skill Objectives

After completing this chapter, you should be able to:

1. Measure blood pressure by palpation.
2. Measure blood pressure by auscultation.
3. Assemble the equipment used to administer oxygen.
4. Administer supplemental oxygen using a nasal cannula and a nonrebreathing mask.
5. Perform bag-valve-mask ventilation.
6. Perform automated external defibrillation.

In some EMS systems, first responders use supplemental skills to enhance the care they give their patients. These skills include taking blood pressure, administering supplemental oxygen, and performing automated external defibrillation. The topics covered in this chapter are not required by the national curriculum, but they may be adopted by some states or first responder systems. Even if these skills are not used by your system, the information contained in this chapter will help you to assist other EMS personnel in providing care for patients

Blood Pressure

Blood pressure is one way to measure the condition of a patient's circulatory system. High blood pressure may indicate that the patient is susceptible to a stroke. Low blood pressure generally indicates one of various types of shock. (See Chapter 12.)

The blood pressure measurement consists of a reading of two numbers (for example, 120 over 80, or 120/80). These numbers represent the pressures found in the arteries as the heart contracts and relaxes. The numbers are determined by the pressure exerted in millimeters of mercury (mm Hg), as shown on the dial.

The higher number (120 in the example of 120 over 80) is called the **systolic pressure**. This measures the force exerted on the walls of the arteries as the heart contracts.

The lower number (80 in the example of 120 over 80) is known as the **diastolic pressure**. It represents the arterial pressure during the relaxation phase of the heart.

systolic pressure The measurement of blood pressure exerted against the walls of the arteries during contraction of the heart.

diastolic pressure The measurement of pressure exerted against the walls of the arteries while the left ventricle of the heart is at rest.

hypertension High blood pressure.

hypotension Lowered blood pressure.

palpation To examine by touch.

Normal Blood Pressure

Blood pressure ranges vary greatly. Excitement or stress may raise a person's blood pressure. **Hypertension** (high blood pressure) exists when the blood pressure remains greater than 146/96 after repeated examinations over several weeks. Hypertension is a serious medical condition that requires treatment by a physician.

Hypotension (severe low blood pressure) exists when the systolic pressure (the higher number) falls to 90 or below. A patient with this condition is usually in serious trouble. Treatment of shock should be started immediately if the patient is also experiencing other signs of shock (for example, cold, clammy, pale skin or dizziness).

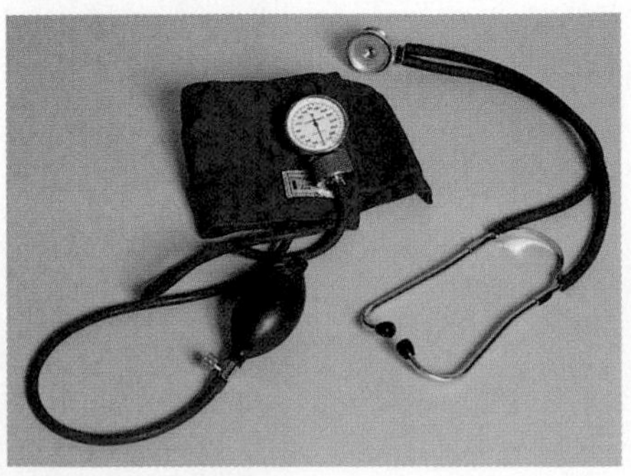

Figure 19.1 Blood pressure cuff and stethoscope.

Taking Blood Pressure by Palpation

To take a patient's blood pressure by **palpation**, apply the blood pressure cuff on the uninjured (or less injured) arm (**Figure 19.1**). Wrap the cuff around the upper arm. The bottom of the cuff should be 1 inch to

2 inches above the crease of the elbow. The arrow should point to the brachial artery, which is located on the medial side of the arm at the crease of the elbow.

Blood pressure cuffs come in different sizes for adults, children, and infants. Be sure to use the appropriate size for your patient, such as a narrow cuff for a child, and an extra-large cuff for an obese adult. Cuffs that are too small may give falsely high readings, and cuffs that are too large may give falsely low readings.

Place the indicator dial in a position where you can easily see the movement of the indicator needle. Turn the control knob on the blood pressure inflator bulb clockwise to close the valve. With the fingers of your other hand, locate the radial pulse at the patient's wrist. Slowly pump up the blood pressure cuff until you can no longer feel the radial pulse. Continue to pump up the cuff for another 30 mm (millimeters) beyond the disappearing point of the radial pulse.

Slowly release the pressure in the cuff by turning the valve counterclockwise (**Figure 19.2**). Continue to feel for the radial pulse, and when you first feel the pulse return, carefully note the position of the indicator needle on the dial. This number is the systolic pressure.

The palpation method of taking blood pressure does not give you a diastolic pressure. You will have only one number, the systolic pressure, instead of the two numbers. Report the results as "the blood pressure by palpation is 90."

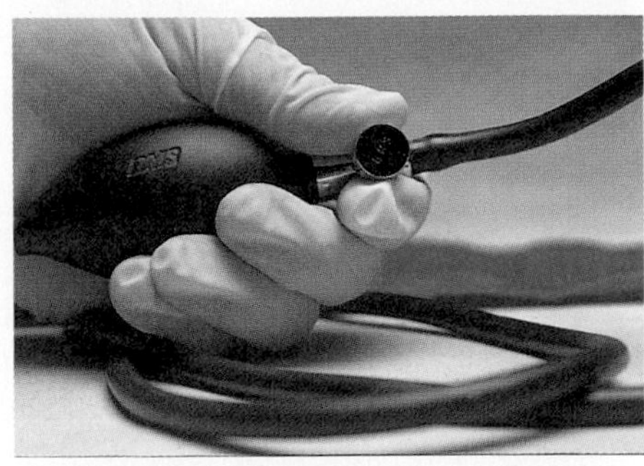

Figure 19.2 Slowly release pressure on the blood pressure cuff by turning the valve counterclockwise.

Taking Blood Pressure by Auscultation

To take blood pressure by **auscultation**, you need both a blood pressure cuff and a stethoscope. Apply the blood pressure cuff in the same manner and position as in the palpation method. After you apply the cuff, locate the brachial artery pulse on the medial side of the arm at the crease of the elbow.

auscultation Listening to sounds with a stethoscope.

Put the earpieces of the stethoscope in your ears with the earpieces pointing forward. Place the diaphragm of the stethoscope over the site of the brachial pulse. Using your index and middle fingers, hold the diaphragm snugly against the patient's arm. Do not use your thumb! If you use your thumb, you may hear your own heartbeat in the stethoscope.

Listen as you inflate the blood pressure cuff. When you can no longer hear the sound of the brachial pulse, note the pressure on the dial.

Continue to inflate the cuff for another 30 mm over the pressure at which the brachial pulse disappeared. Then slowly and smoothly release air from the cuff by opening the control valve, at a rate of 2 to 4 mm per second. Carefully watch the indicator needle, listen for the pulse to return, and note the pressure reading when you can hear the pulse again. This is the systolic pressure.

As the cuff pressure continues to fall (at 2 to 4 mm per second), listen for the moment when the pulse disappears. Note the number when you can no longer hear the pulse; this is the diastolic pressure.

Blood pressure taken by auscultation (**Figure 19.3**) is reported as systolic pressure over diastolic pressure (the larger number over the smaller number) and is always given in even numbers (for example, 120 over 84, 90 over 40, or 186 over 98).

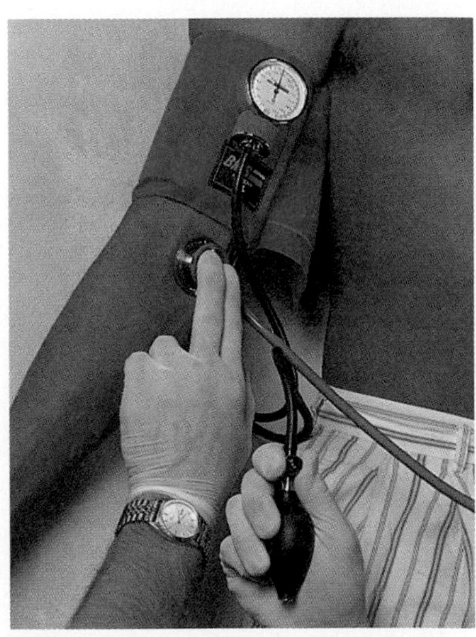

Figure 19.3 Taking blood pressure by auscultation.

It takes practice to become skilled in taking blood pressures. Take every opportunity to practice on as many healthy, uninjured people as possible. Practice on children and the elderly as well as your friends and coworkers. This will help prepare you to measure the blood pressure of a seriously ill or injured patient.

Oxygen Administration

Under normal conditions, your body can operate efficiently using the oxygen that is contained in the air, even though air only contains 21 percent oxygen.

The amount of blood lost after a traumatic injury could mean that insufficient oxygen is delivered to the cells of the body. This results in shock. Administering supplemental oxygen to patients showing signs and symptoms of shock increases the amount of oxygen delivered to the cells of the body and often makes a positive difference in the patient's outcome.

Patients who have suffered a heart attack or stroke or patients who have a chronic heart or lung disease may be unable to get sufficient oxygen from room air. These patients will also benefit from receiving supplemental oxygen.

Not all first responders know how to administer oxygen; however, knowing this skill can be helpful in areas where EMS response may be delayed. By learning this skill, you will be able to assist other members of the EMS team. You should administer oxygen only after receiving proper training and with the approval of your medical director.

THREE COMPONENTS OF OXYGEN EQUIPMENT
(Figure 19.4)

- *Oxygen cylinder*
- *Pressure regulator/flowmeter*
- *Nasal cannula or face mask*

Oxygen Equipment

Oxygen Cylinders

Oxygen is compressed to 2,000 pounds per square inch (psi) and stored in portable cylinders. The portable oxygen cylinders used by most EMS systems are either D or E size. Oxygen cylinders must be marked with a green color and be labeled as medical oxygen. Depending on the flow rate, each cylinder lasts for at least 20 minutes. A valve at the top of the oxygen cylinder allows you to control the flow of oxygen from the cylinder.

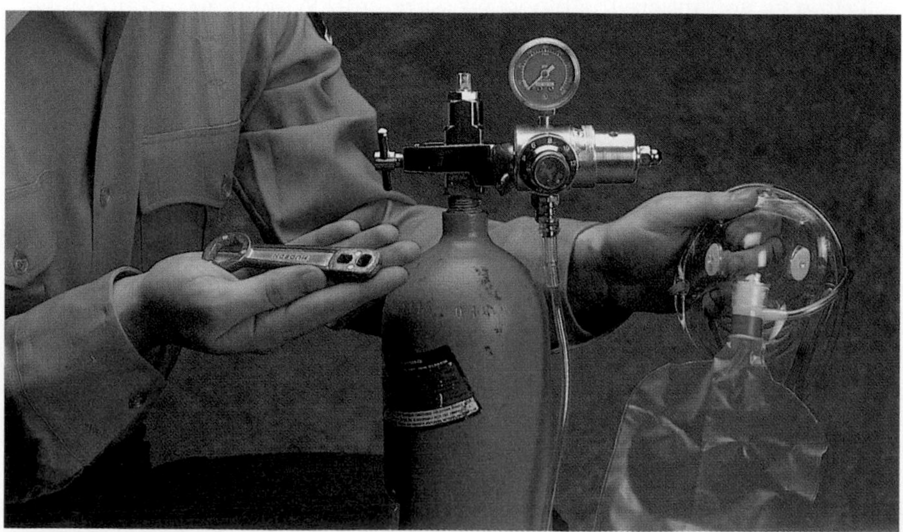

Figure 19.4 Oxygen administration equipment.

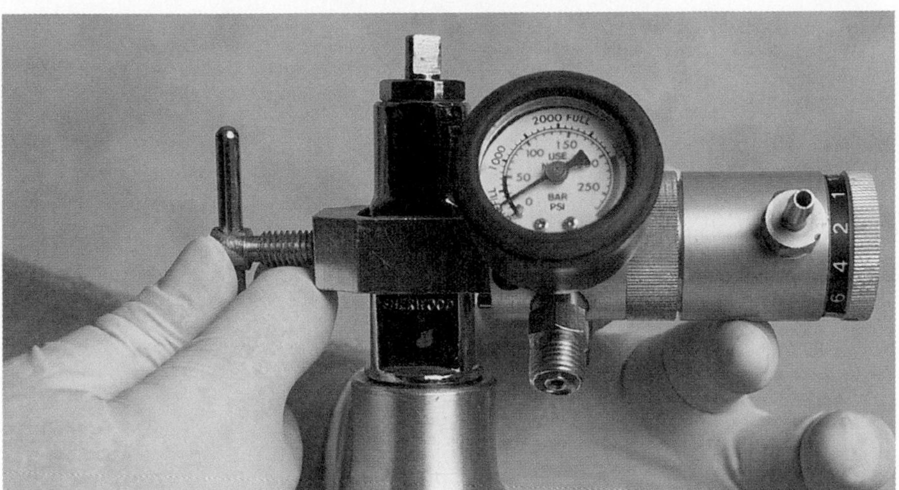

Figure 19.5 Proper position of the pressure regulator/flowmeter on the valve stem.

Pressure Regulator/Flowmeter

Oxygen in the cylinder is stored at 2,000 psi, but it can only be used when the pressure is down to about 50 psi. This is done by the use of a pressure regulator. The regulator and the **flowmeter** are a single unit attached to the outlet of the oxygen cylinder. Once the pressure has been reduced, you can adjust the flowmeter to deliver oxygen at a rate of 2 to 15 liters per minute. Because patients with different medical conditions require different amounts of oxygen, the flowmeter lets you select the proper amount of oxygen to administer. A gasket between the cylinder and the pressure regulator/flowmeter ensures a tight seal and maintains the high pressure inside the cylinder (**Figure 19.5**).

flowmeter A device on oxygen cylinders used to control and measure the flow of oxygen.

nasal cannula A clear plastic tube used to deliver oxygen that fits onto the patient's nose.

face mask A clear plastic mask used for oxygen administration that covers the mouth and nose.

Nasal Cannulas and Face Masks

The third part of an oxygen delivery system is a device that ensures the oxygen is delivered to the patient, and is not lost in the air. **Nasal cannulas** have two small holes, which fit into the patient's nostrils. Nasal cannulas are used to deliver medium concentrations of oxygen (35 percent to 50 percent). **Face masks** are placed over the patient's face to deliver oxygen through the patient's mouth and nostrils. Nonrebreathing masks are most commonly used by first responders. They deliver high concentrations of oxygen (up to 90 percent). These two oxygen-delivery devices are discussed more fully in the section on administering supplemental oxygen.

Safety Considerations

Oxygen does not burn or explode by itself. However, it actively supports combustion and can quickly turn a small spark or flame into a serious fire. Therefore, all sparks, heat, flames, and oily substances must be kept away from oxygen equipment. Smoking should never be permitted around oxygen equipment.

The pressurized cylinders are also hazardous because the high pressure in an oxygen cylinder can cause an explosion if the cylinder is damaged. Be sure the oxygen cylinder will not fall. If the shut-off valve at the top of the cylinder is damaged, the cylinder can take off like a rocket. Oxygen cylinders should be kept inside sturdy carrying cases that protect the cylinder and regulator/flowmeter. Handle the cylinder carefully to guard against damage.

Safety Tips

Avoid using oxygen around fire or flames. Keep oxygen cylinders secured to minimize the danger of explosion.

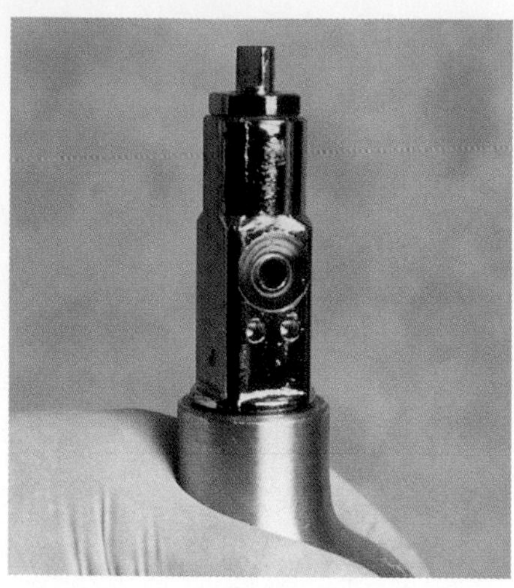

Figure 19.6 A valve stem with pin-index holes.

Administering Supplemental Oxygen

To administer supplemental oxygen, place the regulator/flowmeter over the stem of the oxygen cylinder, and line up the pins on the pin indexing system correctly (**Figure 19.6**). Be sure to check for the mandatory gasket. Tighten the securing screw firmly by hand. With the special key or wrench provided, turn the cylinder valve two turns counterclockwise to allow oxygen from the cylinder to enter the regulator/flowmeter.

Check the gauge on the pressure regulator/flowmeter to see how much oxygen pressure remains in the cylinder. If the cylinder contains less than 500 psi, the amount of oxygen in the cylinder is too low for emergency use and should be replaced with a full (2,000 psi) cylinder.

To administer oxygen, you will need to adjust the flowmeter to deliver the desired liter-per-minute flow of oxygen. The patient's condition and the type of oxygen delivery device you use (a mask or a nasal cannula) dictates the proper flow. When the oxygen flow begins, place the face mask or nasal cannula onto the patient's head.

Nasal Cannula

A nasal cannula is a simple oxygen-delivery device. It consists of two small prongs that fit into the patient's nostrils and a strap that holds the cannula on the patient's face (**Figure 19.7**). A cannula delivers low-flow oxygen at 2 to 6 liters per minute and in concentrations of 35 percent to 50 percent oxygen. Low-flow oxygen can be used for fairly stable patients such as those with slight chest pain, or mild shortness of breath.

To use nasal cannula, first adjust the liter flow to 2 to 6 liters per minute and then apply the cannula to the patient. The cannula should fit snugly but should not be tight.

Nonrebreathing Mask

A nonrebreathing mask consists of connecting tubing, a reservoir bag, one-way valves, and a face piece (**Figure 19.8**). It is used to deliver high flows of oxygen, at 8 to 15 liters per minute. A nonrebreathing face mask can deliver concentrations of oxygen as high as 90 percent. This mask works by storing oxygen in the reservoir bag. When the patient inhales, oxygen is drawn from the reservoir bag. When the patient exhales, the air is exhausted through the one-way valves on the side of the mask.

Nonrebreathing face masks should be used for patients who require higher flows of oxygen. These include patients experiencing serious shortness of breath, severe chest pain, carbon monoxide poisoning, and congestive heart failure (CHF). Patients who are showing signs and symptoms of shock should also be treated with high-flow oxygen from a nonrebreathing face mask.

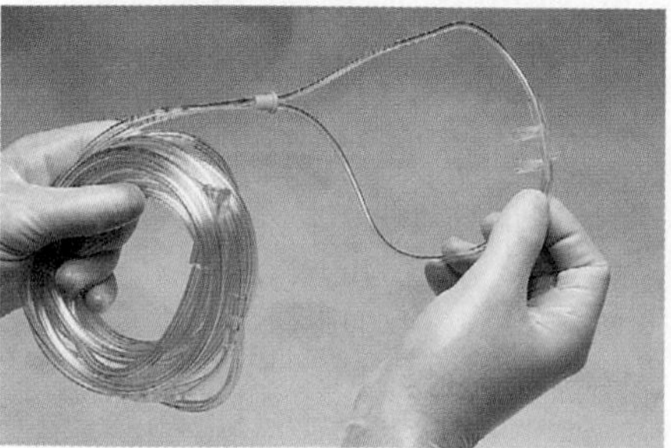

Figure 19.7 A nasal cannula.

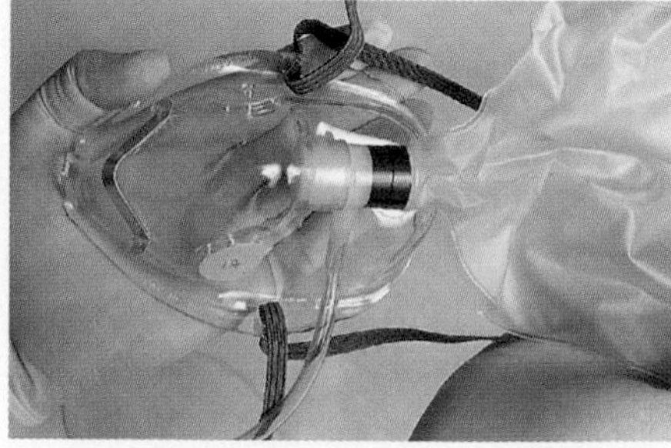

Figure 19.8 A nonrebreathing oxygen mask.

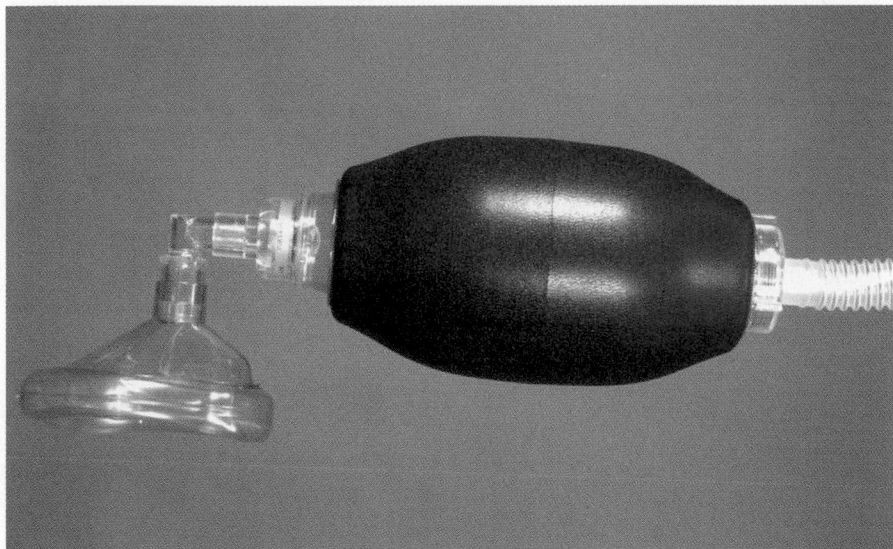

Figure 19.9 A bag-valve-mask device.

To use a nonrebreathing mask, first adjust the oxygen flow to 8 to 15 liters per minute to inflate the reservoir bag before putting it on the patient. After the bag inflates, place the mask over the patient's face. Adjust the straps to secure a snug fit. Adjust the liter flow to keep the bag at least partially inflated while the patient inhales.

Hazards of Supplemental Oxygen

Supplemental oxygen can be life saving, but it must be used carefully in order to be safe. Although this gives you a basic outline on setting up oxygen equipment, you will need additional classwork and practical training before you administer oxygen in emergency situations.

Bag-Valve-Mask Device

The **bag-valve-mask (BVM) device** has three parts: a self-inflating bag, one-way valves, and a face mask (**Figure 19.9**). To use this device, a rescuer places the mask over the face of the patient and makes a tight seal. Squeezing the bag pushes air through a one-way valve, through the face mask, and into the patient's mouth and nose. As the patient passively exhales, a second one-way valve near the face mask releases the air. The self-inflating bag refills when the rescuer releases the pressure on it. Without supplemental oxygen, the BVM device delivers 21 percent oxygen, the percentage of oxygen in room air. Supplemental oxygen is usually added to the BVM device. A BVM device can deliver up to 90 percent oxygen to a patient, if 10 to 15 liters per minute of oxygen is supplied into the reservoir bag. Many BVM devices are designed to be discarded after a single use.

bag-valve-mask (BVM) device A patient ventilation device which consists of a bag, one-way valves, and a face mask, which can deliver 90 percent oxygen to a patient.

The BVM device is used for the same purpose as a mouth-to-mask device, to ventilate a nonbreathing patient. Although the BVM device can administer up to 90 percent oxygen when used with supplemental oxygen, there are two disadvantages to its use. A single rescuer may find it difficult to maintain a seal between the face and mask with one hand. Additionally, the BVM device may be hard for people with small hands to use, because they may not be able to squeeze the bag hard enough to get an adequate volume of air into the patient.

Technique

The beginning steps for using a BVM device are the same steps you use for performing rescue breathing. Check to determine if the patient is unresponsive. Open the patient's airway using the head tilt–chin lift technique or the jaw-thrust technique for patients with suspected neck or spinal injuries. See if the patient is breathing: look at the patient's chest, listen for the sound of air movement, and feel for the movement of air on the side of your face and ear. If the patient is not breathing, consider using an oral or nasal airway. The specific steps for using a BVM device are listed below and shown in the Skill Drill (**Figure 19.10**).

1. Kneel above the patient's head. This position will enable you to keep the airway open, make a tight seal on the mask, and squeeze the bag. Maintain the patient's neck in an extended position. The BVM device does not maintain the patient's airway in an open position. You must continue to stabilize the head and maintain the head either in an extended position for the head tilt–chin lift or in a neutral position for the jaw-thrust technique.
2. Open the patient's mouth and check for fluids, foreign bodies, or dentures. Suction if needed. Consider the use of an oral or nasal airway.
3. Select the proper mask size. The mask should be big enough to seal over the bridge of the patient's nose and fit in the groove between the lower lip and the chin. A mask that is too small or too large may make it impossible to maintain a seal.
4. Place the mask over the patient's face. Start by putting the angled or grooved end of the mask over the bridge of the nose. Then bring the bottom of the mask against the groove between the lower lip and the chin.
5. Seal the mask. Place the middle, ring, and little fingers of one hand under the angle of the jaw. Lift up on the jaw. Make a "C" with the index finger and thumb of the same hand, and place them over the mask. Clamp the mask by lifting the jaw and bringing the mask in contact with the jaw. Continue to hold the mask in position.
6. Squeeze the bag. Using your other hand, squeeze the bag once every 5 seconds. Try to squeeze a large volume of air. Squeeze every 3 seconds for infants and children.
7. Check for chest rise. As you squeeze the bag, watch for a rise in the chest. If you do not see the chest rise, air is probably leaking around the mask or there is an obstruction in the airway. If air is leaking around the mask, try to make a better seal between the mask and the patient's jaw. If you suspect an airway obstruction follow the steps you learned in Chapter 6.
8. Add supplemental oxygen. Using a BVM device without supplemental oxygen supplies the patient with 21 percent oxygen. By adding 10 to 15 liters per minute of oxygen to the BVM device, you can increase the oxygen concentration to 90 percent. Adjust the liter flow on the pressure regulator/flowmeter to deliver between 10 and 15 liters per minute and connect the oxygen tubing from the flowmeter outlet to the inlet nipple on the BVM device. This higher percentage of oxygen is beneficial for a nonbreathing patient.

Skill Drill

Figure 19.10 Using a Bag-Valve-Mask Device with One Rescuer

1
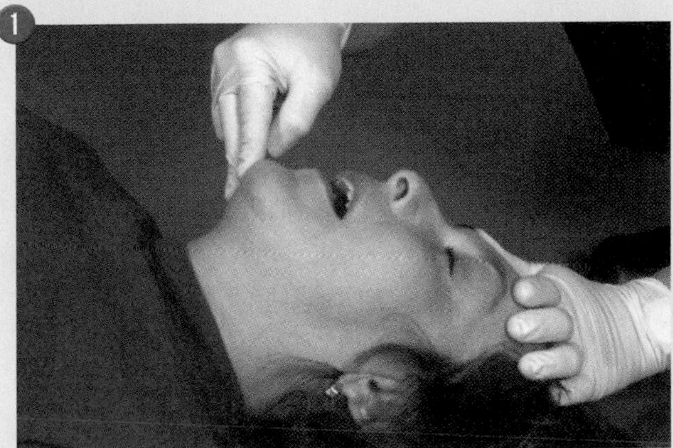
Kneel at patient's head and maintain an open airway. Check the patient's mouth for fluids, foreign bodies, and dentures.

2
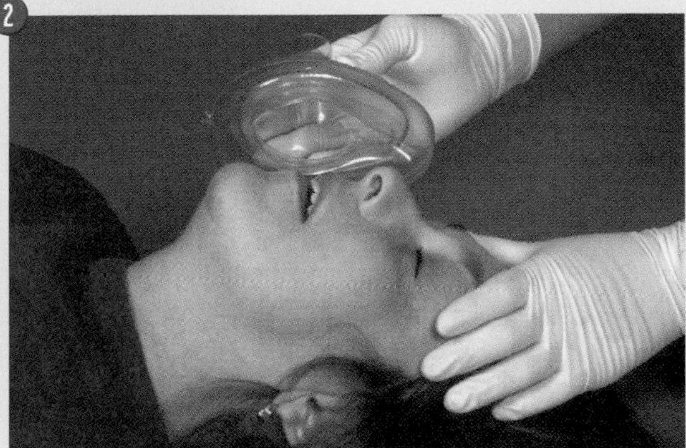
Select the proper mask size.

3
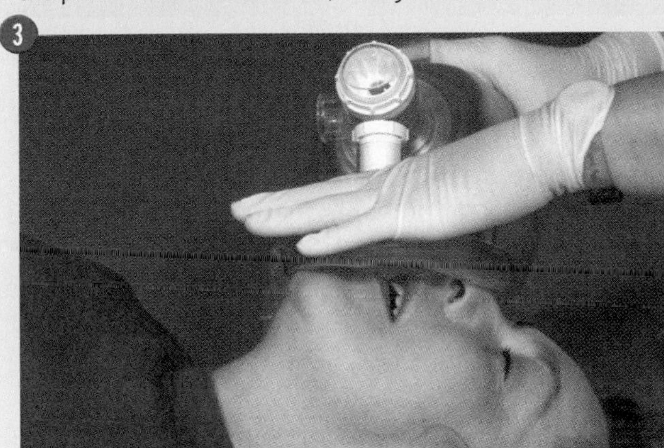
Place the mask over the patient's face.

4
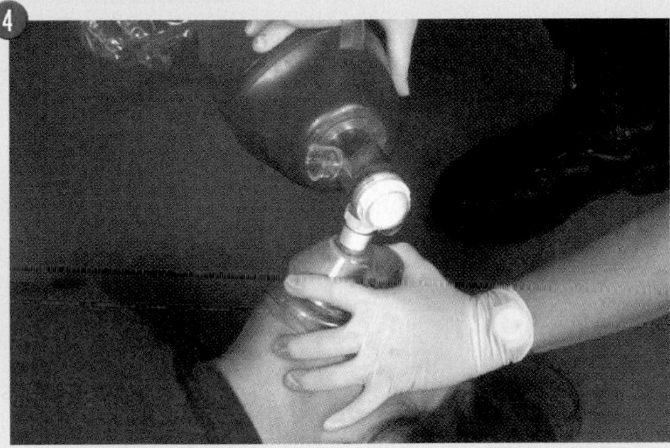
Seal the mask.

5
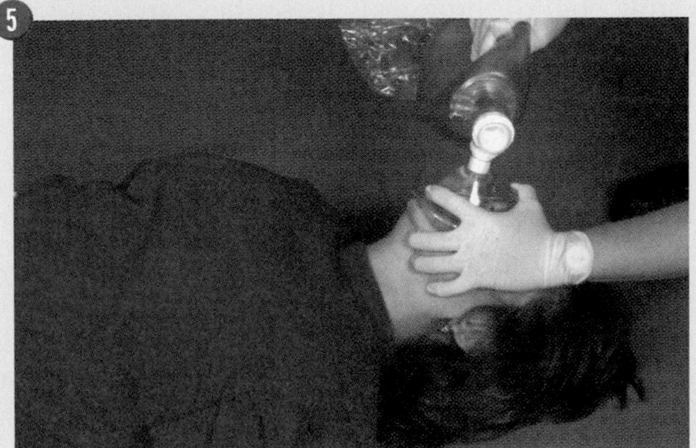
Squeeze the bag with your other hand. Check for chest rise.

6
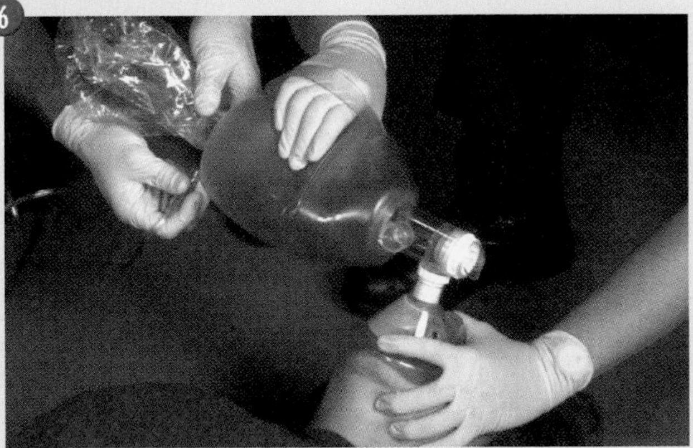
Add supplemental oxygen.

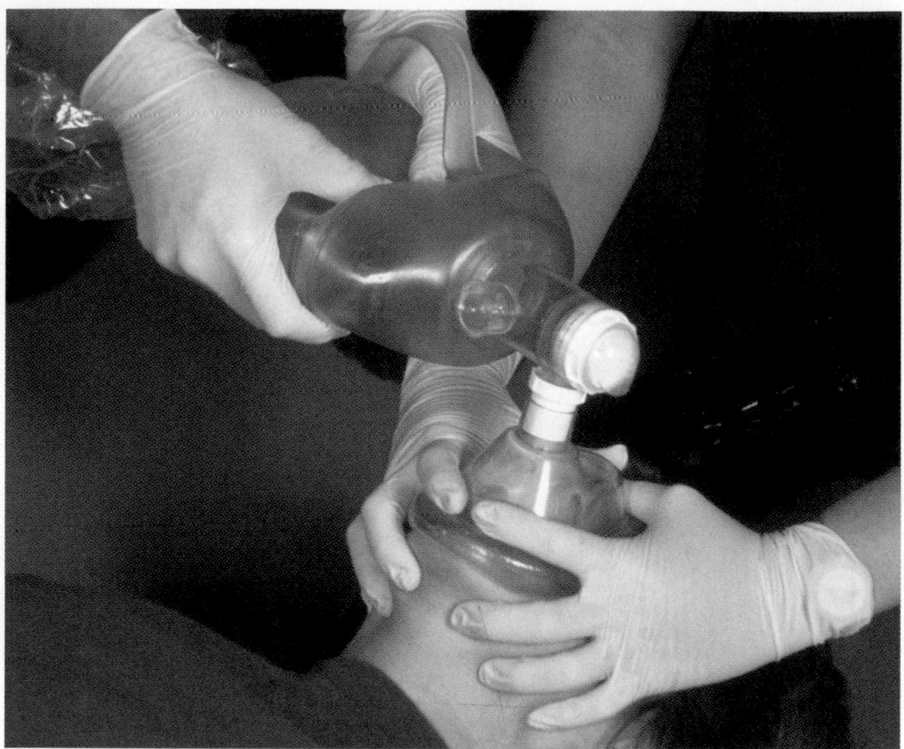

Figure 19.11 Using a BVM device with two rescuers.

Note: If paramedics have inserted an endotracheal tube down the patient's windpipe (trachea), the BVM device is connected directly to the end of the endotraceal tube. In this case no facemask is needed. When you squeeze the BVM device, you force air directly into the patient's lungs. You should receive instruction in this type of ventilation if you will be performing it.

With sufficient training and practice, one person can ventilate a patient using a BVM device. However, it is difficult to maintain a good seal and squeeze the bag with only two hands. A BVM device should be done as a two-person operation if additional rescuers are present (**Figure 19.11**). With two rescuers, one person squeezes the bag and the other person uses both hands to seal the mask to the patient. Use the middle, ring and little fingers of both hands under the angles of the jaw, and use the index fingers and thumbs of both hands to form two "Cs" around the facemask. Most people can seal the mask much more easily using both hands.

Using the BVM device requires proper training and practice. The BVM device can be a life-saving tool. Your EMS service may use BVM devices for nonbreathing patients. Or you may be asked to assist EMT-Bs or paramedics in ventilating nonbreathing patients so they can perform other needed skills. Check with your supervisor or medical director to learn the protocols for your service.

Early Defibrillation by First Responders

ventricular fibrillation An uncoordinated muscular quivering of the heart; the most common abnormal rhythm causing cardiac arrest.

More than 50 percent of all out-of-hospital cardiac arrest patients have an irregular heart electrical rhythm called **ventricular fibrillation**. This condition, often referred to as "V-fib," is the rapid, disorganized, and ineffective vibration of the heart. An electric shock applied to the heart will defibrillate it and reorganize the vibrations into effective heartbeats.

The American Heart Association's chain of survival recognizes the importance of early cardiac defibrillation and advanced life support. This chain includes the early recognition of cardiac arrest and access to

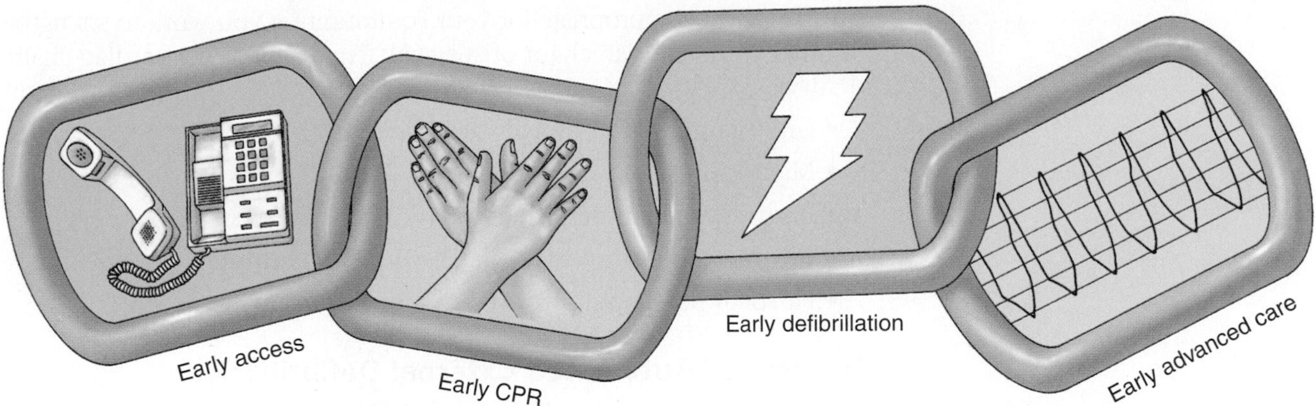

Figure 19.12 Cardiac chain of survival.

EMS, early citizen CPR, early defibrillation by first responders or other EMS providers, and early advanced care. A patient in cardiac arrest stands the greatest chance for survival when early defibrillation is available. The cardiac chain of survival is shown in **Figure 19.12**.

The first responder is often the first emergency care provider to reach a patient who has collapsed in cardiac arrest. The first responder can start CPR and try to keep the patient's brain and heart supplied with oxygen. In many EMS systems, that is all the first responder can do. This can be lifesaving care if paramedics respond promptly with advanced life support.

Increasing numbers of EMS systems, however, are equipping first responders with **automated external defibrillators (AEDs)**. These machines accurately identify ventricular fibrillation and advise you to deliver a defibrillating shock if needed. Such equipment allows the first responder to combine effective CPR with early defibrillation to restore an organized heartbeat (**Figure 19.13**).

automated external defibrillator (AED) Portable battery-powered device that recognizes fibrillation and advises when a countershock is indicated. Delivers an electric charge to patients with ventricular fibrillation.

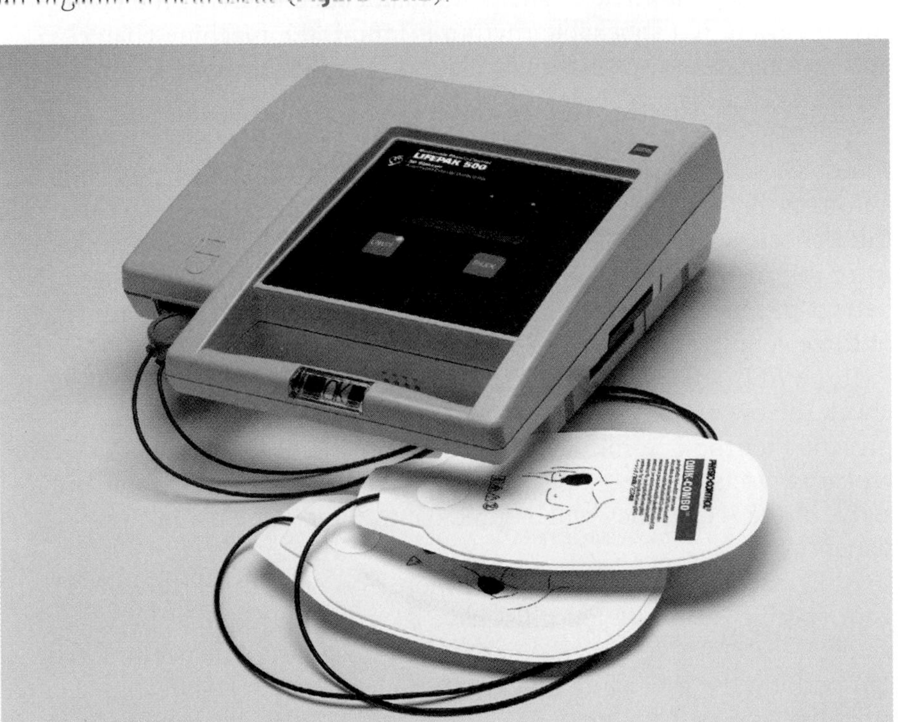

Figure 19.13 An automated external defibrillator.

AEDs may be appropriate for your community if you work to strengthen all links of the cardiac chain of survival. The links of the cardiac chain of survival include:

- Citizens trained to quickly access the EMS system.
- Many citizens trained to perform CPR.
- Early automated defibrillation available from first responders.
- Advanced life support available within 10 minutes.
- Hospital personnel prepared to give prompt cardiac care.

Performing Automated External Defibrillation

If you arrive on the scene before an AED is available, check the patient for responsiveness, airway, breathing, and circulation (**Figure 19.14, step 1**). If the patient is unresponsive, is not breathing, and has no pulse, you should begin CPR, as outlined in Chapters 6, 7, and 8 (**Figure 19.14, step 2**). If you are by yourself and are trained in using an AED, first assess the patient's ABCs. If the patient is in cardiac arrest, begin the AED procedure before starting CPR.

Once the AED is brought to the scene, quickly attach it to the patient (**Figure 19.14, step 3**). Stop CPR and remove your hands from the patient before you turn on the defibrillator (**Figure 19.14, step 4**). No one should touch the patient once the machine has been turned on. The machine analyzes for a shockable rhythm (**Figure 19.14, step 5**). If a shockable rhythm is found, the machine quickly recommends defibrillation (**Figure 19.14, step 6**). You should first say, "Clear the patient" and ensure that no one is touching the patient before you press the "shock" button on the defibrillator.

After the first shock is delivered, immediately press the "analyze" button on the defibrillator. The defibrillator then analyzes the heart rhythm again. If a shockable rhythm is found, the machine charges and recommends a second defibrillation. The first responder should then press the "shock" button a second time.

This procedure of "analyze" and "shock" can be repeated up to three times. These three shocks are called "stacked shocks." Some machines automatically analyze and recommend shocks three times. After the third shock is delivered, some machines time a 60-second interval. After this interval has passed, the AED recommends that you check the patient or push the "analyze" button again and perform a second set of three countershocks.

If the AED advises no shock, check the pulse. If the pulse is present, check the breathing. Support ventilations if necessary. If no pulse is present after the one-minute interval, resume CPR for one minute, and repeat two sets of three shocks. When advanced life support personnel arrive at the scene, they will assume control and responsibility for the patient's care.

AED machines vary in their operation. You need to learn how to use your specific AED and you must have the training required by your medical director in order to practice this procedure. Practice until you can perform the procedure quickly and safely. Because the recommended guidelines for performing AED change, you should always follow the most current American Heart Association guidelines.

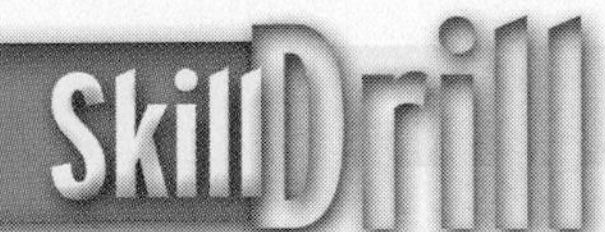

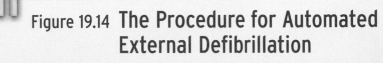

Figure 19.14 The Procedure for Automated External Defibrillation

1

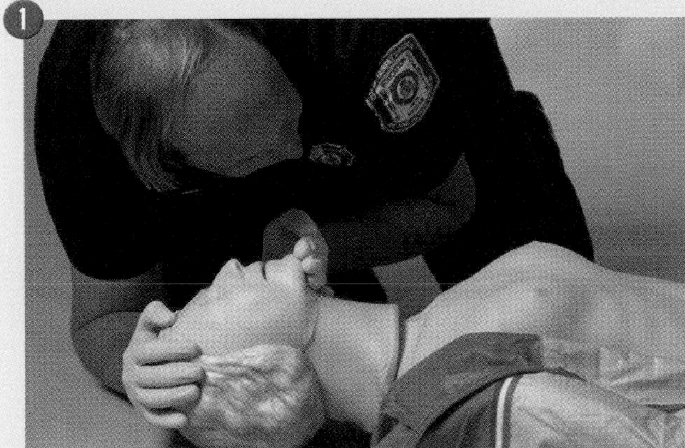

Check ABCs—look, listen, feel.

2

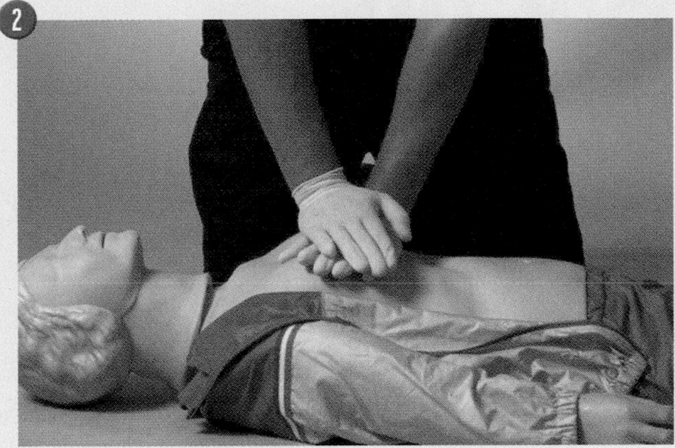

If patient is pulseless and not breathing, begin CPR.

3

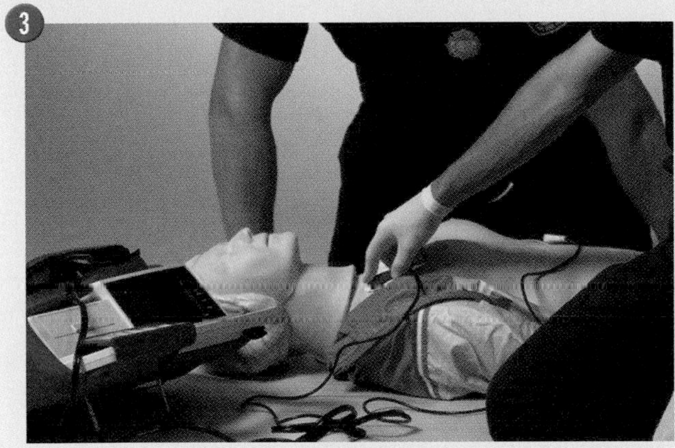

Apply adhesive electrode pads and connect to defibrillator.

4

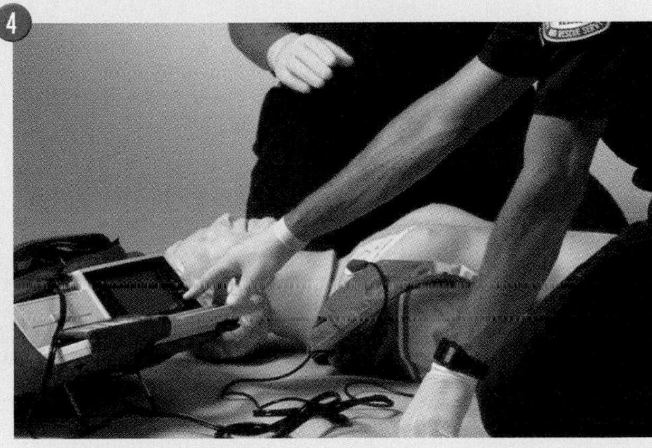

Turn defibrillator on.

5

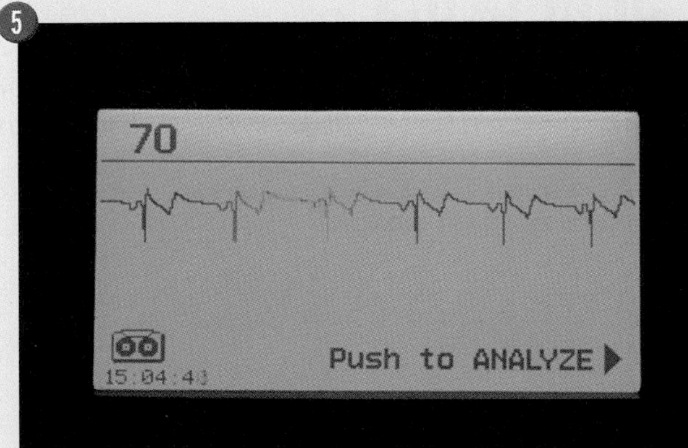

Allow machine to analyze rhythm.

6

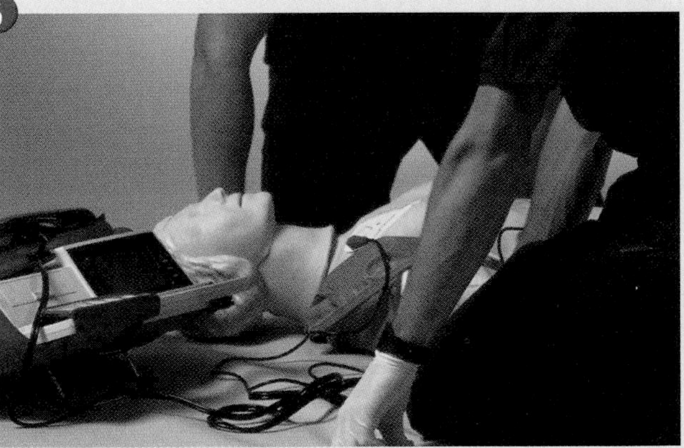

Determine if shock is indicated by the defibrillator. If shock is indicated, defibrillate the patient.

19

Prep Kit

Ready for Review

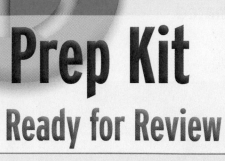

Ready for Review thoroughly summarizes the chapter.

This chapter covers the procedures used to measure blood pressure by palpation and auscultation, to administer oxygen by face mask and nasal cannula, and to perform automated external defibrillation. Depending on the role of the first responder in your EMS system, you may need a special class to practice any or all of these skills.

Vital Vocabulary

The Vital Vocabulary are the key terms for this chapter.

auscultation—*page 439*
automated external defibrillator (AED)—*page 447*
bag-valve-mask (BVM) device—*page 443*
diastolic pressure—*page 438*
face mask—*page 441*
flowmeter—*page 441*
hypertension—*page 438*
hypotension—*page 438*
nasal cannula—*page 441*
palpation—*page 438*
systolic pressure—*page 438*
ventricular fibrillation—*page 446*

Practice Points

The Practice Points are the key skills you need to know.

1. Measuring blood pressure by palpation.
2. Measuring blood pressure by auscultation.
3. Assembling the equipment used to administer oxygen.
4. Administering supplemental oxygen using a nasal cannula and a nonrebreathing mask.
5. Performing automated external defibrillation.

Skill Drills

The Skill Drills provide a visual summary of some of the more complex skills from the skills objectives.

19.10 Using a Bag-Valve-Mask Device with One Rescuer—*page 445*

19.14 The Procedure for Automated External Defibrillation—*page 449*

Ready to Respond

Ready to Respond presents a fictitious scenario to help you review what you learned in this chapter.

You are called to a house for a sick person. When you arrive, you find a 78-year-old man sitting in a chair. You note that he is short of breath and is breathing 42 times a minute. Your partner, who is taking the lead in assessing Mr. Schmidt, asks you to "get a set of vital signs and put him on oxygen."

1. You should

A. Take the vital signs first

B. Administer supplemental oxygen first and then obtain vital signs

2. What device would probably be best for administering oxygen to this patient?

A. Nasal cannula

B. Rebreathing face mask

C. Nonrebreathing face mask

D. Bag-valve-mask device

3. What is the proper flow rate of oxygen for this device?

A. 2 to 4 liters per minute

B. 4 to 6 liters per minute

C. 6 to 10 liters per minute

D. 8 to 15 liters per minute

4. Which means of taking blood pressure would be best?

A. Palpation

B. Brachial

C. Auscultation

D. Femoral

MODULE 8 QuickQuiz

Supplemental Skills

1. Disabilities that occur with age include
   1. decreased hearing
   2. impairment of sight
   3. slowed movement
   4. senility

   A. none of the above

   B. 2, 3, 4

   C. 1, 2, 4

   D. all of the above

2. As you begin to examine an elderly man who is dressed with several layers of clothing you should

   A. remove his clothing only if you can move him to a warm place

   B. do a less than complete examination

   C. remove a much of his clothing as necessary to examine him properly

   D. perform an exam through his clothing

3. A person who points to his ear and shakes his head "no" may be trying to tell you that he:

   A. is senile

   B. wants you to repeat what you said

   C. is deaf

   D. does not understand English

4. When guiding a blind person, you should

   A. walk slightly behind the patient

   B. walk slightly in front of the patient

   C. talk loudly so the patient can hear you

   D. have the patient use their cane

5. If a patient is agitated, disruptive, or violent you should

   A. approach the patient slowly

   B. ask the family or bystanders for help

   C. wait for adequate assistance

   D. be aggressive so the patient will know you are in charge

6. As a first responder, your first goal in special rescue situations is

   A. call for additional resources

   B. prevent bystanders from getting injured

   C. rescue the patient

   D. assessing the scene to ensure your safety

7. List, in order, the four steps you should follow when attempting water rescue.

____

____

____

____

8. Initial treatment of a person in the water includes all but which of the following?

A. support the back and neck and turn the patient face up

B. open the airway using the jaw-thrust technique

C. performing rescue breathing

D. performing chest compressions

9. If you must go onto the ice to attempt a rescue, you should try to spread your weight over a wider area.

A. true

B. false

10. Deadly hazards that may be present in confined spaces include

1. insufficient oxygen
2. darkness
3. poisonous gases
4. danger of collapse

A. 1, 2, 4

B. 1, 3. 4

C. 3, 4

D. all of the above

11. Match each term in the left column with the appropriate definition in the right column.

1. systolic	A. high blood pressure
2. hypotension	B. the lower number in a blood pressure
3. auscultation	C. taking blood pressure by feeling a pulse
4. palpation	D. the upper number in a blood pressure
5. diastolic	E. low blood pressure
6. hypertension	F. pulse sound heard with a stethoscope

Continued.

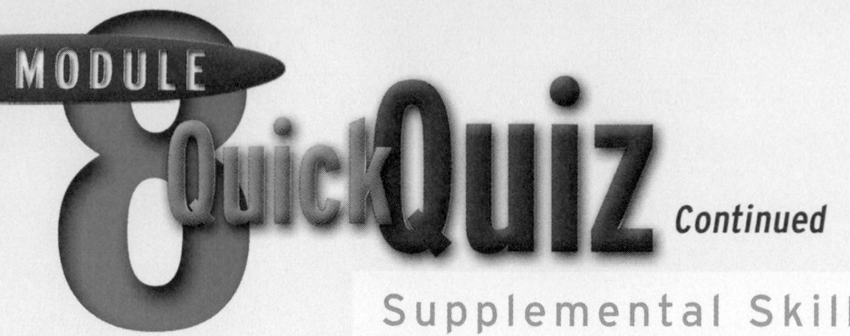

Module 8 QuickQuiz *Continued*

Supplemental Skills

12. Hypotension exists when the systolic pressure falls below

A. 70

B. 80

C. 90

D. 95

13. A patient who has signs and symptoms of shock should have oxygen administered by

A. nasal cannula

B. nonrebreathing face mask

C. bag-valve-mask device

D. mouth-to-mask device

14. A bag-valve-mask device can deliver up to ____ percent of oxygen.

A. 35 to 50

B. 50 to 65

C. 90

D. 100

15. Which of the following statements about defibrillation is true?

A. it is a serious condition of the heart known as "V-fib"

B. it is a procedure that delivers an electrical shock to the heart

C. it is a rapid disorganized ineffective pulsation of the heart that occurs when a person is in cardiac arrest

D. it identifies the ineffective pulsations of the heart in cardiac arrest and reorganizes them into effective heartbeats

1. D **2.** C **3.** C **4.** B **5.** C **6.** D **7.** reach, throw, row, go **8.** D **9.** A **10.** B **11.** 1=D, 2=E, 3=F, 4=C, 5=B, 6=A **12.** C **13.** B **14.** C **15.** B

Additional Photo Credits

Module Opener 1
© Craig Jackson, In the Dark Photography

Chapter Opener 1
© Kenneth Murray, Photo Researchers, Inc.
p. 5 © Craig Jackson, In the Dark Photography
p. 9 © Bob Daemmrich, Stock Boston
p. 9 © Craig Jackson, In the Dark Photography

Chapter Opener 2
© Mike Heller, 911 Pictures
p. 20 © Bill Brent, The Boston Globe
p. 30 © Mark Gibson

Chapter Opener 3
© Audrey Gibson
p. 41 © James Shaffer, PhotoEdit
p. 43 © Hiroyuki Matsumoto, Tony Stone Images

Chapter Opener 4
© Wendy Campbell, Outside Images, Picture Quest

Chapter Opener 5
© Craig Jackson, In the Dark Photography

Module Opener 2
© 2000 PhotoDisc, Inc.

Chapter Opener 6
© Craig Jackson, In the Dark Photography

Module Opener 3
© Tim Parker

Chapter Opener 7
© Craig Jackson, In the Dark Photography

Module Opener 4
© 2000 PhotoDisc, Inc.

Chapter Opener 8
© Mike Heller, 911 Pictures

Module Opener 5
© 2000 PhotoDisc, Inc.

Chapter Opener 9
© Craig Jackson, In the Dark Photography

Chapter Opener 10
© Craig Jackson, In the Dark Photography
p. 226 © Doug Martin, Photo Researchers, Inc.
p. 226 © Howard Paul

Chapter Opener 11
© Craig Jackson, In the Dark Photography
p. 245 Courtesy MIEMSS

Chapter Opener 12
© Craig Jackson, In the Dark Photography
p. 265 © Jones and Bartlett, Inc.

Chapter Opener 13
© Craig Jackson, In the Dark Photography

Module Opener 6
© 2000 PhotoDisc, Inc.

Chapter Opener 14
© Jones and Bartlett Publishers, Inc.

Chapter Opener 15
© Tom Carter, 911 Pictures

Module Opener 7
© 2000 PhotoDisc, Inc.

Chapter Opener 16
© Mike Heller, 911 Pictures
p. 383 © Matthew McVay, Tony Stone Worldwide
p. 395 © Linda Gheen
p. 398 © U. S. Department of Transportation
p. 399 © U.S. Department of Transportation
p. 401 © Mac Medan, Corbis/Sygma

Module Opener 8
© 2000 PhotoDisc, Inc.

Chapter Opener 17
© Mike Heller, 911 Pictures

Chapter Opener 18
© Thomas Gaulke, 911 Pictures
p. 432 © Bill Aaron, PhotoEdit, Picture Quest; © Michael Siluk, The Picture Cube; © Chris Rogers, Rainbow, Picture Quest

Chapter Opener 19
© Craig Jackson, In the Dark Photography

Additional photo research: Carol Wendel

Glossary

abandonment Failure of the first responder to continue emergency medical treatment until relieved by someone with the same or higher level of training.

abdomen The body cavity, lying between the thorax and the pelvis that contains the major organs of digestion and excretion.

abdominal breathing Breathing using only the diaphragm.

abrasion Loss of skin as a result of a body part being rubbed or scraped across a rough or hard surface.

acceptance The fifth stage of the grief process, when the person experiencing grief recognizes the finality of the grief-causing event.

acid A chemical substance with a pH of less than 7.0 that can cause severe burns.

acute abdomen The sudden onset of abdominal pain caused by disease or trauma that irritates the lining of the abdominal cavity and requires immediate medical or surgical treatment.

advanced life support (ALS) The use of specialized equipment such as cardiac monitors, defibrillators, intravenous fluids, drug infusion, and endotracheal intubation to stabilize patients who have experienced sudden illness or injury.

air embolism A bubble of air obstructing a blood vessel.

airway The passages from the openings of the mouth and nose to the air sacs in the lungs through which air enters and leaves the lungs.

airway obstruction Partial or complete obstruction of the respiratory passages resulting from blockage by food, small objects, or vomitus.

alcohol A liquid obtained by fermentation of carbohydrates with yeast.

alveoli The air sacs of the lungs where the exchange of oxygen and carbon dioxide takes place.

amphetamines Stimulants that produce a general mood elevation, improve task performance, suppress appetite, or prevent sleepiness.

anaphylactic shock Severe shock caused by an allergic reaction to food, medicine, or insect stings.

anger The second stage of the grief reaction, when the person suffering grief becomes upset at the grief-causing event or other situation.

anterior The front surface of the body.

angina pectoris Chest pain with squeezing or tightness in the chest caused by an inadequate flow of blood to the heart muscle.

anus The distal or terminal ending of the gastrointestinal tract.

appropriate medical facility A hospital with adequate medical resources to provide continuing care to sick or injured patients who are transported after field treatment by first responders.

arm Part of the upper extremity that extends from the shoulder to the elbow.

arm-to-arm drag An emergency patient move that consists of the rescuer grasping the patient's arms from behind; used to remove a patient from a hazardous place.

arterial bleeding Serious bleeding from an artery in which blood frequently pulses or spurts from an open wound.

aspiration Breathing in foreign matter such as food, drink, or vomitus into the airway or lungs.

aspirator A suction device.

assessment-based care A system of patient evaluation in which the chief complaint of the patient and other signs and symptoms are gathered and the care given is based on this information rather than on a formal diagnosis.

asthma An acute spasm of the smaller air passages marked by labored breathing and wheezing.

atherosclerosis A disease characterized by a thickening and destruction of the arterial walls and caused by fatty deposits within them; the arteries lose the ability to dilate and carry blood.

atrium Either of the two upper chambers of the heart.

auscultation Listening to sounds with a stethoscope.

automated external defibrillator (AED) Portable battery-powered device that recognizes fibrillation and advises when a countershock is indicated. Delivers an electric charge to patients with ventricular fibrillation.

AVPU scale A scale to measure a patient's level of consciousness. The letters stand for Alert, Verbal, Pain, and Unresponsive.

avulsion An injury in which a piece of skin is either torn completely loose from all of its attachments or is left hanging as a flap.

backboard A straight board used for splinting, extricating, and transporting patients with suspected spine injuries.

bag of waters The amniotic fluid that surrounds the baby before birth.

bag-valve-mask (BVM) device A patient ventilation device which consists of a bag, one-way valves, and a face mask, which can deliver 90% oxygen to a patient.

barbiturates Drugs that depress the nervous system; they can alter the state of consciousness so that the individual may appear drowsy or peaceful.

bargaining The third stage of the grief reaction, when the person experiencing grief barters to change the grief-causing event.

basic life support (BLS) Emergency lifesaving procedures performed without advanced emergency procedures to stabilize patients who have experienced sudden illness or injury.

Glossary

behavioral emergencies Situations where a person exhibits abnormal behavior that is unacceptable or cannot be tolerated by the patients themselves or by family, friends, or the community.

birth canal The vagina and the lower part of the uterus.

blanket drag An emergency patient move technique in which a rescuer encloses a patient in a blanket and drags the patient to safety.

blood pressure The pressure of the circulating blood against the walls of the arteries.

bloody show The bloody mucus plug that is discharged from the vagina when labor begins.

body substance isolation (BSI) An infection control concept that treats all bodily fluids as potentially infectious.

bounding pulse A strong pulse (similar to the pulse that follows physical exertion like running or lifting heavy objects).

brachial artery pressure point Pressure point located in the arm between the elbow and the shoulder; also used in taking blood pressure and for checking the pulse in infants.

brachial pulse The pulse on the inside of the upper arm.

breech presentation A delivery in which the baby's buttocks, arm, shoulder, or leg appears first rather than the head.

bronchi The two main branches of the windpipe that lead into the right and left lungs. Within the lungs, they branch into smaller airways.

bronchitis Inflammation of the airways in the lungs.

bruise Injury caused by a blunt object striking the body and crushing the tissue beneath the skin. Also called a contusion.

bulb syringe A rubber or plastic device used for gentle suction in newborns and small infants.

capillaries The smallest blood vessels that connect small arteries and small veins. Capillary walls serve as the membrane to exchange oxygen and carbon dioxide.

capillary bleeding Bleeding from the capillaries in which blood oozes from the open wound.

capillary refill The ability of the circulatory system to restore blood to the capillary blood vessels after it has been squeezed out by the examiner.

carbon dioxide (CO_2) The gas formed in respiration and exhaled in breathing.

carbon monoxide (CO) A colorless, odorless, poisonous gas formed by incomplete combustion, such as in a fire.

cardiac arrest A sudden ceasing of heart function.

cardiogenic shock Shock resulting from inadequate functioning of the heart.

cardiopulmonary resuscitation (CPR) The artificial circulation of the blood and movement of air into and out of the lungs in a pulseless, nonbreathing patient.

cartilage A tough, elastic form of connective tissue that covers the ends of most bones to form joints. Also found in some specific areas such as the nose and ear.

carotid arteries The principle arteries of the neck. They supply blood to the face, head, and brain.

carotid pulse A pulse that can be felt on each side of the neck where the carotid artery is close to the skin.

casualty sorting The sorting of patients for treatment and transportation.

central nervous system (CNS) The brain and spinal cord.

cerebrospinal fluid (CSF) A clear, watery fluid that fills the space between the brain and spinal cord and their protective coverings.

cervical collar A neck brace that partially stabilizes the neck following injury.

cervical spine That portion of the spinal column consisting of the 7 vertebrae located in the neck.

chemical burns Burns that occur when any toxic substance comes in contact with the skin. Most chemical burns are caused by strong acids or alkalis.

chest compression Manual chest-pressing method that mimics the squeezing and relaxation cycles a normal heart goes through; administered to a person in cardiac arrest; also called "external chest compression" and "closed-chest cardiac massage."

chest-thrust maneuver A series of manual thrusts to the chest to relieve upper airway obstruction; used in the treatment of infants, pregnant women, or extremely obese people.

chief complaint The patient's response to a question such as "What happened?" or "What's wrong?"

child Anyone between one and eight years of age.

chocking A piece of wood or metal placed in front of or behind a wheel to prevent vehicle movement.

chronic obstructive lung disease (COLD) A slow process of destruction of the airways, alveoli, and pulmonary blood vessels caused by chronic bronchial obstruction (emphysema). This condition is also known as chronic obstructive pulmonary disease (COPD).

circulatory system The heart and blood vessels, which together are responsible for the continuous flow of blood throughout the body.

clavicle The collarbone.

closed fracture A fracture in which the overlying skin has not been damaged.

Glossary

closed head injury Injury where there is bleeding and/or swelling within the skull.

closed wound Injury in which soft-tissue damage occurs beneath the skin but there is no break in the surface of the skin.

clothes drag An emergency patient move used to remove a patient from a hazardous environment. Performed by grasping the patient's clothes and moving the patient head first from the unsafe area.

cocaine A powerful stimulant that induces an extreme state of euphoria. Legitimately, it is a potent local anesthetic. On the street, it is commonly known as "coke." Synthetic cocaine is known as "crack."

coccyx The tailbone; the small bone below the sacrum formed by the final 4 vertebrae.

coma A state of unconsciousness from which the patient cannot be aroused.

competent Able to make rational decisions about personal well-being.

congestive heart failure (CHF) Heart disease characterized by breathlessness, fluid retention in the lungs, and generalized swelling of the body.

contractions Muscular movements of the uterus that push the baby out of the mother.

cradle-in-arms carry A one-rescuer patient movement technique used primarily for children. The patient is cradled in the hollow formed by the rescuer's arms and chest.

cravat A triangular swathe of cloth that is used to hold a body part splinted against the body.

critical incident stress debriefing (CISD) A system of psychological support designed to reduce stress on emergency personnel after a major stress-producing incident.

croup Inflammation and narrowing of the air passages in young children causing a barking cough, hoarseness, and a harsh, high-pitched breathing sound.

crowning Appearance of the baby's head during a contraction as it is pushed outward through the vagina.

cyanosis Bluish coloration of the skin resulting from poor oxygenation of the circulating blood.

decompression sickness (the bends) A condition seen in divers in which gas, especially nitrogen, forms bubbles in blood vessels obstructing them.

defibrillation Delivery of an electric current through a person's chest wall and heart for the purpose of ending lethal heart rhythms such as ventricular fibrillation.

delirium tremens (DTs) A severe, often fatal, complication of alcohol withdrawal that can occur from one to seven days after withdrawal. It is characterized by restlessness, fever, sweating, confusion, disorientation, agitation, hallucinations, and convulsions.

denial The first stage of a grief reaction, when the person suffering grief rejects the grief-causing event.

depression The fourth stage of the grief reaction, when the person expresses despair—an absence of cheerfulness and hope—as a result of the grief-causing event.

diabetes A disease in which the body is unable to use sugar normally because of a deficiency or total lack of insulin; often called "sugar diabetes."

diabetic coma A state of unconsciousness that occurs when the body has too much sugar and not enough insulin.

diaphragm A muscular dome that separates the chest from the abdominal cavity. Contraction of the diaphragm and the chest wall muscles brings air into the lungs; relaxation expels air from the lungs.

diastolic pressure The measurement of pressure exerted against the walls of the arteries while the left ventricle of the heart is at rest.

digestive system The gastrointestinal tract (stomach and intestines), mouth, salivary glands, pharynx, esophagus, liver, gallbladder, pancreas, rectum, and anus, which together are responsible for the absorption of food and the elimination of solid waste from the body.

dislocation Disruption of a joint so that the bone ends are no longer in alignment.

distal Describing structures that are nearer to the free end of an extremity; any location that is farther from the midline than the point of reference named.

downers Depressants; barbiturates.

dressing A bandage.

drowning Death from suffocation after submersion in water.

duty to act A first responder's legal responsibility to respond promptly to an emergency scene and provide medical care (within the limits of training and available equipment).

dyspnea Difficulty or pain with breathing.

electrical burns Burns caused by electric current.

Emergency Medical Technician-Basic (EMT-B) A person who is trained and certified to provide basic life support and certain other noninvasive prehospital medical procedures.

emergency services dispatch center A fire, police, or emergency medical services (EMS) agency; a 9-1-1 center; or a seven-digit telephone number used by one or all of the emergency agencies to receive and dispatch requests for emergency care.

Glossary

emotional shock A state of shock caused by sudden illness, accident, or death of a loved one.

empathy The ability to participate in another person's feelings or ideas.

entrance wound Point where an injurious object such as a bullet enters the body.

epiglottis The valve located at the upper end of the voice box that prevents food from entering the larynx.

epiglottitis Severe inflammation and swelling of the epiglottis; a life-threatening situation.

epilepsy A disease manifested by seizures, caused by an abnormal focus of electrical activity in the brain.

esophagus The tube through which food passes. It starts at the throat and ends at the stomach.

exhalation Breathing out.

exit wound Point where an injurious object such as a bullet passes out of the body.

expressed consent Consent actually given by a person authorizing the first responder to provide care or transportation.

external cardiac compressions A means of applying artificial circulation by applying rhythmic pressure and relaxation on the lower half of the sternum.

externally rotated Rotated outward, as in a fractured hip.

extremities The arms and legs.

extrication Removal from a difficult situation or position; removal of a patient from a wrecked car or other place of entrapment.

face mask A clear plastic mask used for oxygen administration that covers the mouth and nose.

femoral artery pressure point Pressure point located in the groin, where the femoral artery is close to the skin.

fetus A developing baby in the uterus or womb.

firefighter drag A method of moving a patient without lifting or carrying him or her; used when the patient is heavier than the rescuer.

flail chest A condition that occurs when three or more ribs are broken each in two places, and the chest wall lying between the fractures becomes a free-floating segment.

floating ribs The eleventh and twelfth ribs, which do not connect to the sternum.

flotation device A life ring, life buoy, or other floating device used in water rescue.

flowmeter A device on oxygen cylinders used to control and measure the flow of oxygen.

forearm The lower portion of the upper extremity; from the elbow to the wrist.

fracture Any break in a bone.

frostbite Partial or complete freezing of the skin and deeper tissues caused by exposure to the cold.

full-thickness burns Burns that extend through the skin and into or beyond the underlying tissues; the most serious class of burn.

fusee A warning device or flare that burns with a red color; usually used in scene protection at motor vehicle crash sites.

gag reflex A strong involuntary effort to vomit caused by something being placed or caught in the throat.

gastric distention Inflation of the stomach caused when excessive pressures are used during artificial ventilation and air is directed into the stomach rather than the lungs.

genitourinary system The organs of reproduction, together with the organs involved in the production and excretion of urine.

Golden Hour A concept of emergency patient care that attempts to place a trauma patient into definitive medical care within one hour of injury.

Good Samaritan laws Laws that encourage individuals to voluntarily help an injured or suddenly ill person by minimizing the liability for any errors or omissions in rendering good faith emergency care.

gunshot wound A puncture wound caused by a bullet or shotgun pellet.

hallucinogens Chemicals that cause a person to see visions or hear sounds that are not real.

HazMat Hazardous material or chemical.

head tilt–chin lift Opening the airway by tilting the patient's head backward and lifting the chin forward, bringing the entire lower jaw with it.

heat exhaustion A form of shock that occurs when the body loses too much water and too many electrolytes through very heavy sweating after exposure to heat.

heatstroke A condition of rapidly rising internal body temperature that occurs when the body's mechanisms for the release of heat are overwhelmed. Untreated heatstroke can result in death.

Heimlich maneuver A series of manual thrusts to the abdomen to relieve upper airway obstruction.

hemorrhage Bleeding.

hereditary deafness Deafness present at birth.

hives An allergic skin disorder marked by patches of swelling, redness, and intense itching.

Glossary

hot zone A contaminated area.

hypertension High blood pressure.

hypotension Lowered blood pressure.

hypothermia A condition in which the internal body temperature falls below 95°F after prolonged exposure to cool or freezing temperatures.

illness Sickness.

immobilize To reduce or prevent movement of a limb, usually by splinting.

impaled object An object such as a knife, splinter of wood, or glass that penetrates the skin and remains in the body.

implied consent Consent to receive emergency care that is assumed because the individual is unconscious, underage, or so badly injured or ill that he or she cannot respond.

infant Anyone under one year of age.

inferior That portion of the body or body part that lies nearer the feet than the head.

inhalation Breathing in.

initial patient assessment The first actions taken to form an impression of the patient's condition; to determine the patient's responsiveness and introduce yourself to the patient; to check the patient's airway, breathing, and circulation; and to acknowledge the patient's chief complaint.

insulin A hormone produced by the pancreas that enables sugar in the blood to be used by the cells of the body; insulin is used in the treatment and control of diabetes mellitus.

insulin shock Condition that occurs in a diabetic who has taken too much insulin or has not eaten enough food. (Also referred to as a low blood sugar reaction or just "a reaction.")

intravenous (IV) fluid Fluid other than blood or blood products infused into the vascular system to maintain an adequate circulatory blood volume.

jaw-thrust technique Opening the airway by bringing the patient's jaw forward without extending the head.

joint The place where two bones come in contact with each other.

labor The process of delivering a baby.

laceration An irregular cut or tear through the skin.

larynx A structure composed of cartilage in the neck that guards the entrance to the windpipe and functions as the organ of voice Also called the voice box.

lateral Away from the midline of the body.

leg The lower extremity; specifically, the lower portion, from the knee to the ankle.

ligaments Fibrous bands that connect bones to bones and support and strengthen joints.

living wills Legal documents with specific instructions that the patient does not want to be resuscitated or kept alive by mechanical support systems.

logrolling A technique used to move a patient onto a long backboard.

lumbar spine The lower part of the back formed by the lowest five nonfused vertebrae.

lungs The organs that supply the body with oxygen and eliminate carbon dioxide from the blood.

mandible The lower jaw.

manual suction device A hand-powered device used for clearing the upper airway of mucus, blood, or vomitus.

mechanical suction device An electrically powered device used for clearing the upper airway of mucus, blood, or vomitus.

mechanism of injury The means by which a traumatic injury occurs.

medial Toward the midline of the body.

midline An imaginary vertical line drawn from the midforehead through the nose and the navel to the floor.

miscarriage Delivery of the fetus before it is mature enough to survive outside the womb (about 20 weeks), from either natural (spontaneous abortion) or induced causes.

mouth-to-mask ventilation device A piece of equipment that consists of a mask, a one-way valve, and a mouthpiece. Rescue breathing is performed by breathing into the mouthpiece after placing the mask over the patient's mouth and nose.

mouth-to-stoma breathing Rescue breathing for patients who, because of surgical removal of the larynx, have a stoma.

multiple-casualty incident An accident or situation involving more patients than you can handle with the initial resources available.

nasal airway An airway adjunct that is inserted into the nostril of a patient who is not able to maintain a natural airway. It is also called a nasopharyngeal airway.

nasal cannula A clear plastic tube used to deliver oxygen that fits onto the patient's nose.

nasopharynx The posterior part of the nose.

near drowning Survival, at least temporarily, after suffocation in water.

neck breathers Patients who have a stoma and breathe through the opening in their neck.

negligence Deviation from the accepted standard of care resulting in further injury to the patient.

Glossary

nerves Fiber tracts or pathways that carry messages from the spinal cord and brain to all body parts and back; sensory, motor, or a combination of both.

nervous system The brain, spinal cord, and nerves.

nitroglycerin A medicine used to treat angina pectoris; it increases blood flow and oxygen supply to the heart muscle and reduces or eliminates the pain of angina pectoris.

occlusive dressing An airtight dressing or bandage for a wound.

one-person walking assist A method used if the patient is able to bear his or her own weight.

one-rescuer CPR Cardiopulmonary resuscitation performed by one rescuer.

on-scene peer support Stress counselors at the scene of stressful incidents to deal with stress reduction.

open fracture Any fracture in which the overlying skin has been damaged.

open wound Injury that breaks the skin or mucous membrane.

oral airway An airway adjunct that is inserted into the mouth to keep the tongue from blocking the upper airway. It is also called an oropharyngeal or nasopharyngeal airway.

oropharynx The posterior part of the mouth.

osteoporosis Abnormal brittleness of the bones in older people caused by loss of calcium; affected bones fracture easily.

oxygen (O) A colorless, odorless gas that is essential for life.

pack-strap carry A one-person carry that allows the rescuer to carry a patient while keeping one hand free.

palpation To examine by touch.

paralysis Inability of a conscious person to move voluntarily.

paramedic An emergency medical technician who has completed an extensive course of 800 or more hours and who can perform advanced life support skills.

partial-thickness burns Burns in which the outer layers of skin are burned; these burns are characterized by blister formation.

pathogens Microorganisms that are capable of causing disease.

pelvis The closed bony ring, consisting of the sacrum and the pelvic bones, that connects the trunk to the lower extremities.

physical examination The step in the patient assessment sequence in which the first responder carefully examines the patient from head to toe, looking for additional injuries and other problems.

placenta Life-support system of the baby during its time inside the mother (commonly called the "afterbirth").

plasma The fluid part of the blood that carries blood cells, transports nutrients, and removes cellular waste materials.

platelets Microscopic disk-shaped elements in the blood that are essential to the process of blood clot formation, the mechanism that stops bleeding.

pneumatic antishock garment (PASG) A trousers-like device placed around a shock victim's legs and abdomen and inflated with air. Also called medical antishock trousers (MAST).

pocket mask A mechanical breathing device used to administer mouth-to-mask rescue breathing.

poison Any substance that may cause injury or death if relatively small amounts are ingested, inhaled, or absorbed, or applied to, injected into, or developed within the body.

portable stretcher A lightweight nonwheeled device for transporting a patient. Used in small spaces where the wheeled ambulance stretcher cannot be used.

posterior The back surface of the body.

posterior tibial pulse Ankle pulse.

pre-incident stress education Training about stress and stress reactions conducted for public safety providers before they are exposed to stressful situations.

premature baby A baby who delivers before eight months gestation or who weighs less than 5-1/2 pounds at birth.

pressure points Points where a blood vessel lies near a bone; pressure can be applied to these points to help control bleeding.

prolapse of the umbilical cord A delivery in which the umbilical cord appears before the baby does; the baby's head may compress the cord and cut off all circulation to the baby.

proximal Describing structures that are closer to the trunk.

psychogenic shock Commonly known as fainting; caused by a temporary reduction in blood supply to the brain.

psychotic behavior Mental disturbance characterized by defective or lost contact with reality.

pulmonary edema (right) Congestive heart failure causes fluid to leak from the capillary and build up in the alveolus, impeding oxygen and carbon dioxide exchange.

pulse The wave of pressure that is created by the heart as it contracts and forces blood out of the heart and into the major arteries.

puncture A wound resulting from a bullet, knife, ice pick, splinter, or any other pointed object.

Glossary

pupil The circular opening in the middle of the eye.

rabies An acute viral infection of the central nervous system transmitted by the bite of an infected animal.

radial pulse Wrist pulse.

radius The bone on the thumb side of the forearm.

reach-throw-row-go A four-step reminder of the sequence of actions that should be taken in water rescue situations.

recovery position A sidelying position that helps an unconscious patient maintain an open airway.

redirection A means of focusing the patient's attention on the immediate situation or crisis.

rescue breathing Artificial means of breathing for a patient.

respiratory arrest Sudden stoppage of breathing.

respiratory burns Burns to the respiratory system resulting from inhaling superheated air.

respiratory rate The speed at which a person is breathing (measured in breaths per minute).

respiratory system All the structures of the body that contribute to normal breathing.

restatement Rephrasing a patient's own statement to show that he or she is being heard and understood by the rescuer.

ribs The paired arches of bone, 12 on either side, that extend from the thoracic vertebrae toward the anterior midline of the trunk.

rigid splints Splints made from firm materials such as wood, aluminum, or plastic.

riptide An unusually strong surface current flowing outward from a seashore that can carry swimmers "out to sea."

road rash An abrasion caused by sliding along a highway. Usually seen after motorcycle or bicycle accidents.

Rule of Nines A way to calculate the amount of body surface burned; the body is divided into sections, each of which constitutes approximately 9% or 18% of the total body surface area.

sacrum One of 3 bones (sacrum and 2 pelvic bones) that make up the pelvic ring; forms the base of the spine.

saline Salt water.

SAMPLE history A patient's medical history. S=signs/symptoms, A=allergies, M=medications, P=pertinent past history, L=last oral intake, E=events associated with the illness or injury.

scoop stretcher A firm patient-carrying device that can be split into halves and applied to the patient from both sides.

seizures Sudden episodes of uncontrolled electrical activity in the brain.

self-contained breathing apparatus (SCBA) A complete unit for delivery of air to a rescuer who enters a contaminated area; contains a mask, regulator, and air supply.

shock A state of collapse of the cardiovascular system; the state of inadequate delivery of blood to the organs of the body.

shoulder girdle The proximal portion of the upper extremity; made up of the clavicle, the scapula, and the humerus.

sign A condition that you observe in a patient, such as bleeding or the temperature of a patient's skin.

situational crisis A state of emotional upset or turmoil caused by a sudden and disruptive event.

skull The bones of the head, collectively; serves as the protective structure for the brain.

sling A triangular bandage or material tied around the neck to support the weight of an injured upper extremity.

soft splint A splint made from soft material that provides gentle support.

splinting Immobilizing an injured part by using a rigid or soft support splint.

spontaneous nosebleed A nosebleed with no apparent cause.

sprain A joint injury in which the joint is partially or temporarily dislocated, and some of the supporting ligaments are either stretched or torn.

stair chair A small portable device used for transporting patients in a sitting position.

standard of care The manner in which an individual must act or behave when giving care (often defined by national organizations such as the American Heart Association).

START system A system of casualty sorting using Simple Triage And Rapid Treatment.

sternum The breastbone.

stoma An opening in the neck that connects the windpipe (trachea) to the skin.

straddle lift A method used to place a patient on a back-board if there is not enough space to perform a logroll.

straddle slide A method of placing a patient on a long backboard by straddling both the board and patient and sliding the patient onto the board.

suctioning Aspirating (sucking out) fluid by mechanical means.

sudden infant death syndrome (SIDS) Death from unknown cause that occurs during sleep in an otherwise healthy infant; also called crib death.

suicide Self-inflicted death.

Glossary

superficial burns Burns in which only the superficial part of the skin has been injured; an example is a sunburn.

superior Toward the head; lying higher in the body.

symptom A condition the patient tells you, such as "I feel dizzy."

systolic pressure The measurement of blood pressure exerted against the walls of the arteries during contraction of the heart.

tempered glass Safety glass that breaks into small pieces when hit with a sharp, pointed object.

temporary deafness Deafness that is usually caused by an explosion or loud noise; hearing usually returns after a short time.

tendons Tough, rope-like cords of fibrous tissue that attach muscles to bones.

thermal burns Burns caused by heat; the most common type of burn.

thoracic spine The 12 vertebrae that attach to the 12 ribs; the upper part of the back.

thready pulse A weak pulse.

topographic anatomy The superficial landmarks on the body that serve as location guides to the structures that lie beneath them.

toxic Poisonous.

trachea The windpipe.

traction splint A splint used to immobilize a fractured thigh bone that produces a longitudinal pull on the extremity.

trauma A wound or injury, either physical or psychological.

triage The sorting of patients into groups according to the severity of their injuries; used to determine priorities for treatment and transport.

two-person chair carry Two rescuers use a chair to support the weight of the patient.

two-person extremity carry A method of carrying a patient out of tight quarters using two rescuers and no equipment.

two-person seat carry A method of carrying a patient in which two rescuers link arms behind the patient's back and under the patient's knees; requires no equipment.

two-person walking assist Used when a patient cannot bear his or her own weight; two rescuers completely support the patient.

two-rescuer CPR Cardiopulmonary resuscitation performed by two rescuers.

ulna The bone on the little-finger side of the forearm.

umbilical cord Rope-like attachment between the mother and baby; nourishment and waste products pass to and from the baby and the mother through this cord.

universal precautions Procedures for infection control that treat blood and certain bodily fluids as capable of transmitting bloodborne diseases.

uppers Drugs that stimulate the central nervous system. These include amphetamines and cocaine.

uterus (womb) Muscular organ that holds and nourishes the developing baby.

vagina The opening through which the baby emerges.

venous bleeding External bleeding from a vein, characterized by steady flow; the bleeding may be profuse and life threatening.

ventilation The exchange of air between the lungs and the air of the environment; breathing.

ventricle Either of the two lower chambers of the heart.

ventricular fibrillation An uncoordinated muscular quivering of the heart; the most common abnormal rhythm causing cardiac arrest.

vertebrae The 33 bones of the spinal column: 7 cervical, 12 thoracic, 5 lumbar, 5 sacral, and 4 coccygeal vertebrae.

vital signs Signs of life, specifically pulse, respiration, blood pressure, and temperature.

wooden cribbing Wooden 2 x 4 or 4 x 4 boards used for stabilization or bracing.

xiphoid process The flexible cartilage at the lower tip of the sternum; a key landmark in the administration of CPR and the Heimlich maneuver.

Index

Index

Index

D

Index

Index

Index

Index

Index

Index

Quick Emergency Index